Behavioral Neuroscience

An Introduction

With select illustrations created for this book by

Frank Armitage, Ojai, California

And contributions from

Jay Angevine, Jr., University of Arizona College of Medicine, Tucson
Elliott Blass, The Johns Hopkins University, Baltimore
David Cohen, University of Virginia School of Medicine, Charlottesville
Edward Evarts, National Institute of Mental Health, Bethesda
Michael Gabriel, University of Texas at Austin
William Greenough, University of Illinois, Champaign
John Harvey, University of Iowa, Iowa City
Bartley Hoebel, Princeton University, Princeton
Robert Jensen, University of California, Irvine
Leonard Kitzes, University of California, Irvine Medical Center, Irvine
Rodolfo Llinas, New York University Medical Center, New York
Horace Loh, University of California, San Francisco
Andras Pellionisz, New York University Medical Center, New York
Lewis Petrinovich, University of California, Riverside
Jon Sassin, University of California, Irvine Medical Center, Irvine
David Segal, University of California, San Diego
Kenneth Simansky, Cornell Medical School, White Plains, New York
Larry Squire, University of California, San Diego
Arnold Starr, University of California, Irvine Medical Center, Irvine
Maurice B. Sterman, Veterans Administration Hospital, Sepulveda, California
Michael Stryker, University of California, San Francisco
Timothy Teyler, Northeastern Ohio University College of Medicine, Rootstown
Richard Thompson, University of California, Irvine
Roderick van Buskirk, Stanford University, Stanford
E. Leong Way, University of California, San Francisco
Richard Whalen, State University of New York, Stony Brook
Pauline Yahr, University of California, Irvine

Cover illustration from Fig. 5-8D.

Behavioral Neuroscience

An Introduction

Carl W. Cotman

James L. McGaugh

Department of Psychobiology
University of California
Irvine, California

ACADEMIC PRESS
A Subsidiary of Harcourt Brace Jovanovich, Publishers

New York London Toronto Sydney San Francisco

ACADEMIC PRESS, INC.
111 Fifth Avenue, New York, New York 10003

United Kingdom Edition published by
ACADEMIC PRESS, INC. (LONDON) LTD.
24/28 Oval Road, London NW1 7DX

Library of Congress Cataloging in Publication Data

Cotman, Carl W
    Behavioral neuroscience.

    Bibliography: p.
    1. Neuropsychology. 2. Human behavior.
3. Nervous system. I. McGaugh, James L. , joint
author. II. Title. [DNLM: 1. Behavior––Physiology. 2. Nervous system––Physiology. WL102.3 C844b]
QP360.C67   152   79–50214
ISBN 0–12–191650–3

PRINTED IN THE UNITED STATES OF AMERICA

80 81 82   9 8 7 6 5 4 3 2

To Ann, Adrian, Danna, Daniel and Cheryl
and
Becky, Doug, Jan and Linda

Contents

Preface

Behavioral neuroscience is a new and complex discipline that employs the tools and language of biology, chemistry, physiology, and psychology in the study of behavior. Yet for all its diversity, it is among the most exciting of endeavors. "Behavioral Neuroscience" aims to achieve an understanding of the biological mechanisms that determine our behavior and that of the animal world in which we live. This text provides a basic understanding of what is known about the means by which neurons communicate and about the nervous system which interprets, integrates, and transmits signals into meaningful and appropriate behaviors.

This book originated, in part, from an undergraduate course called "Introduction to Psychobiology" that has been taught at the University of California at Irvine since 1965. At other colleges and universities the course might be called "Introduction to Physiological Psychology," "Introduction to Biological Psychology," "Introduction to Neurosciences," "Introduction to Neurobiology," etc. This course is attended primarily by students who have some background in biology and/or psychology and who often are majors in biology, physiology, or psychology. Many of them plan to attend graduate school or medical school.

"Behavioral Neuroscience" is organized so that it starts with a broad overview presented in Chapter 1. In Chapter 2 we describe the general operation and organization of the nervous system and introduce some of the major types of neurons in the context of their systems. The presentation then moves directly to the cellular level and focuses on neurons, their basic characteristics (Chapter 3), and how they communicate (Chapters 4 and 5). We explore the action at the neuronal membrane and across the synapse. Synapses are plastic, modifiable. We discuss these processes and the basic integrative properties of defined groups of neurons (Chapter 6). Based on the principles and concepts derived we discuss learning in model systems (Chapter 7) and follow this directly with a discussion of complex learning and memory (Chapter 8). We define the problem, present the

xiii

data, and derive the central conclusions. We proceed with a description and analysis of the systems which process sensory stimuli (Chapters 9 and 10) and generate movement (Chapter 11). We describe the operation and upkeep of the body in relation to behavior (Chapter 12) and the performance of certain behaviors necessary for the care of the body, for example, thirst and hunger in Chapter 13 and sleep and activity rhythms in Chapter 14. What factors control these behaviors? We describe the development of the neural circuitry and its plasticity throughout life (Chapter 15) as it is modified in accordance with a lifetime plan. In Chapter 16 we describe the development of behavior, the ever-so-complex product of all that "wiring" during development. Behavior is sometimes abnormal, brought on by mental disorders, drug abuse, and alcoholism, and in Chapter 17 we analyze these from a behavioral and neuroscientific perspective. The final chapter (18) focuses on man, on us, and asks the question, "Why am I what I am?" Certain known aspects of man's nervous system give some of the answers—but in reality these answers raise even more questions. Overall then, in the course of this text, we explore behavior from the perspective of basic neuroscience.

The coverage of behavioral neuroscience is fairly complete. Thus it is unlikely that any quarter or semester course at an undergraduate level will cover the entire book. Most faculty will wish to select from it, depending on their own particular orientation. Those wishing a more biological approach to behavioral neuroscience may prefer to concentrate on the earlier chapters in the text; those wishing a more psychological approach will draw more heavily on the later chapters, more or less along the outline suggested in the instructor's manual.

As an aid to the creation of this text, we have enlisted the help of many experts who have assisted in the preparation of various segments of this book. The contributions of these specialists have enabled us to produce a text which is uniformly accurate and up to date. We are indeed grateful to all the following experts who have given so generously of their time and effort to provide this information: Dr. J. Angevine, Jr. (neuroanatomy, Chapter 2, and cortical lobes, Chapter 18); Drs. J. Harvey and K. Simansky (neurotransmitter circuitry, Chapter 6); Drs. R. Llinas and A. Pellionisz (original figures on dendritic integration, Chapter 6); Dr. R. Thompson (model systems and elementary learning, Chapter 7); Dr. M. Gabriel (neurophysiological correlates of learning, Chapter 8); Dr. L. Squire (human learning and memory, Chapter 8); Dr. L. Kitzes (auditory receptors, Chapter 9); Dr. A. Starr (clinical disorders of hearing, Chapter 9); Dr. M. Stryker (visual system and plasticity, Chapter 10); Dr. E. Evarts (motor system, Chapter 11); Drs. R. Whalen and J. Sassin (neuroendocrinology, Chapter 12); Drs. T. Teyler, R. Jensen and D. Cohen (autonomic nervous system, Chapter 12); Dr. E. Blass (thirst, Chapter 13); Dr. B. Hoebel (contribution on hunger, Chapter 13); Drs. M. Sterman and R. Jensen (sleep, Chapter 14); Dr. R. van

Buskirk (biological rhythms, Chapter 14); Dr. W. Greenough (environmental influences on brain structure, Chapter 15); Dr. P. Yahr (contribution on genetic influences on behavior, Chapter 16); Dr. R. Whalen (hormones and behavior, Chapter 16); Dr. L. Petrinovich (material on language development in birds and man, Chapter 16); Dr. D. Segal (schizophrenia and affective disorders, Chapter 17); Dr. E. Way (drug abuse, Chapter 17); and Dr. H. Loh (endorphins and enkephalins, Chapter 6 and 17).

We acknowledge the aid of these experts; however, we bear the responsibility for the material as it appears in final form. We have made every effort to provide essential introductory background for each section. When concepts are introduced that depend on basic principles derived from chemistry, biology, or psychology, we have provided the appropriate background. Our goal was to see that despite varied backgrounds, students will find this text easy to read. We have also, insofar as possible, written sections to be self-contained so that the instructor can select only parts of the text and still achieve continuity. The list of key terms at the end of each chapter will aid in reading and retaining information contained in the chapter. These plus the outline at the beginning of each chapter and the summary at the end should serve as a helpful study guide.

We are also pleased to acknowledge especially Dr. Robert Jensen who aided us extensively, particularly with Chapters 8, 10, 12, 13 and 14, and Dr. Jay Angevine, Jr., who provided many helpful editorial and content suggestions on numerous chapters. Dr. Jensen played a vital and stimulating role and we are infinitely appreciative of his diligent help and good cheer. Dr. Angevine spent a sabbatical in Dr. Cotman's laboratory; his inspiration and fellowship are very much appreciated. We are also grateful to Dr. W. Greenough and Dr. S. Gerling who read the entire text and provided many helpful critical comments. Finally, we thank Dr. S. Erulkar, Dr. H. Killackey, Dr. J. Swett, Dr. P. Landfield, Dr. M. Nieto, Dr. S. Hoff, Dr. E. Zaidel, J. Ryan, and D. Smith for their discussion, assistance, and critical comments on various chapters.

We were very fortunate indeed to obtain the services of Frank Armitage for the preparation of conceptual sketches and "story boards." Each drawing was developed in close consultation with Dr. Cotman to assure conceptual accuracy. Through this process, Mr. Armitage has been able to provide animated representations of many key concepts. The line drawings were done by Maureen Killackey except for those in Chapter 11 which were done by Christine Bondante. We are also pleased to acknowledge Julene Mueller and Linda O'Shea for their dedicated and invaluable secretarial, editorial, and managerial assistance and Christine Gentry for assistance in photography and reference verification. We also gratefully acknowledge the photographic contributions of M. Weisbrodt (photos in Chapters 11 and 17). Dr. Cotman is grateful to his wife for her exceeding patience and support and her helpful comments on various sections of the text. Dr. McGaugh appreciates the encouragement, understanding and good cheer of his wife. And, finally, thanks are due to the many at Academic Press who have played important roles in the project.

This book is written for students. It is our hope that those reading it will enjoy it and share some of the excitement and enthusiasm we and the contributors have for behavioral neuroscience. We welcome any comments that the users of this book may have. Please write to either of us at the Department of Psychobiology, University of California, Irvine, California. We enjoyed writing the book and hope that you find it both interesting reading and exciting learning.

Carl W. Cotman
James L. McGaugh

Behavioral Neuroscience

An Introduction

1

What Does the Nervous System Do?

I. Introduction

. . . We think of ourselves and others as engaged from moment to moment in doing this or that. That is a convenience of speech. Each of us at any moment of the waking day is a whole bundle of acts simultaneously proceeding. . . . In no case does any other of all the doings of the moment disturb the one focal doing. We are each therefore at any moment a pattern of active doing; a single pattern of pieces all subordinate to one keypiece. No other part of the pattern is allowed to disturb the keypiece of the pattern. Should it do so then the pattern changes and the disturbing piece becomes usually the keypiece of a new pattern which supplants the previous. The keypiece is the crown of the unified doing of the moment (Sherrington, 1946, pp. 172–173).

1

Our responses are the products of the nervous system acting through the body. We walk, talk, touch, look, listen, even laugh, in so many ways that our total responses can only be summed up as behavior—behavior designed for the moment. Our nervous system provides an immense repertoire of specific behavior, together with built-in contingency plans. It is at one and the same time reporter, editor, producer, file clerk and delivery boy for our moment by moment events. It collects critical newsworthy information, analyzes it, modifies it in relation to our interests, keeps a record of all transactions and delivers a report to our muscles and glands so we may act. In our behavior we see reliability, precision and versatility—programs of living designed specifically for us. Yet our reactions to many things are identical, universals of response shared so commonly among all men and women that we are able to analyze the biological basis of behavior from them.

In this text we shall concern ourselves with the biological bases of behavior, the "hows," "whys," and "so whats." How does the nervous system administer that miraculous performance called behavior? What is the role of the subcomponents of behavior in relationship to its overall plan? These questions are challenging ones, and at present we really do not have all the answers. But in behavioral neuroscience we are attaining more and more exciting findings. The prospects for the future are very bright indeed. Neurobiology is still a very young field, and much is happening every day. In this text we shall take you into the nervous system and from within try to show how it pilots our behaviors. However, prior to embarking on this journey and seeking out the ways the nervous system controls behavior, we would do well to put our mission into perspective. Just what does the nervous system do?

II. Functions of the Nervous System

A. The Nervous System Organizes and Directs Motor Responses

We can start at the end—ourselves moving. Much behavior is purposeful movement, and the nervous system is the executor of this movement. As Lord Adrian (1955), a revered neurophysiologist and one of the founding fathers of the study of the brain, once wrote, "The chief function of the nervous system is to send messages to the muscles which will make the body move effectively as a whole." Such effective, unitary movement has extraordinarily diverse components. Embodied in it are some of the simplest and some of the most complex behavioral responses. The simplest of these is a reflex. A tap to the knee elicits a kick of the leg, the prick of a pin on a finger brings its withdrawal. Patterns of movement, whether those of a Mozart playing a concerto or of you and me simply talking, are the integrated result of many influences.

But even holding still is a tremendous motor task. We might not normally think about it, but one of the jobs of the nervous system is simply to maintain posture. The nervous system is constantly at work maintaining our body's posture to keep us upright. It issues a continuing program of signals so that the appropriate muscles maintain the appropriate tensions. No robot yet invented even approximates the skill of our nervous system in moving a body or keeping it erect.

Motion is totally unified: the body moves as a whole in a highly coordinated manner.

> The individual cannot be the seat of two focal acts at once. In the pattern of doing of the moment the focal act has commonly a number of satellite acts contributory to it, the keypiece of the pattern. A score of contributory acts of posture, and of sensory adjustment, secondarily contribute to give speed or steadiness or precision to the focal act, and of these each one can be and probably has been at other moments a centre of awareness. . . . Elsewhere focal mind is exemplified by perception or cognition, but here we see it wedded to motricity, "doing" a motor act (Sherrington, 1946, p. 173).

We can see then that the answer to "so what" and "why" is that motion gives us behavior.

How? Behind the scenes, under our skin so to speak, driving our muscles are teams of nerve cells playing out their patterns of activity from the spinal cord and instructing the muscles, through long nerve fibers, to contract and relax. Those teams prompt muscles to action, pulling on our bones in different ways so smoothly we scarcely realize the underlying structure is bone and muscle. This neuronal activity and the teams of neurons playing it out give us purposeful motion.

B.   The Nervous System Monitors Its Outside World

The nervous system is concerned and inquisitive about what goes on around it. It monitors light, sound, smell and "the feel" of things. In brief, it monitors every physical stimulus known. Where pertinent, it even looks at magnetic fields; birds use such information to migrate.

Such monitoring is carried out by specialized receptors. Eyes capture light and convert it into brain language; ears hear sounds; the nose collects smells; hands, legs, and, in fact, our whole body surface is sensitive to touch, pressure and vibration. The receptors of these body parts report to the brain, and the impressions they bring result in behavior: a simple reflex, an association or perhaps simply a mental note of what has transpired. The job of the nervous system is to make sense of the stimuli which it receives. "Why?" To monitor the environment. "How?" With receptors. "So what?" To adjust behavior in a meaningful way to the world about.

Much of what exists in the external world, even in our immediate surroundings, we never perceive, at least at a conscious level. How do we select certain things for our attention over others? If we become deeply interested in one particular thing, chances are good that we will miss others. Yet at the same time the important things never go unnoticed—they are just too impressive. Try sitting on a tack and not noticing it. Pain, as we are all too aware, emblazons itself upon our brains and calls us to action. The job of the nervous system, then, is to put stimuli in the appropriate perspective. Mind is focal in collecting and integrating stimuli and in producing responses.

C.   Learning and Remembering

Learning is the most important thing we do. What we perceive becomes, in many cases, part of us so that our present is a cumulative function of the past. We must learn or we cannot become even the feeblest masters of our destinies. Creatures, such as an amoeba, for example, unblessed with anything like our powerful memories, meander about looking for morsels of food. Merely eating consumes nearly full time for simple creatures, but occupies only a fraction of our day because of our superior nervous system and physiology. Learning, not eating, is our dominant mechanism of survival, giving self-assurance and economy, as well as sustenance, to daily living. It is what we learn individually and are finally able to put into practice that makes us each so different. It is also our combined efforts that make our society and give us a rich culture. So perhaps we can see why we can say that learning is the most important thing we do.

How do we learn? In many ways, only a few of which are really known, the nervous system builds into its structure relics of its past. In order to study learning and memory, we need to understand the basic cellular operations of the memory system. For now, we can say that somehow neural circuitry encodes the realities it has experienced and the logic and associations that have served us so well.

Despite all we know, everything stamped into the files of our brain, and all we can do from what we have learned, the mind's product is still focal, unitary action, as Sherrington saw. We still strive to make one decision, generate one thought, do one thing; no other part of the pattern is allowed to disturb the focus.

D. Thinking and Personality

We use our brain to generate and relate thoughts. Thinking takes individual events and generates concepts—ideas. Ideas then become their own reality as they are put into practice. Ideas are one of the most important products of our brain. Some people make a living solely on their ideas. The nervous system is working ceaselessly on all it has in its possession and all it takes in, even when we are not conscious of its goings on, in order that individuals may achieve their goals.

Everyone has a unique personality. It, along with our abilities, makes us individuals. We may all respond in the same way to simple stimuli, but we feel and behave in many different ways toward complex situations and to other individuals. Our nervous system is us, making us what we are.

E. Much of the Nervous System Is Devoted to the Care and Upkeep of the Body

The body and nervous system are partners, and each depends on the other. The role of the nervous system in relationship to the external world is obvious. It is at the forefront of our conscious experience. Less well known is the key role the nervous system plays in body function, much of which is outside one's normal conscious experience. The nervous system acts through the body, and it maintains and cares for its home, its avenue of access to the external world. The nervous system not only ties together and unifies the world about but it does so for the internal world as well. As Carrel said, "The body is a unity which has become multiplicity while keeping its unity" (Carrel, 1938). The nervous system draws the organs together to function as a unit, coordinates internal body states, and maintains the body's constancy. The nervous system is, in a sense, the keeper of the greenhouse—the moist healthy environment inside us. It keeps us warm or cool, by directing and promoting heat loss or heat preservation. How does it do this? There are divisions of the nervous system subcontracted specifically for these purposes. As we shall see in Chapter 2, the nervous system is, in fact, composed of many subsystems.

Our bodies have to be renewed, and we require sources of energy and building materials in order to maintain existence. Food and water are needed by all. "To your good health" is the toast, and a well put one it is at that. Our nervous system directs our behavior toward the goals of fulfilling its needs and locating food. It tells us when we are thirsty and when we must eat, and it directs the ensuing course of action. All the more to our delight, it makes this course a rewarding experience. What great pleasure there is in fine food and fine drink!

Our nervous system protects itself and its inseparable partner, the body, from injury. It causes us to scream out in pain when we are hurt. Pain tells us to cease whatever we are doing and change our behavior to relieve that distress. Some responses are high priority reflexes bypassing the brain altogether, other reactions are complex deliberations drawing upon past history and future plans held in the mind's stores. Upon injury, the nervous system also directs reparative responses to aid in the rebuilding of the body.

Furthermore, the nervous system directs adaptive body responses, the reaction to stress, for example. In this way we gain extra psychic and physical energy which we can bring to bear on a particular response. Athletes most frequently break records under the stress of competition, and similarly students often perform miracles in learning before examinations. Recall the last time you were scared! Beyond adaptation to emergencies, however, the nervous system is involved in mating behavior, reproduction and care of the young. It ensures its own future, so to speak, by promoting social behavior and, in particular, by seeing that males and females are attracted to one another.

All of our living is under control of the nervous system. It is a careful and wise planner that knows what it needs to do, and it does it extraordinarily well. Perhaps all the activity, all the daily tasks, are very wearisome for the body and the brain. But rest comes. We fall asleep. Sleep restores our mental and physical states. Yet even in sleep, we see the unitary and focal action of the nervous system. Our stream of waking consciousness leaves, and we find new states. Muscles relax, active movement is depressed, active posture is relaxed, the eyelids fall and the mind drifts off to the unknown to wander in dreams and to return when we awaken. Sleep is indeed a puzzle. As Sherrington commented, "This reaction of falling asleep seems at first sight the pursuance of a vicious circle. Fatigue, tending to incapacitate realizes a mechanism which incapacitates altogether" (Sherrington, 1946, p. 259). At any rate, the nervous system directs sleep: it is commander-in-chief of waking and unwaking states, mind awake–mind asleep, a daily rhythm which paces our life: 16 hours awake–8 hours asleep, 16–8, 16–8, 16–8.

F. Development and Maturation

It is obvious, of course, that the job of the nervous system does not start with the mature person or mature animal. It starts before we are born, when in fact, the nervous system itself is incomplete. The central nervous system (CNS) grows and develops along with other parts of the body. Together with the brain, sexual characteristics develop; attributes and abilities mature.

It is also obvious that the means to function perfectly, reliably, flexibly is stringent at all times. A mistake is a mistake no matter when it happens. The nervous system must deliver the correct responses even when it is immature.

The nervous system is adjusting behavior throughout life and delivering that behavior according to an ever-changing plan. Initially it is learning to move, to eat, to communicate. But it continues in the development and constant refinement of behavior in light of our experiences, capacities and goals. We acquire skills and learn to behave in more and more sophisticated ways. And there again, many of the same changes in nervous system functions continue to unfold, and in the end the twilight years come, with all the nuances of insight that old age brings. Behavior develops against genetic and experiential backdrops, combined in a manner which is seemingly inseparable.

G.   Behavioral Abnormalities

Sometimes, though, the workings go astray, and behavior becomes abnormal. These malfunctions tell us about the normal operation of the brain. We can learn from the variations which occur naturally, as well as those we experimentally create. When the nervous system malfunctions, its product, behavior, does likewise. Behavioral abnormalities may take the form of perceptual or motor deficits, or they may be displayed in personality or thought disorders such as schizophrenia. Here the unity can disappear; the constant workings, the reliability, the precision give way. The nervous system can often be controlled by drugs or, on the other hand, it can be engineered into strange and often unfortunate states through drug abuse. Some drugs have lasting consequences on the activity of the nervous system that far outlive the functional lifetime of the drug.

III.   What the Nervous System Does

We see it does everything, and it does it with precision, unity and versatility. How are all these feats possible? Ironically, although the mind—brain—does it, it does not tell us how. It does not report on how we stand or move, nor is it particularly informative about how we think. Its main assertions are that it is I standing, it is I performing, it is I thinking about this and that. It gives us a startlingly real revelation of the unity of focal mind.

We must rely on discerning observation and detailed measurement to discover how the nervous system operates. Fundamentally the nervous system delivers the same fantastic performance all through life. Through it all, it maintains unity of focal mind. Of course, there is always change, there is ever a new individual; man knows he is forever changing. The nervous system directs and oversees the never-ending changes.

In Chapter 2, we shall begin our exploration of the biological bases of behavior by describing the organizing principles of the nervous system. How is the system put together? What are the main principles underlying its plan? As the story unfolds in Chapter 2 and in subsequent chapters we shall describe our current state of knowledge on how the nervous system monitors the outside world, how it directs motion, learns and stores experiences and maintains and adapts the internal state of the body. We shall describe the various ways in which external and internal influences come together to produce behavior. Near the end of the book we shall describe the way the nervous system develops, and how certain behaviors come about. Finally, in the last chapter we shall explore some of the capacities and properties of our nervous system which distinguish us from animals.

References

Adrian, E. D. (1935). "The Mechanism of Nervous Action." Univ. of Pennsylvania Press, Philadelphia.
Carrel, A. (1938). Foreword to "Methods of Tissue Culture" by R. C. Parker. Harper (Hoeber), New York.
Sherrington, C. S. (1946). "Man on His Nature." Cambridge Univ. Press, London and New York.

2

Organizing Principles of the Nervous System

I. Introduction

Our nervous system is in essence a collection of specialized cells—*neurons*—organized in a highly specific way. Neurons carrying out functions related to a particular task are assembled into groups. These in turn are connected into functional subsystems and ultimately into the complex supersystem that is the nervous system. Some trillion neurons, specialized in innumerable ways, give the nervous system its capacity to pilot our behavior. In this chapter we shall guide you through the intricacies of its operation and attempt to show you the ways in which it makes our lives so rich and full. Without the nervous system, we would be inert, mute, unresponsive—for all purposes, living statues.

The brain is a many-layered edifice containing billions of neurons and untold numbers of connections, thousands of specialized regions and dozens of functionally oriented subsystems. All this is arranged in an interrelated and interdependent scheme of organization. Sight and perception of events in the world, for example, are the special tasks of the visual system. Neurons of the visual system, as any other neural subsystem, are wired into circuits with all the precision of electronic devices—a television set, calculator or computer—but with far more miniaturization of components.

In this chapter we present an overview of the rest of the book, and describe the basic organizing principles of the nervous system. We begin with its five cardinal attributes. It is pervasive, and has oneness, and it works flexibly, rapidly and reliably. These attributes arise out of the complexity of neural structure, most especially of its central components, the brain and spinal cord. We shall then discuss the major substructures of the nervous system and explore the way they are organized and function.

A. The Pervasive Nervous System—Serving and Protecting the Body

The two most striking general features of the nervous system are its *widespread distribution* and its *oneness*. These cardinal attributes allow the system to keep track of events everywhere in the body and to respond in a manner for its general good. To illustrate these simple but paramount features, let us engage for a moment in fantasy.

Imagine that someone you know is almost completely transparent, a ghostly person in whom only the nervous system is visible (Fig. 2-1). Such a flight of fancy may seem better suited to science fiction. But it is more than a daydream. It is an important step in understanding what the nervous system is and what it does. It makes us realize how important the system is in the design and operation of the body.

The central masses and myriad outreaching threads of the nervous system delineate the body, its parts and features. Over 100,000 miles of nerve fibers run through and trace out all our inner and outer parts. It approaches the ubiquity of the vascular system. Both systems are nearly omnipresent, as well as somewhat complementary in function. By means of neural signals and blood-borne substances, the two systems integrate the activities of body parts, protect them in numerous ways, enhance their performances in effort or exercise, promote their growth and maintain their healthy tone and vigor. Both systems look after the body's well-being.

The density of nerve supply varies from place to place according to the needs of body parts. The degree of innervation of a part tells us how much that part needs to send messages to the system. Thus in places liberally supplied with nerve endings (such as the finger tips or lips), stimuli can be especially painful. In other regions (that are largely neglected by nerve fibers), we don't mind an intrusion as much. We would probably rather sit on a tack than step on one!

The nervous system is completely successful in planning and delivering its service. All body regions receive exactly the nerve supply they need, no more, no less. No region is far from an available line over which to send a message, even though messages from that place are seldom sent. And a message may be sent at any time; the lines are always open, the switchboard ever on call.

B. Oneness of the Nervous System—Unifying the Body

We have seen the widespread and effective distribution of the nervous system. Let us now return to the phantom view and consider its oneness. We see that it is like a tree. Its trunk comprises the intricate, graceful mass of the brain and the slender, tubular spinal cord (Fig. 2-1). The important thing to remember about this tree is its continuity, the stringing together of all parts that allows each part to be in touch with every other. And you might pause to think (in case you had not already thought of it), "This tree inside me—this is where I live."

The brain and spinal cord represent the _central nervous system_ (CNS). Extending to either side of this neural tree trunk are numerous pairs of branches, the cranial and spinal nerves from brain and cord, respectively. These nerves, some thick and others thin, divide again and again into smaller and smaller branches. Eventually, they ramify into thousands of fine branchlets, ultimately into millions of terminal twigs and tips too small to be seen with the naked eye (and hence suggested by shading). This tremendous, far-flung system of branches is the _peripheral nervous system_ (PNS). It reaches out everywhere, to the eyes, ears, lips, tongue, torso and limbs, fingers and toes—to the body's periphery.

The nervous system provides total connectivity; it offers bodywide communi-

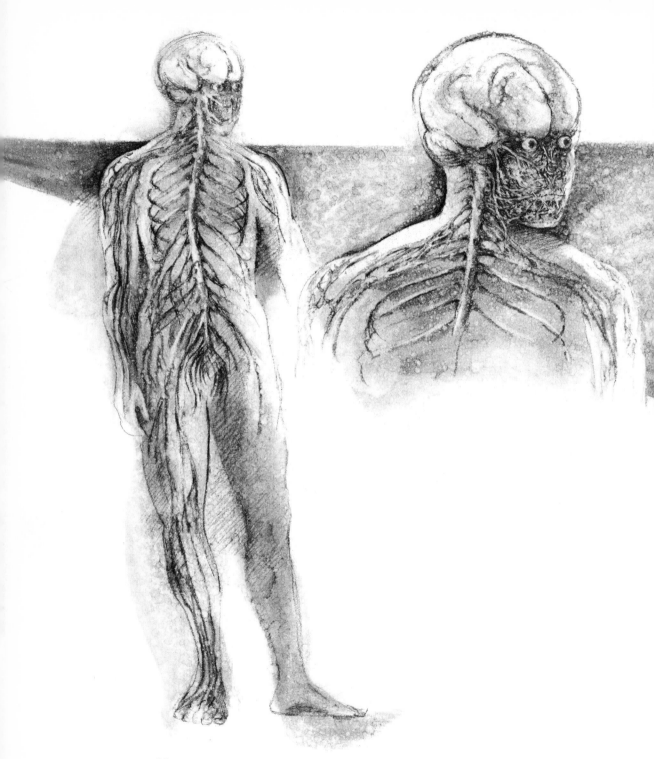

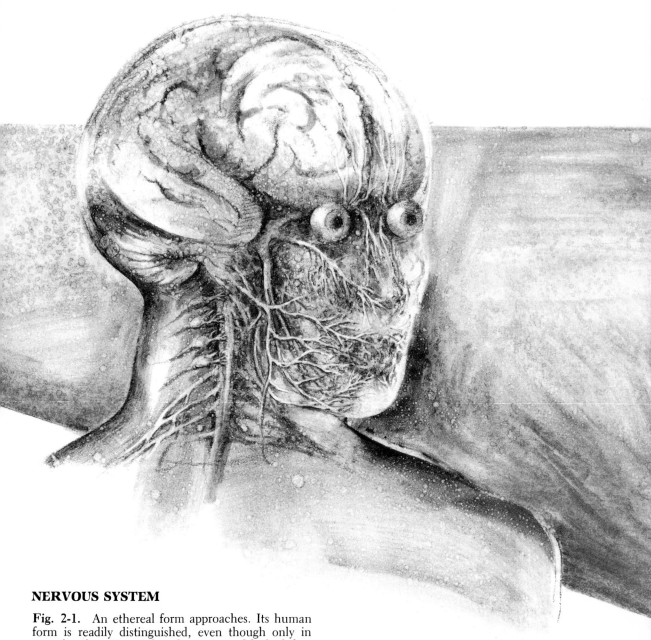

NERVOUS SYSTEM

Fig. 2-1. An ethereal form approaches. Its human
form is readily distinguished, even though only in
neural outline. Except for a few regions of the body less
densely infiltrated by neural threads, the shapes of body
parts—the head, torso and limbs—may easily be seen.
If the finest nerve filaments were visible, the identifying
characteristics of brow, ears, nose, cheeks, lips and
chin could be made out.

cation. A message entering the PNS from any body part travels centrally over that tree of ever-combining, constantly enlarging and frequently interlacing twigs, branchlets and branches until it reaches the trunk—the brain or spinal cord, depending on where the message came from. The nervous system does not provide any direct "hookups" over which, let us say, the ring finger and right big toe could hold a private chat. Every message must go to the CNS. Once inside, the message is received and "studied" there. New signals are then generated and distributed to other places in the brain and cord. Some go to points nearby through local circuits, others to remote locations over long-distance lines. Certain of these places (notably the cerebral cortex) scrutinize the message further, others elaborate appropriate responses. Ultimately, messages are sent back to body muscles. Thus, while extensive deliberation accompanies every transaction, each part of the body, through the nervous system, can affect the activity of the entire body or of any other part of it. One world, one body!

C. Flexibility of the Nervous System—Appropriate and Considered Responses

Great flexibility is noted in the components which handle signals. We know that if we make separate calls in succession from the same telephone, we will probably not get the same operator. Even when placing many calls in a row, we may never get a particular operator more than once. Which operator answers at any moment depends on how busy the switchboard is at that time and who is available to handle the call. Messages to the CNS from sensory neurons may be handled by various central neurons standing by to receive signals from a given body part. A message is processed by a team of neurons, never by a single one. The particular cluster of neurons responding would depend upon the activity of the entire nervous system at that time, as well as upon the activity of its individual cells from one moment to the next. Sometimes, certain cells are "tied up" and other cells nearby must serve in their place. At other times, cells may be under instructions from supervisory cells "higher up" to handle only certain types of messages, perhaps only urgent ones. Occasionally, if the body is in an emergency state of activity or a life-threatening situation, messages (even important ones) may not be studied at all, or responses may be deferred.

There are limitations, of course, in such flexibility. Not every neuron can handle every call. Cells that receive signals from the ear, for example, do not handle messages from the eye. But within any such sensory or motor subsystem, myriad numbers of neurons are receiving and sorting out signals from one moment to the next. At some level of data analysis, each subsystem reviews its messages on a priority basis that is changing constantly over a wide range. Stimuli

2. ORGANIZING PRINCIPLES OF THE NERVOUS SYSTEM

that are pleasurable at certain times may become irritating at others, and vice versa. The entire nervous system, meanwhile, continually scans the reports of its many subsystems.

Such latitude of information processing by nerve cells and their connections shows that more is involved than a multiplicity of elements and circuits. Fixed circuits are employed flexibly. The nervous system offers flexibility in which systems and components come into play. This attribute allows us to function appropriately and intelligently in an ever-changing environment.

D. Speed of Operation of the Nervous System—Instant Service

The nervous system couples flexibility with speed in a way that has no match. Speed and accuracy a computer has, but sometimes it can be anything but flexible! The old expression "as quick as thought" is a tribute to the lightning fast integrative properties of single nerve cells. Thoughts are quick, reflexes instantaneous. Responses are as fast as they need be. We may respond to a stimulus instantly, a short time later or perhaps only after a long period. Just when our response comes (if it comes at all) depends partly on the nature of the stimulus, as well as on the activity of our nervous system at that time or later. But it also depends on such factors as our training and experience, as well as on our personal, societal and genetic backgrounds.

E. Reliability of the Nervous System—A Precise but Delicate Instrument

The reliability of our nervous system, like its flexibility, speed and predictability of response, again must be evaluated in terms of its individual cellular elements and of the entire system.

Nerve cells seldom make mistakes. The cellular specializations, cytoplasmic machinery and electrochemical events that they use to receive signals and generate responses are dependable. Furthermore, there are billions of neurons in the CNS and innumerable routes (including detours) over which they can send their messages. Thus, a loss of substantial portions of a population of neurons may not lead to serious disruption of service. What can happen is that residual neurons and alternative routes of communication are called into service. This service may not be as good as before, but at least it is better than nothing. The principle of redundancy provides reliability.

The nervous system is not always completely reliable. It does not always achieve the "foolproof" quality built into its respective components. Sometimes signals are inaccurate or distorted, messages are lost or misrouted and responses are inadequate or misdirected. Even poor decisions are made. The consequences of mistakes are often minor—a bit of clumsiness here, a wrong number there. The brain may become tired or disordered from overwork, lack of sleep, illness, want of essential nutrient or chemical substances or a variety of other causes. But even in these cases it performs admirably. It can ill afford to bungle emergency messages pertaining to the well-being of the body. It is part of the body itself and thus inseparable from the customers it serves. We see that our nervous system is more than a proficient integrator and regulator of the body's activities. It is a scholar and historian; it has highly developed capabilities for learning and memory. It is a wise planner; it weighs demands on the basis of need and in the framework of experience and constraints. It does more than merely react to and regulate events. Often, it initiates them. The nervous system thus not only "reserves the right to change its services and products at any time" but also "builds for the future." It renews and remodels many of the parts of its cells. The brain indeed has a "mind of its own!"

F. Summary of Cardinal Attributes of the Nervous System—Taking Stock

In a general way, we now see some of the major attributes of the nervous system. The PNS conveys signals from the environment (external and internal) to the CNS. There, with great flexibility, speed and reliability these signals are integrated and evaluated in relation to current and past events. A decision is made, a memory formed or a response initiated. The nervous system is much like a giant corporation: various jobs are assigned to experts, special cells in special structural relationships. It has many subdivisions—particular, highly individualized structures.

We shall turn now to an overview of the larger divisions of the human brain and from there to an analysis of functions of the parts of its marvelous whole.

II. Overview—The General Region of the CNS

Let us remove the dense nerve branches of the PNS and take a better look at the central trunk: the brain and spinal cord (Fig. 2-2, far right). Many of the parts are visible from the surface.

2. ORGANIZING PRINCIPLES OF THE NERVOUS SYSTEM

A. Cerebrum

The largest and most striking structure is uppermost—the _cerebrum_. It is almost completely divided into right and left cerebral hemispheres. The hemispheres look like mirror images of one another, but in many respects they are not completely alike. Each has abilities not as well developed in the other. For example, one hemisphere plays great roles in speech and calculation. The other is necessary for appreciation of spatial relationships and nonverbal ideation. In either hemisphere, however, analysis of environmental features and synthesis of response patterns are carried out to a degree and detail unmatched elsewhere in the nervous system.

B. Cerebellum and Pons

Lower down the neuraxis, we see the _cerebellum_. Its bulk is partly hidden by the overlying cerebral hemisphere. The cerebellum is a sort of computer; it regulates the rate, range and force of movements. It works in concert with the cerebrum, as well as with the spinal cord and other structures. Without the cerebellum, we would still enjoy all our sensations. But its loss would seriously impair the dexterity and smooth execution of our movements, while noticeably diminishing our strength and muscular tone.

Below the cerebellum is the _pons_, a bridge of nerve fibers which appears to cross from one side of the cerebellum to the other. It seems to strap the cerebellum to the brain stem like a backpack around someone's waist. It is a key link between the cerebrum and cerebellum, a massive cable through which the cerebral motor region "plugs in" to the cerebellar computer. This connection allows volitional movements to be carried out in a coordinated, flowing and well-directed manner.

C. Medulla Oblongata

Protruding from the pons, the slender, conical _medulla oblongata_ (often called simply the medulla) tapers smoothly into the spinal cord below. Like many brain regions, it has an importance all out of proportion to its size. Although no larger than a finger, it is crucial to survival. Even small injury to it leads to devastating, if not fatal, consequences. Through it run long cables of nerve fibers, _tracts_ over which the brain and cord communicate in performing different functions. Within the medulla lie clusters of neurons (_nuclei_) that carry out vital activities—breathing, swallowing, adjusting heart rate, regulating the caliber of

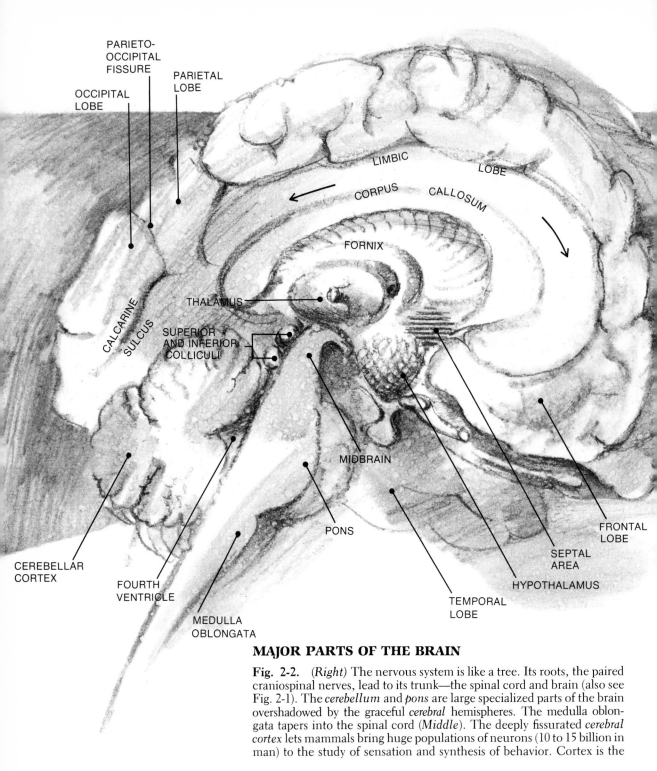

PARIETO-OCCIPITAL FISSURE

OCCIPITAL LOBE

PARIETAL LOBE

LIMBIC LOBE

CORPUS CALLOSUM

FORNIX

THALAMUS

CALCARINE SULCUS

SUPERIOR AND INFERIOR COLLICULI

MIDBRAIN

PONS

CEREBELLAR CORTEX

FOURTH VENTRICLE

MEDULLA OBLONGATA

TEMPORAL LOBE

HYPOTHALAMUS

SEPTAL AREA

FRONTAL LOBE

MAJOR PARTS OF THE BRAIN

Fig. 2-2. (*Right*) The nervous system is like a tree. Its roots, the paired craniospinal nerves, lead to its trunk—the spinal cord and brain (also see Fig. 2-1). The *cerebellum* and *pons* are large specialized parts of the brain overshadowed by the graceful *cerebral* hemispheres. The medulla oblongata tapers into the spinal cord (*Middle*). The deeply fissurated *cerebral cortex* lets mammals bring huge populations of neurons (10 to 15 billion in man) to the study of sensation and synthesis of behavior. Cortex is the

18

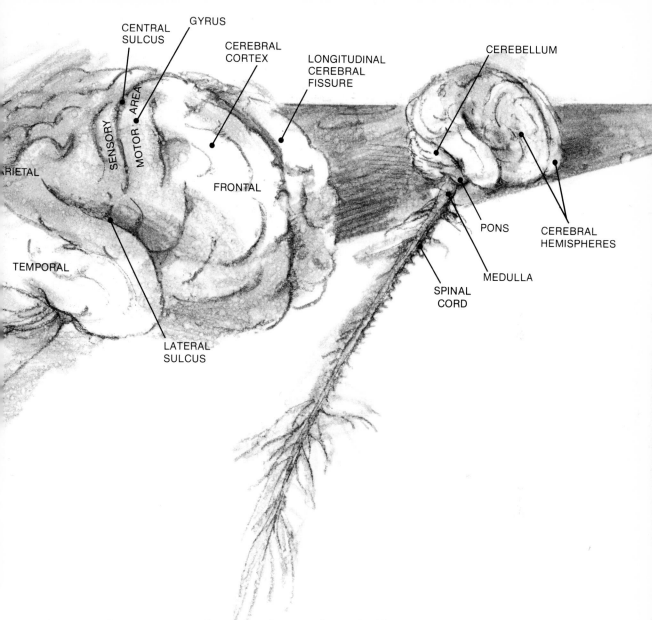

CENTRAL
SULCUS

GYRUS

CEREBRAL
CORTEX

LONGITUDINAL
CEREBRAL
FISSURE

CEREBELLUM

SENSORY

MOTOR AREA

RIETAL

FRONTAL

TEMPORAL

PONS

CEREBRAL
HEMISPHERES

MEDULLA

SPINAL
CORD

LATERAL
SULCUS

highest form of gray matter; its cells are very diverse and organized into layers. (*Left*) Human brain shown in sagittal plane. The cerebral hemisphere, pons, medulla oblongata and spinal cord are evident. The corpus callosum is a massive bridge of fibers interconnecting the cells of the two cerebral hemispheres. Some areas of the brain contain hollow spaces (ventricles) which are partially visible in this illustration. In the center of the hemisphere we see the thalamus, a part of the forebrain, and below that, forming the brainstem, we see the superior and inferior colliculi (parts of the midbrain) and the pons and medulla oblongata (part of the hindbrain).

smaller blood vessels, waking and sleeping, and other critical life functions. Moreover, certain medullary neurons have broad powers over levels of activity in the entire neuraxis. Thus, consciousness and alertness depend upon their upward effects, while the readiness and coordination of spinal reflexes for posture, locomotion and visceral control rely upon their downward influences.

D. Spinal Cord

At last we come to the trunk of the tree, the *spinal cord*. Through its roots, the many pairs of nerves, bodily sensations enter. Over its tracts, sensory messages flow up to the overlying brain. Over other tracts commands from the brain flow down to spinal motor centers, to the motor neurons there or to other nerve cells which assist them. These small cells regulate motor neurons and integrate their activity from one level to another, as well as across the midline. Although such intrinsic spinal neurons are closely supervised by the brain, they accomplish the swift and complex spinal reflexes in an efficient manner on their own. The spinal cord is divided into segments (cervical, thoracic, lumbar, sacral and coccygeal) according to the level of the body it serves.

E. A Closer Look at the Brain

As we move closer to the brain (Fig. 2-2, middle), we see that the cerebrum is highly convoluted. Its rumpled surface is thrown up into many hills (*gyri*) and criss-crossed by numerous valleys (*sulci*). The central sulcus and lateral sulcus are most prominent. Here and there deeper infoldings, canyons called *fissures*, provide boundaries for the lobes of a cerebral hemisphere. But such folding has greater significance. It enormously increases the cerebral surface area. Over two-thirds of this area lies hidden in the many involutions, and visible territories are expanded by the arched convolutions. Many mammals, especially man, the elephant and cetaceans (the whales, porpoises and dolphins) have an extensively convoluted cerebrum; others, such as rats and mice, have a smooth cerebrum. Certain fissures and sulci mark off six arbitrary but accepted cortical regions or lobes: parietal, occipital, temporal, frontal, central and limbic lobes. The *parietal lobe* lies behind the *central sulcus* and above the *lateral sulcus*; it blends to the rear with the *occipital lobe*, from which it is not clearly demarcated (see Fig. 2-2, middle and left). The *temporal lobe* also joins with the occipital; it extends forward beneath the lateral sulcus like the thumb of a boxing glove. The *frontal lobe* is the vast territory above the lateral sulcus and in front of the central sulcus.

In the above four lobes lie the primary sensory and motor areas: the *auditory* cortex, on the temporal bank of the lateral sulcus; the *visual* cortex, surrounding the occipital pole; the parietal *somesthetic* cortex, just behind the central sulcus; and the frontal *motor* cortex, just in front of that sulcus and in fact inseparable from its sensory neighbor. Large regions that surround these specialized areas elaborate sounds, sights, bodily sensations and movements in ways that are very important. But even greater syntheses take place in the association cortex. These regions knit the sensory modalities together.

Cerebral cortex is *gray matter*, in which nerve cell bodies lie, as opposed to *white matter*, in which long threadlike processes (axons) leading out of these cell bodies collect in bundles running this way and that. All parts of the CNS display these two fundamental and contrasting substances. The general arrangement is that the gray forms the central core, which is surrounded by the white.

Let us now turn to a view of the brain that can be obtained only if it is divided down the middle into halves (Fig. 2-2, left). The cerebral hemispheres are almost completely separate to begin with, but other structures are largely continuous across the midline, and must be sliced apart carefully. The surface we see after bisecting the brain is mostly artificial; only that hidden surface of the cerebral cortex facing the midline is present in the living brain. But real or not, this surface is instructive. For the first time we see the entire neuraxis at once and all its parts in natural order from top to bottom.

A large curved structure in the center resembles an overturned canoe. It is the *corpus callosum*, a bridge of white matter containing millions of nerve fibers, long neuronal processes called axons. It connects the cortex of the two hemispheres—important, because as mentioned previously they are not alike. The *limbic lobe* is a wide zone of cortex that borders the callosum (limbic means border). It is implicated in emotion and in stable, purposeful behavior.

Sensory signals reach the cerebral cortex via the *thalamus*, an egg-shaped mass of neurons (its name means inner chamber). Long ago it was thought to be a cavity supplying animal spirits to the cerebral cortex. But it is a nearly solid structure, the major sensory portal to the cerebral cortex. Beneath it the tiny *hypothalamus* (4 gm to the brain's 1400 gm total weight) controls visceral, endocrine and metabolic activities of vital importance.

Beneath the callosum, the brain wall is so thin that cortex and white matter cannot be made out; an almost translucent partition covers a large cavity or lateral ventricle (not shown). The brain is hollow; the lateral ventricles of the two hemispheres communicate with a median space in the thalamus called the third ventricle. Through the slender, cylindrical *midbrain* a narrow conduit (the cerebral aqueduct) leads down to another cavity (the fourth ventricle) roofed by the cerebellum. The brain *ventricles* form a drainage system. Cerebrospinal fluid (produced in the cavities and in the brain itself) percolates through this system to escape through apertures into a space between the brain membranes. In this space (which extends past the tip of the spinal cord) the fluid cushions and supports the heavy brain and dangling cord; the CNS floats "head-up" in this liquid like a deep-sea diver.

The _midbrain_ is a small pipe connected to a huge _forebrain_ which includes the thalamus and cerebral cortex, but it has as obvious and diverse significance as the neck to the head! Numerous tracts pass up and down it. Its injury can have serious results—unconsciouness, if not death. In its roof, the superior and inferior colliculi (small hills) analyze sights and sounds and elaborate reflexes and responses to them. In its floor, motor neurons control eye movements and constrict the pupils. Deeper still, the reticular formation that forms its core exerts excitatory and inhibitory effects upon the forebrain and the _hindbrain_—the pons, medulla oblongata and cerebellum. The midbrain and hindbrain are often referred to collectively as the brain stem.

F.   The Dissected Brain—The Inside View

We need to probe to discover the other major areas of the brain and the interrelationships between parts. We must carefully dissect away parts of the surface.

A lateral view of a dissected brain (Fig. 2-3) reveals a surprisingly ordered internal topography: graceful shapes of gray matter, curling ribbons of white. The cerebral cortex is sharply defined; it crowns each gyrus and forms the banks of the fissures and sulci. In the underlying white matter, myriad nerve fibers follow definite prescribed routes from place to place. Such routings form the major pathways interconnecting brain areas.

We can see the _cortical association fibers_ as they loop from one gyrus to the next. Previously we mentioned that the thalamus is the major sensory portal to the cerebral cortex. In this view we can see the many fibers that provide this link. Many fibers project to the cortex (in a radiating crown, the _corona radiata_) and a similar number return to the thalamus. These fibers provide the reciprocal connections for thalamocortical "discussions" of sensory and other matters.

As part of this discussion, signals from the eye course via the optic nerve, a thick cable of over a million nerve fibers, to a cell group in the thalamus called the lateral geniculate body. The broad and graceful visual radiation carries messages from the lateral geniculate to the visual cortex of the occipital pole. We can tell much about the flow of information from inspection of such tracts.

We mentioned that the cerebellum is a kind of computer, regulating movement, that is "on line" to the cerebrum by way of the pons. The cerebellum works

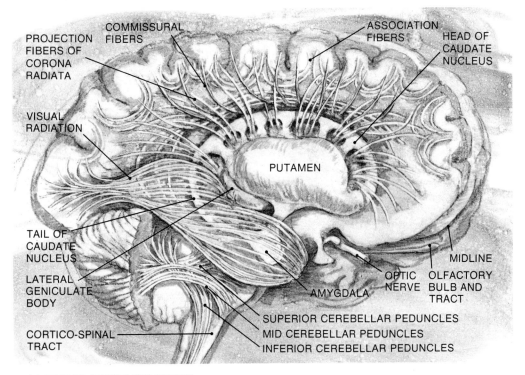

PROJECTION FIBERS OF CORONA RADIATA

COMMISSURAL FIBERS

ASSOCIATION FIBERS

HEAD OF CAUDATE NUCLEUS

VISUAL RADIATION

PUTAMEN

TAIL OF CAUDATE NUCLEUS

MIDLINE

LATERAL GENICULATE BODY

OPTIC NERVE

OLFACTORY BULB AND TRACT

AMYGDALA

CORTICO-SPINAL TRACT

SUPERIOR CEREBELLAR PEDUNCLES
MID CEREBELLAR PEDUNCLES
INFERIOR CEREBELLAR PEDUNCLES

INTERNAL TOPOGRAPHY

Fig. 2-3. Dissected view of the brain in midsagittal plane. Note the position of the midline. Beneath the cerebral cortex association fibers loop from one gyrus to another. Longer ones sweep through the white matter like huge cables and broad fans. Some (commissural fibers) enter the corpus callosum to link the cortex of both hemispheres instead of joining different cortical regions of one. Projection fibers leave the hemisphere and go to other places, some all the way to the spinal cord (corticospinal tract). Fibers from the cerebral cortex end within the pons and in turn pass via the middle cerebellar peduncle into the cerebellum. Spinocerebellar tracts leave the spinal cord and enter the cerebellum through the inferior cerebellar peduncle; still another cerebellar peduncle, the superior, leads up to the thalamus (not shown), ultimately providing a route back to the cerebral cortex. Many fibers interconnect the thalamus and cerebral cortex. Many projection fibers from the thalamus spread like a fan (corona radiata). A nucleus of the thalamus serving vision (the lateral geniculate body) gives rise to the visual radiation. The putamen and caudate nucleus, parts of the basal ganglia, are shown.

closely with the spinal cord and cerebral cortex, as follows. Fibers from the cerebral cortex of one hemisphere end within the pons, interlocking there with other fibers which run across the midline and extend laterally into the cerebellum. Thus cerebral fibers of one side of the brain pass messages to pontine fibers, which then convey them to the cerebellum on the opposite side. Another connection curves into the cerebellum from the medulla; it brings news from the spinal cord regarding stretches and tensions on muscles and tendons. Such information is essential if the cerebellum is to refine movement and posture. Refinement of either is a demanding and unremitting task.

Thus the cerebellum "listens" to the cerebral cortex above it and to the spinal cord below. Its "answers"—how to employ muscles in a coordinated manner at any given moment—are dispatched over another cable largely hidden behind the temporal fibers of the visual radiation. This cable runs to the contralateral thalamus, which passes cerebellar responses back to the motor cortex where this long-range consultation with the cerebellum began. Since the foregoing circuitry involves two crossings of the midline (a "double cross"), we realize that cerebral–cerebellar transactions involve both sides of the brain.

In this dissection, we can see several major structures not readily visible in Fig. 2-3. The far-reaching cortical outputs pass out of sight behind a bulging mass of gray matter, the *putamen*. A companion mass of cells, the *caudate nucleus*, curves behind the fan of fibers. The putamen and caudate nucleus are *basal ganglia*, masses of nerve cell bodies in the core of the cerebral hemispheres. They are joined at several places. In reality, they are two incompletely separated parts of a larger mass of deep gray matter. Together, they resemble a giant boulder partially split by weathering into two fragments. The outer, more bulky fragment is the putamen. The inner curved piece is the caudate; its elongated mass curls around the temporal lobe like a tail. Its shape conforms to the curvature of the brain cavity in which it lies; it is like a fish swimming within the brain (see Fig. 2-3). The basal ganglia are important areas of motor integration.

III.   Elements of the Nervous System

The major parts of the nervous system just described are, in fact, collections of *neurons* organized to form specific functional units. Prior to describing the structure and general operation of specific subsystems we shall introduce the neurons. As the parts of the nervous system are distinct, so are the neurons. They are large or small and shaped in many different ways according to their tasks. We shall see some of the myriad types of neurons in certain of the subsystems. In this way, as we watch function unfold from a general overview, we shall also see the cells "behind the scenes." Then when we come to study neurons in detail (in Chapter 3), we shall recognize them in their functional context.

Most neurons in the mammalian nervous system are multipolar, that is, bearing several processes. Without doubt this type of neuron is the hallmark of our nervous system (Fig. 2-4). The cell body is the part which contains the nucleus and DNA. Several receptive processes extend directly from the cell body. Branching like a tree, these varyingly thick, tapering processes are called

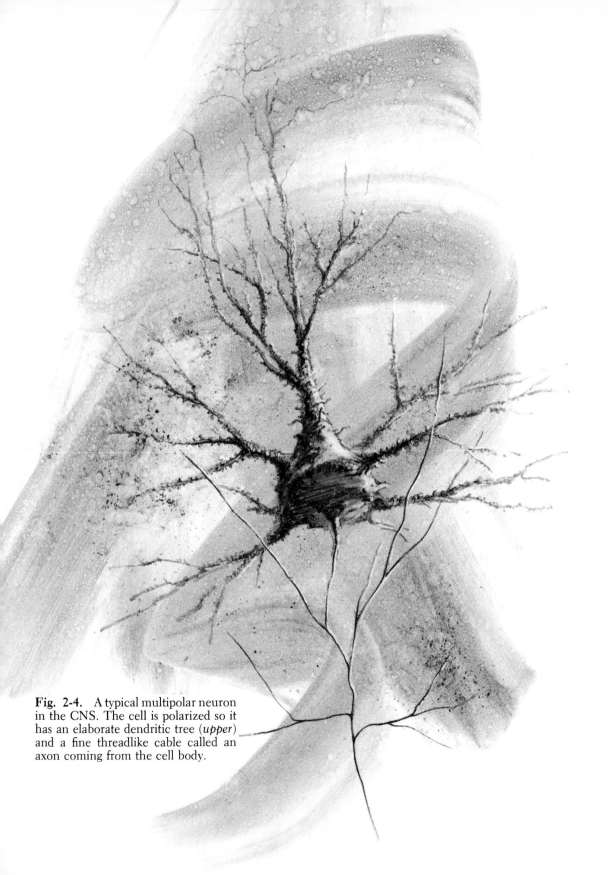

Fig. 2-4. A typical multipolar neuron in the CNS. The cell is polarized so it has an elaborate dendritic tree (*upper*) and a fine threadlike cable called an axon coming from the cell body.

dendrites. Like the bird haven a tree provides, the dendritic arbor offers in its many branches and countless twigs enormous surface on which signals from other neurons can "come to roost." Tall and stately, low and spreading, the shape and luxuriance of dendritic trees say more about the integrative role of a neuron than any other structural feature.

Somewhere around the body of a multipolar cell lies the single cable called the *axon*. Sometimes, it may arise from the stem of a dendrite. Its departure may be direct and ruler straight, indicating a clearly defined route of communication to some distant place. Or the axon may wander about after emerging, as if it were lost or had failed to "make up its mind" where it wanted to go. It may become tangled in the dendrites of the cell from which it came or with those of other cells nearby. Such rambling courses have great importance; they provide the local circuits of the CNS. Over such short, meandering axons communications between neurons in a given region take place. We can obtain a preview of several examples of multipolar neurons in Figs. 2-5 and 2-9.

Neurons can have many shapes. A neuron is extremely versatile in the way it deploys and uses its parts. Any part can perform most any communicative function if special circumstances make it advantageous to the nervous system. Some neurons, for example, have a long axon with the cell body along its course (Fig. 2-5, inset) or slightly offset to one side (Fig. 2-12). These neurons are designed to bring sensory information to the CNS, and their elongated bipolar structure ideally serves this purpose. Such neurons are *primary sensory neurons*: the first nerve cells to get the news of a change in stimulus quality from specialized receptors.

Virtually all primary neurons lie outside the CNS in clusters called *ganglia*. They are sentinels of the nervous system, standing ceaseless guard alongside the neuraxis. Each sentry extends one arm out to the body's frontier, the other back into the CNS.

While the primary neurons live in the ganglia all by themselves, *secondary* or higher neurons cannot. They form clusters also, but since they lie in the CNS they are surrounded by other neurons attending to other matters. A word other than "ganglion" is used. The word ganglion connotes isolation of a crowd of neurons, like a bead along a string. Accordingly, a group of functionally related central neurons, sensory or otherwise, is called a *nucleus*. This term implies a "nucleus of neural activity," and must not be confused with the nucleus of a cell. The neurons which comprise a nucleus mingle with the immense population of CNS neurons in which they reside. Unlike the uniform, dutiful sentinels in the lonely outposts of the ganglia, the neurons in even a single brain nucleus may have many shapes, sizes and functional assignments. Their heterogeneity is reflected in their multipolar design, just as we saw the simple reporting function of a sensory ganglion cell expressed by bipolarity.

Primary neurons report to the dendritic trees of secondary sensory neurons in the CNS, which collect this information along with other news. On their surface membranes secondary neurons integrate all these reports, and through their axons they send the conclusions to other cells in the CNS. In turn, billions of neurons in various brain nuclei consider, reconsider and finally interpret the news for us.

It is the work of the neurons, connected in specific ways and functioning according to strict specifications, which delivers oneness, flexibility, reliability and speed. Organized into subsystems they meet our needs; they determine what we can do.

A.   Functional Subsystems

We shall now examine several subsystems of the nervous system. In the simplest sense the nervous system has three big problems to solve: (1) it must gather environmental stimuli as well as the news from our bodies; (2) it must weigh and consider everything; and (3) it must come forth with an appropriate response, a movement or a feeling, for example. Accordingly, in considering the subsystems we shall first focus on those that gather sensory stimuli (the auditory, visual and somesthetic systems). Then we shall discuss the limbic system, the subsystem most concerned with our feelings. Finally, we shall consider the motor system and spinal cord—the subsystems responsible for operating our glands and making us move and talk.

1.   THE AUDITORY SYSTEM—OUR FIRST TRIP INSIDE THE BRAIN.   The auditory pathway (Fig. 2-5) is a good route to take in our first trip inside the brain. It is long enough for us to see much of the brain along the way. And so much business is transacted up and down the line that we can see many additional organizing principles of the nervous system at work. We shall see the care and scope of information processing in the CNS.

Perception of sound is part of a much larger process of gathering information on physical events affecting the body. This continuing survey of an ever-changing world is a bigger job than most of us realize. The brain, however, treats sound in this broad context right from the start.

Figure 2-5 illustrates the general layout of the auditory system and shows the general flow of signals into it. The pathway travels a long way, from the inner ear through medulla oblongata up to thalamus and cortex and then back down, right out to the inner ear again. The information passes from the *hair cell* (the receptor cell) in the <u>cochlea</u> to the *cochlear and deep auditory nuclei* in the medulla and then to three structures, each of which has a cortical design—the *inferior colliculus* (in the midbrain), the *medial geniculate body* (a nucleus of the thalamus) and the *auditory cortex* itself. In doing so, so much happens to it! So much

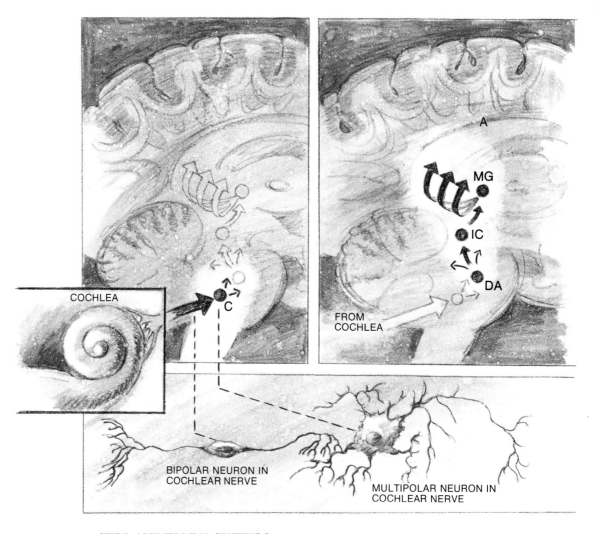

COCHLEA

A

MG

IC

DA

FROM
COCHLEA

C

BIPOLAR NEURON IN
COCHLEAR NERVE

MULTIPOLAR NEURON IN
COCHLEAR NERVE

THE AUDITORY SYSTEM

Fig. 2-5. Just beneath our ears lies a spiral-shaped structure, the *cochlea*. Within this structure lie specialized receptors, the hair cells. Their job is to transform sound into neuronal language, electrical potentials, an energy translation process called transduction. As their first task all sensory subsystems must transduce a stimulus. The primary auditory neurons [bipolar cells (*bottom*)] live in the skull near the cochlea. Their opposing processes are short. The outer process leads to the bony cochlea. There it divides into fingerlike branches that make intimate contact with hair cells, grasping them in several ways. With auditory stimulation, vibration-induced voltage changes in hair cell membranes and subsequent sensory potentials in the fine branches generate action potentials in the outer process. These impulses pass over the cell body and inner process into the brain stem, where secondary sensory neurons in the cochlear nuclei (C) receive and pass along the news. These cells are multipolar (*bottom*). The cochlear nuclei are only the first of many centers along the way. As the impulses travel they reach the *deep auditory nuclei* (DA), *inferior colliculus* (IC) and *medial geniculate* (MG) body of the thalamus are others (*right*). Each center teams with activity as messages flow up and down the system, reporting sounds and seeking more data. Eventually the messages reach the auditory cortex (A).

richness of experience is added, so much extraneous detail left behind and perhaps sent elsewhere. At each level of the upward journey, the messages for cortex are embellished and refined. And at the cortex they receive even more selective study, as features of auditory experience are extracted for further scrutiny and consideration of meaning. The thalamic and midbrain way stations are not just relay points or "whistle stops" along the route to conscious auditory experience.

In any part of the CNS, what goes in is never what comes out. This axiom holds true for single neurons, and especially for clusters of them. Wherever neurons handle information, *integration* takes place.

a. Team operations in processing.   Analysis of hearing is a team operation. The inferior colliculus and medial geniculate work with the auditory cortex, but also with other structures. The deep auditory nuclei are important members of the team. Although not shown in Fig. 2-5, many small cell clusters lie along the short streets, long bypasses, complex interchanges and numerous cross-overs that comprise the auditory pathway. From the interplay of these clusters, inferior colliculus and medial geniculate come discriminations and judgments of sound direction, intensity, volume, pitch and timbre. And, through descending fibers, even the cortex can enter these discussions. The team spirit is everywhere!

b. Dissemination of information.   The auditory brain carries its news in an open or "public" manner up and down its long corridor, for continued study of messages and modified responses to them all along the way. It wastes no time in allowing leaks of information to take place, nor in beginning a thorough, multilevel investigation of the news reported over its lines. This immediate spread of information, even as it is being studied, helps to unify CNS functions.

c. Spatial fidelity in sensory systems.   We do not know how every feature of a sound is analyzed, any more than we can say where such analysis takes place, but frequency or *tone* receives careful handling. Tones are represented in a progressive sequence along the organ of hearing. From the blind end of the cochlea to the end near the ear ossicles, the frequency spectrum is precisely laid out from bass to treble clef. This orderly, successive arrangement is called *tonotopic organization*. In this case, it is the receptors that are so organized: the hair cells and the flimsy membranes on which they are propped up and shaken by vibrations.

Tonotopic organization, however, does not stop at the receptor level. The cells and fibers of many auditory nuclei and tracts also show it. Elements that handle the lowest tones may lie in one part, those concerned with a slightly higher frequency immediately alongside and so forth. At higher levels of the system some tonotopy is lost, or perhaps blurred. Such loss could be due to departure of fibers from the pathway, entrance of others and passage through such busy places as the inferior colliculus, where anything could happen. However, in general, the CNS tries to preserve a "map" of the highly ordered receptive surface of the cochlear duct.

Such *spatial fidelity* of nervous pathways, sensory or otherwise, is an important organizing principle. To judge from their pictures of it, the ancient anatomists viewed the brain as having little internal order—about as much as a pile of spaghetti! The brain, however, is really very neat and methodical in the way it arranges its cells and wires, at least in most places. These admirable qualities are pronounced in the visual, somesthetic and motor pathways, as we shall see.

d. Modulation. We said that the auditory pathway leads from the hair cells all the way up to cortex and back down again. We mentioned also that through such descending fibers the cortex can join in discussions going on below. But why are there so many descending fibers? There are almost as many of them as fibers going up! Why all these downward and outgoing messages along a supposedly incoming sensory path?

The answer is to control and enhance the process of hearing. The descending fibers carry editorial queries and directives from higher offices (the cortex, geniculate and colliculus) to lower offices (the deep auditory and cochlear nuclei), even to the reporters themselves (the bipolar neurons and hair cells). These messages improve the gathering of information. To borrow terms from radio engineering, they increase receptive acuity, filter out "static" or background noise, "squelch" unwanted signals, sharpen contrast and increase the "signal-to-noise" ratio. Each component, including the hair cells, can be "tuned." Such sensory regulation is easier to understand when we remember that we must tune a radio or television set, focus binoculars or a microscope or adjust in some way the various instruments we use to gather information.

Regulation or *modulation* is a key principle in the CNS. In the operation of sensory subsystems, it is an outgoing regulation of incoming signals, but modulation is not confined to sensory pathways. Many neurons of the brain and cord, including the motor neurons firing orders to muscles, are constantly sending back requests for new information or more specific instructions. They report back what they have just accomplished. From such feedback modulation, which is mediated by returning branches of axons, comes heightened sensitivity and more finely graduated response, and from it comes the ability to arrest responses and supplant them with new ones.

We have glimpsed many organizing principles at work along the auditory path. We have seen transduction of stimulus energy, painstaking analysis of features and careful synthesis of response—activities constantly reviewed and adjusted by feedback modulation of input and output. We have noted tasks carried out openly, with a divergence of information to many neurons and places that helps to unify CNS functions. We have witnessed a team effort, in which each neuron in a vast organization of interdependent cells does its job. We have watched this effort consummated by convergence of messages upon clusters of cells and integration of information by the cells in those clusters. We have noted orderliness of design in the intricate avenues of the pathway, the cortical design of stations along the way and the pervasive tonotopic organization. These principles will come in again and again as we examine other subsystems of the nervous system.

2. THE EQUILIBRATORY SYSTEM—SILENT PARTNER OF THE INNER EAR. Deep beneath our ears, along with the receptor cells for hearing, lie those for balance. All the receptors in the inner ear are hair cells. In the equilibratory organ hair cells transduce movements of fluids as in the cochlea. In this case, the movements occur within slender, curved tubules (the semicircular canals) which arch in all three planes of space. In addition, in two places (small, membranous bags, the utricle and saccule) hair cells translate the inertial or gravitational pull on tiny, sandlike particles embedded with the hairs in a gelatinous mass that is free to shift this way and that. Such movements of fluid in the canals or displacements of jelly in the utricle and saccule result from sudden rotation or inclination of the head. Probably any type of head movement has some effect on all the hair cells, wherever they are. In any event, the messages to the brain begin with voltage changes in hair cell membranes.

Normally, we take our precious sense of *stability*, of the space about us and solid ground beneath for granted. Unless, of course, we are so unlucky as to find ourselves in a great earthquake. At such a moment, as eloquent accounts attest, nameless fright seizes a person—a terrifying sensation of profound *instability*, of space gone awry and terra firma lost. Apparently, many animals experience something like it before we do. Flashes of such fear are our sinking sensations in fast elevators, on a roller coaster or in any situation where the world moves unexpectedly and inexplicably out from under us. Other snatches of this deep but ever-lurking apprehension come from sights, as from the edge of a great drop, which lead us to fear that instability is about to become a reality. Thus, in the CNS a "groundless concern" is perhaps the greatest fear of all. At least it can be very difficult to ignore.

What has all this to do with organizing principles? The sensations of stability, sound, motion and contact; of shapes and movements of things around us; of our own posture and locomotion; of all events affecting the body are only parts of a continuing global survey of an ever-changing environment by the nervous system. Every part, every bit of information, must be considered in light of the whole if we are to proceed safely and appropriately in this environment, and to the extent that it brings these two entireties, ourselves and the environment, into accord, the nervous system converts empty space and meaningless surroundings into our biosphere.

3. THE VISUAL SYSTEM. Vision exerts strong and sometimes supreme command over our other senses, as optical illusions demonstrate, and it exercises similar effects upon our posture and locomotion. With one's eyes closed, standing soon becomes difficult, and except by luck threading a needle would be impossible.

Figure 2-6 shows the basic features and circuitry of the visual system—from the eyes, to the *lateral geniculate body*, to the cortex. To the occipital lobes of the cerebrum are entrusted the precious assets of sight. The beautifully organized *visual cortex* scrutinizes images of the world about as they are transmitted, as if by wirephoto, from the eyes. The visual pathway is partially crossed, long, private and precise.

a. Crossed connections. Through partially crossed connections each hemisphere studies the half of the world on the opposite side of the body. The two *optic nerves* exchange fully half their total two million fibers immediately after they enter the cranial vault. At the *optic chiasm*, fibers from the nasal half of each retina (which looks outward past one's temple) cross, while those from the temporal half (which looks inward toward the nose) remain uncrossed. In this partially crossed way, corresponding sides of what each eye sees are combined on one side of the brain. The left hemisphere "looks" to one's right, and the right hemisphere to the left (see Fig. 2-6). In accord, the motor cortex in the left frontal lobe oversees willed movements on the right and vice versa.

THE VISUAL SYSTEM

Fig. 2-6. Although long, the visual pathway is direct and straightforward. We may imagine it "lighting up" in three stages: (A) First the optic nerves trade fibers from the nasal half of each retina (which looks outward past one's temple); fibers from the temporal half (which looks inward toward the nose) remain uncrossed. In this partially crossed way, corresponding sides of the world as seen by each eye are combined on one side of the brain. The optic tracts (continuations of the recombined nerve fibers) carry their congruent representations of the visual field straight back to the thalamus. (B) In each half of the thalamus, retinal impulses are received by a large nucleus bent upon itself like a knee (genu)—the lateral geniculate body. The many neurons in this complex, layered structure extract and analyze features. Much analysis, however, has already been carried out in the retina, that part of the brain that peers from the skull. (C) From the lateral geniculate, the elegant fan of the visual radiation unfolds in a curling manner, first curving forward into the temporal lobe and then (as if with a flourish) looping back again to sweep broadly and gracefully to the occipital pole. Its many neatly arranged fibers end in the visual cortex—along the banks of the calcarine sulcus in orderly array. There, steps toward greater integration will be taken. Thus at three levels—retinal, thalamic and cortical—visual impulses are integrated progressively by neurons extracting more and more complex combinations of features at each level. The visual pathway, flashing its news over two long but direct beams, is crystal-clear. In a dissection (Fig. 2-3) you can trace most of it with the naked eye.

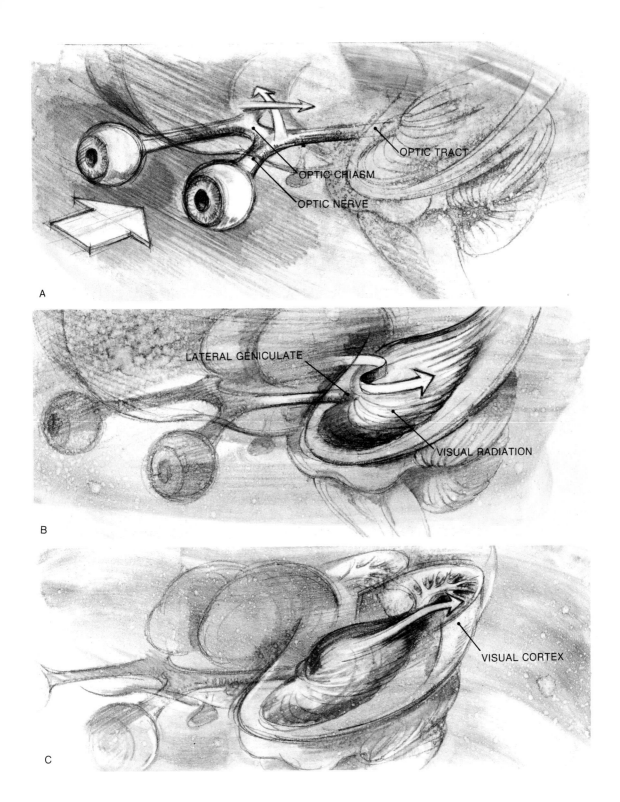

A

OPTIC TRACT

OPTIC CHIASM

OPTIC NERVE

B

LATERAL GENICULATE

VISUAL RADIATION

C

VISUAL CORTEX

This principle of crossed connections appears puzzling and unnecessarily complicated at first. Why does the brain do things the hard way? In reply, we can say that transactions across the median of the neuraxis, some of them partial (as in the visual pathway), others total and still others "double crosses," act to unify neural activity and thus integrate the body. The body would not be "a body" if each side of the nervous system "looked after its own." There would only be two halves of a body with little in common except the axial skeleton, some organs here and there and the blood. The environment would not be a totality, either. In the visual system, for example, there would be two different motion pictures of the world going on, as separate as two films showing currently at the left and right theaters of a double cinema!

b. Length and privacy. The visual pathway is obviously *long.* It runs all the way from the eyes to the back of the head.

It is also *private.* Unlike the auditory routes, which handle many of their affairs openly, little information leaks out of the cable from the eye to thalamus, or from it to cortex. Only high priority messages for the midbrain, to the superior colliculus and regions nearby, depart from it. This information is urgently needed for pupillary and ocular reflexes, conjugate eye movements and complex behavioral patterns that must be initiated without delay, but otherwise the optic nerve, tract and radiation comprise a private line, as far as any monitoring by inquisitive neurons outside it is concerned.

c. Precision. Visual connections are neatly laid out. We might say that the visual brain is the epitome of precision.

The retina has point-to-point projections to the lateral geniculate, as does that nucleus to the visual cortex. In principle, this *retinotopy* is like the tonotopy of the auditory path, but more pronounced. Moreover, photosensitive regions of the retina that are more important to visual acuity receive ever-widening territories. The cortical area concerned with keenest sight is a large region at the occipital pole, even though the place of most acute vision is a mere spot and pit upon the retina. In contrast, the areas that study peripheral vision are narrow bands on the cortical map (little more than the banks of the calcarine sulcus), even though such vision occupies most of the photosensitive surface of the eye.

Such distortions of the retinal map illustrate another principle: the amount of feature analyzing region devoted to a receptive surface is proportional to the *importance* of that surface, not its area. In central analyzers, such as the lateral geniculate or visual cortex, it is the value (not the size) of a body part that counts.

The visual system is *precise* down to the level of its cells. Each cell or group of cells looks for a certain feature in the pattern of visual stimuli and only that feature—onset or cessation of illumination, concentric rings, different colors, a straight bar tipped at a certain angle moving in a given direction, for example.

2. ORGANIZING PRINCIPLES OF THE NERVOUS SYSTEM

The features extracted become more and more specific in going from retina to cortex; specific retinal cells respond only to simple features, while specific cortical cells can respond to specific objects. In the visual system we see important principles of cellular function: (1) hierarchy of analysis at the cellular level and (2) functional specificity of neurons and their consequent individuality. The subsystem assigns specific tasks to its constituent cells, and as a result each cell has some individual role and ability.

Thus from the visual system we have gathered new organizing principles: crossed transactions that help to unify the body and its environment; direct, private and precise circuitry through which to transmit fine-grain images of sensory events; specified assignments of tasks and individualized neurons in specialized regions that carry them out; maps that magnify the importance of sensory surfaces; interdependent but progressive levels of analysis; and (as we shall discuss in Chapter 10) an enduring plasticity, not only to meet challenges from moment to moment, but to adapt continually and frugally throughout life.

4. THE SOMESTHETIC SYSTEM—THE BODY IS A BOOK THE BRAIN CAN READ. Sounds, smells and rays of light come to us from a distance, but many stimuli reach the body from sources close to hand, or originate inside it. On the surface and in the substance of the body events of many kinds follow in ceaseless procession. What is happening on the skin? In the far-flung fabric of connective tissue? In the muscles, tendons and joints, and the heart, lungs and other vital organs? The CNS has to keep track of so many things that it is hard to count and classify them. Of five systems (which monitor sight, sound, smell and taste) only one is left to characterize all the rest that we can feel. It is the somesthetic system.

Light touch (like that of a feather) is an external sensation. Pain, warmth and cold are others. The changes in energy, or stimuli, that produce them affect the skin and tissues immediately underneath. Certain sensations, however, arise more deeply: deep pain, pressure, vibration, sense of position or movement of body parts, judgments of weight, shape and form of objects. Internal sensations, arising from the viscera, are the hardest to put into words and often difficult to locate precisely. They are almost always unpleasant, and seldom can be ignored: fullness of bladder, emptiness (or overfullness) of stomach, distention or stretching of the bowel, abdominal or pelvic cramps, the frighteningly familiar (but fortunately forgettable) feeling of nausea.

How does the nervous system detect and report the diverse stimuli in the spectrum of energy that bathes the body? We first saw the answer in the auditory system: _transduction_. A variety of specialized receptors transduce changes in a wide range of mechanical or thermal forms of energy into electrical potentials that initiate nerve impulses. The auditory hair cells are not true neurons, but modified epithelial cells. They pass their findings on to primary neurons, the bipolar cells of the auditory ganglion. Somesthetic receptors can also be modified surface or "sense" cells, but are usually specializations at the tip of the outer process of the primary neuron itself. Some are quite simple: tiny, unmyelinated nerve branches ramifying in a strategic spot. Others are ingenious arrangements of cells in capsules around a nerve fiber, such that discharge of impulses will vary with different degrees of capsular deformation. Whatever their form, construction and mode of operation, receptors are distributed in greater or less density throughout the body, in almost every place except the nervous system itself. Even though the CNS is insensitive, a number of receptors are found in its covering membranes and along its blood vessels.

All these receptors enable the nervous system to monitor the flow of energy that ebbs and floods around and through the body. As we have already suggested, they are interested in *changes* in this flow, not the flow itself. Their reports of changes (by increased or decreased rates of firing or other coded responses) lead to bodily sensations. The primary neurons that transmit these reports enter the spinal cord or certain cranial nerves.

As shown in Fig. 2-7, body sensations are reported over two contrasting types of pathways, lemniscal and reticular. *Lemniscal pathways* are extremely rapid and reliable. There is little chance for messages to depart for other important destinations that lie along these high-speed routes. The ungarbled reports transmitted over these lines make possible the *discriminative* aspects of somatic sensation. Interruption of lemniscal pathways will impair such critical sensory judgments. Lemniscal pathways are essential to sensory analysis by the cortex, but offer few shorter, alternative routings and do nothing to provide for local traffic of impulses. Yet a spread of information over such short connections is crucial for reflexes that must be carried out quickly, as well as for general activation of the brain, as in arousal and alertness.

Reticular pathways exert greater, longer and more generalized influences on the regions of the CNS through which they run than the lemniscal ones. We depict these differences in our illustration by upward spread of diffuse, persistent luminescence versus ascending flashes of narrow, fleeting beams of light, respectively. Some half-dozen of these diffuse reticular pathways lead upward through the cord and brainstem, usually coursing more deeply than the lemnisci. They convey impulses to the same thalamic and cortical terminals as the fast routes, as well as to other places close by. The information arrives less expeditiously, however, and is distributed less selectively to the neurons awaiting it. It is less detailed, because much has been lost in transit. Nevertheless, what does arrive is a consensus of many brainstem neurons that is crucial to the *affective* aspects of sensation and general awareness. Interruption of these pathways can alter feelings that sensations are agreeable or disagreeable, abolish consciousness or seriously impair alertness and attention.

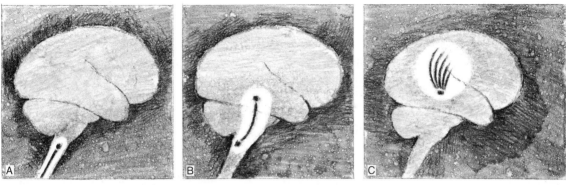

SPECIFIC OR LEMNISCAL PATHWAYS

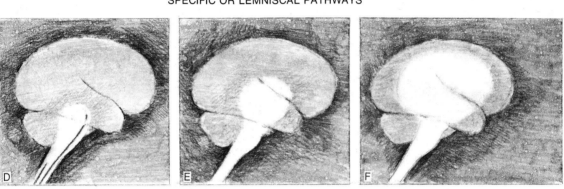

DIFFUSE OR RETICULAR PATHWAYS

SOMESTHETIC SYSTEM

Fig. 2-7. Somesthetic impulses travel up the neuraxis along many avenues but in two different ways, lemniscal pathways (A,B,C) and reticular pathways (D,E,F). Signals go almost directly, through a minimum number of intermediate stops, to specific distant destinations over fast-conducting, clearly defined tracts called lemnisci (ribbons). The optic pathway, as we have seen, shows this design; its messages proceed directly over the rapidly conducting cables of the optic nerve, tract and radiation. Although not as visible, similar cables, the specific lemniscal pathways, lie buried near the surface of the spinal cord and brain stem. They bring information swiftly to the thalamus and cortex, and reliably too, because almost nothing is lost along the way. Signals also proceed upward indirectly, through many intermediate stations, to local as well as distant destinations over more slowly conducting, less clearly defined tracts. From these tracts, fibers or their side branches leave at many points and spread diffusely into places along the way, especially into the reticular formation. The auditory pathway illustrates this type of arrangement, although it offers lemniscal routes also. Some of its messages go quite promptly to the medial geniculate body and auditory cortex, but how many more must get lost somewhere else!

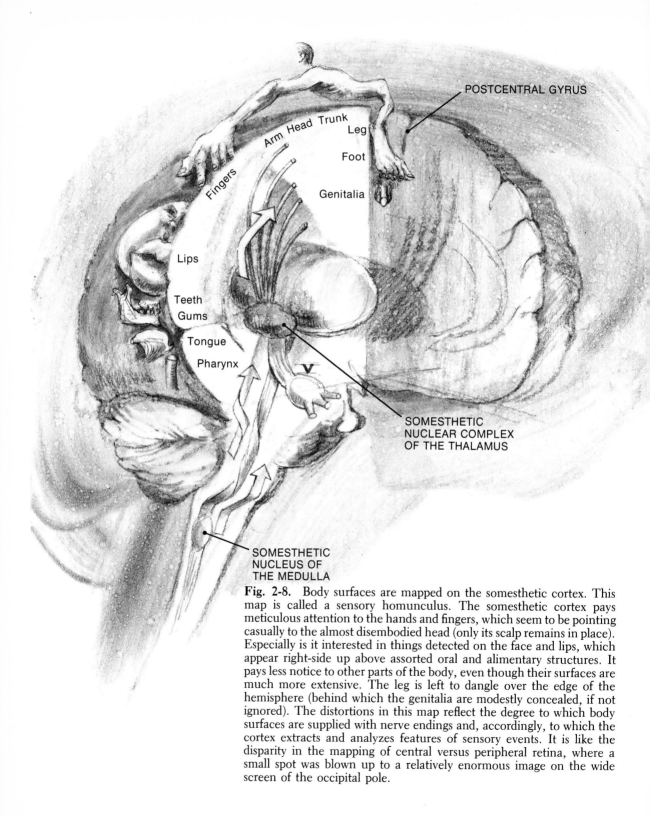

POSTCENTRAL GYRUS

Arm Head Trunk
Leg
Foot
Genitalia
Fingers
Lips
Teeth
Gums
Tongue
Pharynx

V

SOMESTHETIC
NUCLEAR COMPLEX
OF THE THALAMUS

SOMESTHETIC
NUCLEUS OF
THE MEDULLA

Fig. 2-8. Body surfaces are mapped on the somesthetic cortex. This map is called a sensory homunculus. The somesthetic cortex pays meticulous attention to the hands and fingers, which seem to be pointing casually to the almost disembodied head (only its scalp remains in place). Especially is it interested in things detected on the face and lips, which appear right-side up above assorted oral and alimentary structures. It pays less notice to other parts of the body, even though their surfaces are much more extensive. The leg is left to dangle over the edge of the hemisphere (behind which the genitalia are modestly concealed, if not ignored). The distortions in this map reflect the degree to which body surfaces are supplied with nerve endings and, accordingly, to which the cortex extracts and analyzes features of sensory events. It is like the disparity in the mapping of central versus peripheral retina, where a small spot was blown up to a relatively enormous image on the wide screen of the occipital pole.

Eventually, through the lemniscal and reticular routes up the cord and brainstem, information on body sensations reaches the thalamus. It enters the somesthetic nuclear complex, a large region near the medial and lateral geniculate bodies that study sights and sounds, respectively. From the thalamus, fibers pass in precise somatotopic array through the fanlike sensory radiation to the *primary somesthetic cortex*. It lies in the parietal lobe, just behind the central sulcus. It is close to the motor cortex, with which it works closely and is, in fact, inseparable. Here, in keeping with previous principles (mapping sensory regions according to their importance and crossed transactions to promote unity), a functionally appropriate (if anatomically grotesque) picture of the opposite side of the body is represented. This distorted, largely upside-down (and altogether repugnant) image of half a body is the way a cerebral hemisphere sees it. It is the primary _sensory homunculus_ (Fig. 2-8).

a. Multiple representation. We have just examined two kinds of sensory pathways, diffuse and specific. Multiple representation is an organizing principle, an outgrowth of neuronal specificity and individuality. In this logical extension of those principles, entire networks of neurons are given specific jobs to perform. The resulting individuality of such teams is seen in such things as fast and slow tracts or additional functionally different homunculi. In fact, secondary somesthetic, auditory and visual areas have been recognized in the cerebral cortex for some time, even though their functional contributions are not entirely clear.

Thus, the body is mapped, perhaps over and over for different purposes, in the thalamus and cortex, but the many senses must be blended. Touch is only one of them. Pressure, vibration, sense of position and movement are others, and we could list many more, never forgetting pain. Pain is charted less precisely, but more than adequately. All these sensations must be alloyed if the nervous system is to gain meaningful impressions of changes in and on the body and make continuing, appropriate responses. Let us take a closer look at the progressive process.

b. Interdependent hierarchy. The countless somesthetic neurons, like their visual and auditory counterparts, are organized in an interdependent hierarchy. A difference, however, is that unlike the sensations of sight and hearing there are many kinds of cutaneous and deeper stimuli from many places to scrutinize and put together. At the lowest organizational levels, the bits and pieces of information, no matter how quickly and exactly reported, do not mean very much: a sudden signal here, a longer signal there, a faster or slower train of signals somewhere else. When first reported, they are just one or another isolated deviation from the status quo. At higher levels, rough sketches are found: a contact here, a presence there, a cold or hot spot. At still higher levels, pictures begin to form. Now the neurons are looking for certain features in combination: the simultaneous presence, perhaps, of several colder, sharper places on the palm of the hand. At the highest echelons, in the thalamus and cortex, sharp images appear, with fine colorations and also with perspectives on what might come next: two points of a compass close together, a dime in a pocket or purse, finger positions on the neck of a violin. Individuals with injuries to the primary somesthetic area can feel objects handled with their eyes closed, but cannot evaluate their textures, shapes, weights or temperature. In short, they cannot recognize them nor can they correctly and precisely localize sensations, appreciate locations and positions of body parts or sense their movements as easily as before.

As at the retinal, geniculate and cortical levels of visual analysis, at each stage the features selected by somesthetic neurons represent increasingly complex combinations. Selection at each level is signaled by a change in neuronal response; like tiny slot machines neurons "pay off" best when the right combination comes up!

   c. *Appropriate and comprehensive combinations.*   The combination of signals can be as important in determining the nature of a sensation as the labeled lines over which the reports come. In the body lie receptors that signal potentially harmful changes, just as sensors in a building detect smoke, or movement when the premises should be unoccupied. However, interpretation of these changes as pain requires activity by neurons, just as evaluation of smoke as a fire or of movement as an intruder must be made by the watchman. In each case, additional facts must be obtained and considered. Moreover, combinations of signals contribute to the affective quality of a sensation. The experience of pain as severe and calling for emergency measures again necessitates a synthesis of information, much as appraisal of a fire as serious or an intruder as a burglar. We check on everything—all that we receive, all that we know. The great organizing principle is *integration*—all must be appropriately and meaningfully alloyed.

In summary, the somesthetic system illustrates many principles that by now are familiar; efficient cellular design, private and public pathways, somatotopy, an interdependent neuronal hierarchy, division of labor, starting many tasks at once (and never finishing some), progressive feature extraction and analysis, neural specificity and individuality, magnified images and crossed connections, adaptability to loss of parts and perhaps others implied if not stated. It also introduces new ones, or extension of previous ones: receptors looking for changes, for novelty; dual channels for fast, accurate long-distance communications, as well as prolonged local conversations; multiple representations for different tasks and for different purposes; syntheses of data, as well as labeled lines, that define the nature and quality of sensations; and, last but not least, patterns.

Patterns are the essence of neural function, and neurons must report, interpret and recognize those patterns. The wonder of sight notwithstanding, the brain is blind. It cannot look at the energy that fluctuates ceaselessly on and in the body in so many ways and places, not even at that which falls upon the retina. It can only detect changes in electrical signals and their patterns in the secret corridors of its inner space and over fleeting instants of time. Like a blind person, fingering the dots of Braille, the nervous system knows that each new pattern or combination of patterns means something. In this way, the blind brain can read and understand what is written in the body. And, when the writing is on the curved screen of the retina, it believes it can see.

5. THE THALAMUS—PARTNER TO THE CORTEX. The thalamus is the principal terminus of the great sensory subsystems, the central clearing house for all sensations except smell. Previously we noted that auditory signals pass through a nucleus of the thalamus (the medial geniculate), visual signals through another nucleus (the lateral geniculate) and somesthetic signals through the somesthetic nuclear complex of the thalamus. Smell, that often neglected but powerful input, comes directly to the cerebral hemisphere from its smaller and oldest part, the olfactory bulb.

Three kinds of messages come to the thalamus. Only two are directly related to sensation. These are the discriminative and affective messages we noted in somesthesis: what the signals mean and whether they are pleasant or unpleasant. An affective judgment is always possible, if not actually made. The thalamus has much to do with affective judgments.

The third kind of message to the thalamus comes from nonsensory parts of the brain that exploit its strategic central location and magnificent integrative circuitry. Signals from the cerebellum and basal ganglia, as well as from the limbic system (see below), pass through its forward half, just as ones from the eyes, ear and body stream through farther back. These forward connections implicate the thalamus in motor control and emotion. It represents, therefore, a key communications link for many forebrain mechanisms, not only sensory ones. As clinical proof, lesions of the front half of the thalamus may produce the types of tremors and movement disorders seen in cerebellar or basal ganglia disease or the emotional problems and deficits in learning, memory and planning that follow damage to the maze of limbic pathways.

But the thalamus does more than filter and sift out messages, passing abstracts and detailed reports up to the cortex for further review. It is an immensely important structure, if not the dominant one, in maintaining consciousness, alertness and attention. In these elusive but high functions, it works hand-in-hand with the cerebral cortex and the *reticular formation*, the core of the brain stem. Through the thalamus the diffuse reticular pathways (see above) connect with an equally diffuse thalamocortical activating system. In this way, the brain stem, of which the reticular formation and thalamus are parts, "turns on" the cortex, as one would turn on a television set. Upon this diffuse pattern of activation "pictures" of specific sensations arrive and are displayed on the already glowing screens of the auditory, visual and somesthetic areas of the cortical console.

An important corollary to teamwork is that no part of the brain works alone. No part "does anything" except to perform input–output transformations. No place is the "seat" or "center" of a particular activity, any more than a town or city is really the center of business or government it is said to be. Each place depends upon other places in a continuing partnership of activity. Thus the thalamus is a partner to the cortex, as well as to many other structures, and it is associated with many functions, but it is not *where* those functions take place. Especially when the mystery of generalized brain activity is before us, we should heed the words of the neurosurgeon Wilder Penfield who said, "There is no room or place where consciousness dwells" (Penfield, 1975).

6. THE MOTOR SYSTEM—WHERE NEURAL ACTIVITY AT LAST COMES TO MOTION. The *motor cortex* (Fig. 2-9) is a broad and beautifully organized band of frontal gray matter adjoining the central sulcus, immediately in front of the primary sensory homunculus. It also features an inverted representation of the opposite half of the body, a *motor homunculus*. It is so similar to its distorted sensory counterpart that we do not illustrate it. As with the sensory analyzing regions, this area of cortex where movement patterns are synthesized stresses the importance of body parts, not their size. Stimulation of a part of the cortex devoted to fingers brings about contractions in groups of muscles that produce definite, if crude, movements.

The motor cortex is part of a great keyboard only the brain can play upon. Each volitional movement is the result of a meaningful pattern of neuronal activity played upon the different areas of the motor cortex generating patterns of muscle movements in the periphery—an arm reaching out, a finger extending, touching. . . .

The motor cortex is only one part of the motor system. As we see from Fig. 2-9 it stands at the top of an arrangement of fibers leading primarily to the motor neurons in the spinal cord. The cerebellum and basal ganglia send fibers to cortex and work with it as a part of a team. The motor cortex sends the final decisions down to motor neurons in the spinal cord, which in turn drive the appropriate muscles.

The essence of the team play by the three members of the motor system is as follows. The basal ganglia are wired between nearly the *entire* cortex, on one hand, and the *motor* cortex (by way of the thalamus), on the other. The same thing can be said for the cerebellum. It "listens" to each lobe of the cerebral hemisphere

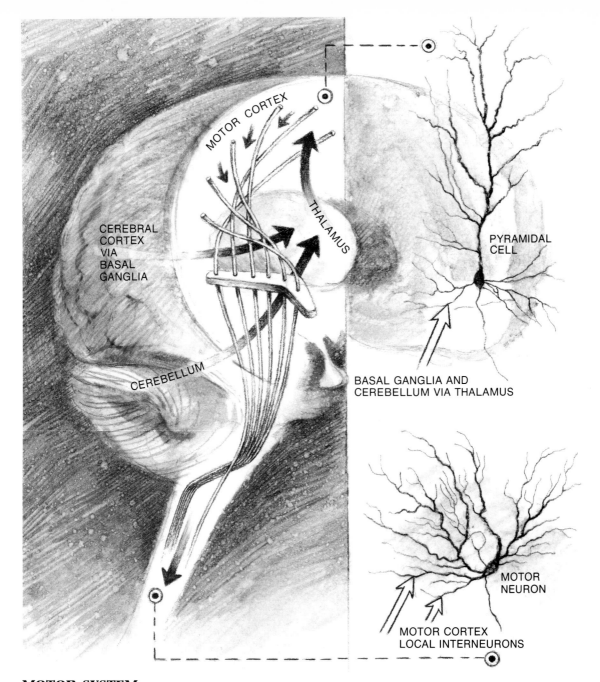

MOTOR SYSTEM

Fig. 2-9. From the motor cortex variously long fibers run directly to their targets, the *motor neurons* or the many small cells nearby that assist these indispensable busy executives whose job it is to drive muscles. These cerebral connections to motor neurons are arranged in parallel, as all cortical outputs are. Cortical *pyramidal cells* collect reports (via the thalamus) from the basal ganglia and cerebellum at various levels on their dendrites. They then adjust their firing rates by feedback circuits through local circuit neurons. The vertical design of these towering, impressive cells enables them to stack all these inputs in an orderly way. What is thus put together is the critical element in motor control.

and "reports back" (again via the thalamus) to motor cortex. Thus, these two members allow almost every region of the cerebral cortex to reinforce, regulate or otherwise modulate commands from the motor homunculus (see Fig. 2-10).

There are many interesting ideas concerning the motor components of the brain, but at present the precise role of the basal ganglia is not well understood. For example, a cat without its cortex has trouble but can relate to its surroundings, but a cat with a large injury of the basal ganglia in addition, as one investigator put it, " . . . will walk out of a third story window with complete unconcern." Perhaps the basal ganglia have never been concerned with movements themselves, but only with their pertinence to a given situation (such as an open third story window). New discoveries in the chemistry and pharmacology of these immense, buried regions of the forebrain are bringing new ideas. Whatever their role, we can be certain of one thing—the principle of teamwork. Each team member—the basal ganglia, cerebellum and motor cortex—plays a role in posture and locomotion, even though these roles are far from clear, and all three huge regions may have other roles and functions of which we know next to nothing.

More partnerships, more principles! How are we to keep track of them? Another homunculus, another map—this one of muscle groups, the movements. A busy and progressive brain, trying to brush aside (yet keep employed) its crowds of cells in getting facts and meeting deadlines, trying always to improve itself, to get ahead—the ever-present teamwork, made possible as before by specialized neuronal design, interdependent connections and constant repartee, and the mystery (as well as the safety) of "dispensable" or electrically unresponsive parts, where the pertinence of our acts may be involved.

Yet something is missing. How does our nervous system define the goals it sees and meets so well? When does it know the appropriate times to carry out its motor functions, however pertinent they may be to some condition or demand? And where does it get that stability, that even posture, over days and years of time? These are challenging questions we shall address next. One of the key subsystems serving these purposes is the limbic system.

7. THE LIMBIC SYSTEM—KEEPING A BODY ON THE BEAM. The limbic system is an elusive one. It is a formidable assortment of components (Fig. 2-11), whose structure and interconnections are incontestable but whose functional roles are difficult to characterize. What does the limbic ensemble do? A popular answer is that it integrates an extraordinarily wide range of inputs, elaborates and maintains complex itineraries of response and thereby provides for correctly scheduled, goal-directed behavior. It keeps us "on the beam."

Whatever its mysteries, its main parts (hypothalamus, hippocampus, limbic lobe, amygdala) are clear, if complex. The tiny hypothalamus lies at the heart of the limbic system. It, therefore, deserves to be described first. After that, we shall characterize the larger parts, the limbic lobe, hippocampus and amygdala. Fi-

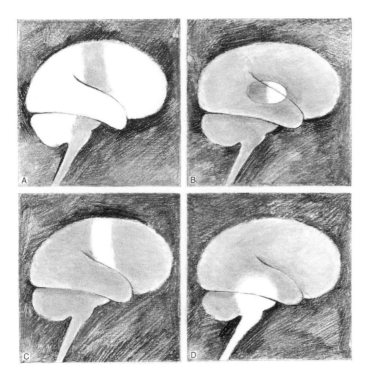

Fig. 2-10. As a willed movement is about to happen, cortex, basal ganglia and cerebellum are illuminated, preparing for activity (A); the motor homunculus, however, is dark. Next (B) only thalamus shines out; it is collecting reports from cerebellum and ganglia, mostly in its forward half. Then (C) the motor homunculus lights up: commands are being sent to motor neurons! Finally (D) the brain stem and spinal cord glow—their motor neurons are firing, and intense supportive activity by local interneurons is in progress. Needless to say, our animation and story are simplified, to put it mildly. All four things are happening at once, and almost never stop.

nally, we shall introduce two others of overriding importance to the whole, the limbic midbrain area and frontal lobe.

The *hypothalamus* is small in size, but packed with tiny clusters of neurons and neurosecretory cells amid a spider web of fibers and a maze of sensing devices. It plays a cardinal role in the short-term and long-range *homeostasis* or stability of the body. It is in a sense like an instrument panel. There the brain watches dials of internal and outward conditions of the body, flicks switches that turn on visceral motor neurons below and advances or pulls back throttles that

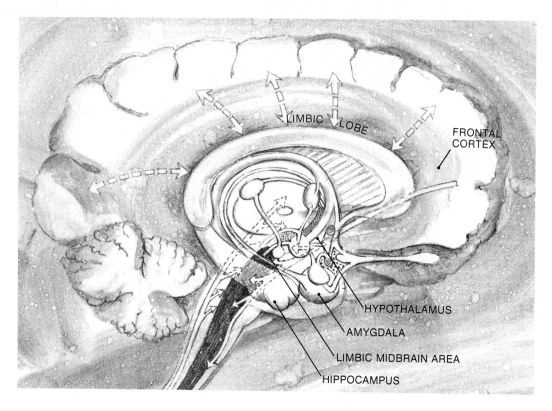

Labels on figure: LIMBIC LOBE, FRONTAL CORTEX, HYPOTHALAMUS, AMYGDALA, LIMBIC MIDBRAIN AREA, HIPPOCAMPUS

LIMBIC SYSTEM AND RETICULAR FORMATION

Fig. 2-11. There are four main parts of the limbic system: the *limbic lobe* (see also Fig. 2-2), a belt of cortex bordering the corpus callosum and brain stem; the intimately related *hippocampus*, a buried gyrus in the temporal lobe; the *amygdala*, a mass of cells also buried in that lobe near its pole; and the diminutive but authoritative *hypothalamus*. A fifth part, the *limbic midbrain area*, is self-defining. It is a portal for chiefly unpleasant events that require activation of bodily defense mechanisms (shivering, adrenal responses and so forth). Impulses that pass through it quickly evoke the correct neural and endocrine measures from the hypothalamus just above it. A large frontal area, the *frontal cortex*, is the sixth part of the limbic system. To this widely connected area comes news from a great many places: other cortical regions, thalamus, the olfactory system, amygdala and limbic midbrain, to name but a few of its myriad inputs. This cortex is extremely well-informed, much more "widely read" than the neighboring motor cortex; the latter concentrates on bulletins relating to movements in the making. Thus, the limbic system communicates with a vast number of brain areas (open arrows).

adjust hormonal power from the underlying pituitary gland. Other limbic structures, in the forebrain above it and in the reticular formation below, have access to this panel. It is thus a compact but key control console. Two huge neuronal assemblies on either side manipulate it, regulating behavior and adjusting endocrine activity; altering external motility and internal state appropriately to meet close-up, sudden and sometimes unanticipated needs, but also aligning them correctly with vectors for specific destinations.

Here we see a principle: there may not be centers of functions, but there certainly are centers of functional *control*. Gram for gram (it weighs only 4 gm), the hypothalamus is the most dramatic example. But we have seen others, in the colliculi and thalamus, as well as elsewhere. The machinery adjusted by the control center, in contrast, is always widely placed—usually almost everywhere about the CNS.

The output of the hypothalamus is both neural and endocrine, through electrical signals and hormones, "by land or by sea," or however we wish to think of it. It is *comprehensive* in its effects upon the body, and that is what the nervous system is all about, and it covers the entire temporal range from *immediate* to *life-long* influences upon our responses. It would be nice to have another gram of it! Yet, as we study the brains of different vertebrates, we find that in this respect we are all alike. The basic plan of the hypothalamus is similar in most animals; its almost universal instrument layout apparently meets most needs efficiently. What we have, however, that other vertebrates lack is more access to it. This higher control is a feature of the human limbic system, as we shall see below.

a. Convergence. The great horseshoe of the <u>*limbic lobe*</u> lies close to the parietal and occipital lobes, where somesthetic and visual pathways terminate. One limb falls in the temporal lobe, where sounds and smells arrive and syntheses of many kinds take place. The other limb covers a region of frontal lobe near the motor cortex (and not far from the frontal pole). This broad ring of cortex collects news on all the body's happenings, on all the plans afoot. It illustrates the principle of *convergence* on the vast scale that we have seen in several other places: cerebellum, thalamus, basal ganglia. The variety of reports the limbic lobe brings together is very great. Its compendium is delivered to the hippocampus that lies beneath and out of sight.

The *hippocampus* represents a paradox. Its internal structure is better known than that of any other limbic component. (In fact, only in the cerebellum do we know more about the design of a piece of cortex.) Its connections are generally clear, but its functions remain the most mysterious. This strange, geometrically arranged yet beautifully landscaped hidden cortex tantalizes investigators. (A few admire its graceful curves.) Many though feel it hides the ultimate limbic secret. We do have some idea of functions that depend on it. Recognition of novelty appears to be one, memory another, learning a third. It seems to make decisions on all the news it scans, not only from other cortical regions above it but also from the brain stem far below. Some of these decisions apparently are whether things represent changes that (for safety's sake) demand scrutiny until explained; whether features match up with others (as in recognizing spaces where one has been); whether to tape and store data (for future reference); and whether to retrieve some long-stored pattern of signals from widely scattered files about the brain (as in recalling "all those old familiar places"). It may inhibit inappropriate behavior. The most recent hypothesis is that the hippocampus serves as a spatial map helping us to remember where we have been.

The *amygdala* is a basal ganglion, closely related to the caudate and putamen. In many vertebrates, the three structures form one large complex and indeed, in our own brain, they maintain anatomical continuity despite their segregation and enlargement. Like the larger basal ganglia, the amygdala listens to the cerebral cortex (including the almost forgotten olfactory bulb) and talks to many other structures, especially the hypothalamus. As to functions of the amygdala we are uncertain. Its activity seems concerned with internal needs of the body—with visceral demands—and their outward expression or gratification in movement and posture.

The *limbic midbrain area*, a midline region in the reticular formation, contains several small but distinctive cell clusters. A definite zone that an anatomist can define and point out, it is a portal for essentially unpleasant events that require unconditional activation of bodily defense mechanisms: the stress responses evoked by pain, cold and certain functional changes in the viscera. It is the only place (in the cat's brain, at least) where electrical stimulation apparently leads to pain. (Such experiments were quickly stopped.) Impulses ascending through it are in a good position to elicit the necessary neural and endocrine countermeasures from the nearby hypothalamus. Thus this area enables the limbic system to monitor the constant needs of the body and to initiate appropriate responses.

By direct lines the *frontal lobes* modulate ("administrate" is too strong) the activity of other limbic components (Fig. 2-11). They affect the mysterious hippocampal decisions, regulate upward traffic through the limbic midbrain portal and display their knowledge somewhere on the hypothalamic instrument panel. Thus the frontal lobes exert control, but not command, over the function and interplay of other limbic structures—at times decisively as in suppressing grief or anger, at other times only temporarily as in postponing responses to visceral demands or gratification of bodily needs. Occasionally (sometimes unfortunately, sometimes not) such frontal lobe control is not exercised, and in certain tragic accidents to the brain (see Chapter 18) it is lost.

Whether the frontal lobes get their way or not, they lie far from the cortical regions that study auditory, visual and somesthetic messages. They are also far removed from the sense of smell, although they know what is going on in the neglected olfactory bulbs nestling in their shadow. They are even many steps away from the vast meeting place of those other three lobes—temporal, occipital and parietal—where sensations are blended into an environmental whole, infused with a sense of self and brought toward understanding. It appears that our frontal lobes are at a great distance from all the bustling places of the cortex, from all the immediate business, from all the ceaseless tumult. They are detached, perhaps serene and musing. They seem to have some lofty view of us, some high overlook on our distant goals and upon the paths of living that should lead to them.

b. Unifications of past, present and future. We have emphasized the oneness of the nervous system—how it offers bodywide communication over the neural "tree" inside us, how it unifies our body, how it unifies our environment. Now, from the comprehensive and continuing activities of the hypothalamus and its limbic affiliates, we can see how it unifies our past and future. Other regions of the CNS, such as the medulla or spinal cord, perhaps contribute more immediately to our necessary stabilities of internal medium and posture, but the limbic system confers our stability of purposeful behavior: our detailed schemes of conduct over time, our itineraries of life.

However, a vertebrate brain, especially our brain, is unpredictable. Sometimes a bell is rung, but no one answers. Perhaps the response may be a long time in coming. In the meantime, the brain answers many other rings at its numerous portals, calls for service that may not be as long delayed. The limbic system is a crucial part of the brain's machinery for assigning priorities to rings or calls. It assigns immediate responses to priority calls, but defers responses to others until later. It has vast capacity for sorting, holding or storing calls. It can answer them simultaneously, as well as promptly, or file them away—for hours or days, sometimes for months and years. Meanwhile, it schedules appropriate responses for the right times and places: a time to do it, a place not to do it. Through its myriad inputs it enables us to keep track of all our goals. Through its universal outputs it enables us to answer all those demanding and competing visceral, bodily and external calls made upon our nervous system—every ring at every door, sometime or someday.

8. THE SPINAL CORD—THE TRUNK OF THE NEURAL TREE. Like some noble standard borne on high, the imposing brain stands forth atop the spinal cord (Fig. 2-12), its graceful mass and austere elegance overshadowing the slender shaft that appears to hold it aloft. One might think from this "cord's-eye" view that the brain's many lordly functions might be far removed from whatever might be going on beneath it. But such is not the case. As we have learned, the nervous system has oneness, like a tree. Here at last we have come to its trunk.

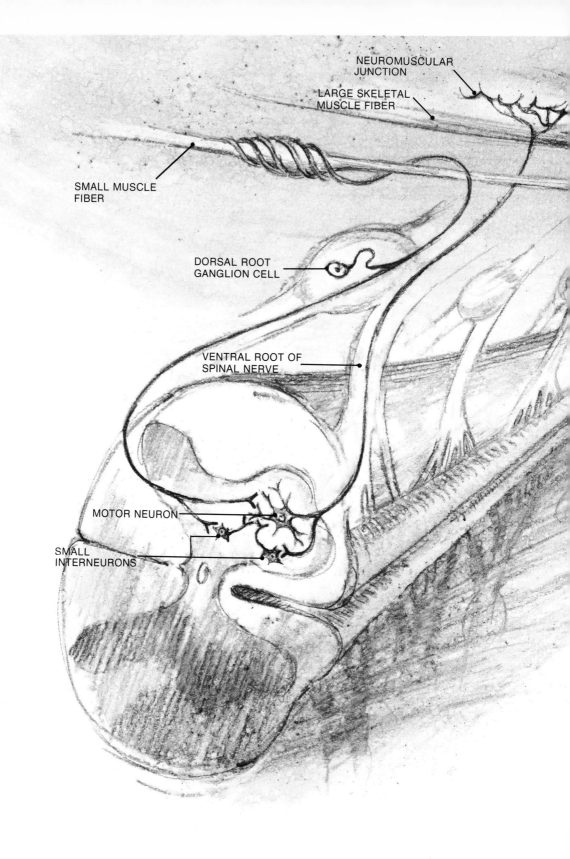

NEUROMUSCULAR
JUNCTION

LARGE SKELETAL
MUSCLE FIBER

SMALL MUSCLE
FIBER

DORSAL ROOT
GANGLION CELL

VENTRAL ROOT OF
SPINAL NERVE

MOTOR NEURON

SMALL
INTERNEURONS

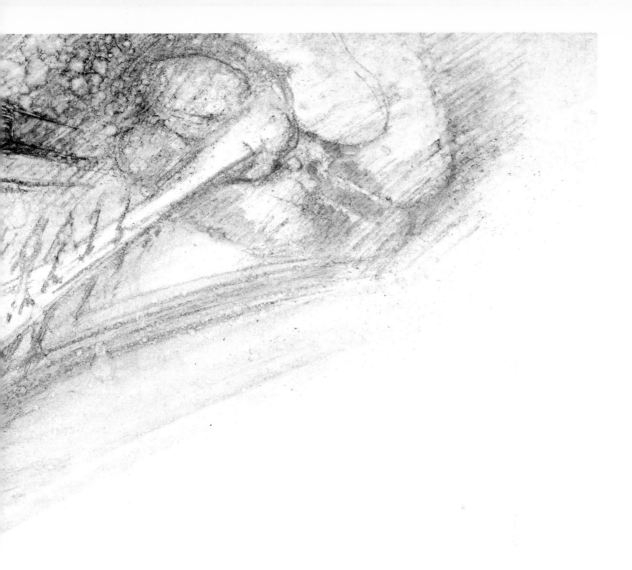

SPINAL CORD

Fig. 2-12. Far beneath the commanding brain, a trusty motor neuron waits for instructions. Through this "final common pathway" pass the orders, not only of the brain, but of the entire nervous system! The long axon of the motor cell leads through the ventral root of a spinal nerve to a skeletal muscle. There the nerve fiber branches to innervate many muscle fibers. Another reliable cell, a primary sensory neuron in a dorsal root ganglion, is quick to report a need for increased muscular activity. It is connected to a stretch receptor, a transducer in a slender muscle fiber arranged in parallel with the powerful contractile elements that lie alongside. It can contract feebly, just enough to keep itself taut and ready. But if the muscle in which it lies is lengthened, it will be stretched. The receptor transduces this elongation to sensory generator potentials that, if strong enough, will trigger an action potential (nerve impulse). The message will flash to the spinal cord, bypassing every central neuron in its way to get the news to the motor neuron as quickly as possible.

Far below the ruling but not omnipotent brain, each large _motor neuron_ in the lumbar cord stands ready, always on duty, to dispatch orders—the orders of the entire nervous system! Its long dendrites, extending from the many angles of its multipolar cell body, collect and integrate all manner of signals, from near and afar. Its long axon leads through the ventral root of a spinal nerve and along that nerve to a skeletal muscle.

  a. Local reflexes for immediate action and posture. Another faithful servant, a primary sensory neuron in a dorsal root ganglion, is quick to report the need for increased activity in the muscle it innervates (see Fig. 2-12). While other such sensory cells have pain, touch or other receptors at the peripheral end of their long T-shaped processes, the one illustrated is connected to a stretch receptor. This clever device lies in a diminutive muscle fiber arranged in parallel with the powerful contractile elements that lie alongside. It can contract only feebly, just enough to keep itself taut and ready to report stretch or to heighten its normal sensitivity. If the muscle in which it lies is lengthened (as our thigh muscle lengthens if our knee buckles or a doctor strikes the patellar tendon with a reflex hammer), such spindly fibers will be stretched. The receptor transduces this pull to sensory generator potentials that, if strong enough, trigger a nerve impulse (action potential). The message flashes to the spinal cord and, once inside, bypasses every neuron in its way to get the news to the motor neuron as quickly as possible. Thus, when stretched, the response of the muscle is to contract. This is called the _stretch reflex_.

Why is stretch of muscles so important? The answer is so simple we do not stop to think of it. Unlike aquatic vertebrates which (when not swimming) float, we must continually fight the pull of gravity. To ignore it for even an instant is to fall in a heap—a crumpled body all but useless except for the organs still working inside. Thus, the stretch of extensor muscles that precedes a fall is critical information in maintenance of erect posture, as well as essential for the reciprocal muscular activity necessary for locomotion. This news is so important to us, therefore, that the nervous system has done a most extraordinary thing: it has routed the sensory message directly to the motor neuron, bypassing the entire interneuronal circuitry of the CNS! The incoming primary fiber leads directly through the gray and white matter of the spinal cord to the only cell through which neural function (no matter how exalted) can be translated into action. This monosynaptic or two-neuron extensor reflex is thought by some to be simple: more primitive than multisynaptic ones, the three-neuron, four-neuron or hundred-neuron reflexes that take place in the spinal cord across its midline and between its segmental levels of integration, but to us it is transcendent in its beauty of design.

Thus, despite all the fast or slow routes that convey spinal sensations up to

      2. ORGANIZING PRINCIPLES OF THE NERVOUS SYSTEM

the brain for feature analysis, all the parallel or serial pathways that bring its masterful synthesis of response patterns down again, all the spinal or higher-level interneurons that process and integrate information from reports of a full bladder to an earthquake—all the inevitable "channels, administrative assistants and red tape" that could get in the way—a single sensory cell far out in its lonely ganglionic outpost can cut through the huge organization and teeming activity of our nervous system to instantly alert a motor neuron of a muscle stretching and an impending fall. Truly remarkable! In the stark simplicity of the two-neuron extensor reflex lies as much triumph for sound organizing principles as in the cerebral cortex, if not more.

b. *Purposeful and efficient design.* We can now see in overview the most general of organizing principles in the nervous system, and realize that its complex cellular design is laid out in the most purposeful and efficient way to meet our needs. It is designed to serve the best interests of its customers—you, us, everyone. The designing principles as we see them are clever, masterful and, all told, rather obvious once they are seen in the perspective of the whole nervous system. It is often our lack of general, not specific, knowledge that makes the organizing principles opaque.

c. *Motor control of viscera.* Not all motor neurons innervate skeletal muscles. A group of small motor neurons in the intermediate gray matter above the ventral horn (above the cells shown in Fig. 2-12) innervate the viscera. Sensations from them are usually unpleasant and compelling. Their activities are greatly regulated by the limbic system and hypothalamus through neural and endocrine influences. The complex task of integrating the work of the vital organs—the heart, lungs, and blood vessels, the digestive and urogenital systems with all their associated glands (not to mention bringing all this into line with outward body activities)—is impressive, to say the least.

The part of the nervous system that looks after these internal activities, these "housekeeping chores" of the body, is the *autonomic nervous system* (ANS). The ANS consists of two major groups of neurons. The small motor neurons do not run directly to the smooth or cardiac muscle, but pass instead to another group of neurons which lie in tiny ganglia en route to their targets. The ANS is responsible for maintaining internal stability. It speeds up heart rate during times of stress, it promotes sweating during times of excessive heat and so forth. It operates more or less automatically through the principle of feedback; a disturbance in body state activates it, and it instructs its target organ or organs to correct the imbalance.

In the end, visceral activities are regulated in a harmonious manner. At many levels in the spinal cord, in the brain stem reticular formation and especially in the limbic system and hypothalamus, visceral and somatic functions are brought together in comprehensive strategies. The coordinated performances of many respiratory and digestive activities provide eloquent examples of total bodily function.

In summary, from the priceless labor of motor neurons comes the contraction of muscle, *motility*. From the scant two million of them in the human nervous system comes *behavior*, the ultimate level of communication the system knows: the secretions and contractions, postures and gestures, movements and sounds—the countless words of motility that express as best they can those mysteries locked in the webbed vaults of the brain.

IV. Overview and Summary

In the beginning of this chapter we said that the pervasive nervous system provided oneness, flexibility, speed and reliability. These capabilities arise from its intricate circuitry. Neurons whose labor is united are organized into common groups (the functional nuclei) and interconnected (by tracts) into precise circuits. The nervous system unifies the body and delivers purposeful responses time and time again. It decides the way in which we relate to our environment, and it oversees our internal states and feelings.

From our surroundings we experience light, sound, odors and objects which we see, hear, smell and touch. We read the patterns of these stimuli (as if in Braille) through our visual, auditory, olfactory and somesthetic systems, and our vestibular system tells us about our body position—Are we upright?—and relates us to the earth. Our sensory systems pick out the significant stimuli, the changing ones, and present them to the brain. There they are analyzed, first singly and then in combination, all in relation to our present situation and past history.

To do these truly awesome things, all sensory systems follow a few general principles. They must transduce stimuli by specialized receptors into neuronal terms: coded electrical signals. All these receptors, no matter where they are, look for differences; what is changing in the environment is what the brain knows best, and the incoming signals are regulated by outgoing modulation, so that the brain may choose the most significant stimuli. It cares most about what we care about most. It is us!

Much sensory processing occurs right at the receptors, in the coding of stimuli. These coded signals are then passed to the brain or spinal cord in an organized, well-defined topographical manner. The cochlea is represented in a tonotopic map in the medial geniculate and again in auditory cortex. The retina is laid out in a spatiotopic map in the lateral geniculate and again in visual cortex.

Receptive areas of the skin form a somatotopic map—an homunculus—in the somatosensory thalamus and again in primary somesthetic cortex. Everything is neat; everything is in its place. Every subsystem has a map, perhaps two or three.

The incoming sensory pathways are always partially crossed, so that both sides of the brain can study a particular receptive region in the periphery. (Even so, one side of the brain may turn out to be the dominant scholar). And the volume of brain devoted to a particular region is largest for the most relevant or useful parts of that region, as it should be.

At each successive station along a sensory pathway, stimuli are displayed in a certain way and integrated by neurons. In the visual system, for example, a line on an object visualized is only a pattern of spots to the retinal cells, but at the other end of the pathway, in the visual cortex, it is recognized as a line by a few special neurons. Stimuli are displayed over and over in this progressive integration. The incoming trains of coded signals are broken down, recoded and sent on somewhere else for further analysis of features that become more and more meaningful as they go along.

The highest level of such obsessive sensory processing is in the cerebral cortex. The cortex analyzes the patterns, as they are displayed yet one more time, reducing and combining the crucial data and synthesizing new patterns of coded signals for some other structure to read, but so much work has already been accomplished elsewhere, right from the start! In all sensory systems, there is great division of labor and a hierarchy of analysis.

While the general principles used by the sensory subsystems are similar, there are differences in the organization of their pathways. In the visual system retinal fibers go first to the thalamus and then directly to cortex. The pathway is direct and private, and is uninterrupted by addition or loss of bits of information. The auditory system, on the other hand, has many stations. It is characterized as public, since it has so many side paths through which to interact with outside structures on the way. These two systems also differ in their dependence on the cortex: loss of visual cortex destroys sight, but destruction of auditory cortex (which is rare) probably has a subtotal (although severe) effect on hearing in humans, if not in carnivores.

The somatosensory system appears to show a big difference: it features *two* pathways, lemniscal and reticular. The first is rapid and reliable. The other exerts greater, longer and more generalized influences. Recently we have begun to see that the visual and auditory systems also have dual pathways—perhaps triple ones! Thus parallel processing or multiple representation seems to be an organizing principle found in all sensory systems, and, in fact, it is used by many neural systems (even local ones) throughout the CNS.

We must monitor our internal state as well as what is outside. Moreover, our reaction to external stimuli will depend partly on how we feel and what we need for our bodies. There is again a division of labor in the way the CNS informs us of inner happenings and meets internal needs. Our "autonomic" nervous system runs the body's internal state on automatic pilot (at least to a degree) and attends to such jobs as adjusting heart rate, maintaining body temperature and providing a burst of epinephrine when necessary. The ANS activates the appropriate bodily responses in times of stress, energy need, rapid changes of temperature and so forth.

The limbic system (consisting of hypothalamus, limbic lobe, hippocampus, and amygdala) attends to our emotions and awareness. It sees that we are motivated to eat, and that we seek pleasure. The hypothalamus is the heart of the system. It sends out chemical signals, hormones, into the bloodstream from which they find their way to various target organs. These hormones serve a vast number of purposes, less quickly perhaps than nerve impulses, but more lastingly. They adjust the internal milieu of the body—to keep it nearly constant or to meet external demands. Indirectly, they also control major aspects of reproduction and maturation.

The hippocampus is the central structure, the star of the limbic system. It recognizes novelty. It tells us where we have been and where we are going. If spatial memory is stored anywhere, it is stored in the hippocampus. The frontal lobes, on the other hand, are withdrawn. From afar they hold a lofty view of the rest of us and work toward distant goals. Limbic activities, like any other brain functions, must be overseen, and the frontal lobes have this responsibility.

In the limbic system we see many related functions all tied together by one intricate, interrelated set of networks. We can say this system keeps us "on the beam" in relation to our internal and external environments and our ultimate goals. It is the supreme example of the principle of convergence: it brings together a vast number of reports from the widest selection of other neural structures.

We are always moving, and changing our behavior. What we do depends on how stimuli, internal or external, affect us. Our responses are complex and often unpredictable. We may alter our internal bodily state or our mental state without appearing to move. Or we may move, and by so doing act on the present.

Movements—walking, running, writing, speaking—are the tasks of the motor system: the basal ganglia, cerebellum, motor cortex and last, but not least, the spinal cord. Control of movement is again hierarchical. It is possible, of course, to bypass the brain's imposing hierarchy in a so-called simple reflex, such as the knee jerk, but controlled movements are a result of many deliberations in which the motor cortex, centrally involved in such actions, seeks the advice of other structures. This area of cortex features an inverted representation of the opposite side of the body, a homunculus similar to that of the somesthetic system. The map is distorted, but extremely detailed. Stimulation of the place allocated to a finger,

2. ORGANIZING PRINCIPLES OF THE NERVOUS SYSTEM

for example, will cause a signal to be sent to the spinal cord—to activate motor neurons, initiate muscular contraction and make that finger move.

Patterns of activity played in the motor cortex underlie initiation and execution of all voluntary movements, but the motor cortex cannot act effectively by itself. The cerebellum and basal ganglia must refine and reinforce the cortical patterns in various ways. The cerebellum deals with precision of movements and smoothes them; the basal ganglia are not as well understood, but perhaps consider their pertinence. At least that is what some say, but there is so much we would like to know. What is certain is that (as in the sensory systems) there is sharing of labor, progressive analysis and integration.

The most important aspects of neural function are versatility and appropriateness of response. "All things considered" must be our way, and so it is for the nervous system. Such confidence and such certainty are achieved by integration.

Integration takes place in every part of the nervous system, but a few integrative structures stand out among the rest. The thalamus, for example, is a major integrating center of the brain. It is a less celebrated but superbly efficient assistant to the renowned cortex. The cortex and thalamus consult on almost every decision—sensory, motor and otherwise. The thalamus often leads the discussion, although we may say that it is not as sophisticated as its studious companion, but where the cortex studies, the thalamus evaluates. The thalamus scans messages to see whether they are good or bad. It also helps to maintain alertness and consciousness (wherever they may lie) through a diffuse thalamocortical activating system. All the while it combines data and brings them to the attention of the cortex, which then may combine them still further, reduce them to abstract form and synthesize plans for response (if any).

Our behavior is the ultimate result of integration, but some patterns of prospective action must be checked against memory before they are allowed to lead to a response. Memories seem to be stored partially in the cerebral cortex, but not in any particular place. Instead, they are probably incorporated in many systems, from the labeled sensory systems to subcellular and macromolecular ones, in line with what those systems did when the event happened the first time.

We are complex and puzzling, and so is the organization of our nervous system. Yet as we study the nervous system we find, time and time again, that these puzzles, seeming inconsistencies and complexities, are not really those at all. Neuronal function is economical and purposeful, and perhaps this above all is the central organizing principle. As the story of behavioral neuroscience is told in the chapters of this text we hope to give a glimmer, a bit of insight into the purposeful magnificence of neural function. We also hope to provide enough knowledge so that in the future we may learn more about ourselves and the animal world around us.

IV. OVERVIEW AND SUMMARY   57

V.   The Next Step—The Study of Neurons

The nervous system is designed to unify the body and deliver purposeful behavior, and it does this flexibly, rapidly and reliably. It does all this through the talents of individual neurons. What are these cells really like? We must take a close look at them, study their minute structure and learn more about their integrative functions. In Chapter 3 we shall examine their cellular and metabolic properties.

Key Terms

Amygdala: A set of nuclei located near the tip of the temporal lobe. It is a part of the limbic system.

Auditory pathway: Sounds activate receptor cells (hair cells). Signals from receptor cells are carried by primary sensory neurons to the cochlear and deep auditory nuclei, then to the inferior colliculus in the midbrain, to the medial geniculate (a part of the thalamus), and finally to the auditory cortex.

Autonomic nervous system: A part of the nervous system supplying the viscera, smooth muscles, glands, heart and skin.

Axon: The process of a neuron which projects to other neurons or their targets and carries the output messages of the neuron, usually over long distances.

Basal ganglia: A mass of nuclei buried deep to the cerebral cortex, which are important in movement. Basal ganglia include the caudate nucleus and putamen.

Caudate: A nucleus of the basal ganglia.

Central nervous system: The brain and spinal cord.

Central sulcus: A deep infolding which runs in a dorso-ventral direction and segregates the parietal lobe from the frontal lobe. It approximately bisects a cerebral hemisphere.

Cerebellum: The large, spherical-shaped and convoluted structure overlying the pons. It is involved in motor coordination.

Cerebrum (cerebral cortex):   The large, outer layer of the brain overlying the thalamus. It consists of two hemispheres, interconnected by the corpus callosum. Each hemisphere is segregated by fissures and sulci into lobes (frontal, limbic, parietal, occipital and temporal).

Cochlea: A spiral-shaped structure which contains the receptor cells for hearing.

Corona radiata: A fan of projection fibers radiating from the thalamus and projecting to the cortex.

Corpus callosum: A bridge of white matter fibers interconnecting the cerebral hemispheres.

Cortical association fibers: Fibers in the cerebral cortex which loop from one gyrus to the next.

Dendrites: Processes of the nerve cell which receive the vast majority of connections from other neurons.

Fissures: The deepest infoldings of the cerebral cortex (e.g., longitudinal cerebral fissures). Less deep infoldings are called sulci.

Forebrain: The most anterior of the three subdivisions of the embryonic vertebrate brain (forebrain, midbrain, hindbrain). The thalamus is a part of forebrain as are the basal ganglia, cerebral cortex and limbic system.

Frontal lobe: A lobe of the cerebral cortex above the lateral sulcus and in front of the central sulcus. It is intimately involved in limbic system functions.

Ganglia: Discrete clusters of neurons in the peripheral nervous system.

Gray matter: The part of the central nervous system that consists primarily of the cell bodies of neurons and their connections. The other major part is the white matter (major axon tracts).

Gyri: Ridges of the cerebral cortex.

Hippocampus: A part of the limbic system that appears involved in the changing of response patterns.

Hind brain: The most posterior of the three embryonic subdivisions of the embryonic vertebrate brain. It consists of pons, medulla and cerebellum.

Hypothalamus: A group of nuclei near the base of the brain which are part of the limbic system. The hypothalamus is involved in the control of visceral, endocrine and metabolic activities, and it controls the pituitary gland.

Lateral sulcus: A deep lateral infolding which segregates the temporal lobe from other cortical lobes.

Limbic lobe: An area of the cerebral cortex which is a part of the limbic system.

Limbic midbrain area: A midline region in the reticular formation which is part of the limbic system.

Limbic system: A collection of various brain areas (mainly the hypothalamus, hippocampus, limbic lobe and amygdala) whose main responsibility is emotional and goal-directed behaviors.

Longitudinal cerebral fissure: The cleft-like separation between the two cerebral hemispheres.

Medulla oblongata (Medulla): A portion of the hindbrain consisting of various nuclei involved in vital functions (breathing, swallowing, etc.). Various fiber tracts pass through it. It tapers into the spinal cord.

Midbrain: The middle of the three subdivisions of the embryonic brain. It contains primarily the superior and inferior colliculi and includes parts of the reticular formation.

Motor homunculus: A representation of the body image on the motor cortex. Areas of the cortex corresponding to areas of the body contain the neurons responsible for controlling the movement of these areas.

Motor neurons: Those neurons which innervate the muscles and control their contraction.

Motor pathway: In essence, the motor cortex drives spinal motor neurons which stimulate muscles to move. The cerebellum and basal ganglia program the motor cortex via the thalamus.

Nucleus: A functionally related group of central neurons. Often a nucleus in the brain is structurally defined by the various fiber tracts which course around it and the arrangements of cells within it.

Optic chiasm: The point of crossing of the optic nerves.

Optic nerve: The nerve which originates from the retina of the eye and projects to the brain.

Peripheral nervous system: All nervous tissue other than the brain and spinal cord.

Primary sensory neurons: Sensory neurons which are the first neurons to convey sensory information from the periphery. Many, but not all, primary sensory neurons travel to the spinal cord in the dorsal roots.

Pons: A region of the brain stem under the cerebellum. It is a key link between the cerebrum and cerebellum.

Putamen: A nucleus of the basal ganglia.

Retina: The light-sensitive part of the eye which contains the receptors responsible for the transduction of light energy into electrical potentials.

Retinotopy: The topographical (point to point) projections of the visual pathway.

Sensory homunculus: A representative of the body surface on the primary sensory cortex.

Somesthetic pathway: Bodily sensations monitored by receptors are converted to nerve impulses and enter the spinal cord and lemniscal pathways rapidly carry information through a couple of relay nuclei to the thalamus. Reticular pathways which also carry bodily sensations are less direct and more diffuse en route to a part of the thalamus. The thalamus projects to the primary sensory cortex where it forms an image of the body surface (the sensory homunculus).

Spinal cord: A large column of nervous tissue which courses most of the length of the body trunk. It receives input from the periphery and provides output to the muscles.

Stretch reflex: A monosynaptic (two neuron) reflex mediated by the spinal cord which causes muscles to contract when stretched.

Sulci: Deep infoldings of the cerebral cortex (e.g., central sulcus, lateral sulcus).

2. ORGANIZING PRINCIPLES OF THE NERVOUS SYSTEM

Thalamus (inner chamber): An egg-shaped mass of neurons at the top of the brain and beneath the cerebral cortex; it is the great sensory portal to the cortex for all sensations except smell. It is also important in affective judgments and in maintaining consciousness and alertness.

Tonotopic organization: A topographic organization of the frequency spectrum in structures along the auditory pathway.

Transduction: The process by which receptors change sensory stimuli (sound, light, pressure, etc.) into electrical potentials that initiate nerve impulses.

Ventricles: The hollow spaces or cavities in the brain.

Visual pathway: The receptor organs in the eyeball (the retina) project to the lateral geniculate nucleus in the thalamus which in turn projects to the visual cortex. Optic nerve fibers partially cross at the optic chiasm so that the left hemisphere "looks" at the right part of the visual world.

Visual radiation: The ribbon-like band of fibers which connect the lateral geniculate (a part of the thalamus) to the visual cortex.

White matter: Part of the central nervous system which consists primarily of major axon tracts.

References

Carpenter, M. B. (1976). "Human Neuroanatomy." Williams & Wilkins, Baltimore, Maryland.
Noback, C. R., and Demarest, R. J. (1977). "The Nervous System." McGraw-Hill, New York.
Penfield, W. (1975). "The Mystery of the Mind." Princeton Univ. Press, Princeton, New Jersey.

3

Neurons

I. Introduction

The design of the brain is in essence the design of its neurons. The complex circuitry discussed in Chapter 2 is made possible through the use of many different neurons. Each neuronal population is specialized to carry out a particular job. Some cells monitor and whisper the local gossip; others receive and carry powerful commands throughout the body. Pyramidal neurons in the motor cortex, for example, listen to the basal ganglia, evaluate their function and inform the spinal cord of their opinion. Bipolar neurons, on the other hand, are no more than a long wire connecting the periphery to the central nervous system. Other neurons, such as Renshaw cells in the spinal cord or basket cells in the cerebellum, are concerned only with local events. Some neurons are 160 cm long, while others are no larger than 10 μm. One truth emerges more than any other: cell structure in the brain is unlike cell structure in any other tissue. Whereas in other tissues cells are highly redundant, like red blood cells in the bloodstream, brain cells are nonredundant. There are many populations, and even within a population neurons express their individualism. Neurons are as specialized as you and I, if not more so.

The very foundation of basic neurosciences is an analysis of cell structure and the connections between cells. Neurons are specialized for reasons. In the most general sense, neurons are made to receive certain specific connections, perform an appropriate computation on what they have heard and pass on their decision to other neurons also concerned with those particular events. A pyramidal cell listens to as many as 10,000 synaptic inputs and from what it hears makes a single decision. On the other hand, a bipolar cell simply picks up sensory information and relays it to integrative centers. Imagine trying to achieve the tasks of specialized neurons with populations of standardized cells. A string of 10,000 cells of universal design end to end in place of one bipolar cell? A pool of 80,000 confused carbon copies in place of a pyramidal cell? Neuronal specialization achieves speed and fidelity and allows integration.

It is through analysis of cell structure that insights come into the operation of the nervous system. The basic clues in the process of breaking down and assembling information originate from analysis of cell structure. Ultimately construction of a model of a particular function depends on knowing the structure of individual cells and their interrelationships. Stated another way, we cannot talk about how a machine works unless we understand its parts and their design. So it is with the brain; we cannot understand its operation unless we understand the structure of its parts and their operation.

In this chapter we will examine the types of neurons and their general and specific structure. We shall sample the great diversity. We shall also examine the ultrastructure of a neuron in terms of its organelles and molecular components. What does the interior of a neuron look like and how does its metabolism maintain it? How does a gigantic cell, such as a pyramidal cell of the motor cortex whose axon courses from the head to the spine, run its daily business and keep house? In discussing the basic principles of neuronal structure we are providing the background for discussing the development of connections between cells in the brain and for understanding information processing on the level of single cells. The neuron is the most complex and fascinating of all cells.

In order to understand such a complex class of cells as neurons, it is helpful to have some means of classification or categorization. There have been many classifications, and each has its limitations because neurons are truly individuals and defy any rigid classification. Nonetheless, it appears purposeful to describe two major classes of neurons: *projection neurons* (those with long axons which course between one region of the CNS and another) and *local circuit neurons* (those with short axons which connect with other cells in the immediate vicinity) (Rakic, 1975). Local circuit neurons are not so classified on the basis of their processes, type of contacts, or cell size; this classification stipulates only their role in local circuits. This subdivision is different from but not inconsistent with the traditional one of sensory, motor and interneurons. It is a return in some ways to the concepts of early neuroanatomists. The Italian histologist Camillo Golgi, for example, faced with the astonishing richness of neuronal types in the CNS, suggested cells be classified according to the length of their processes. Similarly, in Spain, Ramón y Cajal (1899) grouped all neurons into long-axon and short-axon cells.

II. Projection Neurons

Most large neurons are projection neurons and fit into the "classic" mold of a neuron: they have a long axon, dendrites, and a cell body. These cells are *polarized* and have listening ends (dendrites) and a talking end (an axon with synaptic endings) (Fig. 3-1). *Motor neurons, pyramidal cells* in the cerebral cortex or hippocampus and the *Purkinje cell* in the cerebellar cortex are examples. The motor neuron is the last neuron in the chain of nerve cells within the nervous system; it innervates the effector organs—muscle and glands. It is, as Sherrington emphasized, the "final common pathway"; all nervous activity must pass through it and will be expressed as muscle contraction or glandular secretion. It is a true projection neuron.

The *axon* projects to one or many targets, depending on where it goes in the circuit and how many branches it has. Axons form either special enlargements at their terminals, such as in the motor neuron, or small varicosities along the trajectory of the axon as they make contact and communicate with other cells. The trajectory and the extent of elaboration of the axon of a neuron is the address label of its message. It does not say what the message is, but it certainly tells who the message is delivered to—one cell or millions of cells. Branches of the axon are called *collaterals*, and for neurons which communicate with many other cells these can be extensive. The axon often arises from a small elevation of the cell body called the *axon hillock*, but it may originate from the stem of the principal dendrite as well.

The *dendrites* form treelike arborizations, which are often marvelously elaborate; they are the primary receptive surfaces of the neuron. They make a place for the thousands or millions of terminals or endings of passage and act as minicomputing centers to consider and integrate all the different inputs. Den-

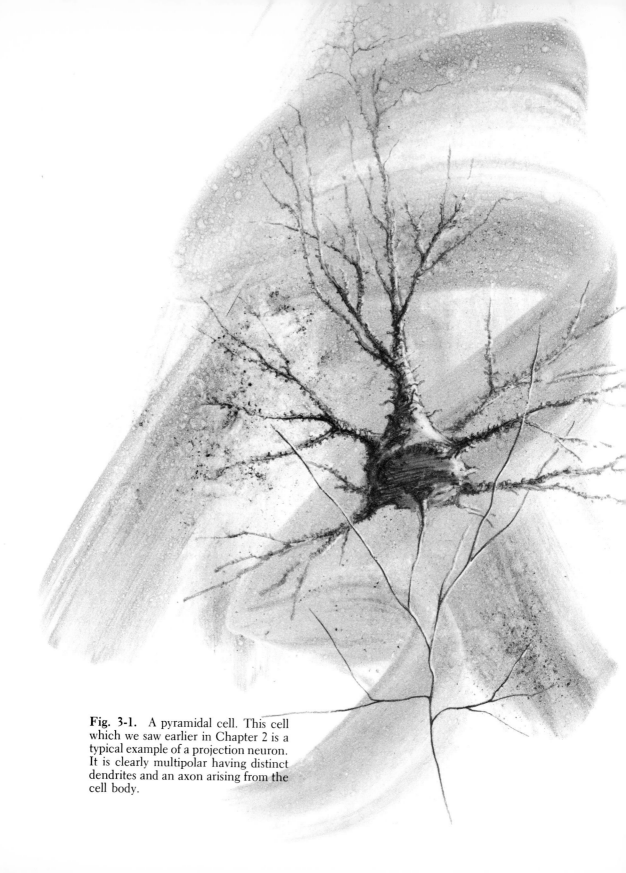

Fig. 3-1. A pyramidal cell. This cell which we saw earlier in Chapter 2 is a typical example of a projection neuron. It is clearly multipolar having distinct dendrites and an axon arising from the cell body.

drites originate from the cell body as one or more primary branches, which then in turn branch and become finer and finer. Most synapses on dendrites terminate on spines—minute thorns of the dendrite's surface. The total volume of the dendrite exceeds that of the cell body many times. The configuration of dendritic branches clearly limits the extent of the cell's receptive field; the neuron can only monitor a field as far as its dendrites reach.

The forms of the largest, most kingly, of the neurons are highly individualistic. Pyramidal cells of the cerebral cortex or hippocampus have a long conically shaped apical dendrite and short conical basilar dendrites radiating in all directions from the apical "hub" (Fig. 3-2A). Purkinje cells have perhaps the most distinctive display of dendrites, a large candelabrum oriented in one plane of space

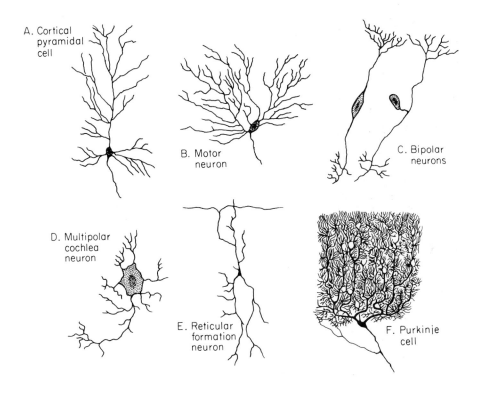

Fig. 3-2. Various types of neurons. Most of these we saw in Chapter 2 in the context of their circuitry. (A) Cortical pyramidal cell. (B) Motor neuron. (C) Bipolar neurons. (D) Multipolar cochlea neuron. (E) Reticular formation neuron. (F) Purkinje cell. Some neurons have similar or even identical dendrites. Others have dendrites which radiate in all directions with only a medium degree of branching. Still others have a main dendritic trunk instead of branches coming off of them. These often possess apical and basilar dendrites. Dendrites may be wavy, tufted or elaborately branched forming extensive arbors.

(Fig. 3-2F). Looked at on one side, it is widely branched and tufted; rotated 90°, it is thin and plumelike. This geometry makes the Purkinje cell ideally suited to monitor the multiple parallel fibers that pass through it. The radially disposed basal dendrites and towering apical dendrite of the pyramidal cell, on the other hand, are ideally suited to gather information within the breadth and height of column-shaped fields in the center. Dendrites are not always so elaborate, sometimes they are "isodendritic"—emanating from the cell body in all directions. Such neurons in the reticular formation, for example, examine the information passing by. Dendrites are individualistic because they are designed for different roles.

Projection neurons form and receive thousands of synapses. The *synapse* is the point of contact and chemical interaction between neurons. (We shall give a rigorous definition of synapses in Chapter 5). The synapses of projection neurons have distinctive sizes and shapes. Motor neurons, for example, arborize and form multiple terminals on muscles. The parallel fibers of the cerebellar cortex which intersect the fanlike dendrites of the Purkinje cell, on the other hand, form *boutons en passage*—swellings of the axon as it proceeds along its course. Similarly climbing fiber inputs on the Purkinje cell have a multiply branched axon, each branch of which climbs a dendritic branch like a vine on a trellis forming a series of boutons. Most of the synapses which are received on the surface of the projection neuron are axodendritic (the axon ends on the dendritic surface). Axosomatic contacts, those made on the cell body or soma, are also common but not nearly as numerous, because the surface area is smaller. Axoaxonic and dendrodendritic synapses, as well as other possible types of contacts, are less often noted on projection neurons, although they are present.

Bipolar neurons (Fig. 3-2C), such as those we saw in Chapter 2 (Figs. 2-5 and 2-12), can be considered along with projection neurons. (They certainly project over long distances.) Traditionally they are considered as sensory neurons in line with their assignment. Bipolar neurons pick up sensory signals at their receptive ends in the periphery and carry the signals to secondary neurons some distance away. Their receptive ends are highly specialized to detect various physical stimuli, such as pressure, which they transform into electrical signals. One might wonder in considering bipolar neurons which end is the axon and which is the dendrite. In fact bipolar neurons in the spinal cord are constructed with the cell body located off to the side so that the axon is on both sides of the cell body. There are no dendrites *per se*, only specialized sensory endings.

III. Local Circuit Neurons

Local circuit neurons—those with no axon or short axons and involved in nearby events within a functional group of cells rather than between groups—are more

numerous than projection neurons. The cerebral cortex has about three times
more local circuit neurons than projection neurons, and in the caudate nucleus,
a large mass of forebrain neurons that taper into a long tail, 95% of the neurons
are local circuit neurons. Such neurons become more abundant in the
phylogenetic elaboration of the brain. For example, in the frog, movements are
relatively crude and stereotyped, and the cerebellar cortex is not elaborate; the
ratio of local circuit neurons (granule cells) to projection neurons (Purkinje cells)
is low, 22 to 1. However, the mouse and human are creatures in which movements are complex and at wide variety; their cerebella are large, and the cortices
are highly elaborate. The ratios of local circuit to projection neurons are 140 to 1
and 1600 to 1, respectively! For every output cell, there are hundreds of local
elements to process information. Similarly, in the cerebral cortex local circuit
neurons are most abundant, and in man there are some 14 billion of them! As
Ramón y Cajal remarked, "The functional superiority of the human brain is
intimately linked with the prodigious abundance and unaccustomed wealth of
forms of the so-called neurons with short axons" (Ramón y Cajal, 1899) (Fig. 3-3).

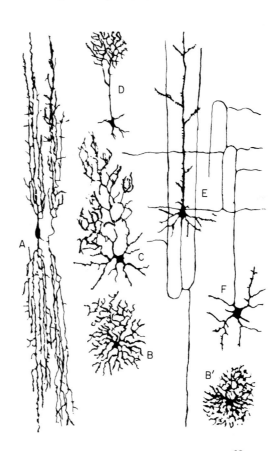

Fig. 3-3. Examples of various local
circuit neurons from the cerebral cortex. (A) Double tufted cell. (B) and (B')
Dwarf element with short axon. (C)
Basket cell. (D) Dwarf element with
axon broken up into a tuft. (E) Pyramid
with recurrent collaterals. (F) Cell with
ascending axon divided into very long
horizontal branches. (From Ramón y
Cajal, 1937.)

Thus, local circuit neurons are of extreme interest, even though we are only beginning to appreciate them and their potential functions. Their general structure has been known for many years, but their function is evasive because few methods exist for their study. They are too small; and there are too many types. Certain select examples, however, are fairly well understood and provide some insight into the nature and role of this class of neurons.

A reasonably well-studied local circuit neuron is the _basket cell_ of the cerebellum. A basket cell has a short axon which trails over the row of Purkinje cell bodies and drops branches which end in a basketlike terminal plexus over each (hence the name basket cell) (Fig. 3-4). This cell's message is one of inhibition. When excited by parallel fibers, it slows down the firing rate of the Purkinje cells, which are also excited by the same parallel fibers. The basket cell dendrites sample the activity of a "beam" of parallel fibers in the vicinity. The basket cell axon projects to Purkinje cells on either side of its beam, where it causes inhibition of Purkinje cell activity. Purkinje cells within the beam of activated parallel fibers are relatively unaffected by this inhibition (see Fig. 3-5). Thus, the basket cell quiets adjacent conversations so that the line of important conversation can be clearly heard.

Not all local circuit neurons are inhibitory, but many are. The shapes of local circuit neurons are numerous, almost unimaginable. In fact, there is much greater wealth of shape in local circuit neurons than there is in projection neurons.

Some local circuit neurons are axonless, the so-called amacrine cells. These cells do not project anywhere and do not fire action potentials, so they are truly local in both respects. Their function can be thought of for the time being in terms of an analogy to heat conduction. They are like heat conductors or sinks, in that they "feel the heat" (the activity) of the local environment and "warm up or cool down" (after their own activity) in accordance with the "temperature" or commotion of the cells that contact them. They in turn influence these other cells to a degree proportional to their own temperature. The unique property of these axonless cells is that their output is completely graded, rather than all-or-none. Cells with axons fire when the signal reaches a critical magnitude. They have a fuse, and like a firecracker discharge in an all-or-none fashion. Amacrine cells get "hotter" or "colder."

Many of the synaptic contacts of local circuit neurons are axodendritic and axosomatic like those of the projection neurons. However, local circuit neurons also make dendrodendritic synapses so that the dendrites of adjacent cells can communicate directly with each other. Influences arriving on one dendrite can in turn be passed directly back to the other dendrite, not by way of the usual sequence of events involving the dendritic tree, cell body, and an axon which might return the message. This is indeed a very local private conversation. We

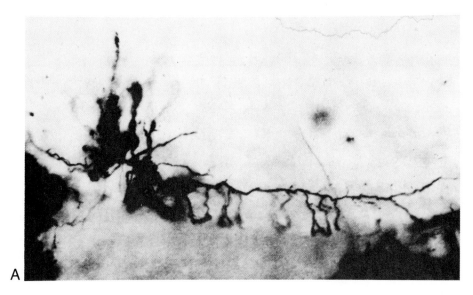

A

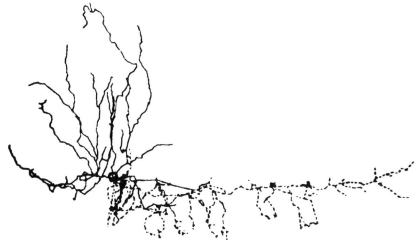

B

Fig. 3-4. (A) Basket cell of the cerebellum Golgi stained basket cell. (B) Three-dimensional computer reconstruction of the cell. (From Llinas and Hillman, 1975.)

shall discuss uses, mechanisms and properties of local circuit neurons in more detail in Chapter 6 on neuronal integration.

In summary, the first determinant of neuronal function is structure. The size, length, and geometry of neuronal processes, axons and dendrites, specify to whom the neuron will listen and to whom it will talk. No other cells in the body are so special and individual.

III. LOCAL CIRCUIT NEURONS

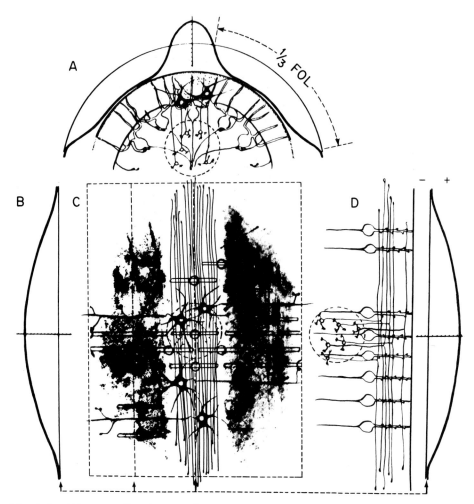

Fig. 3-5. Diagram of local circuit function of basket cells in the cerebellum. Basket cells in the cerebellum (dark cells) project to zones lying outside their own receptive fields. Basket cell activity causes inhibition in cells which receive basket cell synapses. Thus, when a beam of parallel fibers is active Purkinje cells fire in the beam of excitation, but the basket cells inhibit surrounding Purkinje cell excitation as shown by the darkened outlying areas. This emphasizes the parallel fiber excitation. (A), (B) and (D) are side views of a portion of a cerebellar folium. (C) is a top view. (From Szentágothai, 1963.)

IV. Neuronal Ultrastructure

When we take closer and closer views or "zoom" into a neuron and view it at high magnification, we discover another world of structure. We see that the neuron has elaborate, detailed organelles and membrane specializations. The instrument which allows us to examine the neuron at high magnification is the electron microscope. The conventional technique used to prepare tissue for electron microscopy has the following steps.

1. Fix the tissue so as to harden and preserve it.
2. Cut it into small pieces suitable for analysis (since the magnification is so high an area of about 3 mm² is about the largest reasonable sample which can be examined at one time).
3. Embed it in plastic so that very thin sections can be cut.
4. Cut sections with an ultramicrotome and stain them with heavy metals.
5. Examine the tissue in the electron microscope. The electron microscope focuses a beam of electrons through the sample. (Electrons scatter off the heavy metal deposits, otherwise they pass through the tissue undisturbed.) The heavy metals selectively outline the organelles and membranes so that an image is seen which appears like a shaded line drawing.

There are many variations on this general protocol, but the above description should provide an idea of the nature of the material and of why we see what we do. In this section we shall describe the structure and related function of the organelles and the basic fine structure of the synapses and dendrites as viewed in the electron microscope.

A. The Cell Body, Its Organelles and Their Function

Viewed at the level of resolution* provided by the electron microscope the interior structures of the neuron come into view. The cell body is a large arena with a nucleus, mitochondria, lysosomes, polysomes, and rough endoplasmic reticulum floating amongst a network of fine fibers encased by a thin membrane. Figure 3-6 is a three-dimensional representation of a cell body, and Fig. 3-7 is an electron micrograph of a cell body.

The cell body (soma) is the factory of the neuron. It receives copies of the basic macromolecular plans held in the nucleus (see below) to manufacture all cellular components, and it contains specialized organelles to provide the energy and make the parts, as well as a production line to assemble the parts into completed products. The cell body purchases plentiful raw materials (sugars, amino acids, etc.) and converts them into the building blocks of the cell. The external cell membrane contains specific transport systems to pump raw materials into the cell; once inside these materials are converted to other substances by way of the elaborate metabolic pathways in the neuron. These metabolites, along with O_2, are used to supply energy to the cell in order that it can carry out its

*Defined as the ability to recognize structures as separate.

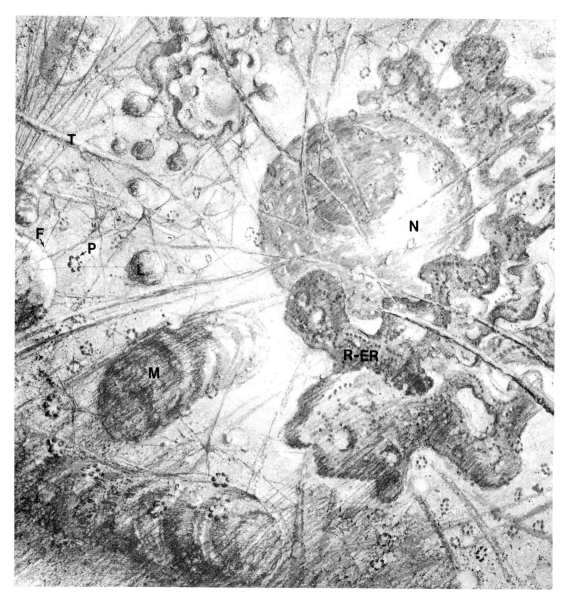

Fig. 3-6. Interior of a neuronal cell body. Lysosomes (L), nucleus (N), rough endoplasmic reticulum (R-ER), polysomes (P), mitochondria (M), microtubules (T) and microfilaments (F).

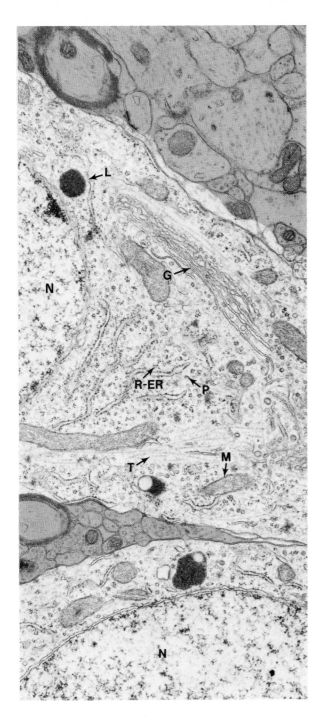

Fig. 3-7. Electron micrograph showing a portion of the cell body of two neurons. The area outside the cell body is shaded. Nucleus (N), rough endoplasmic reticulum (R-ER), mitochondria (M), Golgi apparatus (G), polysomes (P), microtubule (T) and lysosome (L). In most cases there are more examples of each organelle than labeled. Can you identify them?

moment-to-moment metabolic processes and renew its basic structure, which is in a constant state of turnover. Only the DNA in the nucleus is stable. Other molecules and even organelles are constantly destroyed and replaced. The cell body has an enormous task because it must not only produce the macromolecules for itself, but virtually all the proteins for the dendrites, axons and synaptic terminals as well. It has been estimated that the cell body manufactures about one-third of its total protein content each day in order to meet the needs of the entire cell. In general, the complex task of producing macromolecules is controlled and executed by the cell body. The simpler synthetic processes, such as the production of neurotransmitters, are subcontracted to the site where they are used.

The secret of this efficient operation is compartmentalization and division of labor of cellular components; these factors allow the cell to keep reactions separate and organize them into a logical sequence. Membranes are the fundamental unit of the cell. Besides encasing the cell and acting as an interface for intra- and extracellular events, membranes divide the cell into tiny compartments, the cell organelles. Each has a specific job, and the work begins at the plasma membrane.

1. NEURONAL PLASMA MEMBRANE. The entire neuron is surrounded by a dynamic *plasma membrane* about 100 Å thick (10^{-8} m); this unbelievably thin flowing film is all that stands between the extracellular environment and the delicate interior of the neurons. Neurons, as we have seen, are extraordinarily specialized, and the first level of specialization is written in terms of the structure and dynamics of the surface. The plasma membrane with its mosaic of proteins is responsible for cell–cell recognition during development, for keeping certain ions and small molecules out of the cell and letting others in, for accumulating nutrients and rejecting harmful substances, for catalyzing enzymatic reactions, for establishing an electrical potential inside the cell, for conducting an impulse and for sensitizing particular neurons to particular transmitters or modulators.

The plasma membrane, seemingly uniform in electron micrographs, is a world in itself (Fig. 3-8). It is made of lipids and proteins—fats and chains of amino acids. The basic structure of this membrane is a bilayer or sandwich of phospholipids organized such that the polar (charged) regions face outward and the nonpolar regions are inward. This organization maximizes the number of hydrophobic (water-hating) and hydrophilic (water-loving) bonds that can form and makes a relatively durable and ever-so-thin sheet which is impenetrable to most polar molecules or ions. Proteins perforate and organize the bilayer in various specific ways and make it into a functional unit capable of serving the needs of the neuron.

The membrane is dynamic, and the model most frequently used to describe the membrane is the "fluid mosaic" model (Singer and Nicolson, 1972). Lipids diffuse freely in the plane of the bilayer, milling as people in a crowd, and give the membrane a fluidlike quality. The fluid lipid bilayer makes the membrane a two-surfaced sea in which specialized proteins float and perform their functions. Proteins can penetrate the bilayer, forming channels or carriers for the transport of ions and small molecules. Such "integral proteins" (those which deeply penetrate the bilayer) often form intramembranous particles which appear as boulders buried in the bilayer. Other "peripheral" proteins are confined to the edge of the bilayer, facing in or out depending on their task. In the fluid mosaic model, membrane proteins are viewed as adrift in the two-surfaced sea of lipids, and, indeed, experimental evidence on neurons and a vast number of other cells

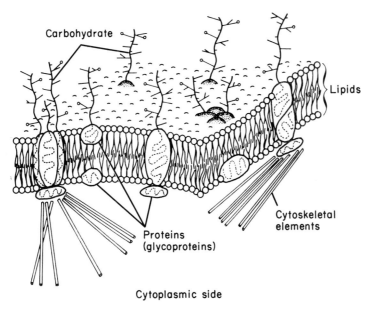

Fig. 3-8. The fluid mosaic model of membrane structure. Certain hypothetical integral membrane glycoproteins are uncoupled and free to diffuse in the membrane plane formed by a fluid lipid bilayer matrix, while others are "anchored" or impeded in their lateral diffusion by cytoskeletal assemblies at the inner membrane surface. (From Nicolson, 1976.)

confirms this for many proteins. However, it is well known that the neuronal membrane is highly specialized. At the cell body it is different from that in the axon, where specialized proteins to generate action potentials are found. Moreover, the membrane at the synapse is also distinctive, where specialized proteins make it sensitive to transmitters. Intramembranous particles are often clustered and immobile at sites of membrane specialization. Thus some proteins drift about and others are immobile.

The neuronal membrane is divided into domains—in the dendrite, at the site of synaptic interaction, in the axon and at presynaptic endings. We are not sure of how many discrete domains there are, but it is certain that the neuron membrane is not uniform in its structure, any more than are different regions of our skin.

The membrane is also asymmetric. Its exterior surface in a neuron, as in most cells, is rich in carbohydrates, particularly sialic acid. Sialic acid is negatively charged, and thus gives the neuronal surface a strong negative charge on its exterior. The carbohydrates appear as complex branched chains (like the fronds of a fern). The fuzzy carbohydrate coat is the furthest outreach of the membrane, and is like a fern forest overlying the bilayer. It is generally believed that the carbohydrate coat is different for different classes of neurons. Frequently, proteins on the external surface of the cell membrane have carbohydrates coupled to them. Very little is known at present about the nature of these surface glycoproteins, but it appears that neurons of the same type (pyramidal cells, Purkinje cells and perhaps even individual neurons of a given type) have distinctive surfaces. The carbohydrate coat is probably used in cell–cell recognition during development and in organizing molecules and ions around the neuronal surface.

2. THE POWER PLANTS—MITOCHONDRIA. Neurons need an enormous amount of energy. The brain is one of the most metabolically active tissues in the body. In man, for example, the brain uses 40 ml of oxygen per minute. A person weighing about 150 pounds consumes about 250 ml of oxygen per minute, so that the brain, which is only about 2% of the total body weight, accounts for almost 20% of the total resting body oxygen consumption!

Mitochondria use oxygen and glucose to produce most of the cell's energy. Mitochondria are small sausage-shaped organelles about 0.10 to 0.50 μm in diameter and several micrometers long. In some neurons mitochondria as long as 20 μm are seen. They have two membranes, an outer one that is smooth and shows no folds and an inner one that is rough and has many folds called cristae. The compartments so created aid in metabolic organization and in using ion gradients for oxidative phosphorylation and other energy-producing processes. Inside the inner compartment is a gel-like semisolid matrix which contains about 50% protein.

In the living neuron mitochondria are not stationary. They move throughout the cell. In the axon, for example, mitochondria zip back and forth in a pulsatile manner. In a later section we shall return to the ways in which mitochondria generate energy.

3. CENTRAL PLANNING—THE NUCLEUS. The *nucleus* is the archivist and architect of the cell. As archivist, it houses the DNA which contains the cell history, the basic information to manufacture all the proteins characteristic of that cell. As architect, it synthesizes RNA from DNA and ships it through its

pores to the cytoplasm for use in protein synthesis. The nucleus is usually situated in or near the center of the cell body. It has a prominent nucleolus and, as in other cells, is bounded by a sievelike membrane whose pores are used for passage of materials between the nucleus and the cytoplasm. The nucleus floats free in the cytoplasm, and from cinematographic observations it appears to rotate.

4. BUILDING PROTEINS—RIBOSOMES, ENDOPLASMIC RETICULUM AND THE GOLGI APPARATUS. Proteins serve as enzymes to catalyze the chemical reactions of the cell and as elements which build the cell's structure as, for example, in membranes. Proteins, like cars, must be replaced after a particular period of use. Without protein synthesis, most neurons would die in a few days. It is the job of the ribosomes, the endoplasmic reticulum and the Golgi apparatus to manufacture and package proteins for use throughout the cell.

In the cytoplasm of the cell body are numerous clusters of *ribosomes*. Ribosomes are about 400 Å in diameter and are made of proteins and ribonucleic acid. Clusters of ribosomes, called *polysomes*, are used primarily in the production of soluble proteins and enzymes. The process of protein synthesis in neurons is essentially identical to that in other cells. The individual ribosomes in polysomes are linked together with messenger RNA (mRNA). mRNA is a long chain of nucleic acids made up of four different nucleotides (adenine, guanine, cytosine and uracil). The sequence of this nucleotide chain is the code for the order of assembly of amino acids into proteins. A specific transfer RNA (tRNA) binds a specific amino acid and "recognizes" a particular mRNA trinucleotide sequence. The tRNA which initiates the synthesis of a protein binds first. As a protein is synthesized, the mRNA moves through the ribosome and is read off by tRNA's carrying different amino acids so that the protein chain grows amino acid by amino acid until the mRNA is completely translated. The chain is then released into the cytoplasm [see Lehninger (1970) for further description].

The synthesis of membrane proteins and their assembly into membranes is carried out by the *rough-surfaced endoplasmic reticulum* (rough ER), *smooth endoplasmic reticulum* (smooth ER) and Golgi apparatus. The system for the production of membranes is like an assembly line with various stations along the line carrying out each step. The rough ER is a labyrinthine system of membranous tubes, vesicles and cisterns whose outer surfaces are studded with ribosomes linked together by mRNA. Hence the name "rough-surfaced." In the case of membrane proteins, the polypeptide chains grow into the lumen of the rough ER; once completed they are transported through the contiguous smooth ER into the third compartment, the Golgi apparatus, where further modifications may be made, such as the addition of carbohydrate if the protein is to be a glycoprotein, and the product is concentrated and "packaged" in membrane vesicles and sequestered for delivery to some other part of the cell.

The smooth ER is continuous with the rough ER but lacks ribosomes. The smooth ER is involved in the distribution of proteins throughout the neuron and appears to extend into the axon and dendrites where it serves as a special channel for the distribution of newly synthesized proteins.

The electron microscope affords incredible power to see structural detail, but sometimes it has too much resolution and important relationships can be missed. When early cytologists used various basic dyes they discovered a very distinctive substance in neurons which was called the _Nissl substance_. We now know that the Nissl substance is in fact the rough endoplasmic reticulum. Basic dyes bind in large quantities to the acidic RNA and so highlight the rough endoplasmic reticulum. The Nissl substance is very distinctive for each type of neuron. In some neurons, such as motor neurons, the Nissl substance appears as large rhombic blocks organized in a regular pattern, while in other neurons, such as sensory ganglion cells, it appears as small dustlike particles. The characteristics of the Nissl substance are very distinct for each type of neuron and are believed to reflect some aspect of their metabolism. For example, after axonal damage the Nissl substance disperses, and then during axon regeneration it goes through a number of structural transformations.

Electron micrographs tell us that the Nissl substance is continuous with other organelles. Thus the Nissl substance is most accurately viewed as a set of "nodal points" in a vast reticulum that pervades almost the entire cytoplasm of the neuron. We might say that the Nissl bodies are minifactories for the manufacture of proteins endowed with an elaborate distribution system for their products.

The _Golgi apparatus_ is a special configuration of smooth endoplasmic reticulum; it has the appearance of broad flattened cisterns piled on top of one another in stacks of five or so. It is a station where proteins destined to become glycoproteins receive their carbohydrates prior to distribution to their final destination. Neurons have a very highly developed Golgi apparatus. In fact, Golgi first described it in neurons, where he called it the "internal reticular apparatus" because of its pervasive quality, arranged as it is in a broad arc or complete circle around the nuclear envelope approximately halfway between it and the plasma membrane.

Overall, the endoplasmic reticulum and Golgi apparatus provide a sophisticated network for the assembly and distribution of proteins throughout the neuron.

5. THE HOUSEKEEPING COMMITTEE—LYSOSOMES. Like old soldiers, old proteins and lipids "never die," but unlike them they do not "fade away." Instead they are actively "liquidated," when their usefulness is past, by lysosomes (Fig. 3-6), small dense spherical or oval bodies, between 0.3 and 0.5 μm in diameter, bounded by a membrane and filled with a finely granular content. _Lysosomes_ are

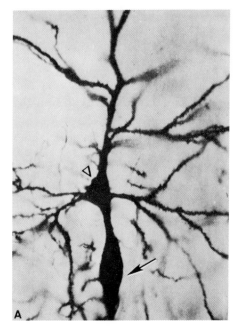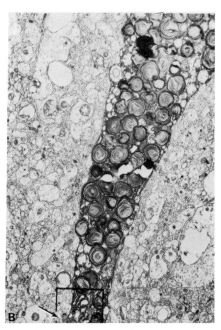

Fig. 3-9. (A) Rapid Golgi preparation of a medium-size layer III pyramidal neuron of the cerebral cortex showing an extensive well-developed apical and basal dendrite and meganeurite arising from the basal pole of the cell and expanding into a large fusiform structure (solid arrow). (B) A meganeurite is shown in this electron micrograph. It is packed with numerous cytoplasmic bodies which represent the accumulated and undigested material due to the enzyme deficiency. (From Purpura and Suzuki, 1976.)

a concentrated mixture of degradative enzymes whose special talent is digesting cellular components. Lysosomes contain enzymes which tear down proteins, lipids and carbohydrates (proteinases, lipases, phosphatases and glycosidases). Lysosomes thus provide a housekeeping-like function in the cell.

All neurons contain numerous lysosomes. A deficiency in one or more of the lysosomes' enzymes is of disastrous consequence to the neuron, and results in a class of illnesses called lysosomal storage diseases, of which _Tay–Sachs disease_ is a common example. Mental retardation and behavioral deterioration are common consequences of such diseases. Specific lysosomal hydrolases are defective in patients with this disease, resulting in accumulation of complex lipids (gangliosides) and other uncatabolyzed substrates within the neuron.

Gangliosides are a class of complex carbohydrate-containing lipids which are normally located primarily on the surface of the neuronal plasma membrane. Patients with Tay–Sachs disease lack the genes to produce the particular enzyme that hydrolyzes a particular ganglioside (GM2). Recently, it has been discovered that cortical neurons in several lysosomal storage diseases display huge neuronal processes called *"meganeurites"* that develop as storage sites for the accumulated and undigestible molecules (Purpura and Suzuki, 1976). Meganeurites appear frequently in the pyramidal neurons of patients with these diseases as a large bulb between the base of the soma and the initial portion of the axon (Fig. 3-9). The abnormal processes are packed with membranous cytoplasmic bodies which have accumulated due to the absence of the lysosomal enzymes. Research in these diseases is now directed toward the use of replacement enzyme therapy so that the deficient enzymes can be reintroduced and can perhaps restore normal metabolism (Desnick *et al.*, 1976).

6. LINKING IT ALL UP—THE CYTOSKELETAL NETWORK. The neuronal cell body and the rest of the neuron has an extensive *cytoskeletal net* consisting of *microtubules, neurofilaments* and *microfilaments*. These course throughout the cell interconnecting all parts. They appear to provide mechanical strength to the cell, probably giving it shape, and also participate in the transport of materials throughout the vast expanse of the neuron. Microtubules in neurons appear in the electron microscope as long tubular elements 200 to 260 Å in diameter, resembling those in all other cells. When cross-sectioned, each tubule shows a dense wall about 60 Å thick and a lighter core. Neurofilaments are about half the diameter of microtubules, about 100 Å in diameter. Microfilaments, which probably represent actin, are even finer, measuring only about 20–30 Å. In the soma, microtubules and neurofilaments occupy most of the space not filled in by the other organelles, curving around these obstacles in broad swaths or "roads" in which they generally run parallel to one another in loose bundles (Fig. 3-7). Their orientation, however, is not completely orderly. These fiber bundles funnel into the bases of dendrites and axons where the microtubules and neurofilaments form parallel arrays.

B.   Dendrites

Dendrites contain the same organelles as the cell body with the exception of the nucleus. There is great variation in the form of the dendritic trees and the shape of the spines, but the internal structure is quite consistent among neurons. Figure 3-10 shows an electron micrograph of a large dendritic branch. Microtubules are extremely prominent in the cytoplasm of large dendrites and are arranged parallel to one another. On the other hand, few neurofilaments occur in dendrites. The mitochondria are usually longitudinally oriented and can reach lengths of 9 μm or more. Rough ER is prominent but appears to decrease as the dendrites extend away from the cell body. Smooth ER is a prominent feature of the dendrite and runs parallel to the microtubules and neurofilaments forming small bulges as it courses.

It is believed that the smooth ER is continuous over long stretches of the dendrite and may provide a channel for the transport of materials. Most proteins are synthesized in the cell body, but some are clearly synthesized in proximal parts of dendrites, where masses of rough ER are found, and are transported distally by way of the cisterns of the smooth ER and along the surface of the microtubular system (Kiss, 1977). Proteins made in the cell body are also transported into the dendrite via the smooth ER.

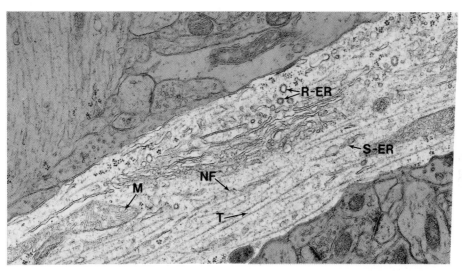

Fig. 3-10. Electron micrograph of a dendrite from a hippocampal pyramidal cell. The area outside the dendrite is shaded. Microtubules (T), neurofilament (NF), mitochondria (M), rough endoplasmic reticulum (R-ER), and smooth endoplasmic reticulum (S-ER) are seen.

Dendrites of most mammalian neurons are studded with small *spines*, upon which most dendritic synapses are located. A pyramidal neuron, for example, has some 4000 spines; these make up about 43% of the total recipient surface of the cell—soma plus dendrites (Mungai, 1967). Besides providing greatly expanded surface area for inputs, spines are also believed to aid in the receipt and integration of synaptic inputs over the dendritic tree.

Each spine consists of two parts, a narrow neck and an ovoid bulb. Most spines are about 2 μm in length, although they may come in widely assorted sizes and shapes depending on the cell type and the position of the spine on the cell. Their cytoplasm is filled with fine filaments and an occasional microtubule. In or near the base of the spine on neurons of the cerebral cortex or hippocampus is a unique fascinating structure called the *spine apparatus*. It looks much like Golgi apparatus consisting of two or three lamellae alternating with dense material (Fig.

3-11). No other neurons have it nor has it been seen in invertebrates or non-mammalian vertebrates. Its distinctiveness has aroused much curiosity and promoted a great deal of speculation as to whether the spine apparatus might have something to do with learning. In actual fact, the role of the spine apparatus is still a mystery. A detailed discussion of the structure of synapses, which are the sites of transmission between neurons, and the nature of other specialized regions which serve as adhesive junctions between neurons will come later.

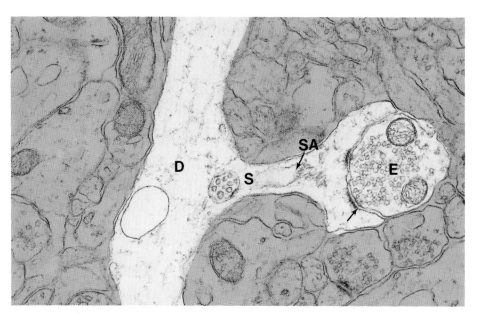

Fig. 3-11. Electron micrograph of a synaptic ending making contact with a dendritic spine. The spine (S) is the small branch extending from the main dendritic shaft (D). The spine forms a cup around a synaptic ending (E). Within the spine a spine apparatus (SA) is seen. The asymmetric synaptic junction of the type shown here (small arrow) is a type 1 junction.

C.   The Axon

The axon, unlike the dendrites, is single (and occasionally absent). It lacks rough ER, but contains mitochondria, numerous neurofilaments (but noticeably fewer microtubules), smooth ER and a few lysosomes. All components display a pronounced orientation along the length of the axon. Ribosomes are nonexistent in a normal adult axon and appear in some way to be confined to the cell body and the dendrites. The means by which their passage into the axon is restricted is unknown at present, but their absence prohibits the axons from synthesizing proteins. Smooth ER lies between the longitudinally oriented neurofilaments and

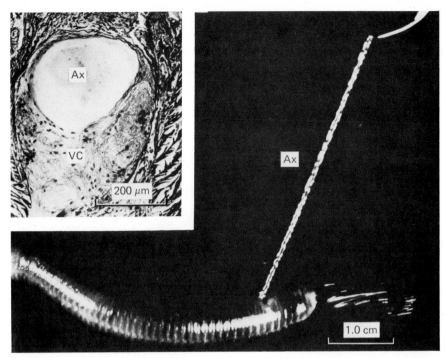

Fig. 3-12. Extraction of axoplasm from the giant seaworm *Myxicola*. A small slit is made in the worm, the axon is exposed and axoplasm (Ax) pulled out with fine forceps. The inset shows a light micrograph of a cross section of the worm. The clear area is the interior of the axon from which the axoplasm was removed. (From Gilbert, 1975.)

microtubules. The irregular-shaped cisternae, part of the smooth ER, are joined together by narrow connections and appear to form a continuous system along the length of the axon. The interior of the axon is filled with *axoplasm*, a gel-like matrix held together by the cytoskeletal network of the axon. In the giant seaworm, *Myxicola*, for example, the axoplasm can be pulled out with care (Fig. (3-12) and it is gel-like probably because of its axonal filaments, which are ordered in a helical manner. Axoplasm in mammalian axons also has a gel-like composition.

The axons of most large neurons which extend over long distances are covered by a sheath called *myelin*. Myelin is unique to the axons; dendrites are never myelinated. Myelin was first described in 1717 by Leeuwenhoek (Fig. 3-13).

> While I was separating from the spinal marrow the strong tunic that surrounds it [spinal meninges], I saw numerous small nervules extending here and there from the spinal marrow; some of these were so minute that very often what I believed to be a simple nervule turned out to be at least five, and each of those five nervules was as small as that which is designated by GAF in Fig. 1. It astonished me that as soon as those nervules had issued from the spinal marrow they were inserted into part of the

hard (*cornea*) tunic which I have said surrounded it, and were, so to speak, united with it. But when they again emerged from that hard part, they seemed to be increased in size and to have acquired a new tunic. I found the nerves which I had severed near their origin here to be so covered with fat and invested with such strong membranes that I was unable to separate them. (From *Epistolae physiologicae super compluribus naturae arcanis* [Delft, 1719], Epistola XXXII, pp. 310–317, found in Clarke and O'Malley, 1968, p. 34.)

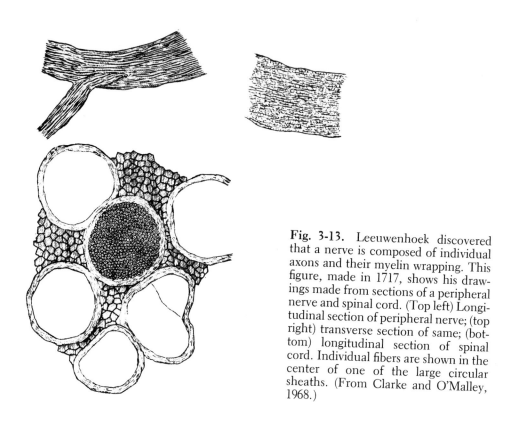

Fig. 3-13. Leeuwenhoek discovered that a nerve is composed of individual axons and their myelin wrapping. This figure, made in 1717, shows his drawings made from sections of a peripheral nerve and spinal cord. (Top left) Longitudinal section of peripheral nerve; (top right) transverse section of same; (bottom) longitudinal section of spinal cord. Individual fibers are shown in the center of one of the large circular sheaths. (From Clarke and O'Malley, 1968.)

It is now known that myelin is made up of the plasma membrane of a glial cell which wraps the axon in a jelly roll-like fashion (Fig. 3-14). In the peripheral nervous system Schwann cells, specialized glial cells, wrap the axon. One Schwann cell wraps approximately a 4 to 5 mm length of one axon. The bare area between the sheaths (wrappings) is called the node of Ranvier. In the central nervous system (CNS) myelin is formed by the oligodendrocytes. In myelinated axons, the action potential travels faster than in an equivalent diameter axon which is unmyelinated. Myelin insulates sections of the axon and forces a propagating action potential to skip from node to node.

86

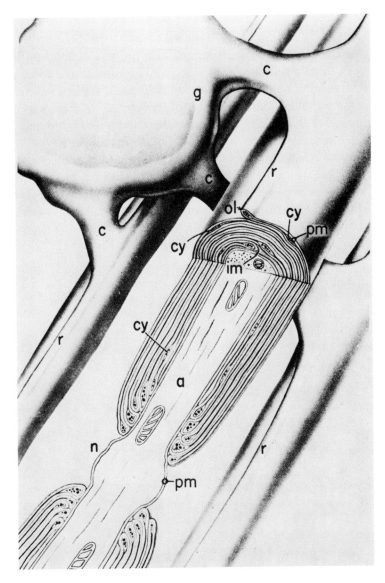

Fig. 3-14. Diagram of myelinated axons showing how processes (c) of a neuroglial cell (g) enwrap axons (a) by means of concentric membranous folds, which ultimately become packed at intervals of 130 to 180 Å units. (cy) "Trapped" cytoplasm of glial cell. (im) Inner mesaxon and inner loop of plasma membrane. (n) Bare portion of axon or node of Ranvier. (ol) Outer loop of plasma membrane. (pm) Plasma membrane. (r) External ridge of myelin sheath. (From Bunge *et al.*, 1961.)

D. Synapses

All synapses have the same general structure. The presynaptic and post-synaptic membranes are highly specialized at their point of contact and form a synaptic junction. In the presynaptic bouton or terminal are secretory vesicles which range in size from about 400 to 2000 nm in diameter. The presence of vesicles at the synaptic junction is one of the most useful criteria for identifying a chemical synapse. The general features are the same at all synapses, but the details of synapse structure depend on the nature of the neuron and its target cell. We shall examine the fine structure of the neuromuscular junction and the structure of CNS synapses. We will see the common structural features of synapses as well as the distinct features which endow them with their specific functions.

1. NEUROMUSCULAR JUNCTION. Figure 3-15 is a three-dimensional re-creation of a neuromuscular junction. This drawing summarizes the findings from many light and electron microscopic studies. Just before reaching a typical

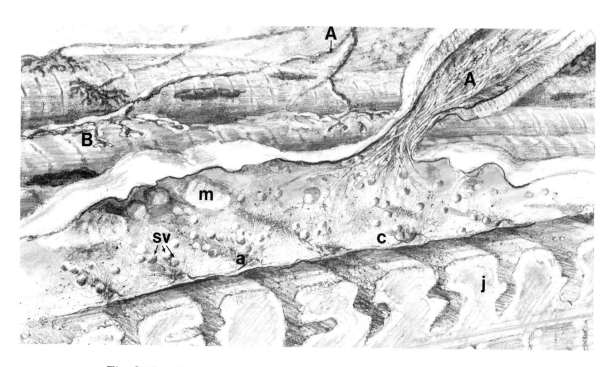

Fig. 3-15. Neuromuscular junction. The axon (A) branches and forms a series of terminal bulbs (B) which contact the membrane surface of the muscle (M). j, junctional folds; c, synaptic cleft; m, mitochondria; sv, synaptic vesicles; a, active zone.

neuromuscular junction, the myelin sheath terminates and the axon, surrounded now only by a thin sheet of Schwann cell cytoplasm, breaks up into a number of tiny terminal branches. At the site of synaptic contact of each branch with the muscle, the muscle membrane is folded into numerous grooves or gutters called *junctional folds*. The space between the pre- and postsynaptic cell membranes is called the *synaptic cleft*. It is broader than between CNS neurons (800 versus 200 Å), and, since all tissues of the body excepting connective tissue are bounded by a complex layer of glycoprotein and other constituents (the basal lamina), the synaptic cleft here includes this fibrous partition, which is not found in CNS synapses. In the synaptic ending are a few mitochondria, a network of fibrous protein, and many small vesicles called *synaptic vesicles*, about 400 nm in diameter and containing a clear core. Some of the vesicles are randomly distributed throughout the terminal, while others are clearly aligned alongside a narrow "mountain range" along the presynaptic membrane—the "active zone" where transmitter is released (see Fig. 3-15). Inside the bilayer of the plasma membrane at the active zone are numerous intramembranous particles, presumably attachment sites for vesicles. Vesicles swarm to these sites when stimulated, fuse with the membrane, and discharge their transmitter stores into the synaptic cleft. If the tissue is treated so the action is stopped during periods of intense stimulation, vesicles can be seen fused with the plasma membrane at the active zone (Heuser *et al.*, 1974; Peper *et al.*, 1974). Opposite the active zone are the junctional folds of the muscle membrane. Intramembranous particles are also numerous at the crest of these folds; here they are believed to correspond to the sites of transmitter interaction with the postsynaptic membrane. On the cytoplasmic side of this membrane, particularly at the crests, a fuzzy undercoating is seen. The general features of a neuromuscular junction are similar in all vertebrates where comparisons have been made.

2. CNS SYNAPSES. Like the neuromuscular junction, CNS synapses have a synaptic cleft and associated secretory synaptic vesicles as well as mitochondria, membrane cisternae, occasional microtubules and numerous fibers. The cleft is narrower (about 200 Å), however, and contact is more intimate owing to the lack of the veil of basal lamina that lies around, but not between, the neurons of the CNS. While the CNS shows wide diversity in its synapses, most synapses can be classified in broad terms as type 1 or type 2 on a structural basis which emphasizes the area of membrane opposition. The area of membrane specialization where the pre- and postsynaptic membranes join is called *synaptic junction*.

The *type 1 synapse* has a highly stereotyped synaptic junction (see Figs. 3-11 and 3-16). The presynaptic axonal membrane has many dense projections on its cytoplasmic side, while the postsynaptic dendritic membrane has a similar but continuous density on its cytoplasmic surface called the postsynaptic density. The

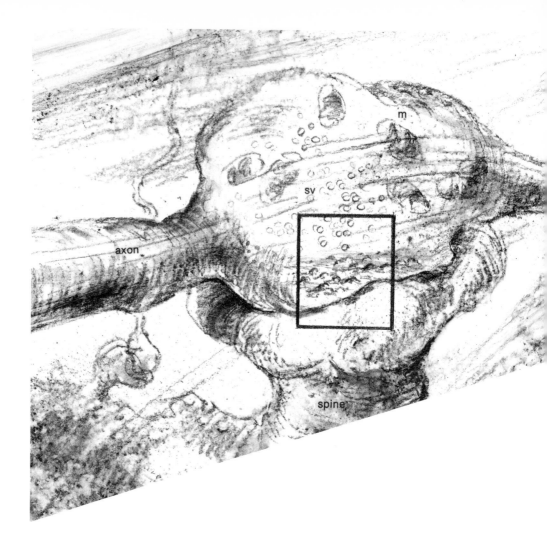

CNS SYNAPSE

Fig. 3-16. Structure of a type 1 CNS synapse. Synapses in the CNS are usually formed as varicosities of the axon and are called *boutons en passage*. One is shown here making contact with a spine of the dendrite. The bouton contains synaptic vesicles (sv), mitochondria (m) and makes a specialized contact with the dendrite called a synaptic junction (shown in detail in the insert). The synaptic junction is the site of membrane specialization. The presynaptic plasma membrane displays a set of dense projections (dp) and the postsynaptic membrane has a prominent postsynaptic density (PSD). Synaptic vesicles contact the membrane at the valleys between the dense projections. The area between the membranes is called the synaptic cleft.

90

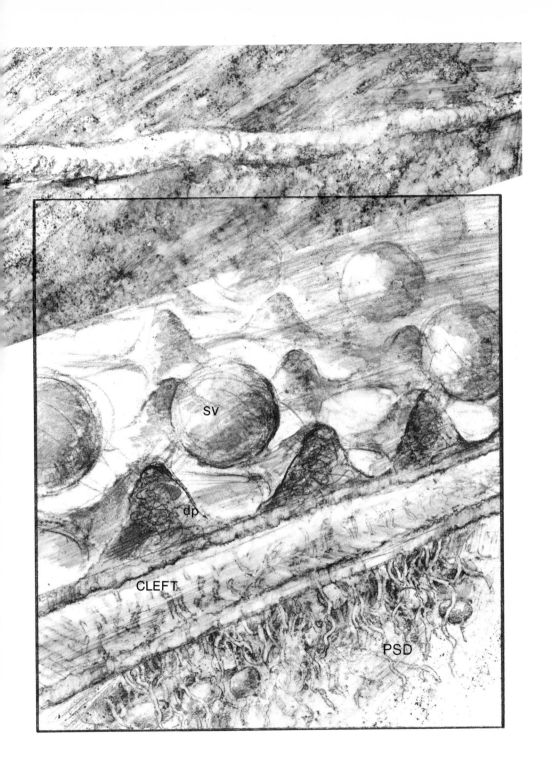

length of a typical synaptic junction is about 0.5 μm. Type 1 synapses account for the vast majority of contacts, are always found on dendrites (usually on spines) and are most commonly excitatory. Type 1 contacts on the cell body are extremely rare.

The *dense projections* of the presynaptic membrane appear as a series of pyramids organized in a hexagonal pattern. These are not seen in all conventional preparations and special stains are required to reveal this elaborate structure. The active zones at a CNS synapse appear to be in the depressions between these pyramids. Synaptic vesicles cluster near the presynaptic membrane and "crash land" between the pyramids during transmitter release. These "valleys" are rich in intramembranous particles.

The *postsynaptic density* stains opaquely in electron micrographs prepared by conventional procedures, hence its name. It is a fibrous matlike material laid up against the postsynaptic membrane. Fine fibers coalesce here and an occasional microtubule is seen to touch, or almost touch, the density, in which small particles are also seen. The postsynaptic density is usually shaped like a disc but sometimes contains a hole. The area of postsynaptic membrane delineated by the density is rich in intramembranous particles. The external surface of the postsynaptic membrane overlying the density is specialized; an array of small bristles and fibers extends into the cleft and some of these join the presynaptic membrane.

Type 2 synapses are never found on spines. They are usually located on the neuronal cell body. They are also usually inhibitory synapses. Figure 3-17 shows a typical type 2 contact made by a basket cell axon on the cell body of a Purkinje cell. The main feature of a type 2 contact is the absence of a prominent postsynaptic density; the area of plasma membrane underlying the synapse has a very light undercoating. The synaptic vesicles appear more susceptible to increased osmotic pressure and often take on a flat or oblong appearance. In the cerebral cortex the distinction between type 1 and type 2 is clear, and in one study it was found that 80 out of 100 synapses fitted into type 1, and 18 of the remainder into type 2 (Colonnier, 1968). In other brain areas, however, these two types seem to be two extremes of a continuum of synaptic types.

Molecular architecture of CNS synapses. The way a synapse operates and develops is a direct consequence of its constituent molecules. What are the constituent molecules of the synapse? In order to analyze the molecules, it is necessary to have pure fractions so that the constituents are available in bulk quantities for chemical characterization. The isolation of a postsynaptic density, a synaptic junction or even an entire synapse for that matter would seem an impossibility in view of the small amount of tissue they occupy and the range of other structures present in the brain. Nevertheless, one of the triumphs of

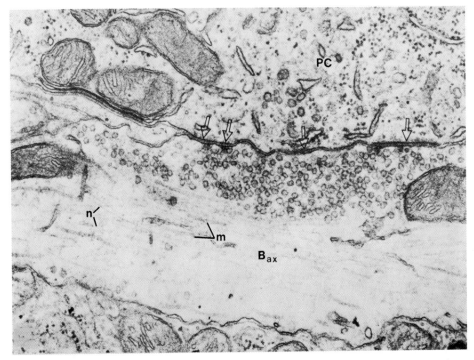

Fig. 3-17. Example of a type 2 contact formed by a basket cell axon (B_{ax}) on a Purkinje cell body. The arrows show point of synaptic contact which on the postsynaptic side is characterized by the absence of a prominent postsynaptic density. Microtubules (m) and microfilaments (n) are also present. (From Palay and Chan-Palay, 1974.)

modern biochemical methodology has been the development of methods to isolate presynaptic endings, synaptic junctions, postsynaptic densities and synaptic vesicles. These achievements are possible because when tissue is disrupted it tends to break up into its component cells and ultimately its cellular organelles, all of which have different sizes and buoyancies. This permits the isolation of organelles as pure fractions (Fig. 3-18). *Subcellular fractionation procedures* yield a pure or nearly pure population of pinched-off nerve endings (synaptosomes) which can be used to study the properties of synapses in the CNS or which can be further subfractionated into component parts. Even the minute synaptic vesicles can be isolated. Synaptic plasma membranes can also be isolated and subfractionated into synaptic junctions and postsynaptic densities for direct analysis.

Studies on isolated synaptic junctions and postsynaptic densities give us the first picture of the molecular architecture of a type 1 central synapse. Isolated synaptic junctions and postsynaptic densities are almost entirely protein with a small amount of carbohydrate. The external surface of the postsynaptic membrane overlying the density displays glycoproteins that pervade the synaptic cleft.

Fig. 3-18. Procedure for the isolation of synaptosomes from brain tissue. (1) Tissue preparation. Brain tissue is removed and cut up into small pieces. (2) Homogenization. The tissue is disrupted by homogenization into subcellular organelles. The homogenizer consists of a glass–Teflon plunger which fits tightly inside a glass vessel. Brain tissue suspended in isotonic sucrose (the tonicity is the same as body fluids) is broken by shear forces into discrete subcellular organelles. M, mitochondria; E, rough endoplasmic reticulum; S, synaptosome; P, polysome; My, myelin; F, membrane fragments; N, nucleus. (3) Differential centrifugation. In a typical subcellular fractionation scheme the particles are first separated according to their size by differential centrifugation. Large particles (nuclei and cell debris) sediment first leaving synaptosomes, mitochondria, myelin, ribosomes and other small organelles in the supernatant. The supernatant (S_1) is separated from the pellet (P_1) and resedimented. The pellet (P_2) contains a mixture of mitochondria, synaptosomes and myelin. (4) Density gradient centrifugation. The P_2 fraction is applied to a gradient and is centrifuged for sufficient time so that the particles sediment to a position in the gradient where the density of the particles is equivalent to that of the gradient medium. Synaptosomes have a buoyant density intermediate between mitochondria and myelin so they are separated from those organelles. (5) Concentration. The fraction is removed from the gradient, diluted with media, pelleted, and then this fraction is resuspended in an appropriate medium for analysis. Synaptosomes can also be further subfractionated into their subcomponents by similar procedures. (After Cotman, 1974.)

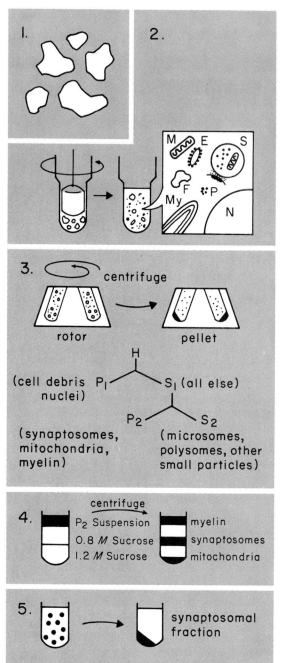

The postsynaptic density is built of only a few proteins (Fig. 3-19), and some of these have been identified. A 45,000 molecular weight protein in postsynaptic densities appears to represent actin, a protein also found in muscle cells (Therien and Mushynski, 1976; Kelly and Cotman, 1977a; Blomberg *et al.*, 1977), and a 55,000 molecular weight component is tubulin, the subunit of the microtubule (Kelly and Cotman, 1977a; Feit *et al.*, 1977; Matus *et al.*, 1975). The major component, which has a molecular weight of 52,000, does not correspond to any identified fibrous protein of the cytoskeletal net (Kelly and Cotman, 1977b; Blom-

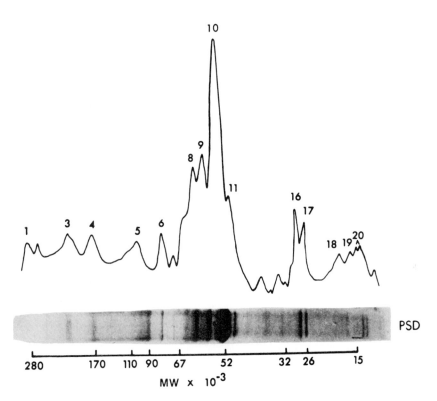

Fig. 3-19. Protein composition of isolated postsynaptic densities. Each dark band corresponds to a protein or class of very closely related proteins. Proteins are separated by polyacrylamide gel electrophoresis in order to determine how many proteins there are and their molecular weight. Polyacrylamide is a porous gel. Isolated synaptic proteins are dissolved in detergent [sodium dodecyl sulfate (SDS)] and applied to the top of the gel. An electric field is applied so that the proteins move into this gel and migrate according to their relative size and charge. The negatively charged SDS, however, binds in large quantities to the proteins so that all proteins have about the same negative charge. Thus they migrate solely according to size or molecular weight. (After Kelly and Cotman, 1977b.)

berg *et al.*, 1977). Thus, the postsynaptic portion of the synaptic junction appears to be a specialized extension of the dendritic cytoskeletal net together with a major unique protein. Intermolecular disulfide bonds (—S—S—) together with hydrophobic interactions appear to unite the PSD polypeptides into supermolecular aggregates and link them to the cytoskeletal network of the dendrite (Kelly and Cotman, 1977b; Cotman and Taylor, 1972; Blomberg *et al.*, 1977).

It appears that the postsynaptic density stabilizes synapses and provides structural support for them (Cotman and Banker, 1974). As described earlier in this chapter, proteins in membranes can drift back and forth in the plane of the membrane unless a means is provided to anchor them in place (Singer and Nicolson, 1972). At the synapse the postsynaptic density may serve as such an anchor, since some proteins at the synapse appear to have a restricted mobility (Kelly *et al.*, 1976). Also, the union of the postsynaptic density to the dendritic cytoskeletal network may aid in controlling the shape of synapses. The presence of actin, an ATPase (Kelly and Cotman, 1977a) and possibly troponin (Blomberg *et al.*, 1977; Wang and Mahler, 1976) suggest that an actomyosin complex may be present at the synapse. In muscle the actomyosin complex is responsible for the contractile properties of muscle, and it is possible and, indeed likely, that the synapse has its own contractile properties.

What is the nature of the contact between pre- and postsynaptic membranes? What kind of molecular bridge lies between neurons at the synapse? Several interpretations have been suggested, including direct covalent attachment, ionic interactions and other nonspecific noncovalent interactions. One way to find out what attaches the pre- and postsynaptic membranes at the synaptic junction is to find out what disrupts the union. Studies in which various chemicals are used to dissociate the junction have shown that synapses are very tough indeed; some of the most harsh treatments dissolve the membrane before they dissociate the cleft! The union is unlikely to depend solely on ionic coordination bonds or weak hydrophobic bonds, and thus it is probably a covalent or a very strong noncovalent interaction (Cotman, 1976). Such studies indicate that proteins are involved in the union of pre- and postsynaptic membranes, but the nature of the union has not been clearly identified.

We have now described many of the general and detailed structural properties of neurons. In subsequent chapters we shall see some of the many ways in which the structure provides neurons with the capacity to carry out their specialized functions. In the remainder of this chapter we shall describe some of the dynamic properties of the neuronal cytoplasm. The cytoplasm of the neuron (neuroplasm) flows throughout the neuron replacing old cytoplasm with new and maintaining metabolic communication throughout the cell. We shall also learn about the energy and nutrient needs of the brain which are required to keep it operating in top condition.

V. The Dynamic Neuroplasm

The *neuroplasm* is a dynamic moving flowing substance; it is not static as electron micrographs or light micrographs make it appear. Proteins, glycoproteins, lipids and even organelles move throughout the neuron with precision and regularity. Even the bulk cytoplasm moves from the soma to the extremities of the neuron; it moves as a column. The neuron contains an elaborate flow mechanism which moves materials throughout the neuron. This system has the responsibility for keeping the different parts of the neuron in metabolic communication and renewing the constituents throughout the cell. All molecules have a finite lifetime and must be renewed. Proteins, for example, are destroyed often within minutes after their production. Some may live for some months, but, in all cases so far studied, all proteins have a finite lifetime and must be replaced. The large surface area and the enormous elongated processes of the axon and dendrites exceed the volume of the cell body many times and present neurons with a particularly unique problem which they solve in a most remarkable way.

The initial breakthrough came in 1948 in a now classic study by Weiss and Hiscoe. It was known that neurons do not divide, and at that time they were thought of as static cells. As Weiss reflected in his lecture to the American Philosophical Society (1969),

> . . . just 25 years ago I stumbled on an observation, quite by chance, which thoroughly upset that placid picture of our nerves. What had been viewed as a static fixture, all of a sudden revealed itself to me as a structure in constant flux. . . . Here is how it came about. It happened during the second world war when I was entrusted by the office of scientific research and development with the task of developing improved methods for the healing of shattered nerves for which my past research on nerve growth offered some promise (Weiss, 1969, pp. 288–289).

Weiss went on to comment on how peripheral nerves will regenerate, but that in practice regeneration is seriously handicapped by the formation of scar tissue in the gap between the severed stumps.

> This scar consists of a pathless fiber jungle in which most of the outgoing new nerve sprouts get stuck and lost. Now in applying some of my earlier results on how to guide nerve sprouts into chosen directions I succeeded in preventing that hurdle from forming by splicing the severed ends together by snugly fitting a segment of artery as a cuff. In elaborating this method . . . some of the arterial sleeves had been too tight partially strangling the enclosed nerve fibers. I shall call that constricted stretch "bottleneck". In cases of this kind I noticed that centrally to the "bottleneck" (closest to the cell body) the nerve fibers were greatly enlarged and contorted, while on the far side they were extremely thin and remained so for life (Weiss, 1969, pp. 290–291).

Constrictions placed on normal nerves created exactly the same asymmetry as those placed on regenerating nerves (Fig. 3-20). Moreover, once the constriction was relieved the bulge disappeared (Fig. 3-20D). Therefore, Weiss concluded, "evidently the mere local narrowing of a nerve fiber has the effect of throttling the traffic of something that is moving down from the cell body continuously even in the intact, functional neuron." This phenomenon was dubbed *axoplasmic flow* and is representative of the processes moving materials throughout the neuron not only down the axon to the synaptic endings but also to the far reaches of the dendrites.

Weiss and Hiscoe (1948) realized that they had observed a movement of the axoplasmic column down the axon. The gelatinous axoplasm moves in mass down the axon! The bulk rate of flow of axoplasm was identified as 1–2 mm/day. This was confirmed later in many laboratories and stood as the constant for the rate of movement of all materials from the soma down the axon to the terminals for many years. But was this fast enough? To move a new protein a mere 4 mm required 2–4 days. As thoughts turned to the considerations of metabolic changes in synaptic endings, which might take place during such events as learning, this rate seemed too slow. Could the rate of axoplasmic flow be the limiting link in the communication between the cell body and the nerve endings? Probably not. In the mid-1960's Lasek (1966) and Grafstein (1967), carrying out basic studies on axonal transport, discovered that transport occurred at two distinctive rates in nerve fibers. There was a slow rate of 1–2 mm/day, but in addition there was a faster rate reaching speeds of up to 400 mm/day. Thus, materials can begin in the cell body and reach terminals 10 mm away in approximately ½ hour. This puts the nerve terminals in close metabolic contact with the soma.

Most studies on axoplasmic flow have utilized a simple paradigm employing radioactive tracers which are injected at the cell body. At various times after injection, nerve or nerve terminals are assayed for their content of radioactive

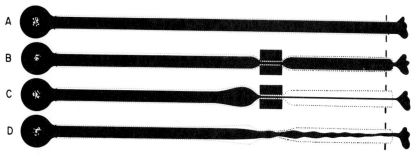

Fig. 3-20. Diagram of the effects of constriction on mature nerve fibers. Constriction causes a damming of flowing materials over time (B,C) on the side of the constriction nearest the cell body. When the constriction is released (D) flow continues and the bulge disappears. (From Weiss, 1969.)

materials. A typical experiment illustrated in Fig. 3-21 shows the flow of radioactive protein in the axon shipped from the cell body after the administration of amino acids at the cell body. Protein moves as an advancing wave depositing material as it flows.

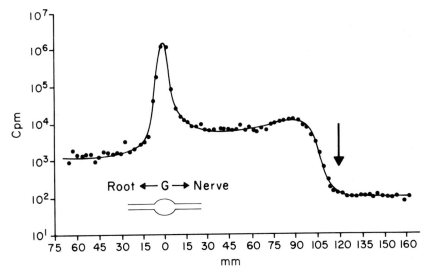

Fig. 3-21. Axoplasmic flow pattern in monkey sciatic nerve. A spinal cord dorsal root ganglion (G) containing the cell bodies was injected with ^{3}H-leucine and, after an incorporation and downflow time of 6 hours, the sciatic nerve, ganglia and dorsal roots were sectioned into 3 mm segments. The activity in each segment is given in counts per minute (cpm) at the indicated distances from the center of the ganglion (G) taken as zero. The downward arrow indicates the intersection of the slope of the advancing crest of activity with respect to the baseline level of activity in the nerve. (Adapted from Ochs, 1972.)

Some components travel with *fast flow* and others with *slow flow* (Grafstein, 1977). Generalizations can be made. The proteins of rapid axoplasmic flow are predominantly membrane bound (McEwen and Grafstein, 1968). Glycoproteins, which are generally membrane bound, move primarily in the fast phase (Forman *et al.*, 1971; Karlsson and Sjöstrand, 1971b). Enzymes related to neurotransmitter biosynthesis appear to flow at a fast rate; however, there is wide variation. Also, gangliosides (Forman and Ledeen, 1972), sulfated mucopolysaccharides (Elam *et al.*, 1970), phospholipids (Miani, 1963) and possibly even calcium (Hammerschlag *et al.*, 1975) are carried by the fast phase. Newly synthesized microtubules, on the other hand, move with the bulk of the axoplasm at a rate of 1–2 mm/day (James and Austin, 1970; McEwen *et al.*, 1971; Karlsson and Sjöstrand, 1971a,b; Feit *et al.*, 1971). In general, it now appears that the cytoskeletal network moves in the slow phase, while other components are largely distributed by the fast phase.

Movement of mitochondria in the axon, however, cannot be conveniently placed in the fast flow or slow flow categories, but rather move at an intermediate rate (Jeffrey and Austin, 1973).

Time lapse photography of neurons in culture shows that their axons contract and dilate (Weiss, 1972). The axon displays a peristaltic wave moving over the axon in a centrifugal direction (Fig. 3-22). The rate of wave propagation was measured as 0.6 μm/minute or about 1 mm/day. Within this moving column a separate reticular system allows the rapid transport of materials. Detailed studies indicate that the smooth endoplasmic reticulum in axons is a continuous intraaxonal pathway which bridges the soma and axon terminals (Droz *et al.*, 1975). This smooth ER appears to be an expressway for the transport of materials by way of fast axonal transport. Fast axoplasmic transport is arrested by drugs, such as colchicine, which disrupt microtubules, leading to the suggestion that microtubules are intimately involved in fast transport (Schmitt, 1968). ATP is required (Ochs, 1974) and appears to drive some type of sliding filament system related to microtubules.

Axoplasmic flow serves to renew the components of the synaptic endings and axon and update the quantity and quality of constituent macromolecules. Proteins, glycoproteins and other molecules turn over within the axon and its terminals, and as they are lost they are replaced by new constituents delivered by axoplasmic flow. Also, as additional enzymes are needed in the terminal to meet low functional states, they are synthesized in the cell body and shipped by way of axoplasmic flow to the terminals. Similar flow mechanisms exist in dendrites, but at present these are not as well studied. As the cell body manufactures new neuroplasm, adds new links to its microtubules and fibers at their roots and gives birth to new mitochondria and other organelles this growing complex continuously moves out.

However, the movement is not only from the cell body toward the synapses. It is bidirectional. Mitochondria, for example, jettison in a retrograde direction. Extracellular proteins, such as horseradish peroxidase (HRP) (LaVail and LaVail, 1974), are captured from the extracellular space by pinocytotic mechanisms at the terminals. Encapsulated in vesicles, HRP and other materials move in a retrograde direction to the cell body. It is as if the nerve terminals provide a taste of their environment and a sample of their business for the cell body. The rate of movement of proteins captured from the extracellular space and transported in a *retrograde* direction is about 22 mm/day in mammalian nerve fibers. Some of the substances transported to the terminal return, after some delay, to the cell body. Estimates of the proportion of material capable of reversing its direction have varied between 10% (Edström and Hanson, 1973) and 50% (Frizell and Sjöstrand, 1974; Bisby, 1976). The fate of the remaining molecules is unknown, but some are probably destroyed and others probably released into the extracellular space.

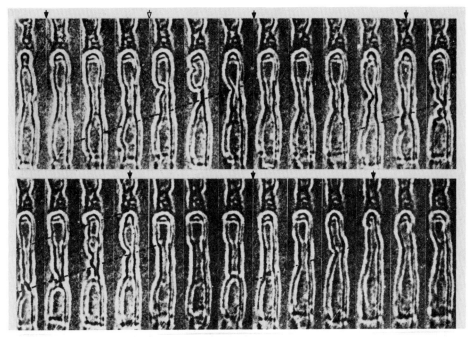

Fig. 3-22. Peristaltic waves in a nerve fiber as seen in a series of photographs taken at 8-minute intervals. The start of each wave is marked by an arrowhead, and its progression is shown by the dotted line. (From Weiss, 1972.)

Molecular traffic in the axon is like a busy thoroughfare. There is an expressway providing fast access to the terminals and there is backward movement. Also the entire road appears to move slowly as the axoplasmic column pulses forward. As Weiss said, "all this is going on perpetually in our nerves beside and beneath the race of functional excitations. *Panta' Rhei*—all is in flux: and so flow our nerves" (Weiss, 1969).

VI. Fueling the Brain: Its Energy and Nutrient Requirements

All the movements, the communication and activity in our "unresting" neurons cost. Neurons cannot be replaced once formed, so their proper maintenance is essential. As noted previously, the brain consumes 20% of the total resting oxygen consumption of the body, even though it is only about 2% of the total body weight. The brain is absolutely dependent on a continued oxidative metabolism for maintenance of its functions. If cerebral blood flow is interrupted, consciousness is lost within 10 seconds—the amount of time required to consume the oxygen contained within the brain and its blood content. Within minutes after cessation of cerebral blood flow irreversible pathological changes occur within the brain.

Neurons use oxygen and glucose to produce adenosine triphosphate (ATP), the major and readily available source of cellular energy. ATP has a high energy phosphate bond, and when split (hydrolyzed) to form ADP and P this energy is released and available to do chemical work.

$$ATP \rightarrow ADP + P_i + energy$$

Many biosynthetic reactions in cells need energy to proceed. Such chemical reactions can be viewed as having a big hill to climb (energy barrier); ATP hydrolysis gives the reactants the big push they need to change into products. ATP can also donate energy to those proteins which live in membranes and have to pump ions uphill, i.e., against their concentration gradients. ATP in brain is used primarily to drive such molecular pumps and to sustain and restore the neuron's ion gradients which run down during neuronal signaling. Mitochondria produce the cell's ATP and also produce other high energy intermediates.

Because of the vital role of energy metabolism in neurons, we shall look for a moment at this process in the brain. Both oxygen and glucose are captured from the bloodstream and find their way into the nerve and glial cells, where these essential substances go through metabolic pathways and produce ATP and other metabolites. Although the brain extracts about 10%, per minute, of the glucose from the blood flowing through it, other potential energy-producing molecules in the blood are not removed to a significant degree. Thus, it has been concluded that in the normal state glucose is the only significant molecule for the brain's energy metabolism. Blood flow through a human brain is approximately 800 ml/minute or approximately 15% of the total cardiac output at basal levels of activity. This level must be maintained within narrow limits or loss of consciousness follows. We will not discuss the regulation of cerebral blood flow, but in general it is achieved by the control of the tone or degree of constriction or dilation of the cerebral vessels. This rate is adjusted to accommodate demands of the brain's metabolic rate.

The steady state level of ATP is high and represents a sum of very rapid synthesis and utilization. On the average all of the terminal phosphates of ATP turn over in about 3 seconds. The level of high energy phosphate bonds is kept constant by the regulation of ADP phosphorylation in relationship to ATP hydrolysis.

Glucose ($C_6H_{12}O_6$) is metabolized primarily via the glycolytic pathway and citric acid cycle to produce carbon dioxide (CO_2) and the necessary cellular energy. The overall reaction is

$$C_6H_{12}O_6 + 6\ O_2 + 38\ ADP + 38\ P_i \rightarrow 6\ CO_2 + 6\ H_2O + 38\ ATP$$

The cell captures approximately 40% of the total potential energy in glucose, the remaining 60% appearing as heat. Moreover, in the process the carbon skeleton of glucose is transformed in many remarkable ways into usable precursors and substrates for cell function.

Thus, the brain lives on a moment by moment basis on O_2 and glucose. The brain manufactures most of the rest of its metabolites, except for the essential amino acids which, like other tissues, the brain obtains from the diet. These enter the bloodstream and are pumped across the *blood–brain barrier* into the brain. With a normal diet, the energy and nutrient requirements are precisely maintained, and the brain has all it needs. When the diet is drastically altered, the brain is the most protected of the organs. It is protected against excessive levels of amino acids, and when there is little food the brain's powerful transport system sequesters what little is available from the blood. As will be discussed in Chapter 15, the brain during its development is particularly dependent on appropriate nutrients. In undernourished animals and people, the brain fails to develop properly. It takes a lot to build a brain and to keep it going.

VII. Summary

Neurons can be considered as projection neurons or local circuit neurons. Projection neurons are large polarized and have dendrites, a cell body and a long, frequently myelinated, axon. They are concerned with long distance interactions. Local circuit neurons are more abundant than projection neurons. They are smaller, have no axon or a short axon and are concerned with local events.

All neurons have elaborate cellular structure and contain many organelles serving specialized functions in much the same way as in other cells. The nucleus contains the genes. In the cytoplasm, ribosomes, endoplasmic reticulum and the Golgi apparatus manufacture proteins and glycoproteins, lysosomes degrade cellular materials and mitochondria provide energy and participate in central metabolism. Proteins of the cytoskeletal network (microtubules, microfilaments and neurofilaments) give the cell mechanical strength and shape and participate in the movement of materials throughout the cell.

Synapses are sites of interneuronal communication. All synapses have a similar general structure, but different detailed structure. A neuromuscular junction displays distinct junctional folds at the synaptic junction with discharge sites arranged in proximity to the crests of the folds. Most central synapses can be considered as type 1 or type 2. Excitatory synapses in the CNS are usually type 1 synaptic junctions, and most frequently those terminate on dendritic spines. Type 1 synapses display a prominent postsynaptic density and presynaptic dense projections. A type 1 junction consists of certain proteins of the cytoskeletal network as well as other specialized proteins. Type 2 junctions are usually inhibitory and are usually located on or near the cell body. A prominent postsynaptic density is absent.

The neuroplasm and most organelles in it are in constant motion. Both axons and dendrites have flow mechanisms. Materials flow in an axon via slow axoplasmic flow (1–2 mm/day) or fast axoplasmic flow (up to 400 mm/day). Slow flow consists primarily of the movement of the axonal column particularly the cytoskeletal network; fast flow carries primarily particulate materials, such as membrane-bound glycoproteins. Material in axons flows in a retrograde manner (back to the cell body) as well; the average rate is about 22 mm/day.

The operation of neurons requires energy for maintaining ion balance, moving materials throughout the cell and interconverting metabolites. Nearly all energy in the brain is derived from glucose. Glucose is metabolized by glycolysis and the citric acid cycle to carbon dioxide, water and ATP. About 40% of the available energy is captured and converted to usable cellular energy.

Key Terms

Axon hillock: A region of the cell body from which the axon arises. It is often the site where action potentials are initiated.

Axoplasmic flow: The flow of materials in axons. Proteins synthesized in the cell body, as well as other materials, flow down the axon. Some move by fast flow (up to 400 mm/day); others by slow flow (1–2 mm/day).

Basket cell: A type of local circuit neuron. It has a short axon which drops branches that end in a basketlike terminal plexus over its target cells. Basket cells are found in the cerebellum and certain other brain areas.

Bipolar neurons: These are usually primary sensory neurons. They have specialized sensory endings at one end and synapses at the other end which convey the information to secondary neurons some distance away.

Boutons en passage: Swellings of the axon where transmitter is discharged in response to stimulation.

Cytoskeletal network: A network of fibers and filaments which course throughout the cytoplasm. The major components are microtubles (200–260 Å tubules), neurofilaments (100 Å) and microfilaments (20–30 Å).

Dendrites: Treelike arborizations of the cell body which form the primary receptive surface of the neuron. Sometimes they emanate from the cell body in all directions (isodendritic); others are radially directed.

Endoplasmic reticulum: The rough endoplasmic reticulum is a membrane-bound sac whose surface is studded with ribosomes; it is involved in the synthesis of proteins. Smooth-surfaced endoplasmic reticulum lacks ribosomes; it is involved in the distribution of newly synthesized proteins.

Golgi apparatus: A special configuration of smooth endoplasmic reticulum. One of its functions is to attach carbohydrates to newly synthesized proteins.

Junctional folds: Infoldings on the muscle membrane at the neuromuscular junction.

Local circuit neurons: Neurons with short axons (or no axons) which connect with other cells in the immediate vicinity. These neurons may or may not be polarized.

Lysosome: A cellular organelle which contains a concentrated mixture of degradative enzymes.

Meganeurites: Large neuronal processes that develop in neurons of patients with lysosomal storage diseases, e.g., Tay–Sachs disease.

Mitochondria: A cellular organelle responsible for the production of energy in the form of ATP, NADH, etc., via the interconversion of cellular metabolites.

Myelin: A sheath which covers portions of axons in certain neurons. It consists of the plasma membrane of a specialized glial cell (a Schwann cell in the peripheral nervous system, and an oligodendrocyte in the central nervous system) which is wrapped several times around the axon.

Nissl substance: The rough endoplasmic reticulum as revealed by certain dyes at the light microscopic level. It is organized in a highly characteristic way for each type of neuron.

Nucleus: A cellular organelle which contains the DNA and synthesizes RNA. It contains the nucleolus.

Plasma membrane: The membrane encasing a cell. Lipids are organized in a bilayer; proteins and glycoproteins may perforate the bilayer or be confined to the edge. The neuronal plasma membrane is very specialized.

Projection neurons: Neurons with long axons which course between one region of the CNS and another. Projection neurons are always polarized.

Purkinje cell: A type of projection neuron found in the cerebellum. Its dendrites are shaped like a large candelabrum, oriented in one plane of space.

Pyramidal cell: A type of projection neuron found in the cerebral cortex and hippocampus which has a pyramid-shaped cell body, cone-shaped apical dendrites and short, conical basal dendrites radiating in all directions.

Ribosomes: Small particles (about 400 Å in diameter) made primarily of proteins and RNA. Clusters of ribosomes (polysomes) are used to produce proteins.

Synapse: The connection between neurons. Most synapses use chemical signals (transmitters); chemical synapses have a presynaptic side where transmitter is released and a postsynaptic side where the transmitter acts on its target cell.

Synaptic junction: The specialized area of the synapse where the presynaptic membrane joins the postsynaptic membrane.

Synaptic vesicles: Small spherical vesicles (about 400 nm in diameter) localized in presynaptic endings (or *boutons en passage*). They are believed to store transmitter and, upon fusion with the presynaptic membrane, discharge it.

Tay–Sachs disease: A hereditary illness characterized by mental retardation and behavioral deterioration. It is a lysosomal storage disease; a lysosomal enzyme which degrades a specific complex carbohydrate (ganglioside GM2) is deficient.

Type 1 synapse: A type of synapse found in the CNS, which has a characteristic asymmetric structure. The presynaptic axonal membrane displays dense projections, while the postsynaptic membrane has a prominent postsynaptic density. Most type 1 synapses terminate on dendrites and are usually excitatory.

Type 2 synapse: A type of synapse found in the CNS, which has a characteristic symmetric structure. Membrane specializations are undeveloped and appear thinner than at a type 1 synaptic junction. Most type 2 synapses are found on the cell body and are usually inhibitory.

General References

Grafstein, B. (1977). Axonal transport; the intracellular traffic of the neuron. *In* "Handbook of Physiology" (E. R. Kandel, ed.), Sect. 1, Vol. I, pp. 691–717. Am. Physiol. Soc., Bethesda, Maryland.

Lehninger, A. L. (1970). "Biochemistry—The Molecular Basis of Cell Structure and Function." Worth Publ., New York.

Peters, A., Palay, S. F., and Webster, H. D. F. (1976). "The Fine Structure of the Nervous System, the Cells and their Processes." Saunders, Philadelphia, Pennsylvania.

Rakic, P. (1975). "Local Circuit Neurons." MIT Press, Cambridge, Massachusetts.

Singer, S. J., and Nicolson, G.L. (1972). The fluid mosaic model of the structure of cell membranes. *Science* **175**, 720–731.

Weiss, P. A. (1969). "Panta' Rhei"—and so flow our nerves. *Am. Sci.* **57**, 287–305.

References

Bisby, M. A. (1976). Orthograde and retrograde axonal transport of labeled protein in motoneurons. *Exp. Neurol.* **50**, 628–640.

Blomberg, F., Cohen, R. S., and Siekevitz, P. (1977). The structure of post-synaptic densities isolated from dog cerebral cortex. II. Characterization and arrangement of some of the major proteins within the structure. *J. Cell Biol.* **74**, 204–225.

Bunge, M. B., Bunge, R. P., and Ris, H. (1961). Ultrastructural study of remyelination in an experimental lesion in adult cat spinal cord. *J. Cell Biol.* **10**, 67–94.

Clarke, E., and O'Malley, C. D. (1968). "The Human Brain and Spinal Cord." Univ. of California Press, Berkeley.

Colonnier, M. (1968). Synaptic patterns on different cell types in the different laminae of the cat visual cortex. An electron microscope study. *Brain Res.* 9, 268–287.

Cotman, C. W. (1974). Isolation of synaptosomes and synaptic plasma membrane fractions. *In* "Methods in Enzymology: Vol. 31, Biomembranes, Part A" (S. Fleischer and L. Pacher, eds.), pp.445–452. Academic Press, New York.

Cotman, C. W. (1976). Lesion-induced synaptogenesis in brain: A study of dynamic changes in neuronal membrane specializations. *J. Supramol. Struct.* 4, 319–327.

Cotman, C. W., and Banker, G. A. (1974). The making of a synapse. *In* "Rev. of Neuroscience" (S. Ehrenpreis and I. J. Kopin, eds.), pp. 2–62. Raven, New York.

Cotman, C. W., and Taylor, D. (1972). Isolation and structural studies on synaptic complexes from rat brain. *J. Cell Biol.* 55, 696–711.

Desnick, R. J., Thorpe, S. R., and Fiddler, M. B. (1976). Toward enzyme therapy for lysosomal storage diseases. *Physiol. Rev.* 56, 57–99.

Droz, B., Rambour, A., and Koenig, H. L. (1975). The smooth endoplasmic reticulum: Structure and role in the renewal of axonal membrane and synaptic vesicles by fast axonal transport. *Brain Res.* 93, 1–13.

Edström, A., and Hanson, M. (1973). Retrograde axonal transport of proteins *in vitro* in frog sciatic nerves. *Brain Res.* 61, 311–320.

Elam, J. S., Goldberg, J. M., Radin, N. S., and Agranoff, B. W. (1970). Rapid axonal transport of sulfated mucopolysaccharide proteins. *Science* 170, 458–460.

Feit, H., Dutton, G. R., Barondes, S. H., and Shelanski, M. L. (1971). Microtubule protein: Identification in and transport to nerve endings. *J. Cell Biol.* 51, 138–147.

Feit, H., Kelly, P., and Cotman, C. W. (1977). The identification of a protein related to tubrilin in the postsynaptic density. *Proc. Natl. Acad. Sci. U.S.A.* 74, 1047–1051.

Forman, D. S., and Ledeen, R. W. (1972). Axonal transport of gangliosides in the goldfish optic nerve. *Science* 177, 630–633.

Forman, D. S., McEwen, B. S., and Grafstein, B. (1971). Rapid transport of radioactivity in goldfish optic nerve following injections of labeled glucosamine. *Brain Res.* 28, 119–130.

Frizell, M., and Sjöstrand, J. (1974). The axonal transport of slowly migrating (^{3}H)leucine labelled proteins and the regeneration rate in regenerating hypoglossal and vagus nerves of the rabbit. *Brain Res.* 81, 267–283.

Gilbert, D. S. (1975). Axoplasm architecture and physical properties as seen in the *Myxicola* giant axon. *J. Physiol.* (London) 253, 257–301.

Grafstein, B. (1967). Transport of protein by goldfish optic nerve fibers. *Science* 157, 196–198.

Grafstein, B. (1977). Axonal transport: The intracellular traffic of the neuron. *In* "Handbook of Physiology" (E. R. Kandel and S. R. Geiger, eds.), Sect. 1, Vol. I, pp. 691–717. Am. Physiol. Soc., Bethesda, Maryland.

Hammerschlag, R., Dravid, A. R., and Chiu, A. Y. (1975). Mechanism of axonal transport: A proposed role for calcium ions. *Science* 188, 273–275.

Heuser, J. E., Reese, T. S., and Landis, D. M. D. (1974). Functional changes in frog neuromuscular junctions studied with freeze-fracture. *J. Neurocytol.* 3, 109–131.

James, K. A. C., and Austin, L. (1970). The binding *in vitro* of cholchicine to axoplasmic proteins from chicken sciatic nerve. *Biochem. J.* 117, 773–777.

Jeffrey, P. L., and Austin, L. (1973). Axoplasmic transport. *Prog. Neurobiol.* 2, 207–255.

Karlsson, J. -O., and Sjöstrand, J. (1971a). Synthesis, migration and turnover of protein in retinal ganglion cells. *J. Neurochem.* 18, 749–767.

Karlsson, J. -O., and Sjöstrand, J. (1971b). Rapid intracellular transport of fucose-containing glycoproteins in retinal ganglion cells. *J. Neurochem.* 18, 2209–2216.

Kelly, P. T., and Cotman, C. W. (1977a). Molecular architecture of CNS synapses: Characterization and possible functions of constituent protein. *Neurosci. Abstr.* (Soc. Neurosci.) 3, 219.

Kelly, P. T., and Cotman, C. W. (1977b). Identification of glycoproteins and proteins at synapses in the central nervous system. *J. Biol. Chem.* **252**, 786–793.

Kelly, P. T., Cotman, C. W., Gentry, C., and Nicolson, G. L. (1976). Distribution and mobility of lectin receptors on synaptic membranes of identified CNS neurons. *J. Cell Biol.* **71**, 487–496.

Kiss, J. (1977). Synthesis and transport of newly formed proteins in dendrites of rat hippocampal pyramid cells. An electron microscope autoradiographic study. *Brain Res.* **124**, 237–250.

Lasek, R. J. (1966). Axoplasmic streaming in the cat dorsal root ganglion cell and the rat ventral motoneuron. *Anat. Rec.* **154**, 373–374.

LaVail, J. H., and LaVail, M. M. (1974). The retrograde intraaxonal transport of horseradish peroxidase in the chick visual system: A light and electron microscopic study. *J. Comp. Neurol.* **157**, 303–358.

Lehninger, A. L. (1970). "Biochemistry—The Molecular Basis of Cell Structure and Function." Worth Publ., New York.

Llinas, R., and Hillman, D. E. (1975). A multipurpose tridimensional reconstruction computer system for neuroanatomy. *In* "Golgi Centennial Symposium: Perspectives in Neurobiology" (M. Santini, ed.), pp. 71–79. Raven, New York.

McEwen, B. S., and Grafstein, B. (1968). Fast and slow components in axonal transport of protein. *J. Cell Biol.* **38**, 494–508.

McEwen, B. S., Forman, D., and Grafstein, B. (1971). Components of fast and slow axonal transport in the goldfish optic nerve. *J. Neurobiol.* **2**, 361–377.

Matus, A. I., Walters, B., and Mughal, S. (1975). Immunohistochemical demonstration of tubulin associated with microtubules and synaptic junctions in mammalian brain. *J. Neurocytol.* **4**, 733–744.

Miani, N. (1963). Analysis of the somato-axonal movement of phospholipids in the vagus and hypoglossal nerves. *J. Neurochem.* **10**, 859–874.

Mungai, J. M. (1967). Dendritic patterns in the somatic sensory cortex of the cat. *J. Anat.* **101**, 403–418.

Nicolson, G. L. (1976). Transmembrane control of the receptors on normal and tumor cells. I. Cytoplasmic influence over cell surface components. *Biochim. Biophys. Acta* **457**, 57–108.

Ochs, S. (1972). Rate of fast axoplasmic transport in mammalian nerve fibers. *J. Physiol. (London)* **227**, 627–645.

Ochs, S. (1974). Energy metabolism and supply of ~P to the fast axoplasmic transport mechanism in nerve. *Fed. Proc., Fed. Am. Soc. Exp. Biol.* **33**, 1049–1058.

Palay, S. L., and Chan-Palay, V. (1974). "Cerebellar Cortex, Cytology and Organization." Springer-Verlag, Berlin and New York.

Peper, K., Dreyer, F., Sandri, C., Akert, K., and Moor, H. (1974). Structure and ultrastructure of the frog motor endplate. A freeze-etching study. *Cell Tissue Res.* **149**, 437–455.

Purpura, D. P., and Suzuki, K. (1976). Distortion of neuronal geometry and formation of aberrant synapses in neuronal storage disease. *Brain Res.* **116**, 1–21.

Rakic, P. (1975). "Local Circuit Neurons." MIT Press, Cambridge, Massachusetts.

Ramón y Cajal, S. (1899). Comparative study of the sensory areas of the human cortex. *In* "Clark University, 1889–1899," Decennial Celebration, pp. 311–382. Clark Univ. Press, Worcester, Massachusetts.

Ramón y Cajal, S. (1937). "Recollections of my life" (E. Horne Craigie, transl.). *Mem. Am. Phil. Soc.* **8**.

Schmitt, F. (1968). The molecular biology of neuronal fibrous proteins. *Neurosci. Res. Program, Bull.* **6**, 119–144.

Singer, S. J., and Nicolson, G. L. (1972). The fluid mosaic model of the structure of cell membranes. *Science* **175**, 720–731.

Szentágothai, J. (1963). [Ujabb adatok a synapsisok funkcionális anatómi ájához.] (New data on the functional anatomy of synapses.) *Magy. Tud. Akad., Orv. Oszt. Kozl.* **6**: 217–227.

Therien, H. M., and Mushynski, W. E. (1976). Isolation of synaptic junctional complexes of high structural integrity from rat brain. *J. Cell Biol.* **71**, 807–822.

Wang, Y., and Mahler, H. R. (1976). Topography of the synaptosomal membrane. *J. Cell Biol.* **71,** 639–658.

Weiss, P. A. (1969). "Panta' Rhei"—and so flow our nerves. *Am. Sci.* **57,** 287–305.

Weiss, P. A. (1972). Neuronal dynamics and axonal flow: Axonal peristalsis. *Proc. Natl. Acad. Sci. U.S.A.* **69,** 1309–1312.

Weiss, P. A., and Hiscoe, H. B. (1948). Experiments on the mechanism of nerve growth. *J. Exp. Zool.* **107,** 315–395.

4

Basic Principles of
Neuronal Signaling

I. Introduction

As we go about our daily activities, we receive many different signals that we put together and evaluate, and, out of this, higher complex behaviors emerge. We respond to a complex array of environmental stimuli, such as light (photons), sound (air vibrations), taste (chemical substances), pressure, and temperature. All of these stimuli must be coded into some type of meaningful signals which the

111

nervous system can process. We respond both to these basic external stimuli and to internal ones, such as memories, wishes, and needs. The nervous system is composed of individual neurons, and these neurons must have the numerous sensory modalities and internal states translated into a limited language so they can deal with all of it. One could imagine a bizarre situation in which light was maintained in fiber optics, sound in sound pipes, and pressure in hollow tubes. The brain would be a miniature "Rube Goldberg" machine. In mixing and integrating the various modalities, it would clearly be an advantage to have some type of general medium into which all information is translated. In everyday experience our language serves that exact purpose. The alphabet has only 26 letters, but the large number of accepted combinations gives us the richness of our language. In language, objects and actions are replaced by words, which transfer information in verbal symbols.

The nervous system is faced with two basic problems: *relaying information* and *integrating* it. Signals from the eyes, ears, and other receptor organs must be transferred to brain centers where they are then processed together with other relevant information. There are two basic solutions to these two problems. Signals are relayed from one part of the nervous system to another in the language of action potentials and are then locally translated and integrated by the conversion of these action potentials to small graded potentials. Action potentials are the delivery messengers, whereas graded potentials are the clerks that bring the messages together and sort them out. The procedure emphasized depends on the distance over which the information must travel. Action potentials are the universal solution of the problem of interneuronal communication over long distances. Graded potentials, usually in the form of synaptic potentials, are the signals generally used over short distances. In addition, graded potentials not only carry information but "weigh" it in a manner called neuronal integration which we shall describe in detail later.

Action potentials can travel the entire length of the axon without change. In addition, they are highly stereotyped events. Each action potential is like all others. In order to carry information, the action potentials must be arranged in some sort of code, such as Morse code, but composed of dots only. One temporal pattern of dots may mean one thing, and another pattern may have a different meaning. The influence of an action potential depends on where and how it contributes to an ongoing temporal pattern of neuronal activity. Action potentials are the elements of neuronal language which carry the news in the pattern of their combinations.

Once an action potential reaches the nerve terminal, a chemical "transmitter substance" is released which then transforms the signal into graded potentials at the next nerve cell, and since many axons converge on a single cell, a spatial pattern of graded potentials on its surface is created, as well as the individual

4. BASIC PRINCIPLES OF NEURONAL SIGNALING

temporal patterns of each axon. The neuron must break the code, weigh the information appropriately, and finally recode it again. Thus, spatial and temporal patterns of action potentials are converted into synaptic potentials which are integrated and finally translated into new patterns of action potentials by which the nerve cell can influence the activity of other neurons and ultimately the effector organs. This local integrative activity is graded and permits extensive interaction between information from many sources. Graded potentials are usually employed for processing within a single neuron; as we shall discover, however, they are also sometimes used between cells, but strictly over short distances.

In this chapter, we will explain how action potentials are generated, and we shall see some of the ways they can code information with the nervous system. In Chapter 5, we will deal with short range interactions and the nature of synaptic potentials, the mode of communications between neurons, and the integration of this wealth of input into a meaningful output.

II.   The "Charged-Up and Ready-to-Go" Neuron

The signals used in information processing are electrical in nature. Action potentials and synaptic potentials are brief, highly distinctive events involving small movements of ions and generation of tiny electrical currents. Even at rest, neurons are "charged up," like batteries, and have a transmembrane potential (called the resting potential) which can be discharged or otherwise changed in the course of signaling. To understand better synaptic and action potentials and how information is processed, we need to describe the source of this electrical potential in neurons.

The electrical potential across the external (plasma) membrane of an inactive neuron is called the *resting potential*. Its role is to provide a stable state of readiness which can be rapidly released so that electrical currents can be used for signaling. Resting potentials make the neuron resemble a battery; both have an available reservoir of energy which can be released upon demand. Nerve cells store electricity and expend it performing their job.

The discovery of electricity in animals began in the eighteenth century with the work of Galvani and Volta. In those days the principal indication of electricity was a spark. Galvani noted that frog muscles contracted when a metal hook piercing the spinal cord made contact with a metal railing. After further experiments, discussion, and controversy, the presence of an electrical potential in nerve and muscle cells was generally accepted. And in 1902, Julius Bernstein proposed a satisfactory explanation for the resting potential—the reservoir of electricity in neurons and muscle cells.

A. Nature of Potentials

It is instructive to begin by defining the nature of voltage and current. A *voltage* develops whenever charges are separated. In metals, charges are carried by electrons but in biological systems, the charges are ions, usually sodium (Na^+), potassium (K^+) or chloride (Cl^-).

A simple circuit serves to illustrate the basic principles. If the negative pole of a battery is connected to the positive pole, electrons flow in the circuit (Fig. 4-1A). The rate of flow of charge is the *current*. In order to describe the flow of the electrons, it is necessary to make a definition. When 6×10^{18} electrons (or units of charge) pass a point, this is called a *coulomb* of charge. When the rate of flow of charge is 1 coulomb per second (C/sec), the quantity of current is called the ampere (A), and it is measured by an ammeter. In nerves the currents are small and are measured in microamperes (10^{-6} amperes).

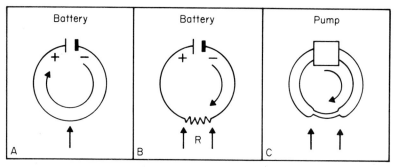

Fig. 4-1. (A) Currents arise from the flow of any charge. Passage of 6×10^{18} units of charge past a point in a circuit is 1 coulomb of charge. The flow of charge at the rate of 1 coulomb/second is 1 ampere. (B) A voltage arises from a separation of charges as, for example, across a resistor. Charges accumulate on one side of the resistor and so create a voltage or potential. The interrelationship between voltage V, current I and resistance R is given by Ohm's law $V = IR$. (C) The development of an electrical potential is like a pressure difference which develops across a constriction in a water line.

Now, suppose a resistor is inserted into the wire. A *resistor* is a device which impedes the flow of current. A simple analogy is the flow of water in a pipe. A resistor in an electrical circuit is like a constriction in a pipe: it causes the charge to accumulate on one side (Fig. 4-1B and C). Now since charges are separated, there is a difference in potential across the resistor. The unit of measure for the potential is the volt (V); 1 volt equals the potential developed by separating 1 coulomb of charge with 1 joule of energy. Since joules are units of energy, then a volt is the amount of energy available per coulomb of charge. The amount of energy in a joule is equivalent to the quantity of heat necessary to raise the temperature of 0.1 ml of water 1°C.

114

The fundamental relationship between voltage, resistance and current is known as Ohm's law. *Ohm's law*, which was at first determined empirically, states that the potential E (in volts) equals current I (in amperes) times the resistance R (in ohms, Ω); that is, $E = IR$. Thus, a current of 1 ampere will flow through a 1 ohm resistor with a potential of 1 volt across it. Ohm's law is very useful in understanding bioelectricity, since it is applicable to the relationship between current voltage and potential in cells as well as in electrical circuits. Often the term conductance is used; it is the reciprocal of resistance ($1/R$) and its unit is the mho (ohm spelled backward). *Conductance* is a measure of the ease with which current flows.

In order to illustrate an essential feature of nerve cells, we must introduce one more electrical device, a *capacitor* (Fig. 4-2). Capacitors are two conducting plates separated by an insulator. Capacitors can hold or store charges as a function of the voltage difference between the conductors. Membranes have a similar capacitance, a result of the insulating properties of the lipid bilayer that separates two conducting aqueous media. The relationship between potential, charge, and capacitance is $V = q/c$, where q is the charge and c the volume of the capacitor. In the circuit described in Fig. 4-2, when the resistor is switched in and out the potential across it changes instantly. However, when a capacitor is present

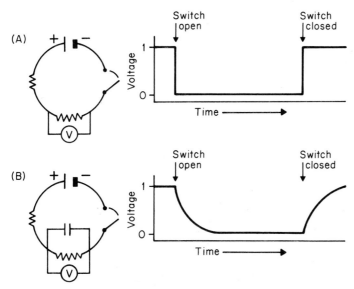

Fig. 4-2. Effect of capacitance on the time course of a potential when the circuit is opened and closed and voltage measured with a voltmeter (V). (A) In the absence of a capacitor the change in potential is instantaneous when the switch is opened and closed. (B) In the presence of a capacitor the change in potential is delayed. The difference in time courses is the time needed to charge or discharge the capacitor.

in parallel with the resistor, there is a gradual increase in potential when the switch opens and a gradual decline when closed. The larger the capacitor, the slower the changes in potential will be. The membranes of excitable cells have circuits equivalent to that pictured in Fig. 4-2. Their membrane capacitances are in parallel with the resistance. If nerve membranes did not have some capacitance, all changes in potential would be instantaneous.

B. Basis of the Resting Potential

Even at rest neurons have a potential across their membrane which makes the interior of the neuron negative relative to the outside. This internal negativity is called the resting potential. In neurons, the resting potential exists because (a) the K^+ ion concentration differs across the cell membrane and (b) the cell membrane is selectively permeable to K^+ ions. These conditions are completely sufficient to produce a membrane potential; nothing else is required. Such ion-based potentials exist across all nerve membranes and are called diffusion potentials.

Bernstein clearly spelled out these fundamental principles in 1902, which is remarkable, since the concept of a cell membrane was not yet clearly formulated and methods to measure bioelectricity were inadequate. Since that time, Bernstein's theory of the resting potential has been amply confirmed and is now well established.

Chemical analysis on a large number of neurons shows that the internal ion concentrations are very different from those of the external environment (Table 4-1). For example, squid axoplasm is high in K^+ and low in Na^+ relative to sea water or squid blood. Motor neurons of a cat also are high in K^+ and low in Na^+, although exact values differ from those of the squid. In general, all excitable cells retain high concentrations of K^+ and exclude Na^+.

Why is a semipermeable membrane required? For an answer, consider an

Table 4-1   Concentration of ions inside a freshly isolated squid axon and in the extracellular fluid[a]

Ion	Axoplasm	Extracellular fluid
Potassium	400	20
Sodium	50	440
Chloride	40–150	560

[a] Data from Hodgkin (1964).

idealized experiment (Fig. 4-3). If the axoplasm of a nerve is removed and the interior filled with KCl and placed in water, K⁺ ions will diffuse out of the axon down their concentration gradient because the membrane is permeable to K⁺. If the membrane were permeable to both K⁺ and Cl⁻ ions, an equilibrium would be reached when the inside and outside ionic concentrations are equal, and there would be no potential. However, the semipermeable quality of the membrane results in a different equilibrium situation. As K⁺ ions leave the interior, they leave Cl⁻ ions inside. This creates an excess negative charge on the inside and thus an electrical potential. When this negative potential becomes sufficiently large, it effectively counteracts the outward flow of K⁺ ions which are attempting to equalize their concentrations. K⁺ ion diffusion is exactly balanced by the electrical attractive forces inside, and so there is no net outward flow of K⁺ ions, even though these ions cross the membrane in both directions. No energy is required to maintain this state. The membrane potential and ion concentrations remain indefinitely. If the membrane were equally permeable to all ions, the ion concentrations would be the same on both sides of the membrane. No charge difference would exist and no potential would be present.

The actual difference between the number of positive and negative charges inside is very small: the squid axon contains only about a 0.000002% surplus of negative charge on the inside. In terms of concentration, this is negligible but sufficient to produce a −70 mV potential! This internal negativity is called the _resting potential_.

The relationship between concentration and membrane potential is given by a mathematical expression known as the _Nernst equation_. The Nernst equation

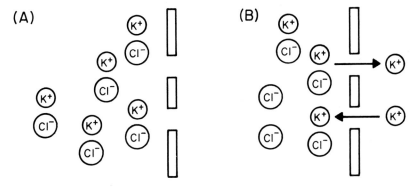

Fig. 4-3. Development of a diffusion potential. (A) If potassium chloride (KCl) is placed on one side of a two-compartment system separated by a membrane selectively permeable to K⁺ ions, K⁺ ions diffuse out down their concentrated gradient until the negative charge from Cl⁻ trapped inside builds up sufficiently to balance the flow of K⁺ ions down their concentration gradient. This results in an excess negative charge on one side and a potential difference (B).

can be derived from equations which describe the ionic diffusional forces and electrostatic forces. When they are equated (as described above) and solved for the *equilibrium potential*, an equation known as the Nernst equation results.

$$E = \frac{RT}{NF} \log \frac{[X]_o}{[X]_i}$$

E is the potential difference across a membrane (equilibrium potential), $[X]_i$ the concentration of permeable ions inside and $[X]_o$ the concentration of ions outside, *T* the absolute temperature (°K) (0°C = +273°K), *N* the charge on the ion, *F* is the Faraday constant (96,500 C of charge) and *R* is a constant (joules/°C-mole) which is necessary in order to make the units compatible. The Nernst equation describes the relationship between the potential difference across the membrane and the concentration of permeable ions across the membrane. The units are in volts. At room temperature for monovalent cations ($N = 1$), the term RT/NF works out to +58 mV. It is essential to emphasize that the potential given by the Nernst equation for a particular ionic concentration gradient is an equilibrium potential. That is, the potential is stable for the parameters given by the equation. There is no net current flow; inward currents and outward currents are equal.

Nernst first described this equation in 1897, and shortly thereafter Bernstein suggested that the Nernst equation described the expected relationship between potential and K^+ ion concentration. However, a direct test was not possible until the potential inside a neuron could be measured. The way to test a hypothesis is to define the variables, vary them and identify the relevant ones. In this case the strategy was to change various ions and see which one, if any, produced a change in the potential as predicted by the Nernst equation. If K^+ is the only ion which alters the resting potential and quantitatively accounts for the measured potentials, then its role would be established.

The simplest experiment was to vary the external ion concentration. Accordingly, a squid giant axon was placed in a bath and the potential inside the axon recorded. The resting potential does not change markedly with changes in the concentration of Na^+ or Cl^- ions. However, it is very sensitive to the external K^+ ion concentration (Hodgkin and Keynes, 1955). It follows from the Nernst equation that a tenfold (1 log unit) change in the ratio of K^+ ion concentrations should produce a 58 mV change in potential. As shown in Fig. 4-4, this is nearly the case over a large range of K^+ ion concentrations. The variance near the resting potential is known to be due to a slight leakiness of the membrane for Na^+ and Cl^- which makes the potential more positive than predicted on the basis of K^+ alone.

A possible criticism of such an experiment where only the external ion concentration is varied is that the concentration of the relevant ionic variable

4. BASIC PRINCIPLES OF NEURONAL SIGNALING

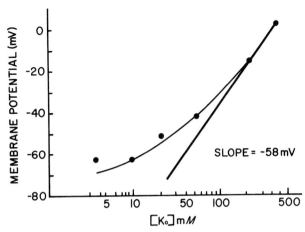

Fig. 4-4. The solid straight line is drawn with a slope of −58 mV, according to the Nernst equation. Because the membrane is also slightly permeable to sodium and chloride, the points deviate from the slope of −58 mV, especially at low external potassium concentrations $[K_0]$ (see text). (After Hodgkin and Keynes, 1955, as adapted by Kuffler and Nichols, 1976.)

inside the axon is unknown. It was discovered that the internal ion concentration can, in fact, be varied (Baker *et al.*, 1962a,b). The axoplasm is squeezed out of the axon by gently rolling it and the axon then reinflated with a perfusion fluid of known composition (Fig. 4-5). In this way, the role of the axon membrane can be investigated with internal and external ion compositions defined.

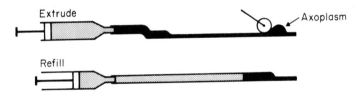

Fig. 4-5. Axoplasm is extruded from a giant squid axon by gently rolling the axon. A syringe is used to refill the axon with a defined media. (After Baker *et al.*, 1962a.)

If the membrane potential of the perfused fiber depends only on the ionic concentration, it should be zero when identical solutions are on both sides of the membrane. Also as predicted, substitution of isotonic K_2SO_4 for KCl gives identical resting potentials, indicating that Cl^- ion concentration is not critical. Indeed, isotonic NaCl does not give any potential (Fig. 4-6). Axons are only very slightly permeable to Na^+ at rest, in accordance with the nature of the resting potential.

What would the potential be if the K^+ ion gradient were reversed so that K^+

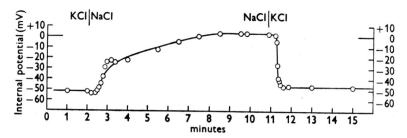

Fig. 4-6. Effect on the resting potential of replacing isotonic KCl with isotonic NaCl inside an axon. The membrane potential changes from the resting potential to 0 potential as NaCl replaces KCl and back again as KCl is restored. (From Baker *et al.*, 1962b.)

was low inside and high outside? Baker and co-workers performed this experiment and recorded a membrane potential of about +70 mV, as expected.

The results clearly establish that the potential of an axon in the resting state is determined by K^+ ion concentration. The selective permeability of the membrane to K^+ sets up a diffusion potential where the relationship between potential and K^+ concentration is described by the Nernst equation. How do we envision the neuron membrane when it is at the level of the resting potential? The membrane is freely permeable to K^+ ions, which pass in and out of a few small holes in the membrane. The tendency of concentrated K^+ ions to flow outward is balanced by the slight excess negative charge inside the axon. There is no ionic current, and the membrane potential is at equilibrium.

Actually, there are many channels but not all are open at any one time. Channels are continually flickering, opening and closing, so that when the membrane is at the resting potential, the same number but different ones are open, on the average, at any instant (Fig. 4-7). Thus the operation of the channels controlling membrane permeability for K^+ is a more or less random affair that may be evaluated on a statistical basis.

We have now described the basic properties of the nerve membrane resting potential and developed a few concepts on its genesis. These concepts provide the basis for understanding other potentials as well. The general principle is that all membrane potentials result from the selective permeability of the membrane to certain ions. The energy value or voltage of the potential is given by the concentration ratio of the permeant ion in accordance with the Nernst equation. For example, muscle cells, like neurons, have resting potentials; in some muscle cells the resting potential is determined by the Cl^- ion concentration instead of K^+. This difference exists because the membrane is permeable to Cl^- ions and relatively impermeable to Na^+ and K^+ at rest. The potential of the membrane is computed, therefore, by inserting internal and external Cl^- ion concentrations into the Nernst equation. If the permeability in a neuron were to instantly shift

4. BASIC PRINCIPLES OF NEURONAL SIGNALING

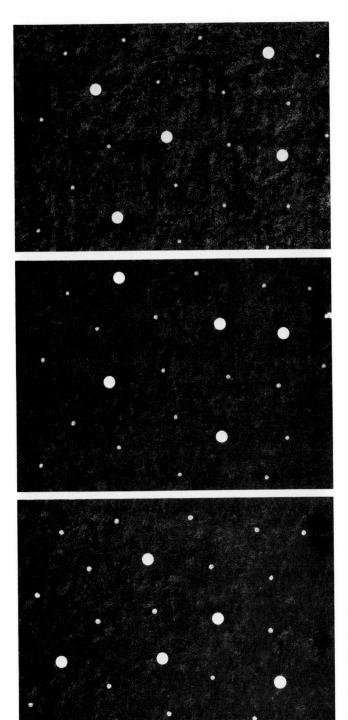

Fig. 4-7. K⁺ channels flicker. Only a fraction of the total K⁺ channels is open when the membrane potential is at the resting potential. On the average, the fraction open is constant, but the individual channels open change from moment to moment. The three panels show the state of the membrane at three instants in time.

from K^+ to Na^+ ions, the membrane potential will adjust all the way from -70 mV to the equilibrium potential for Na ($+50$ mV). As we shall see in the following section, this extraordinary shift, in fact, is the situation during an action potential. The 120 mV spike (from -70 to $+50$) is generated by a transient increase in Na^+ permeability. The membrane moves all the way from the equilibrium potential for K^+ (-70 mV) to the equilibrium potential for Na^+ ($+50$ mV). Synaptic potentials also result from similar changes in membrane permeability evoked by membrane receptors for specific transmitters.

In summary, the resting potential is the reservoir of energy for the neuron which provides for the generation of electrical signals. It is also the standard reference point; all other potentials, action or synaptic, are described in relation to it. A cell is said to be _depolarized_ when its membrane resting potential is reduced toward 0, i.e., its normal negative charge is reduced or removed. Conversely, a cell is said to be _hyperpolarized_ when the resting potential is made more negative, i.e., negative charge is added. Inward currents of cations (positive ions) depolarize cells, whereas outward currents of them hyperpolarize (Fig. 4-8).

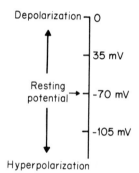

Fig. 4-8. Definitions which describe changes in the level of the membrane potential relative to the resting potential.

C. Electrotonic Properties of Neurons

It was once thought that nerve cells conducted electrical signals only in the way that electricity is conducted in wires. Electric currents travel along a wire in accordance with the ohmic properties of that wire. A wire has low resistance, so that energy, i.e., electrical potential, applied at one end passes with little decrement to the other end. Copper wire is an excellent conductor because of its especially low resistance. Axons, however, are incredibly poor conductors relative to metal wire, even though they manage to conduct potentials all over the body. The electrical resistance of 1 m of small nerve, as Hodgkin has noted, is about the same as a 22 gauge copper wire stretched between the Earth and Saturn 10 times over. Consequently, potentials decay very rapidly with distance in nerves.

4. BASIC PRINCIPLES OF NEURONAL SIGNALING

The passive or *electrotonic conduction* of potential in nerves, then, is similar to but not even remotely as good as a wire. The problem is with the nerve membrane. Nerve axons, as well as dendrites, have a leaky plasma membrane encasing a low resistance cytoplasm (like a poorly insulated wire) (Fig. 4-9). In axons or dendrites during passive current spread, current flows easily in the low resistance interior but dissipates over distance in the membrane, as well as leaking through it.

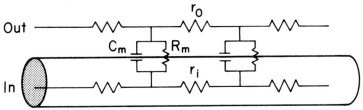

Fig. 4-9. A dendrite or axon has the electrical properties of a tube (or hollow cable). It has a low resistance core (r_i) and a membrane casing which has a high resistance (R_m) and low capacitance (C_m). The external resistance (r_o) is very low. The membrane is relatively leaky to ionic currents so that currents passing through the low resistance core leak out over distance and dissipate.

This passive decay of potential along axons or dendrites is described by a measure called the space constant, which characterizes the rate at which a particular voltage decays with distance. The *space constant* is defined as the distance over which a voltage applied at one point in a neuron (for example, an axon or dendrite) has fallen to 37% of its initial value.

The space constant for a 2 μm diameter nerve fiber of average properties, for example, is about 0.3 mm; a 100 mV signal would decay to 37 mV in this distance if the spread of current were strictly passive. In another 0.3 mm the potential would be only 14 mV. Current spread in dendrites, as we shall see, is largely passive or electrotonic, but in certain areas of the human nervous system axons are over 150 cm long, and similar fibers in the giraffe run more than 4 m between the spinal cord and brain. How, then are messages relayed over such long distances? The answer is that action potentials are used. Action potentials can relay signals over long distances because the signal is boosted as it is propagated.

III. The Action Potential

Action potentials are the basic information units which relay messages along the axon over long distances. They are defined as transient changes in the membrane potential which travel like a wave without change in size along the axon no matter how long it is. The changes are actively self-regenerating, so action potentials do not decay.

Action potentials are so named because they are full of action. They are an electrical disturbance, an ionic storm, traveling along the axon with speeds up to 100 m/second. Their marvelous quality is that they expend the stored energy of the resting potentials so they never tire but go on relentlessly carrying their message along meters of axon with no change from beginning to end. Imagine for a moment we are standing inside the axon as an action potential goes by. Imagine also that Na^+ ions are pink dust particles and K^+ are blue. As the action potential approaches, pink dust begins to blow at us as Na^+ ions herald the advancing storm. Then in a moment, a pink and blue tornado rushes at us along the membrane. Its leading edge is pink, as a result of Na^+ ions entering the membrane, and its trailing surface is blue as a result of K^+ ions leaving the membrane. These ionic movements swirl in the membrane like a great ionic tornado. We never see such events, of course, but a microelectrode does.

Action potentials are recorded from axons by electrodes which pick up the signal. The signal is then amplified and displayed. In a typical experiment an axon is placed in a bath, penetrated with a glass electrode and then stimulated by applying a depolarizing current above a critical value (Fig. 4-10). Right after the stimulus, a transient potential change is recorded which propagates along the axon. The potential has an amplitude of 120 mV and takes only 2–3 msec to pass a given point on the axon. Rising from the resting potential, it shoots to +50 mV and then subsides again to the resting potential. It is of constant voltage amplitude no matter how long the axon, and it travels at speeds of up to 100 m/second (330 ft/second!). At such velocity, the various stages of the process just described would occupy a length of 2 cm along the axon at any moment. The maximal velocity of the action potential travels about one-quarter the speed of a bullet shot from a 22 caliber rifle. It is designed for fast reliable communication.

The value of the membrane potential at which an action potential is initiated is called the _threshold_ value. Threshold is usually about 20 mV above the resting potential. Below threshold, a rise in membrane potential does not lead to an action potential, but should it pass beyond, the action potential explodes with its power and begins its journey along the fiber. Threshold, therefore, is sufficiently above resting potential to ensure that action potentials do not fire spontaneously from small fluctuations in membrane potential. On the other hand, threshold is not so far above that it cannot be reached by the summation of several synaptic potentials.

For a short time after each action potential, the axon is in the _refractory period_. The _absolute refractory period_ is defined as the time after an action potential when a second action potential cannot be initiated. In the frog, the sciatic nerve cannot be reexcited for the first 3 msec, no matter how intense the stimulus; the nerve is in the absolute refractory period (Fig. 4-11). For the next 7 msec, it can be reexcited only with a supranormal stimulus; this interval is called

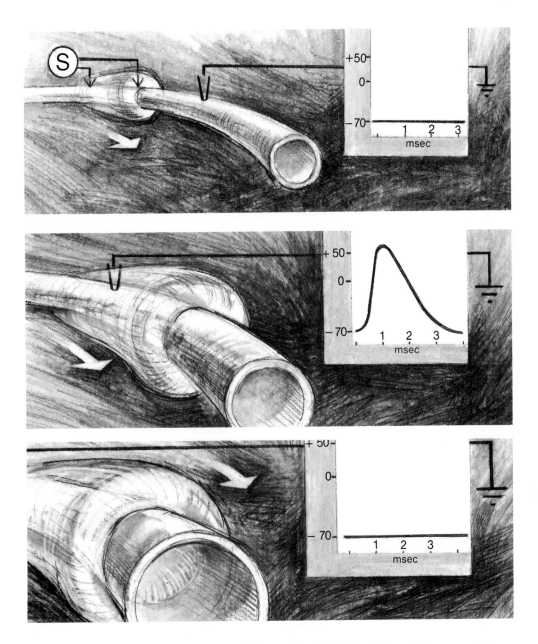

Fig. 4-10. Recording an action potential. Suprathreshold stimulation of the axon at S initiates an action potential, which propagates along the axon. A microelectrode inside the axon is used to measure the change in potential. The sequence of three drawings shows the initiation and passage of an action potential along an axon. The signal is picked up by the electrode, amplified and visualized on an oscilloscope screen (*inset*).

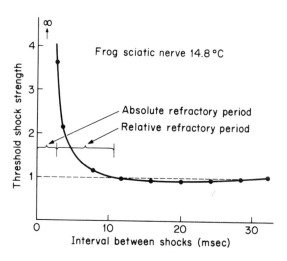

Fig. 4-11. Threshold for a second stimulus versus the time after a first suprathreshold stimulus. The threshold shock is the smallest amplitude shock to the nerve that makes a just detectable twitch in an attached whole muscle. For the first 3 msec the nerve cannot be reexcited and is said to be in the absolute refractory period. For the next 7 msec only a supranormal stimulus will excite and the nerve is said to be in the relative refractory period. (From Hille, 1977).

the *relative refractory period*. Obviously, the refractory period sets an upper limit on the rate of repetitive firing.

Let us examine for a moment the phenomena underlying the generation of the action potential and the way the potential is propagated.

A. Generation of the Wave

For the purposes of understanding the action potential, the axon may be thought of as a long cylinder filled with Na^+ and K^+ ions and encased by a membrane endowed with special properties. A perfused axon reinflated with ionic media consisting of Na^+ and K^+ salts conducts action potentials indistinguishable from those of intact axons. This similarity means that the only requirement for the conduction of action potentials is the plasma membrane and appropriate concentrations of Na^+ and K^+ ions across the membrane.

The axon membrane is a simple and yet most remarkable structure, a phospholipid bilayer penetrated by channels which regulate the flux of Na^+ and K^+ ions across the membrane. The squid axon membrane has about 200 _Na+ channels_ per μm^2 and an equal number or slightly fewer _K+ channels_ per μm^2. The channels are highly selective: Na^+ channels exclude K^+ ions and K^+ channels exclude Na^+ ions. The flux through these channels is very large. When the Na^+ channel is open, approximately 107 ions pass through every second under normal conditions. Na^+ ions, which are about 2 Å in size, must pass single file through the pore. These channels are probably proteins so organized in the bilayer that they span the membrane and form a long aqueous pore (Fig. 4-12). Selectivity is a result of the channel's size and chemical environment (Hille, 1974). The Na^+ channel is funnel shaped, having a wide entrance which tapers to a narrow,

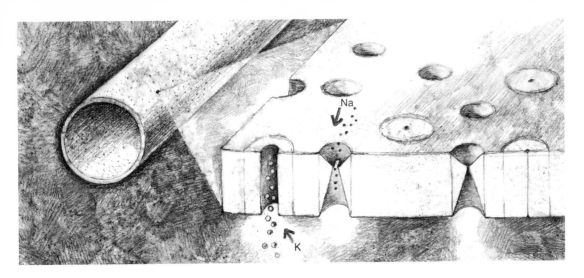

Fig. 4-12. Diagram of a section of the axon membrane and its Na⁺ and K⁺ channels. The structure of the channels is highly schematic, since their exact structure is presently unknown. The key property of the channels is that they are selective to Na⁺ and K⁺ ions and the number open at any instant is controlled by the membrane potential.

approximately rectangular hole 3×5 Å in diameter. The pore has a net negative charge which repels anions and attracts cations. The size of the hole, however, readily excludes large organic cations.

The way the Na⁺ channel excludes K⁺ ions is not well understood at present. It appears as if the geometric properties of the Na⁺ channel as well as short range chemical bonds in the channel exclude K⁺ ions. The investigation of this problem is one of the frontier areas of modern biophysics.

Key properties of these channels are (1) that they open and close, (2) that they allow only Na⁺ or K⁺ ions to pass, and (3) that the average number open at any time is determined by the value of the membrane potential. A depolarization (decrease) of the membrane potential results in an increase in the number of Na⁺ channels open at any one time. Na⁺ as well as K⁺ channels open under orders from the membrane potential. Figure 4-13 illustrates the ionic events in the generation of the action potential.

The action potential is generated by time-locked serial changes in Na⁺ and K⁺ movements—an inward flow of Na⁺ followed by an outward flow of K⁺. At the resting potential most Na⁺ channels are closed. Depolarization, as noted above, opens some Na⁺ channels. The resulting further change in electric field due to entrance of Na⁺ opens more channels and more positively charged Na⁺ ions rush inward. Na⁺ ions thus "storm" the membrane and take control of its potential, raising its voltage to +50 mV, the equilibrium potential for Na⁺. The Na⁺ ions, as we would have expected, have simply run down their

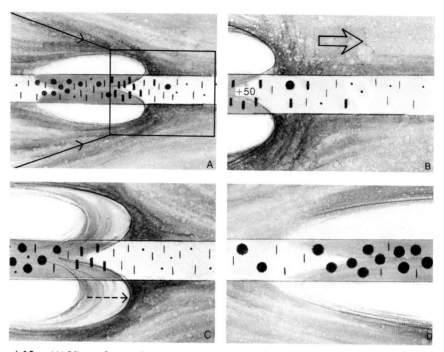

Fig. 4-13. (A) View of axon showing the behavior of the Na and K channels. Na channels are shown by thin bars where the channels are closed and thick bars where the channels are open. (B) At the front of the wave Na channels are open allowing inward Na currents and causing the membrane potential to become +50 mV. (C) Na channels begin to spontaneously close and the wave moves forward. K channels open in the region of membrane where a moment ago Na channels were open. The membrane potential starts to swing back to the resting potential. (D) K channels are fully in command at the tail end of the wave and bring the membrane potential back to the resting potential.

concentration gradient to their equilibrium potential. At E_{Na} (the equilibrium potential for Na), most Na channels are open.

Sodium ion channels, however, can remain open for only a short period, so that at about the time the action potential reaches E_{Na}, Na^+ channels close. In the absence of a significant Na^+ flux, the membrane potential cannot remain at E_{Na}. It starts to decay back to the resting potential, its return accelerated by outward K^+ currents.

At the same time Na^+ channels are closing, there is an increase in the number of K^+ channels opening. Potassium ion channels, like Na^+ channels, are controlled by the membrane potential; thus, the Na^+-generated depolarization generates an increase in available K^+ channels. These channels, however, are sluggish and open very slowly, becoming significant only as Na^+ channels are nearly all closed. Such combined closing of Na^+ and opening of more K^+ channels drives the membrane potential back to the resting potential. (A slight hyper-

4. BASIC PRINCIPLES OF NEURONAL SIGNALING

polarization results because E_K (the equilibrium potential for K) is slightly more negative than the resting potential; later, when fewer K^+ channels are open, the membrane will come back to the resting potential.)

The timing of channel opening and closing is a critical part of the mechanism. For Na^+ and K^+ channels, respectively, these events permit an intense local inward Na^+ current which lasts for about 0.8 msec, followed by an equally intense outward K^+ current which lasts for another 0.7 msec. This interlocked sequence results in an inward–outward current and generates a wave ideally suited for traveling along axon membranes.

What are the events that take place at threshold which initiate an action potential? The ionic part of the story can be envisioned as follows: small depolarizations below threshold result in a slight increase in Na^+ entry, but once such

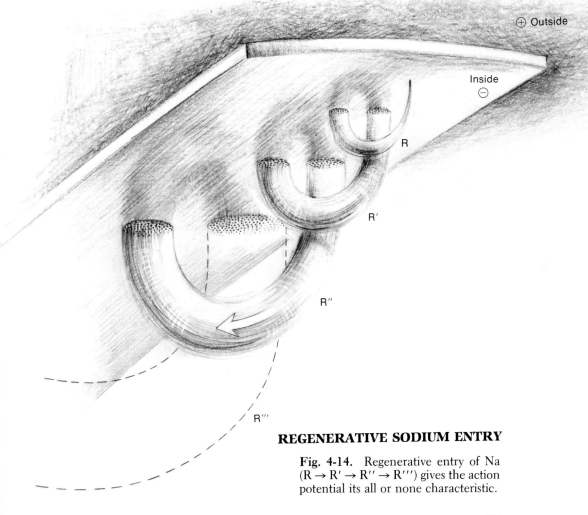

REGENERATIVE SODIUM ENTRY

Fig. 4-14. Regenerative entry of Na ($R \rightarrow R' \rightarrow R'' \rightarrow R'''$) gives the action potential its all or none characteristic.

depolarizations are removed, the potential returns to its resting value because outward K^+ currents override the inward Na^+ flux. Potassium ions have won and kept the axon from firing. At threshold, however, inward Na^+ currents just balance outward K^+ currents, and neither ion gains control. There is no net current, but the membrane potential is "poised" and can go either way with only slight perturbation.

Depolarizations beyond threshold open a sufficiently large number of Na^+ channels so that Na^+ currents overpower K^+ currents, as we have seen. Once threshold is exceeded, a series of regenerative cycles are initiated (Fig. 4-14) that drive the membrane potential to the equilibrium potential for Na^+ ions in a few tenths of a second. We saw that Na^+ entry depolarizes, which increases Na^+ permeability, which permits more Na^+ entry. Thus, Na^+ entry has a positive feedback effect on its own permeability which allows it to gain the upper hand. This effect is illustrated in Fig. 4-15. The regenerative Na^+ cycle is an avalanche-like effect. Once an avalanche starts, it gains more power as it accumulates materials; it will not stop until it spends its energy in the valley below and reaches a new equilibrium. Similarly, once Na^+ entry reaches a critical point, it will not spontaneously stop; it will gain more power running downhill until it reaches a barrier, E_{Na}, at which it has spent its available energy and reaches equilibrium.

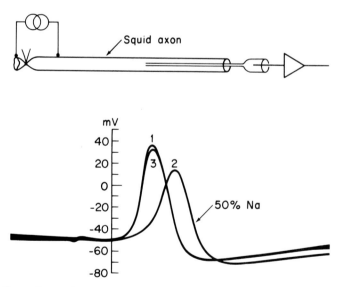

Fig. 4-15. Recording of action potentials made from a squid giant axon with axial micropipet recording electrode in normal seawater and in seawater where the Na^+ concentration is 50%. Records 1 and 3 are of an action potential in seawater and that in 2 is in seawater diluted in half by a mixture of seawater and isotonic dextrose. The axon potential is smaller and rises more slowly when the Na^+ concentration is reduced. (From Hodgkin and Katz, 1949.)

4. BASIC PRINCIPLES OF NEURONAL SIGNALING

The regenerative cycle of Na^+ accounts for the "all-or-none" behavior of action potentials. It is why axons fire.

The voltage-mediated control of permeability is a distinctive property of membranes which generate action potentials; such membranes, therefore, are called _excitable membranes_. Membranes of cells which do not generate action potentials (_inexcitable membranes_) do not possess this ability. If an erythrocyte, for example, is depolarized, no action potential is initiated, since the ion _permeability_ is unaffected. No additional channels open upon depolarization, so the membrane resistance is constant and the membrane behaves in accordance with Ohm's law, i.e., the current is proportional to the applied voltage. When the stimulus is removed, the potential simply returns to the resting level.

B. Experimental Support

Over the past several years a large number of experiments on many different axons have confirmed the Na^+ theory for the generation of the action potential. It is now firmly established that the genesis of the action potential in axons is an inward Na^+ movement. In a key paper in 1949, Hodgkin and Katz tested the Na^+ hypothesis directly by varying the external Na^+ concentration and recording the effect on the peak amplitude of the action potential with intracellular electrodes. It was quite clear from these experiments that the overshoot is less when the external Na^+ is reduced (Fig. 4-15). A decrease to half of the normal concentration of Na^+ made the peak value 21 mV less positive. This result agrees favorably with the 17 mV change predicted from the Nernst equation. Shortly after the Hodgkin and Katz experiment, the Na^+ hypothesis was confirmed by direct measurement of the entry of radioactive Na^+ into axons (Keynes, 1951). The Na^+ gain is small but adequate to account for the potential change observed (the concentration is raised by only 0.005% per impulse in a squid axon).

The key data in analyzing the mechanism of the action potential, however, were not the above but the measurements of the behavior of Na^+ and K^+ channels at different times and voltages. What is the time course of channel opening and closure? What is the exact relationship between potential and these events? At first, analysis seemed impossible, since the changes occurred so quickly and the events were so interrelated. The necessary conceptual and technical breakthrough came from Cole (1968) and associates with the invention of the voltage clamp technique. This technique stops the action potential so that measurements can be made—it takes the "action" out of the action potential! The voltage clamp holds the membrane potential at different values and prevents the spread of the potential so that the ion currents can be measured at defined values of membrane potential. In a typical experiment an electrode is inserted into the axon, and then connected to an electronic device that simply adds sufficient opposing current to counteract the currents of the action potential. If there is no net current, the potential cannot change. The amount of opposing current put out by the device gives an exact measure of the ion currents in the axon. That is, the amount of current that must be applied is a measure of the ion permeability through the channels of the membranes. Since each channel is essentially identical to all the others in the population, the current measured is directly proportional to the number of channels open. The voltage clamp technique is analogous to analyzing the leaks in a bucket of water by measuring the amount of water which must be added to maintain a constant level. The outflow can be deduced from the inflow required to balance it. Voltage clamp records provide us with a picture of the ionic currents and activity of the channels when the potential is unchanging (Hodgkin and Huxley, 1952a–d). In the early experiments of Hodgkin and Huxley, the operation of K^+ channels was studied independently of Na^+ channels by removing the Na^+. The difference in the total currents and K^+ current then allowed them to compute the Na^+ current (Fig. 4-16). The Na^+ current is a strong

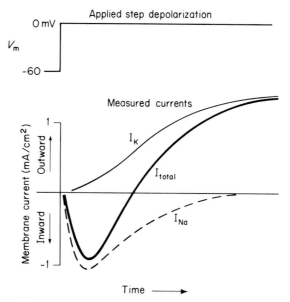

Fig. 4-16. The total current across the membrane during a 60 mV step depolarization is a transient current flowing in through the membrane followed by a delayed and prolonged outward current. The total membrane current (I_{total}) produced by the 60 mV depolarizing potential step can be separated into two components I_{Na^+} and I_{K^+}. With the axon bathed in Na^+-free (choline) seawater or the Na channels blocked by tetrodotoxin, the current generated by the same depolarizing step is due to I_{K^+}. The difference between the total ionic current in seawater and that in Na^+-free seawater (I_{K^+}) reveals I_{Na^+}. I_{Na^+} is also identified by blocking the I_{K^+} by tetraethylammonium ions. (Hodgkin and Huxley, 1952, from Kandel, 1976.)

         4. BASIC PRINCIPLES OF NEURONAL SIGNALING

inward current which begins immediately after clamping and spontaneously decreases at about 0.8 msec. Clearly, since the membrane potential is constant, the channels are closing independent of the change in potential. The K+ current, on the other hand, is an outward current which is delayed and which remains as long as the potential is sustained. Recently, it has been possible to use highly specific drugs to separate the Na+ and K+ currents by blocking their channels selectively. Na+ channels are blocked by *tetrodotoxin* (TTX), and K+ channels by *tetraethylammonium* (TEA) ions.

The individual Na+ and K+ currents have been studied at different membrane potentials in order to describe the relationship between channel opening and the membrane potential. The membrane potential is displaced to various levels intermediate between −60 and +75 mV, and a family of curves generated for each ionic current as a function of potential. Figure 4-17 illustrates a current

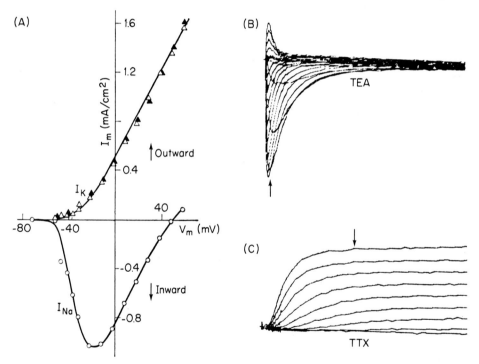

Fig. 4-17. Current–voltage relationships from Na and K current flow in *Myxicola* axon (A). The points are ionic currents during a voltage step from the resting potential to the indicated voltage measured from a family of records for I_{Na} (B) and I_K (C). The family of curves for the Na current are obtained in the presence of tetraethylammonium ions (TEA) to block the K current and the data replotted in the current voltage curve represents the peak early Na current (arrow). The K current is obtained in the presence of tetrodotoxin (TTX) and is the steady state value (arrow). (Adapted from Hille, 1967, Binstock and Goldman, 1969.)

voltage curve plotted from data on the *Myxicola* giant axon. These data show that a decrease in membrane potential causes an increase in the Na$^+$ current and an increase in the number of channels open. This function is graded, and it is greatest between -50 and -20 mV. Depolarization also causes a graded increase in K$^+$, which is not as great as that for Na$^+$ and requires more depolarization.

In summary, the results of *voltage clamp* studies show that Na$^+$ and K$^+$ channels open as a function of increased membrane potential. The Na$^+$ channels open rapidly and close spontaneously; the K$^+$ channels are slower to open and stay open as long as potential is maintained.

C. Propagation of the Wave

As we described in Section II,B, the axon can be considered simply as a conducting fluid encased by a semipermeable membrane. Sodium and K$^+$ gradients exist across this membrane, which contains Na$^+$ and K$^+$ channels that open and close as directed by the membrane potential. We have seen that the action potential wave is generated by a transient inward current of Na$^+$ ions followed by a delayed outward current of K$^+$ ions An action potential can be thought of as a wave rolling along in the axon membrane in the act of breaking; Na$^+$ ions, moving down through the membrane at the breaking edge, are followed by K$^+$ ions moving outward on the trailing slope of the wave. These coordinated currents carry the membrane potential to E_{Na} and back to E_K. The question we now address is, how does the wave travel along the axon?

The key factor in such spread is the low resistance of the axoplasm and of the external environment. The axoplasmic resistance is about 10^9 times less than that of the membrane. Currents follow the path of least resistance, so that the inward Na$^+$ currents will spread electrotonically within the axon core and depolarize adjacent regions in advance of the wave. In front of the advancing impulse, where the membrane potential is still subthreshold, positive ions accumulate on the inside surface. The accumulation results in a discharge of membrane capacitance and depolarization. When threshold is reached, the membrane current reverses and inward Na$^+$ now dominates. This, as we have stressed in our preceding discussions, will drive the membrane to E_{Na} in accordance with the properties of a membrane now primarily permeable to Na$^+$ ions. As Na$^+$ channels close, the membrane is again polarized by K$^+$ ions moving outward. The hyperpolarizing K$^+$ current is powerful and far exceeds the depolarizing effect of current spreading back from the active region, which is now moving ahead to new lengths of the axon for conquest. Thus, the basis of propagation is the electrotonic spread of current within the axon preceding the action potential.

A useful way to think of the spread of the action potential is to consider the events that take place when one lights a fuse. The fuse burns vigorously and in doing so gives off sufficient heat to ignite an adjacent segment. In this way, the flame races along the fuse train. Similarly in an action potential, currents from the commotion of ions spread and "ignite" the nearby membrane. The spread is passive, like that of the fuse, but serves to transport the potential undiminished along the fiber. The wave proceeds in an "all-or-none" manner; if anywhere along the length of the axon it did not so proceed, propagation of the impulse would cease as surely as would the flame sputtering toward a wet segment of fuse.

Some axons, again like some fuses, conduct very slowly while others conduct very rapidly (Table 4-2). Conduction velocity in unmyelinated fibers reaches its zenith in the giant squid and the sea worm, *Myxicola*, where the axons are 0.15–1.0 mm in diameter and speeds are up to 25 m/second. Speed is not due to the properties of the axon membrane or the axoplasm itself, since all membrane properties which affect velocity are essentially identical, but it is related to fiber caliber. As the ratio of volume to surface area increases with larger diameter fibers, the resistance of the axoplasm decreases relative to the membrane resistance so that the currents spread further ahead of the action potential and the potential moves faster. Moreover, for a given diameter of fiber, the rate of passive current spread is about 10 times the speed of propagation of the action potentials. The internal resistance of an axon decreases with greater diameter because the greater volume offers more paths for flow of current. The resistance of its axoplasm is the same, but there is more of that axoplasm (i.e., the sum of

Table 4-2 Conduction velocities in nerve and muscle[a]

Tissue	Temperature (°C)	Myelinated (M)[b] or unmyelinated (U)	Fiber (μm)	Velocity (m/second)
Cat myelinated nerve fibers	38	M	2–20	10–100
Cat unmyelinated nerve fibers	38	U	0.3–1.3	0.7–2.3
Frog myelinated nerve fibers	24	M	3–16	6–32
Prawn myelinated nerve fibers	20	M	35	20
Crab large nerve fibers	20	U	30	5
Squid giant axon	20	U	500	25
Frog muscle fiber	20	U	60	1.6

[a] From Hodgkin (1964). Courtesy of Charles C. Thomas, Publisher, Springfield, Illinois.
[b] For myelinated fibers the figure given is the external diameter of the myelin.

resistance for identical resistors in parallel is less than the resistance of a single one). By analogy, there is much less resistance to the flow of liquids in large pipes than small ones.

The rate an action potential will travel is given by

$$\text{Rate} = C\sqrt{r}$$

where r is the radius of the axon and C is a constant which depends on membrane properties (resistance and capacitance) and the specific axoplasmic resistance. The resistance, capacitance and specific axoplasmic resistance are relatively constant in most axons. Thus, the speed of the action potential for an unmyelinated fiber is proportional to the square root of the axonal radius. Doubling the size of the fiber does not result in a twofold increase in speed, but in a 1.4-fold increase.

It would be clearly impractical to use giant axons whenever speed is required. In the ventral root of a spinal nerve there is simply no room for the thousands of giant axons that would be necessary to carry the multiple signals to muscles at high speed. To carry impulses at 100 m/second, the conduction velocity of most ventral root fibers, an unmyelinated fiber would need to be about 4 mm in diameter! In actuality, an entire nerve, consisting of thousands of fibers, can be somewhat smaller than 4 mm. In the vertebrate nervous system, the solution for providing fast conduction without utilizing giant fibers is that axons are encased by myelin, which greatly increases the conduction velocity to the point where even relatively thin axons can conduct quite fast. A 30 μm myelinated axon conducts at about 20 m/second, whereas a nonmyelinated axon of that size would conduct at about 5 m/second.

Myelin is the plasma membrane of a glial cell wrapped many times around the axon (see Chapter 2). The areas between the wrappings where axon membrane is exposed are called _nodes_. In the peripheral nervous system the nodes are about 0.4 mm apart in a 16 μm fiber, but in smaller fibers they are usually closer. Myelin has a very high resistance and low capacitance, so it is an excellent insulator. The encased portion of the axon is insulated, so ion flow is restricted to the nodes. Thus an action potential initiated at a node "jumps" to the next node (Fig. 4-18). This process is called _saltatory conduction_. The currents flow through the axoplasm until they reach the low resistance node, where they then depolarize the membrane past threshold in the usual manner and initiate an action potential. Between nodes the action potential diminishes slightly, like the flame in a damp fuse, but at the node it is boosted back to full power. The area at the node is very small and rich in channels (100,000 Na^+ channels per μm^2 as opposed to perhaps 20–500 channels per μm^2 on the surfaces of unmyelinated fibers), thus providing a low resistance, high density pathway for the influx of Na^+ during the

4. BASIC PRINCIPLES OF NEURONAL SIGNALING

action potential. At rest, 25 channels are open, and at threshold 300–400 channels open at these nodes. Usually, more than one node is active at once. If the action potential lasts 0.5 msec, travels at 10 m/second, and the internodal length is 1.5 mm, the total wavelength of the action potential is about 6 mm and four consecutive nodes would be in various stages of firing at any instant.

In summary, the high resistance of myelin prevents the loss of currents over distance so that it greatly lengthens the space constant. Furthermore, the low capacitance of myelin minimizes diminution of charges normally consumed in polarizing the membrane. Moreover, the small area of the node and its great density of Na^+ channels allow for rapid depolarization and production of strong currents which can spread to the next node. All these features increase the speed of conduction.

The addition of myelin to axons not only speeds up the action potential, but it makes axonal metabolism more efficient. The high resistance membrane minimizes leakage of substances through the membrane. A frog sciatic nerve, for example, gains about 4000 times fewer Na^+ ions per impulse than the giant squid axon. Since fewer ions enter the membrane during an action potential, fewer must be removed to maintain the ion gradients.

IV. Recovery of Ion Gradients

Eventually, the accumulation of Na^+ and loss of K^+ would result in an axon incapable of generating action potentials. The average optic nerve axon in a human fires about 10^{11} times in 60 years, yet maintains the same Na^+ and K^+ concentrations in old age as in youth. The maintenance of Na^+ and K^+ gradients is accomplished by an enzyme in the membrane called Na^+,K^+-ATPase (Skou, 1957; Hodgkin, 1964). This enzyme pumps Na^+ ions out and K^+ in. Since these ions are moved against their concentration gradients (uphill), work must be done, and energy is required. The energy which stokes the ATPase is ATP, a major source of energy in cells. Like a fuel when burnt, it gives off energy which can be captured for various uses.

Early work in which nerves were placed in solution and stimulated many times showed that axons loaded with radioactive Na^+ could pump the Na^+ back out again. The pumping action was totally dependent on ATP. Axons in which ATP production had been experimentally inhibited stopped pumping. The pump operates continuously; but its activity is increased when more Na^+ enters the cell. As we shall see, this is easily understood from consideration of molecular mechanisms. Careful analysis of ion fluxes shows that the outward movement of Na^+

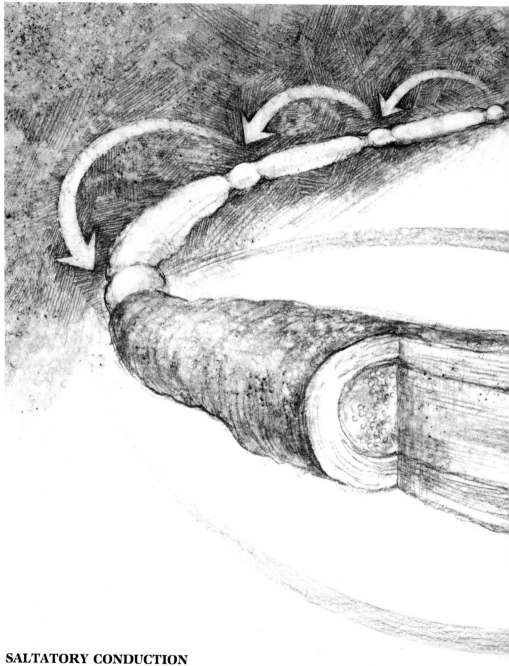

SALTATORY CONDUCTION

Fig. 4-18. The path of an action potential as it jumps from node to node is shown as the curve of the arrow going from the tail to the head of each arrow.

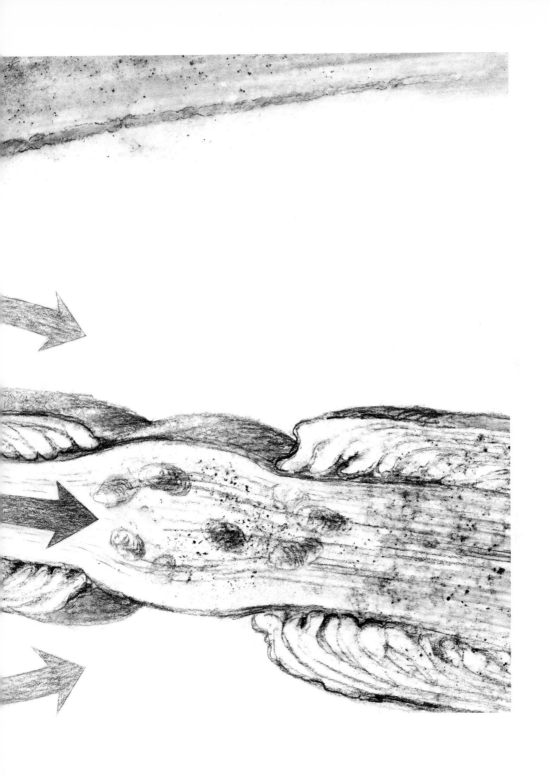

ions is loosely coupled to the inward movement of K^+. In the absence of internal Na^+, the pump slows down.

For each molecule of ATP consumed, three Na^+ ions and two K^+ ions are transported in most fibers. This trade results in more positive charges being removed from the inside. As described previously, when a difference in diffusible charges exists across a semipermeable membrane, the potential changes. Since the action of Na^+,K^+-ATPase results in a net loss of positive charge inside the cell, the inside is made slightly negative when the pump operates. Thus, after a period of high activity the membrane potential hyperpolarizes briefly. This hyperpolarization has been suggested to be a clever mechanism for moving the membrane potential, which is somewhat run down after intense action, away from threshold while ion gradients are being restored.

It is now known that Na^+,K^+-ATPase is a large complex of two unequally sized proteins (Dahl and Hokin, 1974; Hokin, 1974, 1977). The larger has a molecular weight of 100,000, which means it is composed of a chain of approximately 800 amino acids. This protein is folded and organized in the membrane so that part is on the inside and part on the outside. The part inside has a site which reacts with ATP and binds Na^+, while that outside has a site which binds K^+. The other, smaller protein has a molecular weight of about 50,000 in vertebrates. It is required for the enzyme to function, but its exact role is not understood.

In essentially all models, Na^+ and K^+ transport is accomplished by a sequence of conformational changes in the enzyme. These conformational states are generated by the action of ATP and an interaction of Na^+ and K^+ ions. The scheme in Fig. 4-19 illustrates the essence of such a model. The overall reaction is a cycle, starting with the binding and reaction with ATP, progressing through a series of pumping steps and returning to the initial state of the enzyme. This diagram is highly schematic, since the exact native state of the enzyme in the membrane and its altered conformations are not precisely known.

Chloride ions, like Na^+ and K^+ ions, also exist in a gradient. However, in squid axon at least, a chloride pump is not necessary. Cl^- ions distribute passively, according to the Nernst equation, so that E_{Cl} is near the resting potential of the neuron. This is an efficient means of maintaining an ion gradient without expending additional cellular energy. However, in mammalian nerves E_{Cl} is more negative than the resting potential so Cl^- must be constantly pumped out.

Neuronal membranes also have pumps for Ca^{2+}, choline and various amino acids. We shall discuss some of these in later sections. These pumps are sodium dependent and derive their energy from the Na^+ ion gradient. An amino acid from the outside of the cell, for example, will move in along with Na^+ down the sodium concentration gradient. The Na^+,K^+-ATPase then removes the excess Na^+.

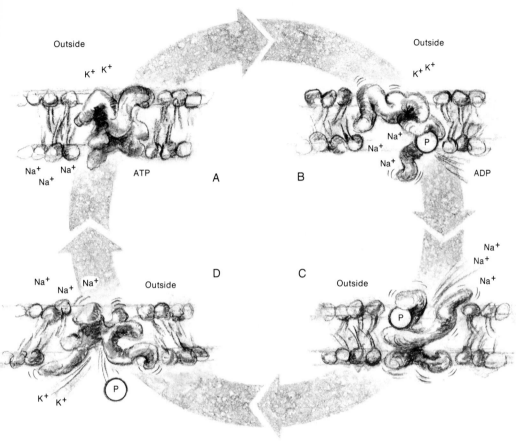

K, Na PUMP

Fig. 4-19. (A) The inactive state of the enzyme ready to pump. The ATP reaction site and the Na binding sites are inside the cell and the K binding site is on the outside. (B) The activated state of the enzyme. The enzyme reacts with ATP and becomes phosphorylated: a phosphate P forms a covalent bond with the enzyme. Reaction with ATP enhances the desire for the enzyme to bind Na and energizes the enzyme to a new and unstable conformation. (C) The second conformation state. The energized enzyme rapidly relaxes to a second conformation which carries Na to the outside of the cell and at the same time causes the enzyme to bind K. It is still phosphorylated and partly energized. (D) The enzyme when it binds K alters its conformation to a third state, deposits K on the inside of the cell and loses its phosphate through reaction with water ($-P + H_2O \rightarrow -OH + P$). The enzyme then returns to its inactive state and is ready to begin a new cycle.

V. Coding

What is a neuronal code? The easiest place to begin to examine neural codes and to discover their diversity is within the sensory systems. Consider the possible ways in which the nervous system can represent changes occurring in the external environment. We have special receptors for receiving and encoding (transducing) the various sensory modalities, whereby each receptor type is best suited and responds maximally to a particular type of stimulus. Thus, for example, eyes are sensitive to light, ears to sound, and skin receptors to pressure, pain, or temperature. Each of these sensory modalities is handled within the nervous system in anatomically clear-cut regions, at least initially. Eventually, pathways from these separate regions converge in association areas, as we have seen. But in the first stages of analysis, rather than having one part of the brain devoted exclusively to a particular body region and receiving all types of information (touch, pain, etc.) from that region, the nervous system instead devotes a particular component to one modality.

The first dimension of neural coding, although obvious, is determined by which group of receptors is activated. At this point, information is already coded as to sensory modality. In turn, within each sensory subsystem information is further coded in terms of which particular neurons within the cell clusters (nuclei) and which axons within their routes of intercommunication (tracts) become active. This topographic activation is called _place coding_. For example, touching a part of the body surface activates certain pressure receptors. These receptors project (as noted in Chapter 2) through a topographically arranged system of several interposed nerve cell bodies and axons to the thalamus and then to a particular region of the somatosensory cerebral cortex. Thus, a spatial pattern of activation of the body surface is preserved in the spatial pattern of activation in all components of the sensory subsystem and, ultimately, in the somatosensory cortex. The cortex "maps out" the activated regions of the body surface by its own spatial patterns of activity.

Place coding is readily demonstrated in all the sensory modalities. An essential prerequisite for place coding is an anatomically precise, topographically organized structure of nerve cells and their axons. In fact, a high degree of somatotopy (preserving the arrangement of body parts) in the fibers connecting sensory nuclei within the CNS is a general finding of neuroanatomy. By inference, therefore, place coding in some form is widely used throughout the nervous system. Just as important to proper functioning, however, is the nature of the information the wires carry.

Other dimensions of neural coding lie in the temporal pattern of action potentials fired by cells within this spatially organized or place coded ensemble of neurons. Many possible _temporal codes_ might be employed by specific neurons, but the problem of finding which codes are being used is difficult. We can record the timing or frequency of action potentials with precision, but to determine the code more information is necessary. Imagine the difficulty that would be experienced by a cryptographer given a sample of neuronal activity to decode. Unless we gave him certain facts, he would not know the nature of the encoded message, the language of that message, or even if he had a complete message or a partial sample. Often our own understanding of these temporal codes as neuroscientists is directly proportional to our knowledge of what is being coded, and so is largely limited to sensory systems where we are sure of stimulus characteristics. No single type of temporal code seems to have won universal acceptance in the nervous system. Even within primary sensory systems, many types of different temporal codes have been shown to exist, depending on the specific types of neurons and peripheral stimuli involved. Little is known about the nature of coding by brain neurons farther removed from the periphery.

In general, however, the temporal codes carried by action potentials can be of a limited number of types (Bullock, 1973). Figure 4-20 illustrates some of the possibilities by which a fish electroreceptor can signal a change in stimulus input.

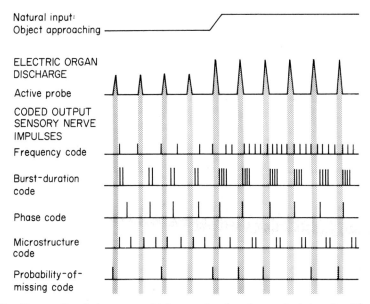

Fig. 4-20. Types of coded output which can signal a change in intensity. The example shows an increase in the discharge intensity of the electric organ of an electric fish when an object is interposed in the electric field emitted into the water by the fish. The electric organ spontaneously discharges and an increase in the amplitude (intensity) of its discharge signals the presence of an object in the electric field. The hypothetical sensory nerve afferents can carry this information to the brain by any one of the codes shown. As discussed in the text, however, the codes apply to many situations. (From Bullock, 1973.)

In this case, the receptor (second trace), is continuously active or oscillating for endogenous reasons, but the amplitude of its oscillation is directly proportional to the magnitude of the external stimulation, which in this case is an approaching object (top trace). There are five possible codes, judging from monitoring the activity of the axons which lead from this receptor to the brain (lower traces).

1. *Simple frequency code* seems to be the most commonly used. Frequency of firing is often related to intensity of stimulation. For example, skin receptors respond with increased firing rates to increases in pressure or temperature. For another example, muscle length is sensed by stretch receptors in the muscle and again is coded by frequency of firing. For a third example, the discharge frequency of certain joint receptors is mathematically related to the angle of the joint, so that such information on body position appears to be frequency coded.

2. *Burst duration code* is also relatively common. In this example an increased amplitude of oscillation of the receptor results in an increase in the time it takes each burst to quiet back down after the high point of the oscillation. This sort of code is well suited to represent transient temporal changes in the stimulus. For example, burst duration coding enables directionally sensitive neurons in the visual subsystem to report motion of a visual stimulus, and in the somesthetic subsystem, as we move our limbs the duration and repetition of movements are encoded by bursts of different length and variable numbers of action potentials.

3. *Phase coding* is more subtle; it involves the time interval elapsing between two ongoing, repetitive, and rhythmic signals arriving at the same location. In the diagram, the phase code is evident in a decreased delay of response following increased amplitude of the oscillation. In the auditory system, we use such a code. It is used to code information on the frequency of sound. It is also used to gather information on where sounds are coming from by comparing the time between arrival of air vibrations in one ear and at the other. The delay between nerve impulses originating in the inner ear that is closer to the sound and those from the other ear is a time function of the angle the sound source makes with respect to the two ears. Thus, sound localization is a kind of "triangulation" by central auditory neurons which base their "sightings" on signal delay.

4. *Microstructure codes* are similar to the familiar Morse code. Figure 4-20 illustrates an instance in which the rate of firing averaged over a full oscillation cycle is constant, but in which at higher stimulus intensities the pulses are no longer evenly spaced across the cycle. Instead, they tend to clump in the center of the cycle. Microstructure codes are less common in sensory systems than the codes described earlier. They are more frequently found in those central neurons which integrate a variety of inputs and which discharge in patterns of signals that are quite different from any single pattern of all those received, i.e., nonlinearly with respect to input. This type of code is what one would expect to find in cells which do much

4. BASIC PRINCIPLES OF NEURONAL SIGNALING

more than relay information in carbon-copy fashion. It is probably very important in the functioning of the CNS.

5. *Stochastic codes*, sometimes referred to as "probability of missing" codes, make use of changes in the probability of firing. This last class of codes is unusual in that it distributes the information widely over many fibers. In contrast, most of the codes discussed above are complete within themselves, and may be decoded from a single fiber. The only exception was the phase code where two inputs are required for decoding. In the example illustrated, the probability of firing of the single hypothetical afferent nerve fiber increased from 50 to 83% with the increase in electrical organ discharge, which is to say the probability of missing decreased by an inverse amount. If this effect took place in many fibers simultaneously, an increased stimulus could be coded in the average number of afferent fibers which fired, rather than by which fibers were activated at any given time. Stochastic codes have two properties that are consistent with findings from recordings of central neurons responding to peripheral stimulation. The first property has already been mentioned: the cells using such a code do not work alone. Hence, the reliability of firing of a given cell after a stimulus is often lower than the reliability of behavioral responses elicited by that stimulus. Such a greater order of events is guaranteed by the number of cells involved. Second, such codes, involving as many cells as they do, would be expected to be highly resistant to malfunction following nerve cell loss. The common failure of experimenters to disrupt higher-order functions with specific lesions is consistent with a widespread use of this code. Such a code is frequently invoked to explain such global functions in the CNS as learning and memory.

VI. Decoding

The above descriptions exemplify the types of codes most probably in use in the nervous system. Now that we have seen how information may be encoded, we shall briefly consider how it can be decoded.

A nerve cell receives many different afferents from various other neurons; each brings its own temporally coded message in the form of action potentials. These are translated into synaptic potentials, which in turn are integrated spatially and temporally within the neuron to yield a constantly fluctuating, graded transmembrane potential which is then recoded into a new series of efferent action potentials. Decoding then is the conversion of afferent action potentials into graded postsynaptic potentials suitable for integration within a neuron. On decoding different inputs, the neuron applies its own "weighting" factors to each. Thus, the ultimate influence of each afferent as to whether an action potential may be generated depends on the immediate past history of excitation of the target neuron, the magnitude of all of its locally generated synaptic responses, and the position of the afferent on the dendrite. All these factors play a role in determining how effective a given afferent will be in helping to fire that particular cell. The sum total of all these inputs, each appropriately weighted, determines the output response of that neuron. Operationally, integration is simply an extension and a dependency of the decoding mechanism used by a neuron. A central problem in neurobiology is the analysis of principles determining the input–output relationships of various anatomical types of neurons, as well as of neurons produced at different times during development of the nervous system.

The final consequence of coding is the individual's repertoire of immediate behavior and stored events. The activity pattern of a motor nerve determines how long and how hard a muscle will contract, and such patterns played over the musculature of a whole limb determines how that limb moves. We take in auditory, visual, and somesthetic information, code it, and generate highly complex behavior.

VII. Summary

Signals are relayed from one part of the nervous system to another in the language of action potentials. Action potentials travel in particular temporal patterns which are used to code for particular events. A particular frequency of action potential, for example, played onto a muscle determines the force of contraction.

Neurons generate action potentials because they have a -70 mV resting potential which provides an available store of energy and because neurons have very special membranes. At rest the membrane is permeable to K^+ ions. Because K^+ ions are higher inside the cell than outside, a resting potential exists which makes the interior of the neuron more negative than the exterior. The resting potential in neurons is fundamentally the equilibrium potential for the K^+ ion gradient. During an action potential, the resting potential is broken down. A suprathreshold depolarizing stimulus signals the voltage sensitive Na^+ channels to open. Sodium ions enter the axonal interior and change the potential to $+50$ mV, which is the equilibrium potential for Na^+. Sodium ion channels rapidly close; however, additional K^+ channels open and restore the membrane potential to its resting level. In the course of signaling, this process repeats many times. The neuron interior gains Na^+ ions and loses a few K^+ ions. The ion gradient is restored and maintained by a Na^+–K^+ pump which uses cellular ATP to drive the ions against their gradients and maintain the ionic gradients across the neuronal membrane.

While action potentials are the language neurons use to pass signals along their length, they use synaptic potentials to talk to other neurons or cells. In Chapter 5 we shall look at the nature of synaptic potentials.

Key Terms

Action potential: A transient all-or-nothing change in the membrane potential which propagates along the axon like a wave. Action potentials, unlike electrotonic potentials, do not decay because they are self-regenerative.

Burst duration codes: Information is contained in a short-lived burst of action potentials.

Capacitance of the membrane: A property of the membrane which allows charge to be stored and separated. It introduces a distortion in the time course of passively conducted signals. Without capacitance all changes in potentials would be instantaneous.

Coulomb: A unit of electrical charge. When 1 coulomb of charge flows for 1 second the quantity of current is called an ampere.

Current: The rate of flow of charge. The unit of measure is the ampere.

Depolarization: Reduction of the membrane potential from resting value toward zero.

Electrotonic potentials: Localized, graded potentials that are determined by the passive electrical properties of cells. The measure of this passive decay is the space constant.

Equilibrium potential: The potential at which, for the given ion gradient across the membrane, there is no net current flow. The relationship between a particular ionic gradient and its equilibrium potential is given by the Nernst equation.

Excitable membranes: Membranes which generate action potentials. Such membranes contain ionic channels whose permeability characteristics are voltage-dependent.

Hyperpolarization: An increase in the membrane potential from its resting value.

Microstructure codes: Information that is contained in the structure of action potentials in a given cycle.

Myelin: The plasma membrane of a glial cell wrapped many times around the axon. It serves to increase the metabolic efficiency of the nerve and increase the speed of action potential propagation.

Nernst equation: The relationship between the concentration of ionic species which permeate the membrane and the membrane potential: $E = 58 \log ([X]_o/[X]_i)$, where X_i and X_o, respectively, are the internal and external ion concentrations.

Node: Localized areas of the axon where myelin does not wrap the axon. Nodes occur at regular intervals.

Ohm's law: Relates voltage V to current I and resistance R: $V = IR$.

Permeability: The property of the membrane that allows ions to diffuse through it. Ions permeate through specific channels.

Phase codes: Information is contained in the time interval elapsing between two ongoing repetitive and rhythmic signals arriving at the same location.

Place coding: A type of coding whereby information at one defined place is presented to another defined place along defined neuronal pathways.

Potassium channel: A pore which allows K^+ ions to pass through it but which excludes other ions not closely related (in size and charge) to potassium.

Refractory period: The time following each action potential during which a stimulus cannot initiate a second action potential.

Resting potential: The electrical potential across the plasma membrane of neurons or muscle cells in the quiescent state. The resting potential (approximately -70 mV in most neurons) results from a very slight excess of negative charge on the inside of the neuron. At rest the membrane is selectively permeable to potassium ions and the difference in potassium ion concentration (high inside, low outside) establishes a diffusion potential.

Saltatory conduction: Conduction of action potentials along myelinated nerves whereby action potential currents leap from node to node.

Simple frequency codes: Information is contained in the frequency of action potentials.

Sodium channel: A pore which allows Na^+ ions to pass through it but which excludes dissimilar ions. Excitable sodium channels in axons open and close in response to changes in membrane potential.

Sodium potassium ATPase: The enzyme located in membranes responsible for translocating sodium and potassium ions across the membrane against their ionic concentration gradients.

Space constant: The distance over which a localized graded (electrotonic) potential decreases to $1/e$ (37%) of its original size in an axon or muscle fiber. The value of the space constant is directly proportional to the square root of the fiber diameter.

Stochastic codes: Information is contained in changes in the probability of firing as a result of a stimulus. Such information is distributed widely over many fibers.

Temporal codes: A type of general code whereby information is contained in the temporal pattern of action potentials.

Tetraethylammonium (TEA):   A quaternary ammonium compound that selectively blocks potassium channels in neuronal and muscle membranes.

Tetrodotoxin (TTX):   A poison which selectively blocks excitable sodium (regenerative) channels.

Threshold: The value of the membrane potential or depolarization at which an action potential is initiated.

Voltage clamp: A technique for displacing the membrane potential to a defined value and holding it there while measuring the currents.

General References

Hille, B. (1977). Ionic basis of resting and action potentials. *In* "Handbook of Physiology" (E. Kandel, ed.), Sect. 1, Vol. 1, Part 1, pp. 99–136. Am. Physiol. Soc., Bethesda, Maryland.

Hodgkin, A. L. (1964). "The Conduction of the Nervous Impulse." Thomas, Springfield, Illinois.

Kandel, E. (1977). "Cellular Basis of Behavior." Freeman, San Francisco, California.

Katz, B. (1966). "Nerve Muscle and Synapse." McGraw-Hill; New York.

Kuffler, S. W., and Nicholls, J. G. (1976). "From Neuron to Brain—A Cellular Approach to the Function of the Nervous System." Sinauer Assoc., Sunderland, Massachusetts.

References

Baker, P. F., Hodgkin, A. L., and Shaw, T. I. (1962a). Replacement of the axoplasm of giant nerves fibres with artificial solutions. *J. Physiol. (London)* **164**, 300–354.

Baker, P. F., Hodgkin, A. L., and Shaw, T. I. (1962b). The effects of changes in internal ionic concentrations on the electrical properties of perfused giant axons. *J. Physiol. (London)* **164**, 355–374.

Bernstein, J. (1902). Untersuchungen zur Thermodynamik der bioelektrischen Ströme. *Pfluegers Arch. Gesamte Physiol. Menschen Tiere* **92**, 521–562.

Binstock, L., and Goldman, L. (1969). Current- and voltage-clamped studies on *Myxicola* giant axons. Effect of tetrodotoxin. *J. Gen. Physiol.* **54**, 730–740.

Bullock, T. H. (1973). Seeing the world through a new sense: Electroreception in fish. *Am. Sci.* **61**, 316–325.

Cole, K. S. (1968). "Membranes, Ions and Impulses," A chapter of classical biophysics. Univ. of California Press, Berkeley.

Dahl, J. L., and Hokin, L. E. (1974). The sodium-potassium adenosine triphosphatase. *Annu. Rev. Biochem.* **43**, 327–356.

Hille, B. (1967). The selective inhibition of delayed potassium currents in nerve by tetraethylammonium. *J. Gen. Physiol.* **50**, 1291–1296.

Hille, B. (1974). Ionic selectivity of Na and K channels in nerve. *Membranes* **3**, 255–323.

Hille, B. (1977). Ionic basis of resting and action potentials. *In* "Handbook of Physiology" (E. Kandel, ed.), Sect. 1, Vol. 1, Part 1, pp. 99–136. Am. Physiol. Soc., Bethesda, Maryland.

Hodgkin, A. L. (1964). "The Conduction of the Nervous Impulse." Thomas, Springfield, Illinois.

Hodgkin, A. L., and Huxley, A. F. (1952a). Currents carried by sodium and potassium ions through the membrane of the giant axon of *Loligo*. *J. Physiol. (London)* **116**, 449–472.

Hodgkin, A. L., and Huxley, A. F. (1952b). The components of membrane conductance in the giant axon of *Loligo*. *J. Physiol. (London)* **116**, 473–496.

Hodgkin, A. L., and Huxley, A. F. (1952c). The dual effect of membrane potential on sodium conductance in the giant axon of *Loligo*. *J. Physiol. (London)* **116**, 497–506.

Hodgkin, A. L., and Huxley, A. F. (1952d). A quantitative description of membrane current and its application to conduction and excitation in nerve. *J. Physiol. (London)* **117**, 500–544.

Hodgkin, A. L., and Katz, B. (1949). The effect of sodium ions on the electrical activity of the giant axon of the squid. *J. Physiol. (London)* **108**, 37–77.

Hodgkin, A. L., and Keynes, R. D. (1955). Active transport of cations in giant axons from *Sepia* and *Loligo*. *J. Physiol. (London)* **128**, 28–60.

Hokin, L. E. (1974). Purification and properties of the (sodium + potassium)-activated adenosine triphosphatase and reconstitution of sodium transport. *Ann. N.Y. Acad. Sci.* **242**, 12–23.

Hokin, L. E. (1977). Purification and properties of Na^+, K^+-ATPases from the tectal gland of *Squalus Acanthias* and the electric organ of *Electrophorus Electricus* and reconstitution of the $Na - K$ pump from the purified enzyme. *FEBS Symp.* **42**, 374–388.

Kandel, E. (1977). "Cellular Basis of Behavior." Freeman, San Francisco, California.

Keynes, R. D. (1951). The ionic movements during nervous activity. *J. Physiol. (London)* **114**, 119–150.

Kuffler, S. W., and Nicholls, J. G. (1976). "From Neuron to Brain—A Cellular Approach to the Function of the Nervous System." Sinauer Assoc., Sunderland, Massachusetts.

Skou, J. C. (1957). The influence of some cations on an adenosine triphosphatase from peripheral nerve. *Biochim. Biophys. Acta* **23**, 394–401.

5

Synaptic Transmission

I. Introduction

An understanding of synaptic transmission is the key to understanding the basic operation of the nervous system at a cellular level. Without transmission, there is no direct communication between cells—there would be only individual isolated

151

cells. The whole point of the nervous system is to control and coordinate body function and enable the body to respond to, and act on, the environment. Synaptic transmission is the key process in the integrative action of the nervous system.

Synaptic transmission is the process at synapses by which a chemical signal (a transmitter) is released from one neuron and diffuses to other neurons or target cells where it generates a signal which excites, inhibits or modulates cellular activity. By means of synaptic transmission, an electrical signal in one neuron passes from the terminal of its axon into another cell and starts in that cell an impulse having characteristics different from its own (Palay and Chan-Palay, 1976).

The term synapse (Greek for connection) was introduced by Foster and Sherrington in 1897 in their "Textbook of Physiology" and defined as "the mode of nexus between neuron and neuron." Foster and Sherrington recognized that at the connection between nerve cells something happened that was different from the conduction along nerve fibers; there was a slight delay, for example. So they gave this connection a special name. Subsequently Sherrington, in his now famous lecture series, "Integrative Action of the Nervous System," presented in 1906 at Yale University, powerfully argued that synapses are very distinctive elements in the nervous system and the key element in the integration of neural information. Sherrington's ideas had a profound impact on understanding the operation of the nervous system, and central to his ideas was the synapse. Initially the synapse was only an abstraction, defined by a word, but over the years the study of synapses—their structure, operation and modifiability—has become the dominant focus in cellular and molecular studies of the nervous system.

Over the next decade, the processes by which signals passed between neurons at synapses intrigued many, but evaded clear analysis. Some thought transmission was chemical. Others were positive it was electrical, a simple jump of the action potential. At scientific meetings there were many great debates. Then in 1921, Otto Loewi established that synaptic transmission was chemical. The story behind his experiment is fascinating. One night Loewi had a dream in which he conceived of an experiment to prove definitely whether transmission was chemical or electrical. In the morning he remembered he had had such a dream but could not recall the experiment. Conveniently, the dream returned the next night and so as not to take any chances Loewi went to the laboratory in the middle of the night and performed the experiment!

Loewi knew that stimulation of the vagus nerve innervating the heart causes the heart to beat more slowly. He reasoned that if vagal nerve endings released a chemical transmitter it should be possible to collect it. Then if the collected solution were applied to a second heart, and the solution contained a chemical that mimics the action of vagal nerve stimulation, the solution should slow the

152

beating of the heart. He performed the experiment and discovered that indeed the vagus nerve released a substance which caused a slowing of heart rate. This experiment provided the first clear evidence that synaptic transmission was chemical.

It was later found that the substance was _acetylcholine_ (ACh), which was already suspected to be the transmitter at this synapse. In retrospect, Loewi's experiment was really a long shot. It is amazing that sufficient transmitter was released and sufficiently concentrated to mimic the action of nerve stimulation. As Loewi remarked, "On mature consideration, in the cold light of the morning I would not have done it." Subsequent experiments in many laboratories have shown that transmission is strictly chemical at the vast majority of synapses in the mammalian nervous system. Electrical synapses exist but are uncommon in the mammalian CNS. However, particularly in some invertebrates and lower vertebrates, synaptic transmission can be chemical and/or electrical. At electrical synapses the cell membranes are electrically coupled and currents pass directly between nerve cells.

It is now known that there are many transmitters. Besides acetylcholine, γ-aminobutyric acid (GABA), glutamate, glycine, serotonin and a class of subtances referred to as catecholamines are known to be transmitters. The nervous system is very rich in the diversity of its transmitters. As we shall discuss in Chapter 6, transmitter types are organized in brain in discrete pathways that interconnect various parts of systems or dart between systems. The pattern of connectivity is highly specific, and different transmitters seem specialized to carry out particular roles. It is not altogether clear why there are so many different transmitters, but it seems that while all transmitters carry out the same function—interneuronal communication—each one or class of transmitters provides a significantly different message. Some shout loudly and elicit fast responses, and others speak softly and have a slow but profound influence on their partners.

In this chapter, we examine the amazing process of synaptic transmission. Synaptic transmission is specialized in subtle but very important ways so that these properties, more than any other, provide the nervous system with the most sophisticated means of intracellular communication in any tissue. Through the action of chemicals, squirted onto other cells organized in specific circuits, emerges a capacity to process signals that is beyond that of any computer yet constructed and probably in fact that ever will be constructed. In order to describe synaptic transmission, we first present an overview of the process and then will select two different classes of synapses which illustrate the fundamental process as well as distinctive regulatory and functional properties. It is now clear that synaptic transmission must be considered in terms of classes of synapses. These classes appear related to the type of transmitter used, since it is the unique chemistry which dictates distinctive function. Accordingly we will direct our discussion to a description of synapses which use ACh as a transmitter (*choliner-gic synapses*) and those which use catecholamines as transmitters (*catechol-aminergic synapses*).

Acetlylcholine is characteristic of a class of transmitters which act fast and change the permeability of the postsynaptic membrane so that the receptive cell is quickly excited or inhibited. The majority of synapses in the CNS and peripheral nervous system fit this class. The cholinergic synapse is also a suitable synapse for study because more is known about its operation than any other and because its basic mechanisms apply in general to other synapses, with certain key exceptions. The important exceptions at present are illustrated by a class of synapses which use catecholamines as transmitters. These synapses have a slow onset and cessation of activation and generate as one of their primary actions a metabolic change in their target cells. Such synapses also appear to be highly modifiable. In Section IV of this chapter we shall analyze the cardinal features of catecholaminergic synapses.

II. Overview of Synaptic Transmission

What are the properties that a chemical synapse must have in order to carry out its functions? There are four basic properties that all synapses share: (1) the presynaptic endings must store the transmitter; (2) the ending must rapidly release the transmitter in response to stimulation by an action potential or more generally by depolarization; (3) the transmitter must reach the target cell and cause a response; and (4) the action of the transmitter must be terminated promptly and the synapse must quickly prepare for a new stimulus.

In general all synapses use the same basic mechanism to release transmitter and activate the target cell (Fig. 5-1). When an action potential arrives at a synaptic ending (Fig. 5-1A), it causes the release of transmitter which is stored inside tiny vesicles called *synaptic vesicles*. A subpopulation of these vesicles are concentrated on the inside of the plasma membrane facing the synaptic cleft. The action potential stimulates an influx of Ca^{2+}, which causes synaptic vesicles to attach to the release sites, fuse with the plasma membrane and expel their supply of transmitter (Fig. 5-1B). The transmitter diffuses to the target cell, where it binds to a *receptor* protein on the external surface of the cell membrane. The interaction of the transmitter and receptor stimulates the cell (Fig. 5-1C). After a brief period the transmitter dissociates from the receptor and the response is terminated. In order to prevent the transmitter from rebinding to the receptor and repeating the cycle, the transmitter is either destroyed by the degradative action of an enzyme or it is taken up, usually into the presynaptic ending (Fig. 5-1D).

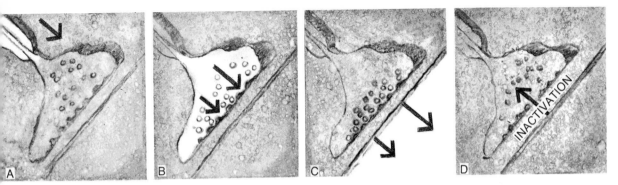

Fig. 5-1. Basic mechanisms of synaptic transmission. (A) Action potential arrives, (B) causes transmitter release, (C) transmitter acts on postsynaptic cell and (D) transmitter action is terminated.

At present, it is generally believed that each neuron type has a single transmitter and is highly specialized to synthesize and metabolize only that transmitter. Catecholaminergic neurons which use dopamine as their transmitter, for example, cannot synthesize acetylcholine, since the necessary enzymes are absent. Other compounds are released along with the transmitters as coordinated secretory products, but the general rule is that only one transmitter is released from all the terminals of a neuron. The receptive properties of the target cell are very specific to the transmitter that is naturally used. Other, "foreign" transmitters are usually without influence.

The effects of the transmitter on the target cell may be excitatory, inhibitory or modulatory. The typical or classic postsynaptic response is a fast local change in the electrical properties of the postsynaptic membrane that is mediated through a change in the ionic permeability of the membrane. The response at a synapse is inhibitory or excitatory but never both in the mammalian nervous system. If the cell is depolarized by the transmitter it is excited, and when the depolarizing stimulus is of sufficient magnitude it initiates action potentials. A cell is inhibited when the transmitter stimulus makes it harder to excite the cell and generate action potentials. In some cases, the transmitter alters the metabolism of the target cell so that it modulates cellular properties. Usually the electrical signal accompanying metabolic modulation is slow in onset.

In the vertebrate CNS a transmitter usually has one primary mode of action at any given synapse. Acetylcholine, for example, is usually excitatory, but can also be inhibitory. The exact nature of the postsynaptic response depends on the properties of the postsynaptic cell. To illustrate, ACh is the transmitter at a skeletal neuromuscular junction that excites these muscles, and it is also the transmitter of vagal input to the heart that inhibits heart rate. The most striking illustration that the properties of the target cell, and not those of the transmitter, determine the response is seen in the sea hare (*Aplysia*, a mollusk). In this invertebrate the same neuron will excite one of the cells with which it connects and inhibit another (Fig. 5-2).

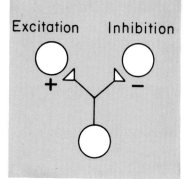

Fig. 5-2. The basic properties of the postsynaptic response are determined by the postsynaptic cell. In *Aplysia californica*, for example, one neuron is inhibited and another excited by a single identified neuron. The same transmitter is released at each synapse, so that the difference must be due to the responsive characteristics of each postsynaptic cell. (Adapted from Gardner and Kandel, 1972.)

Synaptic transmission is also highly modifiable. Synapses apparently modify their output as a function of their previous stimulus history. Following rapid repetitive stimulation, for example, the size of the response often grows larger. The capacity of synapses to alter their input–output relationship appears to depend markedly on the type of synapse. A neuromuscular junction is less modifiable than certain synapses in brain. This property of synaptic plasticity appears related to the nature of the transmitter. Indeed, it may be one reason why different transmitters exist.

III. Cholinergic Synaptic Transmission

Cholinergic synaptic transmission is well suited for detailed study because it is representative of the class of transmitters which act rapidly by causing specific permeability changes in the membrane. The basic mechanisms of synaptic transmission are also best known for this synaptic type. Acetylcholine is a molecule of acetate and choline joined by an ester bond.

$$H_3C-\overset{\overset{\displaystyle CH_3}{|}}{\underset{\underset{\displaystyle CH_3}{|}}{N^+}}-CH_2-CH_2-O-\overset{\overset{\displaystyle O}{||}}{C}-CH_3$$

Acetylcholine

Cholinergic synapses are very common. They are the type of synapse at skeletal neuromuscular junctions and they are used widely in the autonomic nervous system and in the brain (see Chapter 6). Most studies on cholinergic synaptic transmission have been carried out on the spinal innervation of the sartorius muscle of the thigh.

The basic experimental paradigm used in investigations on the neuromuscular junction is shown in Fig. 5-3A. In a typical experiment the leg muscle from a frog and its attached spinal nerve is dissected out and set up in a bath. A recording electrode is inserted into the muscle, and a stimulating electrode is placed on the nerve. The recording electrode is connected to an amplifier where the electrical potential is amplified. The signal is then displayed on an oscilloscope.

A postsynaptic potential recorded at a synapse in response to presynaptic activation is shown in Fig. 5-3B and is called a *synaptic potential*. Originally, the potential at a nerve muscle junction was named an "end-plate potential" and is still frequently called by that name. However, it is now clear that there is no difference between end-plate potentials at nerve–muscle junctions and synaptic potentials at nerve–nerve junctions so this distinction is no longer necessary. In accordance with the recent text by Kuffler and Nicholls (1976) we shall refer to end-plate potentials as synaptic potentials.

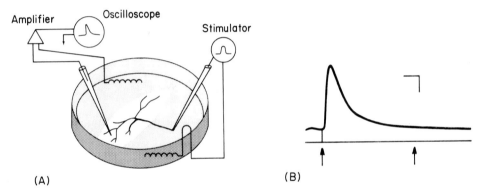

(A)   (B)

Fig. 5-3. (A) Recording a synaptic potential at a neuromuscular junction. A frog sartorius muscle is pinned to wax in the bottom of a dish. The recording glass microelectrode (*left*), which is inside a muscle cell, and a reference wire (ground) in the dish gives the membrane potential of the muscle cell. The recorded potential is amplified and displayed on an oscilloscope. The nerve is stimulated by passing current through a stimulating electrode (*right*). (B) Stimulation of the nerve indicated by the sharp vertical line or "shock artifact" (*arrow*) evokes a synaptic potential. The synaptic potential is a slow depolarization of the muscle membrane.

Figure 5-4 shows a record of a synaptic potential and corresponding *synaptic current*. At the neuromuscular junction a synaptic potential is a rapid depolarization which begins about 0.5 msec after the action potential arrives at the nerve ending and decays to baseline in 2–3 msec. Note the much faster time course of the synaptic current. The slower onset and longer duration of the synaptic potential represents the charging and passive decay of charge from the muscle membrane due to its capacitance. The true index of transmitter action is the

III. CHOLINERGIC SYNAPTIC TRANSMISSION   157

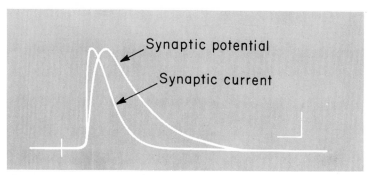

Fig. 5-4. Synaptic potential and underlying synaptic current at a neuromuscular junction: horizontal bar: 2 msec; vertical bar: 1 mV for the synaptic potential and 40 nA for the synaptic current. (Adapted from Barrett and Magleby, 1976.)

synaptic current, since it represents the movement of ions through the membrane.

In the normal physiological situation once the depolarization exceeds the muscle's membrane threshold for spike generation (about 20 mV above resting potential), the muscle initiates an action potential and contracts. In this way the signal is relayed via neurotransmitters from nerve action potentials to muscle action potentials.

In the sections which follow, we shall describe our current understanding of pre- and postsynaptic mechanisms. We shall first describe the mechanism by which ACh is released and then the mechanism of action of ACh on the postsynaptic membrane.

A. Characteristics of Transmitter Release

What triggers the release of transmitter? That is, how is the stimulus of the action potential coupled to the secretion of the transmitter? Some mechanism must exist whereby the action potential causes the transmitter stored in synaptic vesicles to be expelled into the cleft.

In 1952 Sir Bernard Katz, a physiologist awarded the Nobel Prize for his research on synaptic transmission, and his colleague, Professor Paul Fatt, discovered one of the key principles of transmitter release. Working with electronic equipment which was more sensitive than that previously used, these investigators noticed in the unstimulated muscle small "blips" near the region of the synapse (Fig. 5-5). These blips behaved pharmacologically like synaptic potentials in all ways except they were much smaller. Therefore, they were called miniature end plate or _miniature synaptic potentials_. They had the interesting property that they appeared randomly with time and were all of nearly the same basic unit size.

5. SYNAPTIC TRANSMISSION

In the presence of Ca^{2+} ions the rate of the miniature synaptic potentials was greatly accelerated by depolarizing stimuli.

These observations and others led to the formulation of the *"quantal hypothesis"* of transmitter release: each miniature synaptic potential corresponds

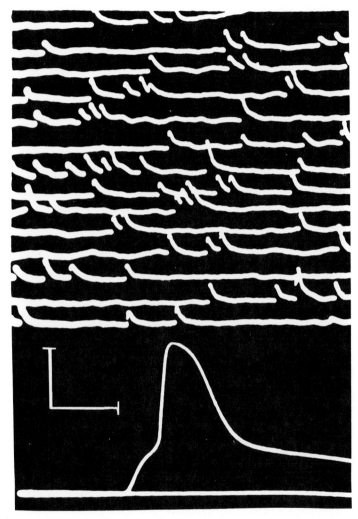

Fig. 5-5. The top tracings are intracellular records from a frog neuromuscular junction taken at high amplification and slow sweep speed. The small deflections are the miniature synaptic potentials which appear randomly over time. The bottom record, taken at lower amplification and high sweep speed, shows a synaptic potential elicited by stimulation of the nerve. The inset gives the voltage calibration (*y* axis) and time calibration (*x* axis): 3.6 mV and 47 msec for the top record; 50 mV and 2 msec for the bottom record. (From Fatt and Katz, 1952.)

to the release of one quantum of transmitter (they were called *quanta* because of their constant size). Action potentials greatly increase the probability that quanta are released so that a synaptic potential is generated by the simultaneous discharge of many quanta. Individual quanta obscure one another in the full-sized synaptic potential, but if transmitter release is suppressed by lowering the Ca^{2+} ion concentration and elevating the Mg^{2+} ion concentration, it is possible to show individual quanta (Fig. 5-6). At low levels of release the number of quanta released varies randomly. Each quantum is now known to consist of about 10,000 ACh molecules (Hartzell *et al.*, 1976), and it is generally believed that a quantum is the expulsion of the contents of a single synaptic vesicle. The quantal hypothesis of transmitter release is well established, and as far as we know at present applies to every synapse. However, even a decade after it was proposed that quanta correspond to the discharge of synaptic vesicles, this notion continues to stir much controversy. Even today it has evaded a rigorous proof (see Martin, 1977).

One fact provided the critical clue necessary for understanding the mechanism of quantal release—Ca^{2+} ions are absolutely essential. In the absence of Ca^{2+}, action potentials will not cause release. In its presence any type of depolarizing stimulus will support release. This and other evidence led to the _Ca hypothesis_ of transmitter release: depolarization causes Ca^{2+} channels to open,

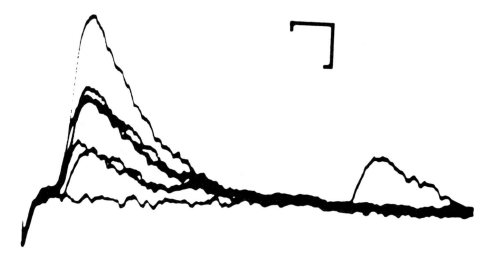

Fig. 5-6. Intracellular records illustrate the quantal nature of transmitter release when output is greatly reduced by lowering Ca and raising Mg in the bath. The nerve was stimulated seven consecutive times, and the responses recorded. The amplitude of the synaptic potential fluctuates from trial to trial and these fluctuations occur in discrete "quantal" steps which are the same size as the miniature synaptic potential. Vertical bar: 0.3 mV; horizontal bar: 2.5 msec. (From Barrett and Magleby, 1976.)

5. SYNAPTIC TRANSMISSION

Ca²⁺ enters the terminal and catalyzes quantal transmitter release (Katz and Miledi, 1967). At high Ca²⁺ concentrations, it is now known that about 1–2 Ca²⁺ ions are needed to trigger the release of 1 quantum (Llinas *et al.*, 1976).

Much evidence has been marshalled in support of the Ca hypothesis. We will mention two particularly powerful arguments. (1) If Ca is injected directly into the terminal, transmitter release immediately follows (Miledi, 1973). Magnesium has no such effect. (2) Voltage clamp studies on the presynaptic terminal show a direct relationship between the presynaptic membrane potential, presynaptic Ca currents and transmitter release (Katz and Miledi, 1967; Llinas *et al.*, 1976) (Fig. 5-7). The resulting data will quantitatively account for release (Llinas *et al.*, 1976).

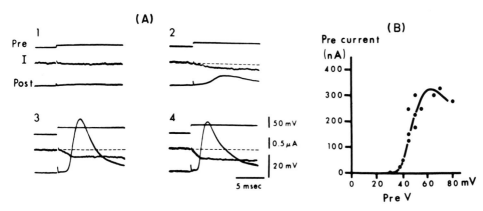

Fig. 5-7. Relationship between presynaptic depolarization and the inward Ca²⁺ current at the giant squid synapse obtained by voltage clamp measurements. A current injecting electrode and a recording electrode were inserted into the presynaptic terminal, and another recording electrode was placed in the postsynaptic fiber. Na⁺ and K⁺ current are pharmacologically blocked so the presynaptic current represents I_{Ca}. (A) Records 1–4 are of different levels of presynaptic potential (pre), the corresponding presynaptic currents (I) and postsynaptic response (post). As the presynaptic depolarization increases (1–4) the size of the presynaptic current also increases. These data show that the entry of Ca²⁺ ions is voltage-dependent and that the amount of transmitter release (post) is proportional to the inward Ca²⁺ current (I). (B) Plot of peak presynaptic current at different values of applied potential. The inward Ca current increased markedly as a function of presynaptic potential. (From Llinas *et al.*, 1976.)

Thus, the basic stimulus of transmitter release is the influx of Ca²⁺ ions into the presynaptic bouton. Calcium ions through a presently unknown mechanism promote the fusion of vesicles with the membrane and the *exocytosis* of transmitter.

Figure 5-8 portrays the process of transmitter release as it is envisioned to occur, and Fig. 5-9 depicts the temporal events intervening between an action potential and the postsynaptic response. These events appear to apply in general to all types of synapses.

III. CHOLINERGIC SYNAPTIC TRANSMISSION

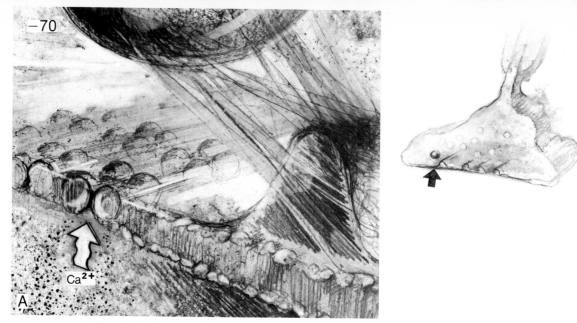

Fig. 5-8. Stages in the release of transmitter. (A) At rest Ca^{2+} cannot enter the terminal because the channels are closed as symbolized by the arrow. *Inset:* Dark arrow points to a release site. (B) The action potential commands Ca channels to open, and Ca^{2+} enters the terminal (*light arrow*). (C) Synaptic vesicles fuse with the membrane and expel their transmitter stores. (D) The vesicle membrane flows into the plasma membrane. It will eventually be recovered by a process called endocytosis (see Fig. 5-17).

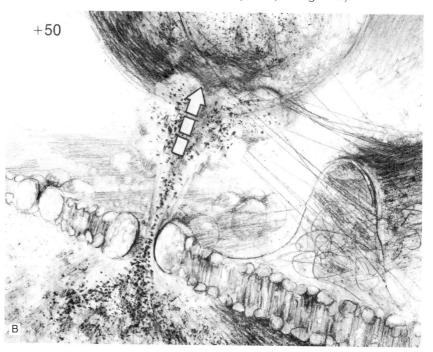

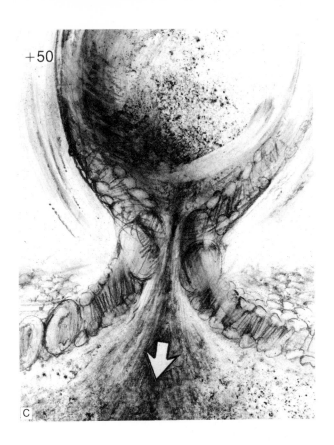

+50

C

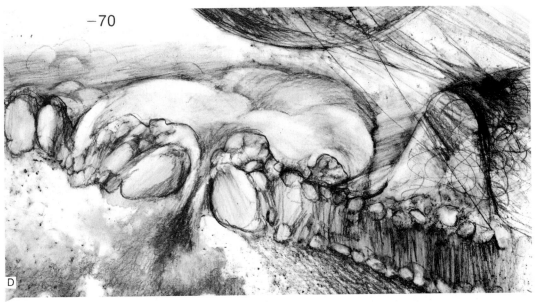

−70

D

163

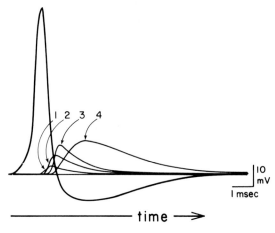

Fig. 5-9. Events during synaptic transmission and their kinetic relationships derived from an analysis of synaptic currents at the giant squid synapse and a computer model based on the data. The initial large peak is the action potential. The four curves represent (1) time course of Ca^{2+} gate formation; (2) time course of Ca^{2+} current; (3) time course of postsynaptic current; and (4) postsynaptic potential (arbitrary scale). (From Llinas *et al.*, 1976.)

B. Nature of the Postsynaptic Response

1. PERMEABILITY EVENTS UNDERLYING EXCITATION OR INHIBITION. Acetylcholine released from the terminal diffuses to the postsynaptic membrane, binds to the receptors, and causes specific changes in the membrane ion permeability. Ion movements which depolarize are *excitatory*, and those which hyperpolarize are *inhibitory*.

At excitatory fast acting ionic synapses, such as cholinergic neuromuscular junctions, a transmitter causes depolarization by increasing the membrane permeability simultaneously to Na^+ and/or K^+ ions. At the neuromuscular junction the permeability to Na^+ is somewhat greater being 1.3 times that of K^+. For a moment these ions flow freely and reduce the resting potential to near zero. The membrane is in effect short circuited by the action of ACh on the membrane. It appears as if Na^+ and K^+ ions pass through a single channel at the neuromuscular junction (Dionne and Ruff, 1977). Thus the channels at the postsynaptic membrane are distinct from those which support action potentials.

At some excitatory ionic synapses, the nature of the ionic mechanism can vary, but it always results in depolarization, and in all cases studied, so far, involves Na ions. The type of ionic permeability change generated is evaluated by measuring the equilibrium potential due to the action of the transmitter. Recall that an *equilibrium potential* is the potential at which the net inward flow of all ions balances the net outward flow. Each synapse has a particular equilibrium potential which characterizes the action of its transmitter. The equilibrium potential is measured at a synapse from voltage clamp experiments (Fig. 5-10), and the relevant ions can be identified by varying their concentration in the bath and determining the effect on the equilibrium potential. If Cl^- ions, for example, are

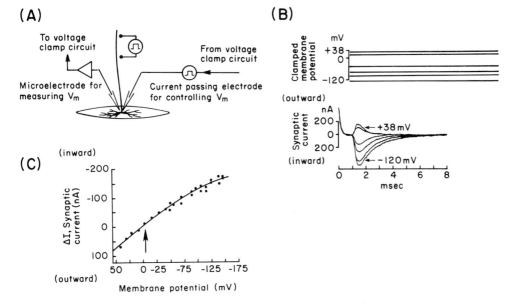

Fig. 5-10. Synaptic currents caused by nerve released ACh at a neuromuscular junction. (A) Recording scheme for voltage clamp at the motor end plate. (B) Representative synaptic currents obtained when the muscle membrane is changed from −120 mV step-wise to +38 mV. (C) Plot of peak synaptic currents at various values of membrane potentials. The membrane current is zero at a membrane potential of about −5 mV, which represents the equilibrium potential for the transmitter. (Redrawn from Kuffler and Nicholls, 1976, as adapted from Magleby and Stevens, 1972a,b.)

unimportant, varying their concentrations will not affect the synaptic equilibrium potential.

Inhibition results when the transmitter increases the membrane permeability to K and/or Cl. In principle, an increase in Cl ion or K ion permeability could hyperpolarize the membrane because the equilibrium potential of these ions is more negative than the resting potential. At the vagal synapse, ACh increases the permeability of the smooth muscle membrane to K ions. With more K channels open, the membrane potential is slightly hyperpolarized and less excitable. The hyperpolarization, however, is only slight because the resting potential is very near the K equilibrium potential (−80 mV). In the mammalian CNS, fast acting inhibitory transmitters (such as γ-aminobutyric acid) often act by increasing Cl ion permeability (Baker, 1976) and possibly also K ion permeability. In CNS neurons the chloride equilibrium potential is close to that of potassium. When the permeability to Cl increases, Cl ions rush into the cell since their concentration is higher outside than inside, and the inward anionic current causes a hyperpolarization. Figure 5-11 summarizes the behavior of the postsynaptic membrane during excitation and inhibition.

III. CHOLINERGIC SYNAPTIC TRANSMISSION

The purpose of inhibition is to counteract the effects of excitation. The powerful K and/or Cl currents hold the potential near the resting potential by counteracting the excitatory action of the Na currents. In the absence of inhibition inward depolarizing currents of Na ions have full control over the membrane

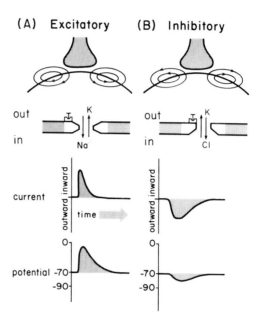

Fig. 5-11. Ionic events at the postsynaptic membrane at classic excitatory and inhibitory synapses. (A) At excitatory synapses the transmitter always increases the permeability to Na$^+$ and, in some cases, to other ions. Depolarization results, since Na$^+$ currents drive the membrane potential toward E_{Na}. K$^+$ is also sometimes involved as, for example, at the neuromuscular junction. (B) At inhibitory synapses transmitter increases the permeability of the membrane to K$^+$ and/or Cl$^-$ ions. The potential hyperpolarizes slightly or changes very little, depending on the equilibrium potential for the permeable ions. If this equilibrium potential is more negative than the resting potential, the cell hyperpolarizes; but if the equilibrium potential is the same as that of the permeable ions, there is no net current flow since the potential is already at its equilibrium state. Inhibition results since increases in ionic currents with equilibrium potentials near the resting potential stabilize the membrane potential against depolarizing currents.

potential. However, during inhibition their effectiveness is reduced because an increase in the number of open K and/or Cl channels "superstabilizes" the membrane potential at, or slightly more negative than, the resting potential.

All fast acting transmitters cause excitation or inhibition by opening particular channels in the postsynaptic membrane. Each transmitter unlocks ion channels so that ion currents flow across the membrane and disturb the resting state of the cell. They challenge the membrane potential toward a new equilibrium state.

166

In actual practice whether or not the synaptic potential arrives at the equilibrium state depends on how much transmitter reaches the postsynaptic receptors. Small quantities of transmitter, such as the 10^4 acetylcholine molecules in a quantum at the neuromuscular junction, cause a change of only about 0.4 mV. Few channels are open so that the net current flow is insufficient to drive the recorded postsynaptic membrane potential more than a few millivolts from its resting value. At synapses, then, responses are graded. The magnitude of the response depends on the amount of transmitter which reaches the receptors and the types of channels activated.

2. TERMINATING THE RESPONSE: THE INACTIVATION MECHANISM. What is the mechanism which terminates the action of a transmitter? Normally ACh remains bound to the receptor for only a few tenths of a millisecond, then it spontaneously dissociates from the receptors and the channels close. In order to prevent ACh from reactivating receptors, it is destroyed by an enzyme called _acetylcholinesterase_ (AChE). This enzyme degrades excessive acetylcholine by hydrolyzing the ester bond giving rise to the products acetate and choline, neither of which will significantly activate the receptors.

$$\text{Acetylcholine} \xrightarrow{\text{acetylcholinesterase}} \text{acetate} + \text{choline}$$

Acetylcholine is split in two by the action of acetylcholinesterase. If acetylcholinesterase is inhibited, the duration of the falling phase of the synaptic potential is longer and the amplitude is larger (Fig. 5-12). In the absence of degradation, molecules of ACh reactivate the receptor many times before they eventually diffuse away. All cholinergic synapses use AChE to inactivate ACh.

Many poisons are inhibitors of acetylcholinesterase. Diisopropyl fluorophosphate (DFP), a compound produced during World War II as a nerve gas, is an

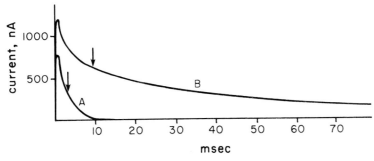

Fig. 5-12. Effect of an anticholinesterase on the time course and magnitude of the synaptic current at a neuromuscular junction. Curve A is the normal response and curve B is the response in the presence of an anticholinesterase. Note the increase in magnitude and time course of the synaptic current. Arrows indicate time of half-maximal response amplitude. (After Hartzell *et al.*, 1975.)

example of an anticholinesterase. Analogues of DFP are contained in many garden variety pesticides. Anticholinesterases act as poisons because they arrest muscle movement; ACh accumulates and keeps the muscle depolarized so it cannot contract under the command of the nerves. Paralysis and asphyxiation result.

3. PROPERTIES OF THE SINGLE CHANNEL AT THE POSTSYNAPTIC MEMBRANE. Let us now move in for a closer look at the postsynaptic membrane and investigate the nature of the molecular events. How do channels open and close and what are they? It is now possible to study the action of single channels through the analysis of ACh-induced noise. As Katz and Miledi (1970), who pioneered this work, stated, "it seemed possible that during steady application of ACh to a motor end plate the statistical effects of molecular bombardment might be discernible as an increase in membrane noise superimposed from the maintained average depolarization." In order to explore this rather remote but exciting possibility, a steady concentration of acetylcholine was applied to a neuromuscular junction so as to produce a few millivolt depolarization. As illustrated in Fig.

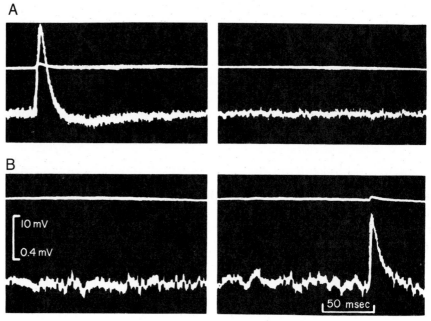

Fig. 5-13. Intracellular recordings of ACh noise from the synaptic region of a frog muscle fiber. (A) Control (no ACh). The upper trace shows low gain tracing and the lower trace shows a high gain tracing. (B) Membrane noise during ACh application. The ACh depolarizes the membrane slightly and generates a marked increase in random fluctuations in potential (*lower trace*). These fluctuations, called ACh noise, are produced by the statistical opening and closing of a few hundred individual channels. The large deflection is a spontaneous miniature synaptic potential. (From Katz and Miledi, 1970.)

168

5-13, ACh generated graded small fluctuations of the potential riding on the depolarization. These small fluctuations were called "_ACh noise_." Each fluctuation corresponded to random statistical variations in the opening and closing of a few hundred channels superimposed on the baseline of about 10^6 open channels. It was found that the current carrying capacity of a channel was about 10^{-15} A, and the channel was open for approximately 1 msec which allowed a net transfer of about 5×10^4 ions. For a depolarization of about 10 mV then, about 4×10^6 channels would open and close every second (Anderson and Stevens, 1973; Katz and Miledi, 1970)!

After more than a decade of research, we now have the first true picture of the action of acetylcholine on the postsynaptic membrane. The model describes three states of the receptor [unbound (R), closed (ACh-R_c), or open (ACh-R_o)] and rate constants for the transitions between these states.

$$ACh + R \underset{k_2}{\overset{k_1}{\rightleftharpoons}} ACh\text{-}R_c \underset{\alpha}{\overset{\beta}{\rightleftharpoons}} ACh\text{-}R_o$$

Released ACh diffuses to the receptors; some of it binds (ACh-R_c) and causes receptors to undergo a conformational change to ACh-R_o and flip open to the flow of ions. This step, described by the rate constant β, is fast and corresponds to the peak of the postsynaptic current. The remaining "unbound" ACh is hydrolyzed by AChE and is gone by the time of the peak synaptic current. The slower falling phase of the synaptic current corresponds to the closing of channels at a rate given by α. The rate of closing appears to be primarily set by a conformational shift of the receptor back to state ACh-R_c.

4. PHARMACOLOGY OF THE POSTSYNAPTIC RESPONSE.   Many drugs which act on the nervous system have their major effect on sympatic transmission. Usually, drugs act on particular systems identified by the neurotransmitter, since the drugs are most commonly variants of the structure of the transmitter. In this section we shall describe the general terminology and provide a brief description of how drugs act on cholinergic receptors in the central and peripheral nervous system. Drugs are classified as agonists or antagonists depending upon whether they activate or inactivate receptors. _Agonists_ activate receptors, thus mimicking the action of the transmitter, whereas _antagonists_ inactivate receptors.

How do various cholinergic drugs act on the receptor? Based on the current understanding of the receptor, it is possible to describe the ways ACh agonists and antagonists affect a single channel. In accordance with the reaction given above the effectiveness of an agonist depends on the ease with which it binds to the receptor (k_1/k_2), the rate at which it opens the channel (β), the conductance of the open conformation, and the mean lifetime of the open conformation ($1/\alpha$). In general, ACh agonists increase the mean lifetime of a single open channel over about a twofold range (Colquhoun _et al._, 1975). The stronger the agonist the longer the channel remains open. On the other hand, a reversible antagonist (such as curare) or irreversible ones (such as α-bungarotoxin) act by the all-or-none inactivation of the receptor molecules (Katz and Miledi, 1973). They simply compete with ACh for the receptor and once bound block those channels.

5. ORGANIZATION AND MOLECULAR CHARACTERISTICS OF THE ACh RECEPTOR. *Acetylcholine receptors* are not uniformly distributed along the surface of the target cell. For example, at the neuromuscular junction receptors are concentrated at the active region of the synapse. There are about 1×10^4 to 3×10^4 receptors per μm^2 at the end plate depending on the species of muscle (Hartzell *et al.*, 1976; Fertuck and Salpeter, 1976). The receptor density is greatest at the crest of the junctional folds which underlie the sites of vesicle discharge. Outside of the synapse, the receptor density is about five per μm^2. The localization of synaptic receptors to the area of the membrane at the synapse appears to be characteristic of all synapses so far studied.

What is the ACh receptor? In order to study the receptor it must be isolated. The key breakthrough came when it was discovered that a small polypeptide called *α-bungarotoxin* in the venom of certain snakes binds specifically and very tightly to the ACh receptor (Lee, 1972). The specific affinity of α-bungarotoxin for the receptor has made it possible to assay the receptor. Figure 5-14 illustrates the procedure for isolating ACh receptors.

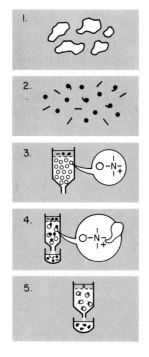

Fig. 5-14. Procedure for isolating ACh receptors. 1. Isolate membranes by centrifugation procedures. The most common source of isolated receptor is the electric organ of *Torpedo californica* or the electric eel, *Electrophorus*, since the synaptic input to the electric organ is solely cholinergic and the terminals cover about 50% of the innervated surface. 2. Dissolve membranes to free the receptor protein. Postsynaptic membranes are disssolved in detergents so that the receptor ( ) is released from other membrane proteins and lipids (—). 3. Prepare an affinity column with an ACh agonist linked to the column beads. The mixture of solubilized membrane proteins is added to the column, which is made of very small beads to which a quaternary ammonium ligand is complexed. 4. When the mixture of soluble ACh receptors and other molecules infiltrate the column the receptors bind to the agonist while other proteins and lipids pass through the column. The receptor proteins stick because they bind to the ligand, while the other components have no affinity for the agonist. 5. Receptor is eluted or displaced from the column by adding high concentrations of an ACh agonist. The agonist displaces the receptor by outcompeting the agonist on the column for the receptor binding sites. In this way pure receptors can be isolated. Yields of pure ACh receptor are quite good and give 40 to 80% of the total number of α-bungarotoxin binding sites in the original homogenate.

The isolated receptor is a protein complex with a molecular weight of about 390,000. The complex is oligomeric, consisting of four distinct subunits with apparent molecular weights of 40,000, 50,500, 59,700 and 64,300 in a ratio of 4 : 2 : 1 : 1 (Fig. 5-15). Each subunit contains some carbohydrate so the subunits are glycoproteins. All of the toxin binding appears to be associated with the 40,000 subunit. The complex contains no AChE activity so the receptor and acetylcholinesterase are distinct molecules. The receptor appears shaped like a crinkled doughnut with a hole in the center and a wrinkled edge. Recently, it has been possible to incorporate purified ACh receptor into artificial membranes and upon addition of an ACh agonist an increase in Na efflux can be observed (Kasai and Changeux, 1971; Michaelson and Raftery, 1974; Hess and Andrews, 1977). This

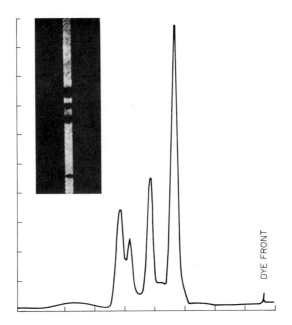

Fig. 5-15. The ACh receptor is a protein complex which consists of four distinct subunits. These four subunits can be resolved from each other by polyacrylamide gel electrophoresis in the presence of the detergent, sodium dodecyl sulfate (SDS). Isolated receptor is dissolved in SDS, applied to the top of the polyacrylamide gel and resolved on the basis of the relative mobility of the individual subunits in an electric field applied across the gel. SDS polyacrylamide gel electrophoresis is one of the most widely used techniques in the study of membrane proteins. A polyacrylamide gel consists of a polyacrylamide matrix which partially retards the migration of proteins. In the presence of SDS, proteins separate according to their molecular weight. Since the SDS binds in large quantities to proteins, its negative charges obscure the intrinsic charge of the protein so that the mobility of the protein in an electric field is determined by its size which, it has been shown, is directly proportional to its molecular weight. Protein–SDS complexes are very negatively charged so they migrate to the anode in an electric field. (Data from Raftery *et al.*, 1976.)

type of experiment, called a reconstitution experiment, allows one to recreate a postsynaptic membrane and study the properties and mechanism of receptor action.

C. Recovery Processes

1.   REPLENISHING ACh STORES: ACh SYNTHESIS.   At rest a neuromuscular junction releases about 0.01% of its total ACh stores per second. This increases to 0.43% per second during stimulation at 20 per second which is about 0.02% per impulse (Potter, 1970). Thus the ACh stores in the nerve terminal are theoretically adequate for about 2300 impulses, which at a stimulus rate of 5 per second would last for 13 minutes before the stores are exhausted. Of course, the stores do not run down. ACh is synthesized constantly even at rest, and during stimulation the rate of synthesis is increased so that only at the most rapid rates of stimulation is the synthetic machinery unable to maintain ACh supplies for release. ACh is synthesized inside the nerve ending from choline and acetyl-coenzyme A

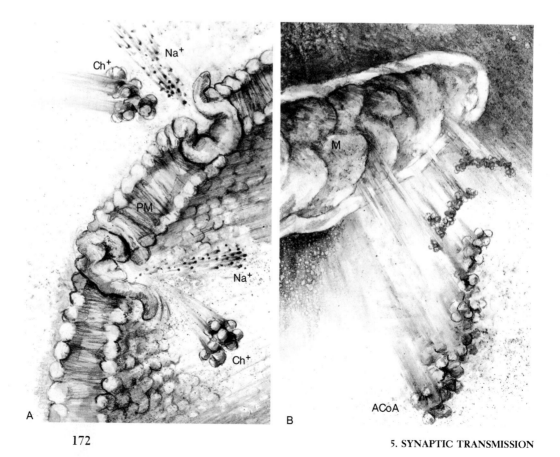

(ACoA). The enzyme which catalyzes the reaction is *choline acetyltransferase*. The sequence of events is illustrated in Fig. 5-16.

All nerve cells as well as other cells accumulate choline, primarily in order to manufacture phospholipids, but in cholinergic neurons the *choline transport system* is unusual. In cholinergic nerve terminals, the transport is characterized by having a very high affinity for choline and being Na dependent. The affinity of

EVENTS IN THE SYNTHESIS OF ACh

$$ACoA + Ch \rightleftharpoons ACh + CoA$$

Fig. 5-16. (A) Neurons do not synthesize choline so the nerve ending recaptures the choline (Ch) generated from the hydrolysis of ACh by AChE. A specific and powerful transport mechanism in the membrane (PM) pumps choline into the nerve ending. (B) Mitochondria (M) inside the nerve ending produce acetyl-coenzyme A (ACoA) as one of their metabolic products. (C) Choline and acetyl-coenzyme A react and form ACh and CoA. The reaction is catalyzed by the enzyme, choline acetyltransferase, which is probably located on the surface of the synaptic vesicles. (D) Recharged vesicles. Each vesicle is loaded with about 10^4 ACh molecules. Once loaded, they move into position for discharge.

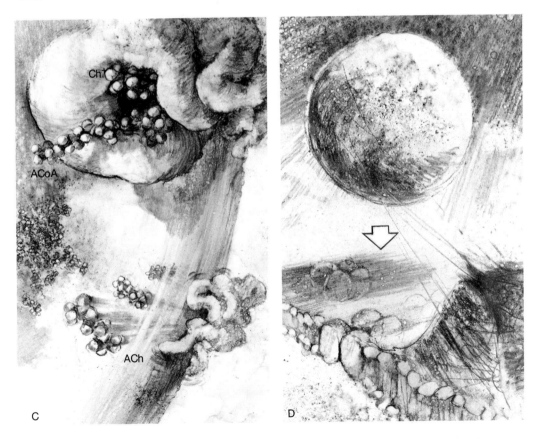

C   D

a transport system is described by a constant K_m which is defined as the concentration of choline which produces one-half maximal velocity of transport. For cholinergic nerve terminals, K_m is 1–2 μM ($10^{-6} M$) as compared to noncholinergic neurons where K_m is the millimolar ($10^{-3} M$) range. Thus the high affinity transport system for choline is maximally active at extremely low concentrations of choline. This system appears to provide good assurance that every bit of choline outside the nerve terminal is captured for use in ACh synthesis.

How is ACh production regulated? The rate-limiting step in ACh synthesis might be either the availability of choline or ACoA, or the activity of the enzyme choline acetyltransferase. If the external choline supply is removed or if choline transport is inhibited by a choline analogue (hemicholinium), ACh production abruptly stops. This and other data show that choline transport is rate limiting in the biosynthesis of ACh (Barker and Mittag, 1975). Thus ACh production might be increased during stimulation if choline transport is increased. In order to test this possibility, the septum was stimulated, and the uptake of choline into isolated hippocampal nerve endings was measured (Simon *et al.*, 1976). The septum projects to the hippocampus, and this pathway is cholinergic. After stimulation, choline uptake and the amount of ACh produced increase; they decrease when the activity of the pathway is reduced by pentobarbital anesthesia (Table 5-1). Thus cholinergic nerve terminals regulate ACh synthesis mainly through the transport of choline.

Once formed ACh is stored in at least two different compartments within a nerve terminal: a readily releasable pool and a storage pool. Studies on the kinetics of acetylcholine synthesis have shown that the readily releasable pool is released in preference to the storage pool (Potter, 1970). Thus an active terminal uses the choline most recently accumulated to produce ACh for immediate release. Neurotransmitter metabolism operates mainly from outside resources: the newest molecules are discharged first.

Table 5-1 Effects of electrical stimulation on ^{3}H-choline uptake into hippocampal synaptosomes[a]

Treatment	Uptake (% of control)
Septal stimulation	210
Pentobarbital anesthesia	25

[a] From Simon *et al.* (1976).

2. REBUILDING SYNAPTIC VESICLES.   Vesicles must not only be refilled with transmitter in order to sustain release, but they must be replaced. A typical neuromuscular junction has a reserve of about 30,000 synaptic vesicles. Each

action potential causes the fusion of about 200 vesicles with the surface membrane so that in 150 impulses the supply would be depleted unless replaced. Moreover, the continual addition of vesicle membrane would cause the terminal to swell excessively. The nerve terminal has a clever conservation mechanism to replace vesicles and maintain terminal volume constant (Heuser and Reese, 1973; Ceccarelli *et al.*, 1973). The series of illustrations portrays the cycle (Fig. 5-17). Membrane is recaptured by *endocytosis* and vesicles are reformed.

D.   Pathology and Disease

Sometimes advances in basic research lead to advances in understanding certain human diseases. *Myasthenia gravis* is one of these cases. It is a disease of the neuromuscular junction in which synaptic transmission fatigues very rapidly so that normal movement and breathing are impossible. The initial breakthrough came quite by accident during experiments on the preparation of an antibody to the ACh receptor (Patrick and Lindstrom, 1973). Pure ACh receptor was injected into rabbits in order that the rabbits' immune system might build an antibody to receptor protein. A few weeks after immunization animals developed a condition closely resembling myasthenia gravis in humans. It was suggested that perhaps receptor-specific antibody was binding to the receptors and causing a reduction in the number of functional receptors. This idea was put to test. Serum from human myasthenia gravis patients was examined to see if factors were present which affected receptors. A fraction was found which blocked α-bungarotoxin binding and which inactivated functional ACh receptors (Bender *et al.*, 1976; Almon *et al.*, 1974). Moreover, in a muscle biopsy sample from patients in the early stages of myasthenia gravis, virtually all junctional folds were intact but the receptor-rich crests were covered by tufted particles which closely resembled antibodies. As the disease progressed, the junctional fold crests were destroyed and in place of the crests were small membrane fragments coated with tufts (Rash *et al.*, 1976). It appears as if myasthenia gravis is an autoimmune disease initially involving an apparent antibody attachment to one or more components of the functional ACh receptor complexes, followed by a systematic destruction and removal of junctional folds by both humoral and cell-mediated autoimmune responses. Thus, in myasthenia gravis patients become immune to their own ACh receptors which causes their destruction.

E.   Summary of Cholinergic Synaptic Transmission

At rest transmitter is discharged in quanta, each of which give rise to miniature synaptic potentials about 0.4 mV in amplitude. These miniature synaptic

RECOVERY OF VESICLES

Fig. 5-17. (A) By a process called exocytosis, vesicles fuse with the presynaptic membrane and become a part of it. Vesicle membrane flows into synaptic plasma membrane.

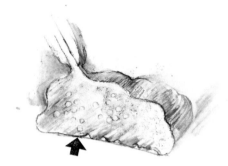

(B) A section of plasma membrane is recaptured by a process called endocytosis. A netlike coat forms on the inside surface of the plasma membrane and plucks off a section of membrane.

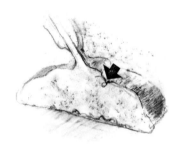

(C) Recaptured membrane forms large cisternae inside the ending which fragment into new synaptic vesicles.

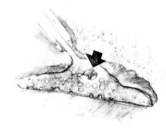

176

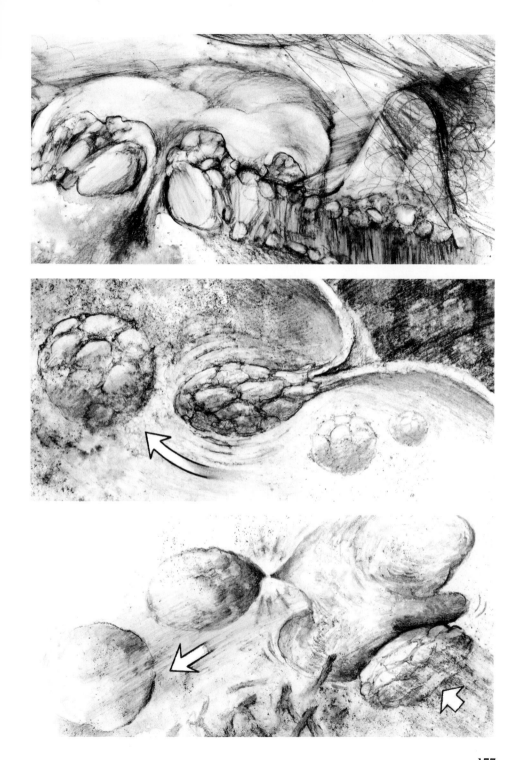

potentials are random in time and represent the resting discharge of synaptic vesicles. The signal for transmitter release is the action potential. The presynaptic membrane has special voltage-sensitive Ca channels. The basic message of the action potential is the voltage change it brings. This stimulates the opening of Ca channels and allows the entry of Ca^{2+} ions. Calcium ions serve as the signal which couples the stimulus of the action potential to the secretion of transmitter. Calcium ions catalyze the fusion of synaptic vesicles with release sites on the presynaptic membrane by a process called exocytosis. An action potential evokes the simultaneous discharge of about 200 quanta (about 10,000 ACh molecules per quanta) within a period of about 200 μsec once Ca^{2+} enters the terminal. The slow step in the stimulus secretion coupling process is the opening of the Ca^{2+} channels. Acetylcholine diffuses across the synaptic cleft to the postsynaptic membrane and binds to a receptor which is a membrane protein complex consisting of four subunits. Acetylcholine causes the receptor to alter its conformation so that at the neuromuscular junction the Na^+ and K^+ permeability increases for about 1 msec. This inward flow of cationic current depolarizes the membrane, and if the current is powerful enough it causes the muscle to fire and contract. Bound ACh spontaneously dissociates from the receptors and the ion channels close. The time course of channel opening and closing parallels the overall time course of the synaptic current. Acetylcholine is hydrolyzed by AChE to acetate and choline so that it is prevented from reactivating the receptor. Acetylcholine can also transmit an inhibitory signal, in which case the permeability of the postsynaptic membrane increases to K^+ and/or Cl^- but not to Na^+.

In the recovery phase, choline is recaptured by a high affinity transport process, and this choline plus acetyl-coenzyme A produced by synaptic mitochondria binds to the enzyme choline acetyltransferase which catalyzes the synthesis of ACh. The transport of choline is the rate-limiting step in the production of ACh. Acetylcholine refills available vesicles which then move into position in preparation for a new stimulus. Synaptic vesicles reform by a process of endocytosis: a section of plasma membrane pinches off and recreates a new synaptic vesicle.

IV. Catecholaminergic Synaptic Transmission

A. Organization of Catecholaminergic Terminals

Catecholaminergic synapses (those synapses where catecholamines are transmitters), as noted previously, typify a type of synapse with a slow action which modulates postsynaptic metabolism. Catecholaminergic neurons in the brain and periphery appear involved in mind, mood and aggression, and are often singled out for their role in mental disorders (Antelman and Caggiula, 1977; Snyder, 1976). As we shall describe in detail in Chapter 17, one of the metabolic errors in schizophrenia, for example, appears to reside in catecholamine metabolism and synaptic transmission. Also catecholaminergic synapses are the targets of many well-known drugs—amphetamine, cocaine, imipramine and reserpine, for example.

Catecholamines are a class of molecules that contain a catechol nucleus (a benzene ring with two adjacent hydroxyl substituents) and one amine group (Fig. 5-18). The term catecholamine usually refers to *dopamine* (DA, dihydroxy-

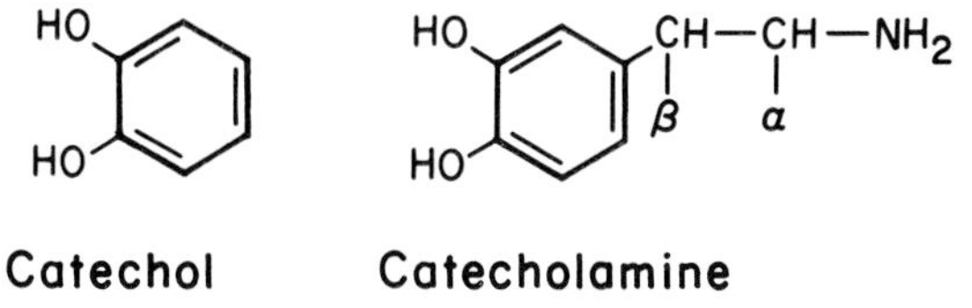

Catechol   Catecholamine

Fig. 5-18. Structure of catecholamine. When hydrogen (H) occupies the α and β positions, the molecule is called dopamine. When a hydroxyl group (OH) is at the β position, it is norepinephrine. Epinephrine (or adrenaline) is norepinephrine with a methyl group (CH_3) added onto the amine.

phenylethylamine) and its metabolic products, *norepinephrine* (NE) and epinephrine (E). The terminology used to describe each type of catecholaminergic synapse is given in Table 5-2.

Table 5-2 Subclasses of catecholaminergic synapses

Transmitter	Synonym	Synapse type
Dopamine	None	Dopaminergic
Norepinephrine	Noradrenaline	Noradrenergic
Epinephrine	Adrenaline	Adrenergic

B. Discharge of Catecholamines

Catecholamine synapses release their transmitter by mechanisms like those at other synapses. An action potential causes an influx of Ca ions which in turn triggers the exocytotic release of transmitter from storage vesicles. Noradrenergic vesicles (those which store NE) contain, besides NE, the enzyme dopamine β-hydroxylase, Mg^{2+} ion, ATP and a protein called chromogranin A. All these are released along with the NE. Thus, after stimulation there is an increase in the quantity of each of these substances in the surrounding medium. Since dopamine β-hydroxylase is released along with the neurotransmitter, the analysis of the levels of the enzyme in the bloodstream has been put to practical use as an assay for the state of the sympathetic nervous system in various disease states (Weinshilboum and Axelrod, 1971).

A few drugs specifically interfere with the storage of catecholamines. _Reserpine_, for example, prevents catecholaminergic synaptic vesicles from storing catecholamine. Reserpine is used relatively frequently to relieve high blood pressure. Noradrenergic nerves treated with reserpine store less catecholamine so they release less upon stimulation. This results in less vasoconstriction and a decrease in blood pressure.

C. Nature of the Postsynaptic Response

Catecholamines signal target cells to carry out a very special series of events which are both electrical and chemical. Stimulation of NE or DA fibers appears to result in primarily inhibitory responses in the majority of CNS neurons. For example, after stimulation of the locus coeruleus, the noradrenergic input to cerebellar Purkinje cells inhibits the spontaneous activity of these cells (Siggins _et al._, 1969). Iontophoretically applied NE creates a slow hyperpolarization and mimics the effect of locus coeruleus stimulation (Siggins _et al._, 1971a). The noradrenergic input to hippocampal and cortical pyramidal cells is also inhibitory (Segal and Bloom, 1974). Activation of the DA nigrostriatal pathway appears to inhibit discharge of most caudate neurons (Siggins, 1978). However, there is evidence, albeit controversial, that some striatal neurons are excited by dopaminergic fibers (Kitai _et al._, 1976). At present, however, the bulk of evidence argues in favor of a primarily slow inhibitory action for DA in the CNS (see Siggins, 1978).

Catecholaminergic synapses typically cause a response which is more prolonged than the classic inhibitory response of the type described in Section III,B,1. In the sympathetic ganglia, for example, activation of the catecholaminergic interneuron causes a slow, inhibitory response (Libet and Tosaka, 1970; Libet and Kobayasi, 1974). Similarly, when NE is directly applied to hippocampal pyramidal cells the latency of its effect is 5 to 30 seconds and the duration of the effect is 10 seconds to 6 minutes. Stimulation of the presynaptic pathway is accompanied by a 150–200 msec latency and a 5 to 120 second duration (Segal and Bloom, 1974, 1976). The action of NE appears to slow down the discharge rate of these neurons.

In Purkinje cells and in sympathetic ganglion neurons of the frog, catecholamines hyperpolarize the cell through a *decrease* in membrane permeability. This is quite an unusual type of change. In Section III,B,1 we saw that ACh mediates inhibition through an *increase* in K or Cl permeability or conductance. In the frog sympathetic ganglia the slow inhibitory postsynaptic potential appears due to a *decrease* in Na conductance (Weight and Padjen, 1973). As Na conductance decreases, the equilibrium potential of the membrane is dominated more by the Cl and K ion conductances and, since these ions have equilibrium potentials more negative than the resting potential, the cell hyperpolarizes. The depolarizing influence of Na at rest is lessened. The nature of the conductance decrease in Purkinje cells is unknown at present. In the sympathetic ganglia of some animals, particularly mammals, there is very little, if any, conductance change, and it has been suggested that the change in the membrane potential is due to the action of an active electrogenic transmembrane ionic pump (like the Na pump) rather than a simple passive channel (see Libet and Kobayshi, 1974).

It is now clear that catecholaminergic neurons also change postsynaptic cellular metabolism. In fact, it has been suggested that this metabolic signal may be an even more essential message than the initial potential change. Dopamine and NE appear to stimulate an enzyme called *adenylate cyclase* which in turn synthesizes *cyclic adenosine monophosphate* (cAMP) from adenosine triphosphate (ATP) (Fig. 5-19).

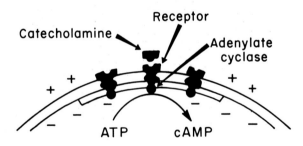

Fig. 5-19. Catecholamines bind to specific receptors on the postsynaptic membrane. The interaction is a "lock–key"-like interaction. There are two consequences of catecholamine receptor interaction: A slow hyperpolarization of the membrane which produces inhibition and a chemical change in which the catecholamine signals a transmembrane activation of adenylate cyclase and the synthesis of more cAMP. cAMP then acts to modulate cellular metabolism in highly specific ways.

Cyclic AMP is called the "second messenger." Transmitters (or hormones) are the first messengers. Inside the cell, cAMP picks up the message from the transmitter and tells the cell that it must change by altering its metabolism or excitability in specific ways. In the pineal gland, for example, stimulation of the noradrenergic input causes a large rise in cAMP which induces an increase in the production of melatonin, the hormone product of the pineal gland. The increase in cAMP can be specifically blocked by propranolol, a β-adrenergic antagonist, so the effect is clearly initiated by the action of NE (Axelrod, 1974a,b).

In a variety of cells where NE and DA are neurotransmitters, they stimulate receptors that stimulate adenylate cyclase and cause an elevation in cAMP levels. In direct support of a role of cAMP in modulating cellular responses, iontophoretically applied cAMP or inhibitors of phosphodiesterase, an enzyme which degrades cAMP, mimic the action of applied NE or DA (Siggins et al., 1971a,b; Siggins, 1978) (Fig. 5-20). The general hypothesis is that an increase in cAMP levels activates protein kinases that (1) phosphorylate certain membrane proteins and alter the permeability characteristics of the membrane and (2) alter the metabolic properties of the cell by activating and inducing certain enzymes and proteins. It is generally felt that cAMP somehow sets the level of excitability in its target cells (Nathanson, 1977; Nathanson and Greengard, 1977).

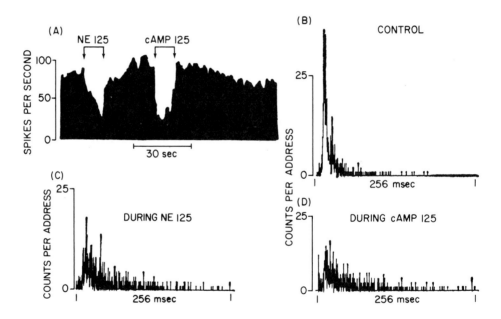

Fig. 5-20. Effects of microelectrophoretic application of NE and cAMP on spontaneous Purkinje cell discharge. (A) Effects of drug application on mean discharge frequency. Duration of drug application is indicated by arrows. Numbers after each drug indicate ejection current in nanoamperes. (B)–(D) Interspike interval histograms of the same cell during the control period and during application of NE and cAMP, respectively. The peak of each histogram indicates the most probable interspike interval in single spike discharge. There is a large decrease in mean frequency, but there is little change in the most probable interspike interval (15.4 msec). (From Siggins et al., 1969, copyright by the American Association for the Advancement of Science.)

5. SYNAPTIC TRANSMISSION

D. Pharmacology of Adrenoceptors

A large number of drugs act on *adrenoceptors* (a term used to refer to the class of receptors for catecholamines) (Iversen and Iversen, 1975). Adrenergic antagonists and agonists are often classified as α or β according to their action. The classification appears so frequently in medicine and neurobiology that a brief discussion is merited. In the 1940's physiologists carried out extensive surveys on the action of the available adrenergic analogues on smooth muscle and other tissues. In view of the types of action discovered, Ahlquist (1948) proposed the classification α and β receptors as two types of receptors which have different agonist or antagonist specificities. Both α and β adrenoceptors respond to NE, E and an agonist called isoproterenol (IsoPr), but the order of potency is different for each class: NE > E > IsoPr for α adrenoceptors and IsoPr > E = NE for β adrenoceptors. Antagonists such as phenoxybenzamine, dibenamine and phentolamine act selectively on α adrenoceptors while propranolol acts on β adrenoceptors. Either adrenoceptor can mediate inhibition or excitation. For example, β adrenoceptors mediate the action of NE which stimulates the contraction of heart muscle or causes the relaxation of smooth muscle in the intestine and bronchi. The α and β classification has proved useful for the peripheral nervous system, but in the CNS the distinction is much less applicable, since α and β agonists or antagonists can have similar actions on the same system. In the CNS such drug actions are best considered in the context of their own action. DA receptors, for example, differ from both α and β adrenoceptors in their pharmacological properties.

Table 5-3 summarizes the action of some of the common drugs which act on catecholamine receptors and their general use. The α and β antagonists listed are

Table 5-3 Some common drugs which act on catecholaminergic receptors and their general use[a]

Drug class	Examples	Use
DA antagonist	Chloropromazine (Thorazine) Haloperidol (Haldol)	Antipsychotics
α Antagonist	Phentolamine Phenoxybenzamine Tolazoline Clonidine (Catapres)	Cardiovascular Hypertension Shock, peripheral vascular disease Hypertension
β Antagonists	Propranolol	Cardiac arrhythmias, angina pectoris, hypertension

[a] Goodman and Gilman (1975).

very commonly used in animal studies in order to manipulate catecholaminergic systems and discern their involvement in various body functions and behaviors (see Iversen and Iversen, 1975; Antelman and Caggiula, 1977).

E.   Inactivation by Reuptake

Catecholamines can be degraded by certain enzymes (monoamine oxidase or catechol-O-methyltransferase) but neither of these enzymes is responsible for inactivation of transmitter, since inhibiting these enzymes has no effect on the rapid termination of the response. How then are catecholamines inactivated?

Axelrod and co-workers suspected that catecholamines might be removed from the cleft by reuptake into presynaptic boutons, and they set out to investigate this possibility in a series of very simple and direct experiments. As Axelrod (1974b) states,

> In order to track down such a mechanism we injected a rat with radioactive noradrenaline. The labeled transmitter persisted in tissues that were rich in sympathetic nerves for many hours, long after its physiological actions were ended, indicating that radioactive noradrenaline was taken up in the sympathetic nerves and held there. My colleagues and I designed a simple experiment to prove this. Sympathetic nerves innervating the left salivary gland in rats were destroyed by removing the superior cervical ganglion on the left side of the neck; about seven days after this operation the noradrenaline nerves of the salivary gland on the right side were intact, whereas the nerves on the left side had completely disappeared. When radioactive noradrenaline was injected, the transmitter was found in the right salivary gland but not in the left one. We also found that in cats injected with radioactive noradrenaline the transmitter was released when the sympathetic nerves were stimulated electrically. The experiments clearly demonstrated that noradrenaline is taken up into, as well as released from, sympathetic nerves. As a result of these experiments we postulated that noradrenaline is rapidly inactivated through its recapture by the sympathetic nerves; once it is back in the nerves, of course, the neurotransmitter cannot exert its effect on postjunctional cells.

In studying the properties of CNS synapses such as the reuptake of transmitter it is desirable to have a preparation which consists only of synapses. As discussed previously (see Chapter 3), CNS synapses or _synaptosomes_ (synaptic bodies) can be isolated by the techniques of subcellular fractionation. Research using synaptosomes has shown that reuptake systems are membrane transport systems which are highly specific for NE, DA and related compounds. The transport system for DA will not, in general, distinguish between DA and NE, but it does not accumulate other transmitters such as γ-aminobutyric acid or ACh. The transport systems used for reuptake are characterized as being Na dependent and having a high affinity for their substrate. A typical K_m is about 1 μM. This means that the velocity of transport is half-maximal when the concentration of extracellular catecholamine is 1 μM. Thus even at the lowest concentration of transmitter, the system operates at near full velocity to keep the extracellular concentration of transmitter very low. Like the transport system for choline, catecholamine systems use the Na ion gradient as a source of energy to accumulate transmitter against its concentration gradient. Sodium must enter the cells along with the transmitter so that in the absence of Na there is no high affinity transport. This newly accumulated transmitter is stored inside nerve terminals and is rapidly released along with endogenous stores (Cotman *et al.*, 1976a,b).

Many drugs block reuptake and can prolong the synaptic action of catecholamines (Fig. 5-21). *Cocaine*, *amphetamine* *and* *imipramine* are but a few which have such action. Cocaine and imipramine are quite specific uptake blockers, whereas amphetamine also stimulates the efflux of catecholamine, apparently from pools outside of storage vesicles.

Reuptake of transmitter from the extracellular space into cellular compartments appears to be a widely used mechanism for transmitter inactivation. Sodium-dependent high affinity transport systems exist not only for catecholamines but for other transmitters or transmitter candidates as well—

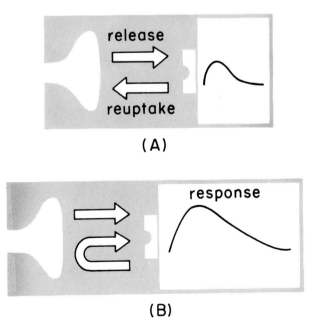

Fig. 5-21. (A) The action of catecholamines on the postsynaptic cell is inactivated by reuptake into the terminal. (B) Drugs which block reuptake on the postsynaptic response potentiate the response by prolonging the life time of transmitter in the synaptic cleft. More transmitter can reactivate the receptor more times.

GABA, glutamate, aspartate, glycine, proline, etc. (Snyder *et al.*, 1973). Initially it was assumed that all such transport systems were present in synaptic boutons, but it has been found that glial cells also have a Na-dependent high affinity transport system for some transmitter candidates such as glutamate (Henn *et al.*, 1974).

F.   Synthesis of Catecholamines

Catecholamines are synthesized from tyrosine, an essential amino acid, by a multistep reaction involving four enzymes (Fig. 5-22). Tyrosine is supplied to

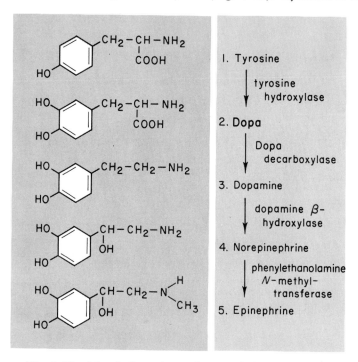

Fig. 5-22.   Metabolic pathway for catecholamine synthesis.

nerve terminals from the blood and is accumulated by a powerful transport system. Tyrosine is converted to dopa via *tyrosine hydroxylase*, an enzyme which requires molecular oxygen, a pteridine cofactor and iron (Fe^{2+}) for its activity. Dopa is decarboxylated by *dopa decarboxylase* to form dopamine which itself is a transmitter in certain neurons. Dopamine is converted to norepinephrine by another hydroxylation enzyme, *dopamine β-hydroxylase*. Dopaminergic neurons (neurons which use dopamine as a neurotransmitter) do not have dopamine β-hydroxylase so that no NE is synthesized in these cells. In the adrenal gland the

5. SYNAPTIC TRANSMISSION

reaction is carried one more step and a methyl group is added via _phenylethanolamine-N-methyltransferase_ to produce epinephrine (also called adrenaline). Note that the names of the enzymes are descriptive of the reaction— hydroxylase for the addition of a hydroxyl group, decarboxylase for the removal of a carboxyl group, etc., so that complete reliance on memory is not necessary.

The complete metabolic machinery to synthesize catecholamines is present in the nerve terminals. The enzymes are organized in discrete subcellular compartments (Fig. 5-23). Tyrosine hydroxylase and dopa decarboxylase are soluble enzymes located outside the synaptic vesicles of noradrenergic neurons. Thus dopa and dopamine are synthesized in the cytoplasm and dopamine then enters the storage vesicle where it is β-hydroxylated (Rutledge and Weiner, 1967).

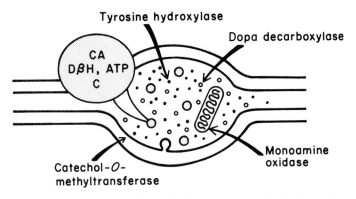

Fig. 5-23. Organization of a noradrenergic bouton. Tyrosine hydroxylase and dopa decarboxylase are soluble enzymes in the cytoplasm, while dopamine β-hydroxylase (DBH) is present inside the storage vesicles. In addition to catecholamine (CA), DBH, ATP and a soluble protein chromogranin A (C) are present inside the storage vesicles. Monoamine oxidase, an enzyme which degrades CA, is present inside the bouton and is associated with mitochondria. Catechol-O-methyltransferase (COMT), another enzyme which degrades CA, is present in the extracellular space.

G. Regulation of Catecholamine Synthesis

Catecholamine neurons, like cholinergic neurons, must have elaborate regulatory mechanisms to control neurotransmitter synthesis at the nerve ending. Despite large fluctuations in the activity of sympathetic neurons and the amount of neurotransmitter released, the level of catecholamine within the nerve endings of these cells can be maintained quite constant (von Euler, 1956).

How are catecholamine stores regulated? In metabolic pathways, control is usually exerted at the initial reaction where the pathway becomes unbranched. The entry point is generally _rate limiting_ so that the rate constant of the initial reaction determines the overall rate of synthesis of the end product of the pathway. The rate-limiting step in the pathway for the synthesis of catecholamines is tyrosine hydroxylase. Tyrosine hydroxylase has a much lower activity than dopa decarboxylase or dopamine β-hydroxylase and so it governs the overall rate of catecholamine synthesis (Levitt et al., 1965). At equivalent concentrations, tyrosine is a much less effective precursor for norepinephrine than dopamine. Increasing the concentration of dopamine leads to an increase in norephinephrine biosynthesis, but increasing the concentration of tyrosine beyond a certain level does not increase the amount of norepinephrine produced (Table 5-4). Tyrosine hydroxylase has a very high affinity (low K_m) for tyrosine so it is normally saturated and rate limiting. Tyrosine hydroxylase acts as a "bottleneck" for the biosynthesis of catecholamines.

Table 5-4 The effect of varying the concentration of tyrosine or dopamine on the rate of norepinephrine synthesis[a,b]

Precursor concentration	Norepinephrine synthesis rate (ng/gm/hour)			
	10^{-5}	5×10^{-4}	10^{-4}	5×10^{-3}
Tyrosine	0.07	0.17	0.19	0.19
Dopamine	0.60	0.80	1.00	1.20

[a] Data from Levitt et al. (1965).
[b] Sympathetic ganglia were removed and perfused with solutions containing various concentrations of tyrosine or dopamine and the amount of norepinephrine synthesized in the ganglia measured.

The activity of tyrosine hydroxylase provides the moment by moment regulation of catecholamine levels. When stores are low after stimulation, the enzyme speeds up and converts more tyrosine to dopa; when stores are adequate, it slows down and synthesizes very little dopa. Regulation is achieved in a very simple way: Tyrosine hydroxylase is sensitive to the concentration of its end products, DA and NE. High levels inhibit the activity of the enzyme so that less DA and NE are then synthesized; low levels relieve the enzyme from inhibition so that more DA and NE can be produced. A number of lines of evidence both in vivo and in vitro support this model (Costa et al., 1974; Weiner et al., 1972). The most direct is that activity of isolated tyrosine hydroxylase is inhibited when high concentrations of DA and NE are included in the assay (Undenfriend et al., 1965). Feedback is probably most important for limiting catecholamine production, and so it is referred to as end product inhibition.

Calcium ions and cAMP are also regulatory signals. These mechanisms involve an activation of tyrosine hydroxylase by an alteration in the affinity

5. SYNAPTIC TRANSMISSION

constants of the enzyme for substrate. These changes are probably allosteric in nature; that is, tyrosine hydroxylase has a special site where activators may bind and alter the interaction of the enzyme with its substrate at the catalytic site. The increase in affinity for tyrosine allows the enzyme to bind a greater fraction of available substrate so that more dopa is synthesized. Isolated enzyme is stimulated by Ca or cAMP, and electrical stimulation of NE cell bodies in the vas deferens or locus coeruleus produces a transient increase in the affinity constants of tyrosine hydroxylase in the nerve endings (Morgenroth *et al.*, 1974; Roth *et al.*, 1975; Harris *et al.*, 1974). It is believed that Ca influx during depolarization elevates cAMP levels.

Thus, the presynaptic bouton regulates internal catecholamine levels via end product inhibition and allosteric activating mechanisms. These regulatory mechanisms are summarized in Fig. 5-24.

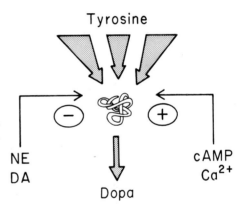

Fig. 5-24. The enzyme tyrosine hydroxylase is primarily responsible for regulating the synthesis of catecholamines. The activity of the enzyme is inhibited by the end products of the pathway, DA and NE. The activity of the enzyme increases when the levels of DA and NE fall, thereby relieving the enzyme from inhibition. Most importantly, however, it appears that Ca or cAMP stimulate tyrosine hydroxylase by allowing it to bind more of the tyrosine available so that more dopa is produced. Once bound the reaction is instantaneous so that activity is set by the amount of substrate bound. This is determined by the affinity of the enzyme for its substrate. Calcium ions and cAMP change the affinity of the enzyme so it binds a greater portion of its available substrate. Thus the reaction is faster.

H.   Summary

Catecholamines are stored in vesicles. An action potential causes Ca influx and the exocytosis of the entire contents of the storage vesicle into the extracellular space. Catecholamines bind to receptors, activate adenylate cyclase and increase cAMP levels in target cells. In most cells so far examined, dopamine and norepinephrine inhibit cellular firing. The response is terminated by reuptake of the catecholamine through powerful transport systems in the synaptic endings.

Recaptured transmitter and that which is newly synthesized both replace the stores.

Catecholamines are synthesized from tyrosine. Tyrosine hydroxylase is the first enzyme in the pathway. It catalyzes the hydroxylation of tyrosine to dopa, which in turn is decarboxylated by dopa decarboxylase to DA. In noradrenergic neurons DA is β-hydroxylated to produce NE, but this enzyme is absent in dopaminergic neurons. Tyrosine hydroxylase is the rate-limiting enzyme in all adrenergic terminals and controls the production of DA and NE. In short-term regulation its activity is inhibited by its end products, NE and/or DA (feedback inhibition). Tyrosine hydroxylase is activated by reduced levels of its end products which relieve the enzyme from inhibition and by Ca^{2+} and cAMP which stimulate enzyme activity by increasing the affinity constants for the substrate so that the enzyme binds more tyrosine and synthesizes more dopa.

Drugs are available which affect nearly every aspect of synaptic transmission unique to catecholaminergic neurons (Table 5-5). Drugs exist which block reuptake, the storage of transmitter, the degradation of transmitter via monoamine oxidase and various receptor agonists and antagonists. Reuptake blockers, monoamine oxidase inhibitors and receptor agonists potentiate the response, while reserpine and receptor antagonists depress the catecholaminergic responses.

Table 5-5 Summary of drugs acting at catecholaminergic synapses

Drugs	Site of action
Reserpine	Depletes storage granules of CA stores
Haloperidol; chlorpromazine	DA receptor antagonist
Phentolamine	α Adrenergic antagonist
Propranolol	β Adrengeric antagonist
Cocaine; imipramine	Reuptake blocker
Amphetamine	Reuptake blocker, stimulates CA efflux from nongranular pools
α Methyl-p-tyrosine	Inactivates tyrosine hydroxylase
Pargyline	Monoamine oxidase inhibitor

V. Synaptic Plasticity

What changes take place in the nervous system which allow us to learn and remember and to adapt our behavior to meet a changing environment? Something must change, and it is a widely held premise in neurobiology that changes in the functional capacities of the nervous system are due to changes in the properties of its synapses. The synapse was targeted as a site of modification almost immediately after it was discovered, and the hypothesis that synapses are modifiable has fared well. Other changes occur, no doubt, but the most fundamental are synaptic changes which alter the communication between neurons or between neurons and other cells.

Synaptic transmission displays plasticity: it is a function of previous stimulus history, strengthening or weakening under different conditions. In this section we will discuss both short- and long-term aspects of synaptic plasticity. First, we will discuss short-term plasticity of synaptic transmission in a monosynaptic pathway. Changes in the frequency of stimulation, for example, alter the magnitude of the synaptic potential over a short term. Then we will turn to catecholaminergic systems in order to examine long-term plasticity. Catecholaminergic systems have the ability to synthesize different amounts of the enzymes responsible for the synthesis of transmitter, and they display a long-term regulation of receptor properties.

A. Synaptic Transmission and Short-Term Plasticity

At a monosynaptic pathway there are three general forms of short-term plasticity: facilitation, depression and potentiation. Figure 5-25 shows these processes at a neuromuscular junction during repetitive stimulation. At stimulation rates of one stimulus every 10 seconds, the amplitude of the synaptic potential remains constant (control level). Increasing the rate of stimulation to 100 per second for a period of 90 seconds results in an immmediate short-term increase in the synaptic potential which is called facilitation. A depression in the synaptic potential is seen very quickly at this stimulation rate. After the 100 per second stimulus train is stopped, and the efficacy of the synapse is tested at the original rate of one stimulus every 10 seconds, the amplitude quickly returns to control and eventually increases beyond control. This is potentiation.

These forms of plasticity can be defined as follows.

Facilitation is a relatively short-term (<1 second) increase in the amplitude of the synaptic potential seen during repetitive stimulation.

Depression is a decrease in the synaptic potential amplitude.

Potentiation is a relatively long-term increase in the synaptic potential amplitude observed during repetitive stimulation.

Variations in stimulus frequency result in different degrees of facilitation, depression and potentiation. For example, when the evoked output of transmitter is large, depression is nearly always seen, but when evoked output is reduced (by a decrease in the rate of stimulation or suppression of output by high Mg^{2+}),

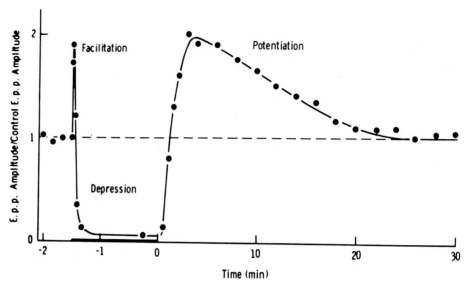

Fig. 5-25. The effect of repetitive stimulation on the amplitude of the synaptic potential (E.p.p.) at a frog neuromuscular junction. The nerve was stimulated once every 10 seconds to establish a baseline response (first four data points). A tetanic train at 100 per second was delivered for 90 seconds (between −1.5 and 0 minutes heavy line). The synaptic potential shows a rapid facilitation about two times over the control response, followed by marked depression until the train is stopped. After the train a test response delivered once every 10 seconds shows that the synaptic potential rapidly recovered and then showed about a twofold potentiation. Potentiation decayed back to control levels in about 20 minutes. (From Barrett and Magleby, 1976.)

depression can be minimal or nonexistent. Thus depression, facilitation and potentiation may phase in and out depending on the exact pattern of impulse traffic and the plastic properties of the synapse.

All synapses do not have the same plastic properties and overall capabilities. Synapses are custom designed. Some synapses show marked facilitation and potentiation while others show very little. At the neuromuscular junction of a rat, for example, potentiation lasts for a few minutes, whereas potentiation in the rat hippocampus induced by a few conditioning stimuli can last for hours, even days! It is believed that the hippocampus serves memory functions, so it is reassuring that its connections have a more accentuated recall of previous stimuli than the more hard-wired neuromuscular junction. Still other synapses work without change over a wide range of conditions. The insect neuromuscular junction of fast flight muscle reliably follows frequencies of 100 per second. Insects beat their wings very rapidly so the nerve must work reliably at high frequencies in order for the insect to fly. Nearly all other synapses fatigue at that rate.

What are the mechanisms that allow synapses to perform in different ways? What properties build into synapses a capacity to modify their output as a

5. SYNAPTIC TRANSMISSION

function of their input? Plasticity mechanisms which serve to modify an established synapse might involve pre- or postsynaptic processes or both (Table 5-6). In practice most of the possible changes listed do occur in one situation or another depending on the system, the time of onset and the duration of the change. In order to illustrate the nature of the mechanisms and the analyses used, we shall focus our discussion on an analysis of the mechanisms of potentiation. This is quite appropriate since to some degree facilitation and potentiation share the same mechanisms (Martin, 1977).

Table 5-6   Mechanisms which might modify synaptic transmission

I.   Presynaptic changes
  A.   Quantity of transmitter released
       (number of quanta discharged per stimulus)
    1.   Changes in the size of the stimulus
    2.   An increase or decrease in Ca available to activate discharge
    3.   Change in the number of full vesicles available
    4.   Increase or decrease in the probability that a given number of available vesicles will discharge
  B.   Decrease or increase in reuptake processes which change the quantity of transmitter available to receptors
II.   Postsynaptic changes
  A.   Increase or decrease in available receptors
  B.   Changes in permeability processes
  C.   Changes in inactivation processes
  D.   Modification in metabolism which alters transmitters effect on cell metabolism

1.   MECHANISM OF POTENTIATION.   At the neuromuscular junction, potentiation is a presynaptic process since the size of quanta recorded from the muscle does not change during the period of potentiation (del Castillo and Katz, 1954; Liley, 1956). Thus potentiation must be due to an increase in the number of quanta released. In some way the system is primed so that a stimulus is more effective in releasing those quanta available. What is the nature of the priming? It is not an increase in the amplitude of the action potential, since records from presynaptic terminals show it does not change (Martin and Pilar, 1964).

A number of lines of evidence point to a role of Ca in potentiation (Martin, 1977). For example, the amount of potentiation depends on the amount of Ca present during the conditioning stimulus. Reducing the Ca concentration during the conditioning stimulation train and returning immediately to the control Ca level results in potentiation of a magnitude and time course expected for a lower Ca level (Rosenthal, 1969). This means that the Ca concentration during the conditioning stimulus is the factor which determines the amount of potentiation and not that before or after the stimulus. Moreover, the rate of spontaneous miniature synaptic potentials is greatly increased after repetitive stimulation (Martin and Pilar, 1964; Liley, 1956), and this increase is dependent on extracellular Ca (Miledi and Thies, 1971). Thus the most likely explanation for potentiation at the neuromuscular junction is that intracellular Ca accumulates and in some way increases evoked quantal release. It has also been suggested that transmitter stores may be more effectively mobilized during potentiation (Schlapfer *et al.*, 1976) and this is probably also involved. For example, there may be a closer clustering of vesicles at release sites so the probability that more vesicles discharge is increased (Fig. 5-26). Facilitation also appears to involve an increase in intracellular Ca.

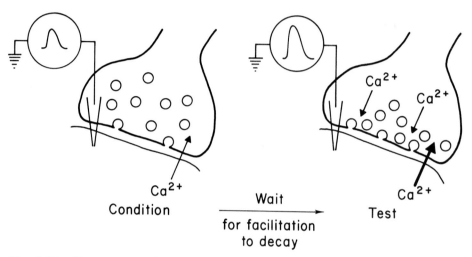

Fig. 5-26. Potentiation. A long-lasting increase in the amplitude of a synaptic potential following repetitive stimulation. Potentiation appears to result from increased intracellular Ca and an increased mobilization of transmitter stores.

Potentiation is particularly long lasting at some synapses in the CNS. For example, in the hippocampus after only a single conditioning stimulus, the second stimulus is markedly increased and after a brief train (15 and 100 per second) potentiation lasting for many hours has been described (Fig. 5-27) (Bliss and Lømo, 1973; Bliss and Gardner Medwin, 1973). Potentiation of this duration has not been reported outside the brain, so the brain may have a particular capacity to develop long-term potentiation. The mechanisms have not been analyzed in detail, but many of the same processes modulating presynaptic release at the neuromuscular junction no doubt apply in the hippocampus. However, evidence is growing that there is a postsynaptic component as well (Fig. 5-27).

It appears as if the neck of dendritic spines is enlarged after potentiation (van Harreveld and Fifkova, 1974; Fifkova and van Harreveld, 1977). This may increase

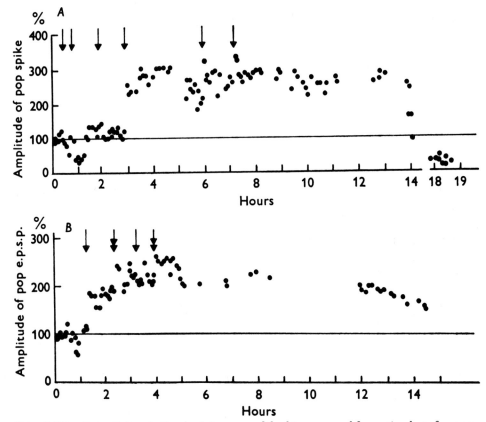

Fig. 5-27. Potentiation in the dentate gyrus of the hippocampal formation lasts for many hours after stimulation of entorhinal input. Six trains of stimuli were given alternately at 15 per second for 10 seconds (single arrows) and 100 per second for 3 seconds (double-headed arrows) and the amplitude of population excitatory synaptic potential (pop e.p.s.p.) and population spike (pop spike) was tested at various times (closed circles). The response grew to 150% of its preconditioned level. When the response was tested at various times as long as 10 hours later it remained elevated. Population synaptic potentials and spikes represent the summated responses of groups of neurons reacting together. (From Bliss and Lømo, 1973.)

the synaptic response because it lowers the input resistance between the synapse and the main dendritic shaft so that more synaptic current reaches the cell body. It is likely that spine configuration changes or other postsynaptic modifications augment presynaptic changes in the CNS during potentiation.

2. SYNAPTIC DEPRESSION. Synaptic depression results from a rundown of one or more of the processes sustaining the synaptic potential. Not unexpectedly, the process which fails to sustain itself depends on the stimulus frequency. At very high rates of stimulation, vesicles are lost faster than they can be replaced; at moderate rates of stimulation, transmitter availability is limiting. It has also been

shown that with repetitive stimulation an increase in extracellular K due to stimulus evoked K efflux can contribute to depression (Erulkar and Weight, 1977).

In summary, traffic across synapses depends on the character of the stimulus: the postsynaptic response can rise or fall depending on the synapse and the stimulation paradigm. Each of the changes is relatively short in duration, lasting at most a day and usually lasting only a few minutes. We have looked at the short-term plastic properties of synapses. Such phenomenon are believed to play an underlying role in short-term memory, for example. However, for more lasting changes other, more durable, mechanisms are required. Synapses do change more permanently, and at the biochemical level research has focused on the induction of neurotransmitter enzymes and receptors.

B. Long-Term Synaptic Plasticity

1. ENZYME INDUCTION.   What is the effect of prolonged use on a synapse? Repetitive stimulation increases the amount of transmitter released and so more must be produced. Do cells make more of the necessary enzymes in order to meet these demands? The most interesting and complete studies are on catecholamines in sympathetic ganglion neurons and adrenal cells.

Increasing the activity of catecholaminergic cells for a period of 1 hour or more causes an increase in the quantity of certain enzymes within a few hours (Thoenen *et al.*, 1969; Thoenen, 1970; Molinoff *et al.*, 1970, 1972; Guidotti *et al.*, 1975). A large increase is found in tyrosine hydroxylase, the rate-limiting enzyme in the pathway entrusted with synthesizing dopa from tyrosine. Dopa decarboxylase, which synthesizes DA from dopa, does not change, and dopamine β-hydroxylase, which produces NE from DA, increases but to a lesser extent than tyrosine hydroxylase (Mueller *et al.*, 1969; Molinoff *et al.*, 1970; Thoenen, 1970; Hanbauer *et al.*, 1973). Most any stimulus which increases activity will induce the enzymes (Kvetňanský *et al.*, 1971; Axelrod *et al.*, 1970; Thoenen *et al.*, 1971; Zigmond, 1976).

The term used to describe an increase in the quantity of particular enzymes in response to a particular stimulus is _enzyme induction_. Enzyme induction is distinct from short-term regulation previously described (see Section IV, F) in which the enzymes are rapidly activated but not increased in quantity. Enzyme induction in response to increased activity in neurons readies the cells so they can more adequately sustain their output the next time they are repetitively activated.

The signal for the induction of tyrosine hydroxylase and dopamine β-hydroxylase is trans-synaptic (Molinoff *et al.*, 1970; Thoenen *et al.*, 1969). In some way synaptic activity tells the postsynaptic cell to synthesize more proteins. If incoming afferents are cut or the receptors are blocked, there is no enzyme induction. Hormonal signals, such as glucocorticosteroids, may augment tyrosine hydroxylase induction (Guidotti *et al.*, 1975). Following hypophysectomy, for example, there is a marked fall in tyrosine hydroxylase (Mueller *et al.*, 1970) and dopamine β-hydroxylase (Weinshilboum and Axelrod, 1970). The reduction in dopamine β-hydroxylase can be reversed by administration of steroids.

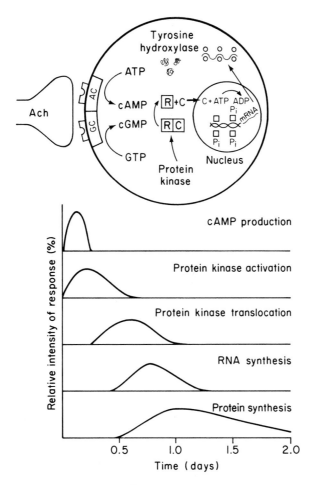

Fig. 5-28. Transsynaptic induction of tyrosine hydroxylase. (A) Flow chart showing the relationship between stimulation of membrane receptors and increase in tyrosine hydroxylase synthesis. ACh stimulates the enzymes, adenylate (AC) and guanylate (GC) cyclase, causing an increase in cAMP and cGMP levels in the cell. cAMP activates a protein kinase (RC) by release of free catalytic subunits (C). The catalytic subunits translocate from the cytoplasm to the nucleus, phosphorylate chromatin and stimulate the production of tyrosine hydroxylase mRNA. The mRNA migrates to the cytoplasm where it binds ribosomes and codes for the synthesis of additional tyrosine hydroxylase. (B) The time relationships of these events are given in the bottom of the figure.

It appears that the transmitter stimulates receptors and activates adenylate cyclase, causing an increase in cAMP and probably cGMP (cyclic guanosine monophosphate) (Fig. 5-28). The cAMP levels (or cyclic nucleotide ratios) rise and when this persists for at least 1 hour the cell responds within 10 hours with a specific activation of protein synthesis. The events of the intervening period are not well established, but it appears cAMP causes an increase in RNA synthesis mediated by a cAMP-stimulated protein kinase translocated from the cytoplasm to the nucleus. The stimulation of tyrosine hydroxylase and dopamine β-hydroxylase protein synthesis is long lasting, but ceases about 40 hours after stimulus application (Guidotti *et al.*, 1975). The enzyme levels, however, remain elevated for much longer.

2.   RECEPTOR INDUCTION.   Catecholamine receptors and receptor-mediated events also appear to show relatively long-term changes. Studies on the pineal gland nicely illustrate the basic features of receptor plasticity in the normal physiological adjustments of a system (Kebabian *et al.*, 1977). The pineal hormone, melatonin, and the enzymes and intermediates involved in its biosynthesis show a marked circadian rhythm which is under the influence of environmental lighting. The highest levels of melatonin, as well as the enzyme regulating its synthesis (serotonin N-acetyltransferase), are present at night. Norepinephrine receptors and adenylate cyclase also show a rhythm (Table 5-7). These rhythms

Table 5-7   Effect of environmental lighting on adenylate cyclase activity and ³H-alprenolol binding in the pineal gland[a,b]

Condition	Adenylate cyclase activity[c]	³H-Alprenolol binding[d]
12 hours in dark	103	6,500
12 hours in light	225	10,500

[a] After Kebabian *et al.* (1975).
[b] Alprenolol binding serves as an index of the number of NE receptors present.
[c] Picomoles of cAMP synthesized per milligram of protein per minute.
[d] Counts per minute of ³H-alprenolol bound per milligram of protein.

are apparently controlled by 24 hour rhythms in the turnover of NE in the sympathetic terminals innervating the gland. Increased receptor stimulation is believed to cause a rapid decrease in the number of receptors resulting in subsensitivity, whereas reduction in NE stimulation produces *supersensitivity* by increasing the number of receptors (Romero and Axelrod, 1975; Kebabian *et al.*, 1975). Thus it appears as if pineal noradrenergic receptors and adenylate cyclase go through sensitivity changes as part of natural circadian rhythms.

5. SYNAPTIC TRANSMISSION

Chronic drug treatment may cause changes in the number of brain receptors and produce significant behavioral affects. In the treatment of schizophrenics, haloperidol is often given over long periods of time. With prolonged treatment, however, complications set in causing abnormal movements of facial muscles and the extremities (tardive dyskinesia). Lowering the dose or terminating the drug worsens these symptoms, while raising it alleviates them. Why? Haloperidol acts on dopamine receptors in the brain. Perhaps the drug supersensitizes these receptors, and this leads to the abnormal and exaggerated movements.

Dopamine receptors can be assayed by measuring the binding of ^{3}H-haloperidol to brain membranes. By using this assay it was found that the amount of bound drug increases by about 20% after 3 weeks of drug treatment (Table 5-8).

Table 5-8 Effect of chronic drug treatment on ^{3}H-haloperidol binding[a,b]

Injected drug	Increase over untreated controls (%)	P
Haloperidol	19 ± 4	0.005
Fluphenazine	27 ± 12	0.05
Promethazine	3 ± 7	N.S.[c]

[a] After Burt *et al*. (1976).
[b] Rats were injected with haloperidol (Haldol) or fluphenazine (Prolixin) daily for 3 weeks and sacrificed 5 to 7 days later. Membranes were prepared from the corpora striata and were assayed for binding of ^{3}H-haloperidol. Samples were incubated, rinsed extensively to remove unbound drug and then counted by liquid scintillation to measure the bound drug.
[c] N.S., not significant.

This increase persists at least 12 days after drug treatment is stopped. Promethazine, a similar drug but lacking DA antagonist properties, fails to enhance binding. Thus prolonged inactivation of DA receptors stimulates the production of more receptors. It is quite possible that such increased receptor activity is one of the fundamental biochemical changes underlying abnormalities associated with withdrawal of the drug. The additional receptors result in hyperactive responses to released DA when the dosage is reduced. Dopamine receptors become supersensitive (Burt *et al*., 1976).

There is also evidence that supersensitivity results when dopamine synaptic activity is reduced by inhibiting dopamine synthesis with α-methyl-p-tyrosine (Moore and Thornburg, 1975), depleting DA storage with reserpine (Moore and Thornburg, 1975; Ungerstedt *et al*., 1975) or making lesions in the nigrostriatal DA pathway (Ungerstedt *et al*., 1975; Iversen and Creese, 1975). Thus, under certain conditions, as in denervation or chronic antagonist treatment, receptors and receptor-mediated events can be induced.

VI. Conclusion and Summary

The effect of a transmitter on a cell is to start or generate a message having characteristics different from its own. Indeed we have seen how rich and diverse these messages can be. The typical or classical response exemplified by a cholinergic synapse is a fast local change in the ionic permeability of the membrane. Such changes excite cells, and when they depolarize them, the depolarization is always mediated by a change in Na ion permeability. Permeability changes inhibit cells when they stabilize the membrane potential near the resting potential or hyperpolarize it. Inhibition is always mediated by an increase in K and/or Cl permeability or a decrease in Na permeability. Other synapses typified by catecholaminergic synapses change the membrane potential more slowly and bring about a profound change in the metabolism of their target cells. This influence is more than a transient ionic permeability change. This metabolic sequel to synaptic activity is long lasting and outlives the transmitter itself. In part, the metabolic influence is probably no more than the engagement of cellular metabolism, adjusting it from the resting level to a state able to deal with the synaptic artillery fire which drives holes in the membrane. In order to respond and continue responding the cell must step up its metabolism. However, there may be other purposes as well. Metabolic influences may change the general state of the cells excitability and set its subsequent response characteristics. While this sequel to synaptic action is most prominent at catecholaminergic synapses, it may not be strictly confined to this class. Other synapses (GABA-nergic and even cholinergic) appear in some cases to increase the levels of cGMP in their target cells; cGMP is a cyclic nucleotide which like cAMP can also act as a second messenger. At present little is known about such changes, but this will be a key area for future research.

All transmitters carry messages, but the messages appear as rich and diverse as the neurons themselves and their particular tasks. At the neuromuscular junction synaptic transmission brings a moment by moment message which is rapidly forgotten. This is really as it should be. Each movement of the muscle is a separate event which cares little about previous movements. The message is transferred and rapidly erased. In the CNS, however, the message surpasses the electrical disturbance at least in some cases. The nature of these messages is now being revealed as an electrical and chemical one, but much of what synapses are telling their target cells is still unknown.

Synapses are highly plastic: their message is dependent on previous stimulus history. Synaptic potentials can increase as during facilitation or potentiation, or decrease as during depression. Potentiation can last for minutes or hours. It depends on the stimulus conditions and importantly on the particular synapse. Other changes, such as enzyme induction or receptor sub- or supersensitivity, may persist for days. Studies on synaptic plasticity illustrate the basic capacity of synapses to generate graded responses and encode information in accordance with other past experience. These elementary forms of physiological plasticity are a very simple form of learning and information storage. Indeed, they form the foundation for a cellular analysis of learning and memory. Synapses are very adaptable, and there is much more to learn about the process and what is achieved by it. Only a few years ago synaptic transmission was viewed as an inhibitory or excitatory electrical disturbance, but in recent years the range of influences and knowledge of the plastic properties of synapses has expanded. In the future years it will no doubt continue to expand as we probe deeper into the mysteries of the mind at this fundamental level.

In Chapter 6 we shall look at a higher property of synaptic transmission. All the inputs to a cell need to be processed into an output. We shall explore the integration of synaptic activity. Then we shall explore the different elementary forms of behavioral plasticity and examine the underlying mechanisms. We shall see how neuronal networks function in a variety of situations.

Key Terms

Acetylcholine (ACh):   The transmitter released by vertebrate motor neurons, preganglionic sympathetic neurons and certain central neurons. The molecule is synthesized from choline and acetyl-coenzyme A by choline acetyltransferase.

Acetylcholinesterase: The enzyme which hydrolyzes ACh to form choline and acetate as products.

ACh noise: Small fluctuations of potential produced by ACh which correspond to random statistical variations in the opening and closing of a few ACh-activated channels.

ACh receptor: A protein complex which binds ACh and mediates the change in ion permeability at the postsynaptic membrane.

Adenylate cyclase: The enzyme which synthesizes cAMP from ATP. Its activity can be stimulated by certain transmitters.

Adrenoceptors: The term used to refer to the class of receptors for catecholamines.

Agonist: A molecule which activates synaptic receptors mimicking the action of the transmitter at that synapse.

Amphetamine: A drug which appears to act in part by promoting the efflux of catecholamines and to a lesser degree blocking their reuptake.

Antagonist: A molecule which inactivates synaptic receptors and decreases the effectiveness of the natural transmitter.

α-Bungarotoxin: A toxin from the venom of a snake which binds with very high affinity to the ACh receptor and acts as a powerful antagonist.

Calcium hypothesis: A hypothesis which states that depolarization of the presynaptic terminal causes calcium channels to open, which allows the entry of a few ions of calcium and catalyzes quantal transmitter release.

Cyclic adenosine monophosphate (cAMP): The second messenger; cAMP levels change in response to transmitter or hormones and cause changes in cellular metabolism.

Catecholamines: A class of molecules that contain a catechol nucleus and an ethylamine group. Catecholamines include dopamine, norepinephrine and epinephrine.

Catecholaminergic: Adjective used to refer to systems which employ catecholamines as transmitters (catecholaminergic neurons, etc.).

Choline acetyltransferase: The enzyme responsible for the synthesis of ACh.

Cholinergic: Adjective used to refer to systems which employ ACh as transmitter (cholinergic neurons, etc.).

Choline transport: The process by which choline is accumulated inside cells from the outside. Choline transport is the rate-limiting process in the biosynthesis of ACh.

Cocaine: A drug which has as one of its actions the ability to interfere with the reuptake of catecholamines.

Depression: A decrease in the amplitude of a synaptic potential as a result of repetitive stimulation.

Dopa decarboxylase: The enzyme which catalyzes the synthesis of dopamine from dopa.

Dopamine: A transmitter found primarily in the CNS.

Dopamine β-hydroxylase: The enzyme that converts dopamine to norepinephrine. It is present in norepinephrine storage vesicles and is released along with the transmitter.

Endocytosis: The process by which portions of the plasma membrane are withdrawn into the cell to form intracellular cisternae and vesicles. Synaptic vesicles are reformed, in part, by the endocytosis of the presynaptic plasma membrane.

Enzyme induction: A process which brings about an increase in the quantity of certain enzymes in response to a particular stimulus. Enzyme induction involves protein synthesis and the production of additional enzyme molecules.

Excitatory synaptic potential: A type of synaptic potential which depolarizes the cell and increases its excitability. At fast acting synapses the transmitter causes particular channels to open; sodium ions are always involved but others may be as well.

Exocytosis: The process by which intracellular vesicles fuse with the plasma membrane and dispel their contents from the cell. Transmitter release occurs by exocytosis.

Facilitation: A relatively short-term increase in the amplitude (< 1 sec) of the synaptic potential during repetitive stimulation.

Inhibitory synaptic potential: A type of synaptic potential which decreases the excitability of a target cell. At fast acting synapses inhibitory transmitters open ion channels which usually cause a slight hyperpolarization.

Miniature synaptic potential: A small change in the postsynaptic membrane potential caused by the spontaneous liberation of a single quantum of transmitter from the presynaptic terminal.

Myasthenia gravis: A disease of neuromuscular junctions characterized by extreme muscular fatigue. It is an autoimmune disease in which patients develop an immune reaction against their cholinergic receptors.

Norepinephrine: A transmitter liberated by most sympathetic neurons and certain central ones.

Phenylethanolamine-*N*-methyl transferase: The enzyme responsible for the synthesis of epinephrine from norepinephrine.

Potentiation: A relatively long-term increase in the synaptic potential observed during repetitive stimulation.

Quantal hypothesis: Each miniature synaptic potential corresponds to the release of one quantum of transmitter.

Quantal release: Secretion of packets of transmitter (quanta) by the presynaptic terminal. One quanta is presumed to correspond to the discharge of one synaptic vesicle.

Reserpine: A drug which interferes with the storage of catecholamines.

Supersensitivity: An increase in the sensitivity to chemical transmitters as a result of chronic drug treatment, denervation or other causes.

Synaptic potential: A postsynaptic potential recorded at a synapse in response to presynaptic activation.

Synaptic transmission: The means by which an electrical signal in one neuron passes from the terminal of its axon into another cell and initiates in that cell a signal having characteristics different from its own. In the mammalian CNS synaptic transmission is primarily chemical.

Synaptosomes: Isolated synaptic boutons which can be isolated from nervous tissue by subcellular fractionation procedures.

Tyrosine hydroxylase: The enzyme which converts tyrosine to dopa. It is the rate-limiting enzyme in the synthesis of catecholamines; its activity is decreased by the end products of the pathway in catecholamine synthesis (end-product inhibition) and is increased by cAMP or Ca^{2+}.

General References

Barrett, E. F., and Magleby, K. L. (1976). Physiology of cholinergic transmission. *In* "Biology of Cholinergic Function" (A. M. Goldberg, ed.), pp. 29–100. Raven, New York.

Cold Spring Harbor Symposia on Quantitative Biology (1976). "The Synapse," Vol. 40. Cold Spring Harbor Lab., Cold Spring Harbor, New York.

Kandel, E. (1977). "Cellular Basis of Behavior." Freeman, San Francisco, California.

Kuffler, S. W., and Nicholls, J. G. (1976). "From Neuron to Brain—A Cellular Approach to the Function of the Nervous System." Sinauer Assoc., Sunderland, Massachusetts.

Martin, A. R. (1977). Junctional transmission. II. *In* "Handbook of Physiology" (E. Kandel, ed.), Sect. 1, Vol. 1, pp. 329–355. Am. Physiol. Soc. Bethesda, Maryland.

References

Ahlquist, R. P. (1948). A study of the adrenotropic receptors. *Am. J. Physiol.* **153**, 586–600.

Almon, R. R., Andrew, C. G., and Appel, S. H. (1974). Serum globulin in myasthenia gravis: Inhibition of α-bungarotoxin binding to acetylcholine receptors. *Science* **186**, 55–57.

Anderson, C. R., and Stevens, C. F. (1973). Voltage clamp analysis of acetylcholine produced end-plate current fluctuations at frog neuromuscular junction. *J. Physiol. (London)* **235**, 655–691.

Antelman, S. M., and Caggiula, A. R. (1977). Norepinephrine-dopamine interactions and behavior. *Science* **195**, 646–653.

Axelrod, J. (1974a). The pineal gland: A neurochemical transducer. *Science* **184**, 1341–1348.

Axelrod, J. (1974b). Neurotransmitters. *Sci. Am.* **230**, 58–71.

Axelrod, J., Mueller, R. A., Henry, J. P., and Stephens, P. M. (1970). Changes in enzymes involved in the biosynthesis and metabolism of noradrenaline and adrenaline after psychosocial stimulation. *Nature (London)* **225**, 1059–1060.

Baker, R. (1976). Pharmacological profile of inhibition in the vestibular and ocular nuclei. *In* "Drugs and Central Synaptic Transmission" (P. B. Bradley and B. N. Dhawan, eds.), pp. 227–234. Macmillan, New York.

Barker, L. A., and Mittag, T. W. (1975). Comparative studies of substrates and inhibitors of choline transport and choline acetyltransferase. *J. Pharmacol. Exp. Ther.* **192**, 86–94.

Barrett, E. F., and Magleby, K. L. (1976). Physiology of cholinergic transmission. *In* "Biology of Cholinergic Function" (A. M. Goldberg and I. Hanin, eds.), pp. 29–100. Raven, New York.

Bender, A. N., Ringel, S. P., and Engel, W. F. (1976). Immunoperoxidase localization of alpha-bungarotoxin: A new approach to myasthenia gravis. *Ann. N.Y. Acad. Sci.* **274**, 20–30.

Bliss, T. V. P., and Gardner-Medwin, A. R. (1973). Long-lasting potentiation of synaptic transmission in the dentate area of the unanaesthetized rabbit following stimulation of the perforant path. *J. Physiol. (London)* **232**, 357–374.

Bliss, T. V. P., and Lømo, T. (1973). Long-lasting potentiation of synaptic transmission in the dentate area of the anaesthetized rabbit following stimulation of the perforant path. *J. Physiol. (London)* **232**, 331–356.

Burt, D. R., Creese, I., and Snyder, S. H. (1976). Antischizophrenic drugs: Chronic treatment elevates dopamine receptor binding in brain. *Science* **196**, 326–327.

Ceccarelli, B., Hurlbut, W. P., and Mauro, A. (1973). Turnover of transmitter and synaptic vesicles at the frog neuromuscular junction. *J. Cell Biol.* **57**, 499–524.

Colquhoun, D., Dionne, V. E., Steinbach, J. H., and Stevens, C. F. (1975). Conductance of channels opened by acetylcholine-like drugs in muscle-end plate. *Nature (London)* **253**, 204–206.

Costa, E., Guidotti, A., and Zivkovic, B. (1974). Short and long term regulation of tyrosine hydroxylase. *In* "Neuropsychopharmacology of Monamines and their Regulatory Enzymes" (E. Usdin, ed.), pp. 161–175. Raven, New York.

Cotman, C. W., Haycock, J. W., and White, W. F. (1976a). Stimulus-secretion coupling processes in brain: Analysis of norepinephrine and gamma-aminobutyric acid release. *J. Physiol. (London)* **254**, 475–505.

Cotman, C. W., Haycock, J. W., and Levy, W. B. (1976b). On the functional coupling of neurotransmitter uptake and release in brain. *Br. J. Pharmacol.* **58**, 569–572.

del Castillo, J., and Katz, B. (1954). Quantal components of the end-plate potential. *J. Physiol. (London)* **124**, 560–573.

Dionne, V. E., and Ruff, R. L. (1977). Endplate current fluctuations reveal only one channel type at frog neuromuscular junction. *Nature (London)* **266**, 263–265.

Erulkar, S. D., and Weight, F. F. (1977). Extracellular potassium and transmitter release at the giant synapse of squid. *J. Physiol. (London)* **266**, 209–218.

Fatt, P., and Katz, B. (1952). Spontaneous subthreshold activity at motor nerve endings. *J. Physiol. (London)* **117**, 109–128.

Fertuck, H. C., and Salpeter, M. M. (1976). Quantitation of junctional and extrajunctional acetylcholine receptors by electron microscope autoradiography after ^{125}I-α-bungarotoxin binding at mouse neuromuscular junctions. *J. Cell Biol.* **69**, 144–158.

Fifkova, E., and van Harreveld, A. (1977). Long lasting morphological changes in dendritic spines of dentate granular cells following stimulation of the entorhinal area. *J. Neurocytol.* **6**, 211–230.

Foster, M., and Sherrington, C. S. (1897). "A Textbook of Physiology," 7th ed., Part III. Macmillan, New York.

Gardner, D., and Kandel, E. R. (1972). Diphasic postsynaptic potential: A chemical synapse capable of mediating conjoint excitation and inhibition. *Science* **176**, 675–678.

Goodman, L. S., and Gilman, A., eds. (1975). "The Pharmacological Basis of Therapeutics," 5th ed. Macmillan, New York.

Guidotti, A., Hanbauer, I., and Costa, E. (1975). Role of cyclic nucleotides in the induction of tyrosine hydroxylase. *Adv. Cyclic Nucleotide Res.* **5**, 619–639.

Hanbauer, I., Kopin, I. J., and Costa, E. (1973). Mechanisms involved in the trans-synaptic increase of tyrosine hydroxylase and dopamine-β-hydroxylase activity in sympathetic ganglia. *Naunyn-Schmiedeberg's Arch. Pharmacol.* **280**, 39–48.

Harris, J. E., Morgenroth, V. H., III, Roth, R. H., and Baldesarini, R. J. (1974). Regulation of catecholamine synthesis in the rat brain *in vitro* by cyclic AMP. *Nature (London)* **252**, 156–158.

Hartzell, H. C., Kuffler, S. W., and Yoshikami, D. (1975). Post-synaptic potentiation: Interaction between quanta of acetylcholine at the skeletal neuromuscular synapse. *J. Physiol. (London)* **251**, 427–463.

Hartzell, H. C., Kuffler, S. W., and Yoshikami, D. (1976). The number of acetylcholine molecules in a quantum and the interaction between quanta at the subsynaptic membrane of the skeletal neuromuscular synapse. *Cold Spring Harbor Symp. Quant. Biol.* **40**, 175–186.

Henn, F. A., Goldstein, M. N., and Hamberger, A. (1974). Uptake of the neurotransmitter candidate glutamate by glia. *Nature (London)* **249**, 663–664.

Hess, G. P., and Andrews, J. P. (1977). Functional acetylcholine receptor–electroplax membrane microsacs (vesicles): Purification and characterization. *Proc. Natl. Acad. Sci. U.S.A.* **74**, 482–486.

Heuser, J. E., Reese, T. S. (1973). Evidence for recycling of synaptic vesicle membrane during transmitter release at the frog neuromuscular junction. *J. Cell Biol.* **57**, 315–344.

Iversen, S. D., and Creese, I. (1975). Behavioral correlates of dopaminergic supersensitivity. *Adv. Neurol.* **9**, 81–92.

Iversen, S. D., and Iversen, L. L. (1975). "Behavioral Pharmacology" Oxford Univ. Press, London and New York.

Kasai, M., and Changeux, J. P. (1971). *In vitro* excitation of purified membrane fragments by cholinergic agonists. *J. Membr. Biol.* **6**, 1–23.

Katz, B., and Miledi, R. (1967). A study of synaptic transmission in the absence of nerve impulses. *J. Physiol. (London)* **192**, 407–436.

Katz, B., and Miledi, R. (1970). Membrane noise produced by acetylcholine. *Nature (London)* **226**, 962–963.

REFERENCES

Katz, B., and Miledi, R. (1973). The effect of α-bungarotoxin on acetylcholine receptors. *Br. J. Pharmacol.* **49**, 138–179.

Kebabian, J. W., Zatz, M., Romero, J. A., and Axelrod, J. (1975). Rapid changes in rat pineal β-adrenergic receptor: Alterations in l-[³H]alprenolol binding and adenylate cyclase. *Proc. Natl. Acad. Sci. U.S.A.* **72**, 3735–3739.

Kebabian, J. W., Zatz., M., and O'Dea, R. F. (1977). Modulation of receptor sensitivity in the pineal: The role of cyclic nucleotides. *Soc. Neurosci. Symp.* **2**, 376–398.

Kitai, S. T., Sugimori, M., and Kocsis, J. D. (1976). Excitatory nature of dopamine in the nigro-caudate pathway. *Exp. Brain Res.* **24**, 351–363.

Kuffler, S. W., and Nicholls, J. G. (1976). "From Neuron to Brain—A Cellular Approach to the Function of the Nervous System." Sinauer Assoc. Sunderland, Massachusetts.

Kvetňanský, R., Gewirtz, G. P., Weise, V. K., and Kopin, I. J. (1971). Enhanced synthesis of adrenal dopamine β-hydroxylase induced by repeated immobilization in rats. *Mol. Pharmacol.* **7**, 81–86.

Lee, C. Y. (1972). Chemistry and pharmacology of polypeptide toxins in snake venoms. *Annu. Rev. Pharmacol.* **12**, 265–286.

Levitt, M., Spector, S., Sjoerdsma, A., and Udenfriend, S. (1965). Elucidation of the rate-limiting step in norepinephrine biosynthesis in the perfused guinea-pig heart. *J. Pharmacol. Exp. Ther.* **148**, 1–8.

Libet, B., and Kobayashi, H. (1974). Adrenergic mediation of slow inhibitory postsynaptic potential in sympathetic ganglia of the frog. *J. Neurophysiol.* **37**, 805–814.

Libet, B., and Tosaka, T. (1970). Dopamine as a synaptic transmitter and modulator in sympathetic ganglia: A different mode of synaptic action. *Proc. Natl. Acad. Sci. U.S.A.* **67**, 667–673.

Liley, A. W. (1956). An investigation of spontaneous activity at the neuromuscular junction of the rat. *J. Physiol. (London)* **132**, 650–666.

Llinas, R., and Nicholson, C. (1975). Calcium role in depolarization–secretion coupling: An aequorin study in squid giant synapse. *Proc. Natl. Acad. Sci. U.S.A.* **72**, 187–190.

Llinas, R., Steinberg, I. E., and Walton, K. (1976). Presynaptic calcium currents and their relation to synaptic transmission: Voltage clamp study in squid giant synapse and theoretical model for the calcium gate. *Proc. Natl. Acad. Sci. U.S.A.* **73**, 2918–2992.

Loewi, O. (1921). Uber humorale Übertragbarkeit der herznervenwirkung. *Pfluegers Arch. Gesamte Physiol. Menschen Tiere* **189**, 239–242.

Magleby, K. L., and Stevens, C. F. (1972). The effect of voltage on the time-course of end-plate currents. *J. Physiol.* **223**, 151–171.

Magleby, K. L., and Stevens, C. F. (1972). A quantitative description of end-plate currents. *J. Physiol.* **223**, 173–197.

Martin, A. R. (1977). Junctional transmission. II. *In* "Handbook of Physiology" (E. Kandel, ed.), Sect. 1, Vol. 1, pp. 329–355. Am. Physiol. Soc., Bethesda, Maryland.

Martin, A. R., and Pilar, G. (1964). Presynaptic and post-synaptic events during post-tetanic potentiation and facilitation in the avian ciliary ganglion. *J. Physiol. (London)* **175**, 17–30.

Michaelson, D. M., and Raftery, M. A. (1974). Purified acetylcholine receptor: Its reconstitution to a chemically excitable membrane. *Proc. Natl. Acad. Sci. U.S.A.* **71**, 4768–4772.

Miledi, R. (1973). Transmitter release induced by injection of calcium ions into nerve terminals. *Proc. R. Soc. London, Ser. B* **183**, 421–425.

Miledi, R., and Thies, R. (1971). Tetanic and post-tetanic rise in frequency of miniature end-plate potentials in low calcium solutions. *J. Physiol. (London)* **212**, 245–257.

Molinoff, P. B., Brimijoin, S., Weinshilboum, R., and Axelrod, J. (1970). Neurally mediated increase in dopamine-β-hydroxylase activity. *Proc. Natl. Acad. Sci. U.S.A.* **66**, 453–458.

Molinoff, P. B., Brimijoin, S., and Axelrod, J. (1972). Induction of dopamine-β-hydroxylase and tyrosine hydroxylase in rat hearts and sympathetic ganglia. *J. Pharmacol. Exp. Ther.* **182**, 116–129.

Moore, K. E., and Thornburg, J. E. (1975). Drug-induced dopaminergic supersensitivity. *Adv. Neurol.* **9**, 93–104.

Morgenroth, V. H., III, Boadle-Biber, M., and Roth, R. H. (1974). Tyrosine hydroxylase: Activation by nerve stimulation. *Proc. Natl. Acad. Sci. U.S.A.* **71**, 4283–4287.

Mueller, R. A., Thoenen, H., and Axelrod, J. (1969). Inhibition of transsynaptically increased tyrosine hydroxylase activity by cycloheximide and actinomycin D. *Mol. Pharmacol.* **5**, 463–469.

Mueller, R. A., Thoenen, H., and Axelrod, J. (1970). Effect of pituitary and ACTH on the maintenance of basal tyrosine hydroxylase activity in rat adrenal gland. *Endocrinology* **86**, 751–755.

Nathanson, J. A. (1977). Cyclic nucleotides and nervous system function. *Physiol. Rev.* **57**, 157–256.

Nathanson, J. A., and Greengard, P. (1977). "Second messengers" in the brain. *Sci. Am.* **237**, 108–119.

Palay, S. L., and Chan-Palay, V. (1976). A guide to the synaptic analysis of the neuropil. *Cold Spring Harbor Symp. Quant. Biol.* **40**, 1–16.

Patrick, J., and Lindstrom, J. M. (1973). Autoimmune response to acetylcholine receptor. *Science* **180**, 871–872.

Potter, L. T. (1970). Synthesis, storage and release of [^{14}C]acetylcholine in isolated rat diaphragm muscles. *J. Physiol. (London)* **206**, 145–166.

Raftery, M. A., Vandlen, R. L., Reed, K. L., and Lee, T. (1976). Characterization of *Torpedo californica* acetylcholine receptor: Its subunit composition and ligand-binding properties in the synapse. *Cold Spring Harbor Sym. Quant. Biol.* **40**, 193–202.

Rash, J. E., Albuquerque, E. X., Hudson, C. S., Mayer, R. F., and Satterfield, J. R. (1976). Studies of human myasthenia gravis: Electrophysiological and ultrastructural evidence compatible with antibody attachment to acetylcholine receptor complex. *Proc. Natl. Acad. Sci. U.S.A.* **73**, 4584–4588.

Romero, J. A., and Axelrod, J. (1975). Regulation of sensitivity to Beta-adrenergic stimulation in induction of pineal N-acetyltransferase. *Proc. Natl. Acad. Sci. U.S.A.* **72**, 1661–1665.

Rosenthal, J. (1969). Post-tetanic potentiation at the neuromuscular junction of the frog. *J. Physiol. (London)* **203**, 121–133.

Roth, R., Morgenroth, V., III, and Salzman, P. U. (1975). Tyrosine hydroxylase: Allosteric activation induced by stimulation of central noradrenergic neurons. *Naunyn-Schmiedeberg's Arch. Pharmacol.* **289**, 327–343.

Rutledge, C. O., and Weiner, N. J. (1967). The effect of reserpine upon the synthesis of norepinephrine in the isolated rabbit heart. *J. Pharmacol. Exp. Ther.* **157**, 290–302.

Schlapfer, W. T., Tremblay, J. P., Woodson, P. B. J., and Barondes, S. H. (1976). Frequency facilitation and post-tetanic potentiation of a unitary synaptic potential in *Aplysia californica* are limited by different processes. *Brain Res.* **109**, 1–20.

Segal, M., and Bloom, F. E. (1974). The action of norepinephrine in the rat hippocampus. II. Activation of the input pathway. *Brain Res.* **72**, 99–114.

Segal, M., and Bloom, F. E. (1976). The action of norepinephrine in the rat hippocampus. III. Hippocampal cellular responses to locus coeruleus stimulation in the awake rat. *Brain Res.* **107**, 499–511.

Sherrington, C. (1961). "The Integrative Action of the Nervous System." Yale Univ. Press, New Haven, Connecticut.

Siggins, G. R. (1978). Electrophysiological role of dopamine in striatum: Excitatory or inhibitory? *In* "Psychopharmacology: A Generation of Progress" (M. A. Lipton, A. Di Mascio, and K. F. Killam, eds.), pp. 143–157. Raven, New York.

Siggins, G. R., Hoffer, B. J., and Bloom, F. E. (1969). Cyclic adenosine monophosphate: Possible mediator for norepinephrine effects on cerebellar Purkinje cells. *Science* **165**, 1018–1020.

Siggins, G. R., Hoffer, B. J., and Bloom, F. E. (1971a). Studies on norepinephrine-containing afferents to Purkinje cells of rat cerebellum. III. Evidence for mediation of norepinephrine effects in cyclic 3′,5′-adenosine monophosphate. *Brain Res.* **25**, 535–553.

Siggins, G. R., Oliver, A. P., Hoffer, B. J., and Bloom, F. E. (1971b). Cyclic adenosine monophosphate and norepinephrine: Effects on transmembrane properties of cerebellar Purkinje cells. *Science* **171**, 192–194.

Simon, J. R., Atweh, S., and Kuhar, M. J. (1976). Sodium-dependent high affinity choline uptake: A regulatory step in the synthesis of acetylcholine. *J. Neurochem.* **26**, 909–922.

Snyder, S. H. (1976). The dopamine hypothesis of schizophrenia: Focus on the dopamine receptor. *Am. J. Psychiatry* **133**, 197–202.

Snyder, S. H., Young, A. B., Bennett, J. R., and Mulder, A. H. (1973). Synaptic biochemistry of amino acids. *Fed. Proc., Fed. Am. Soc. Exp. Biol.* **32**, 2039–2047.

Thoenen, H. (1970). Induction of tyrosine hydroxylase in peripheral and central adrenergic neurons by cold-exposure of rats. *Nature (London)* **228**, 861–862.

Thoenen, H., Mueller, R. A., and Axelrod, J. (1969). Transsynaptic induction of adrenal tyrosine hydroxylase. *J. Pharmacol. Exp. Ther.* **169**, 249–254.

Thoenen, H., Kettler, R., Burkard, W., and Saner, A. (1971). Neurally mediated control of enzymes involved in the synthesis of norepinephrine: Are they regulated as an operational unit? *Naunyn-Schmiedebergs Arch. Pharmakol.* **270**, 146–160.

Undenfriend, S., Zaltzman-Nirenberg, P., and Nagatsu, T. (1965). Inhibitors of purified beef adrenal tyrosine hydroxylase. *Biochem. Pharmacol.* **14**, 837–845.

Ungerstedt, U., Ljungberg, T., Hoffer, B., and Siggins, G. (1975). Dopaminergic supersensitivity in the striatum. *Adv. Neurol.* **9**, 57–65.

van Harreveld, A., and Fifkova, E. (1974). Involvement of glutamate in memory formation. *Brain Res.* **81**, 455–467.

von Euler, U. S. (1956). "Noradrenaline." Thomas, Springfield, Illinois.

Weight, F. F., and Padjen, A. (1973). Slow synaptic inhibition: Evidence for synaptic inactivation of sodium conductance in sympathetic ganglian cells. *Brain Res.* **55**, 219–224.

Weiner, N., Cloutier, G., Bjur, R., and Pfeffer, R. I. (1972). Modification of norepinephrine synthesis in intact tissue by drugs and during short-term adrenergic nerve stimulation. *Pharmacol. Rev.* **24**, 203–221.

Weinshilboum, R., and Axelrod, J. (1970). Dopamine-β-hydroxylase activity in the rat after hypophysectomy. *Endocrinology* **87**, 894–899.

Weinshilboum, R., and Axelrod, J. (1971). Reduced plasma dopamine-β-hydroxylase activity in familial dysautonomia. *N. Engl. J. Med.* **285**, 938–942.

Zigmond, R. E. (1976). The role of preganglionic nerve activity in the regulation of tyrosine hydroxylase in the superior cervical ganglion. *In* "Catecholamines and Stress" (E. Usdin, R. Kvetnanský, and I. J. Kopin, eds.), pp. 283–291. Pergamon, Oxford.

6

Integration: Putting It All Together

I. Introduction

In the brain the computational capacities are so immense that they are difficult to even imagine. A single thought can be elaborated in less than a second, and it engages many millions of nerve cells. Initially, probably only a few thousand neurons would be activated, but each in turn would quickly activate others so that almost instantly millions become engaged in a scintillating spatiotemporal pattern. There is a moment by moment pulsation of events as single neurons and colonies of them examine patterns of activity and distribute their summaries to other parts of the circuit. The Nobel prize-winning physiologist, Sir Charles Sherrington, envisioned the activity patterns going on in the brain as "an enchanted loom." This loom, he wrote in 1947, weaves ". . . a dissolving pattern . . . always a meaningful pattern though never an abiding one. . . . a shifting harmony of subpatterns. . . ."

How is a pattern of information computed and translated into a meaningful output? In order to understand information processing in the nervous system we need to know the circuitry: not every wire and connection, but the general rules of the game. Who talks to whom? We need to know the language: what one set of neurons says to another to impart information and to get a response. In its simplest form we need to know how a single neuron integrates specific inputs and generates a specific output. The essence of signal processing lies in understanding the transactions at the level of a single cell. How does one neuron view the whole business? Given the answer to this key question we could at least theoretically reconstruct the details of the entire operation.

It is not possible at present, however, to build up the nervous system from its basic units. Integration exists at a number of levels—a monosynaptic reflex, a volitional movement, a thought. It is very complex. Accordingly, integration must be studied at a number of levels. It is a convergence of inputs on a single cell; it is groups of cells mixing their input with other groups of cells and coming out with particular messages; it is the operation of discrete systems in their totality (the auditory system, visual system, motor system, etc.) elaborating a response, or a thought; and finally it is the emergence of the total function of the nervous system bringing forth movements from particular parts of the body and not others as we shift our behaviors in a meaningful pattern. Patterns of activity grow in particular groups of neurons, while others dissolve in the background and await their turn perhaps in the next moment. In this chapter we will begin to study integration. We will analyze the interactions of synaptic inputs at the level of the single neuron.

We will also describe the organization and general functions of particular neurotransmitter systems in the CNS. Is the brain chemically coded so that particular chemicals serve particular functions? Are there specific transmitters for pleasure, for pain, for certain behaviors or behavioral abnormalities? Is there coding and integration in terms of particular chemical systems? Much contemporary research into the mechanisms of behavior depends on an understanding of the chemical coding of brain circuitry.

II. Neuronal Integration at the Level of a Single Neuron

The basic unit of integration is the neuron. Every single neuron computes, integrates, and records signals into a pattern of action potentials. Many different types of inputs converge and tell their story, coded in excitatory and inhibitory synaptic potentials, to the surface of the neuron. Each millisecond throughout its life the neuron experiences fluctuating patterns of excitation and inhibition due to the individual activity of thousands of synapses. The job of each neuron (and a motor neuron is a good example) is to integrate all signals, decide when to fire its own action potential, and thus pass a signal on to the next element in the circuit, which for the motor neuron is a muscle. A spinal motor neuron, for example, receives input from peripheral sources, intraspinal connections, and descending channels from the brain. All these bits of information, urgings, and commands must be integrated in a precise way. Since these are the last neurons to process information before the decisive orders flow back out of the nervous system to the effector organs, errors in computation leading to an inappropriate response could cost the animal its life.

The basic mechanisms used in integrating synaptic potentials are generally the same in all neurons, but the details are now known to depend on the exact neuronal type. *Projection neurons* (see Chapter 3), such as motor neurons, are polarized; they receive inputs on their dendrites and soma and transmit action potentials via axons. Integration in dendrites is either passive (electrotonic) or active (involving patches of membrane capable of firing action potentials). On the other hand, *local circuit neurons*, which are nonpolarized and do not have axons, have another means of integration. These cells receive inputs on dendrites and the soma, but the fibers and synapses that bring in these inputs to the target cell are also the ones that take the latter's output away. Therefore, since the presynaptic elements of these two-way junctions are located very close to the outgoing postsynaptic activity (in fact, side by side), the graded electrotonic and summation decay of the postsynaptic potentials is sufficient to modulate the output of these axonless cells. These axonless or *amacrine* neurons are really curious to contemplate; in a sense, they have to listen and talk through their dendrites, and the conversations held there are much more subdued than the decisive "all-or-none" commands other neurons shout down their axons.

A. Projection Neurons with Passive Dendrites

Since the time of Sherrington, the accepted function of dendrites in most CNS neurons has been to integrate spatiotemporally the afferent activity impinging on a cell, in order to "decide" whether and when the axon hillock will initiate an action potential. Dendritic trees, and their spines when present, provide an extensive surface upon which thousands of individual synapses may be accommodated. Individual synapses work on dendrites as they do on any other part of a nerve cell or a muscle cell; activation of receptors at the synaptic junction punches specific holes in the membrane, allowing particular ions to flow in and out of the dendrite thus creating currents. Once the total synaptic activity of the neuron rises to a level that is great enough to depolarize the axon hillock membrane past the threshold for an action potential, the neuron fires.

The spread of synaptic activity within the dendrites and over the somatic membrane is the central issue to grasp in understanding the principles underlying the summation of afferent signals. The spread of current away from a synapse depends upon (1) the time course and magnitude of current flow occurring at the synapse and (2) the cable properties of the dendrites.

Most dendrites are _inexcitable_ and do not generate action potentials. In this case the dendritic tree can be modeled as an arrangement of interconnected cylinders (Fig. 6-1) which individually behave like leaky cables. Thus a given segment of dendrite behaves in accordance with the same cable properties previously described for the _electrotonic_ spread of an action potential; the spread of potential is determined by the space constant, which is inversely proportional to the square root of the dendritic diameter (see Chapter 4), and by the time

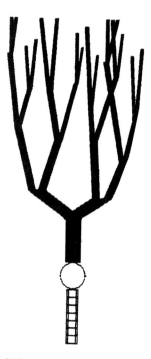

Fig. 6-1. Model of a dendritic tree of a frog Purkinje cell. The dendrite can be reconstructed from cylinders with specified diameters, membrane properties and core resistances. (From Pellionisz and Llinas, 1977.)

6. INTEGRATION: PUTTING IT ALL TOGETHER

constant of that particular patch of membrane. The extent of spread within a branch is a function of the geometry and membrane characteristics of the entire tree. Currents supplied to one part of a dendrite behave electrotonically, spread through the low resistance axoplasm of the dendrite, and with distance dissipate through the leaky membrane.

Computations within a classical neuron, like deliberations of a committee, are carried out by consensus, but with an important difference. Each synaptic input has a vote, but unlike the vote of a committee member, that vote is weighed by how powerful it is. A synapse casts its vote in terms of an electrical current. The current-injecting power of a synapse and its location on the neuronal surface contribute to its efficacy by virtue of the fraction of its current which can reach the axon hillock. Overall, the dendrite is a mosaic of excited synapses, each of which injects tiny currents. These currents all add up like small tributaries flowing into the main dendritic stream (Fig. 6-2). The process of integration over space and time that results from this confluence of signals is called *spatiotemporal summation*.

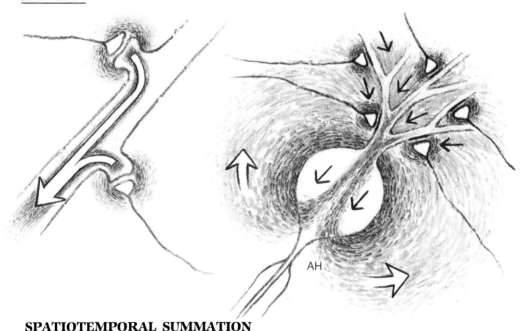

SPATIOTEMPORAL SUMMATION

Fig. 6-2. Activated dendritic synapses start an inward current which flows toward the cell body in accordance with the cable properties of the dendrites. Currents originating from different places and at different times all summate. The total current which reaches the axon hillock (AH) determines whether or not the cell will fire. The threshold for initiating an action potential is lowest at the axon hillock, so when the depolarizing current is strong enough to move the membrane potential past threshold an action potential fires. Arrows show the direction of positive ion flow.

It is important to note that the individual synaptic potentials that impinge on a neuron in the CNS are smaller than those at the neuromuscular junction. For example, synaptic potentials generated within motor neurons of the spinal cord can be studied by stimulation of a single dorsal root muscle afferent (group IA) fiber. Recorded at the cell body, each synaptic potential is only a few microvolts. A synaptic potential would be a few millivolts at the synaptic junction, but synaptic potentials are attenuated due to the cable properties between the synapses and cell body (Redman, 1973). Each group IA synaptic potential is generated by the release of only a few quanta, probably in fact only one (Kuno, 1971). This is probably the case at most CNS synapses. The release of 200–300 quanta typical of the neuromuscular junction would be most unfortunate for central neurons. It would allow a CNS neuron to be fired by a few synapses; there could be no integration. It would be like a committee of, say, 30 people, where only three votes were enough to carry a motion. This is an anarchy not a democracy! Thus, the reduced transmitter output in the CNS, together with dendritic attenuation of signals after receipt, are significant design features that allow many synaptic inputs to be processed simultaneously and meaningfully.

In most neurons it appears that distal synapses are somewhat less influential than proximal ones. It is impossible at present to record synaptic potentials at all levels of dendrites to the same applied current, but the behavior of synaptic potentials can be simulated by a computer model using the geometric and electrical properties of actual neurons. Figure 6-3 shows how synaptic potentials are affected by their dendritic location. We see that the synaptic potential which activates the outer dendritic tree further from the cell body (Fig. 6-3A) is a few millivolts and shows a steep rise to its peak amplitude. As the potential is passively conducted to the cell body it decreases in amplitude and its rate of rise is slower, due to the electrotonic properties of the dendrites. The closer to the cell body the synapse is located, the less the synaptic potential is attentuated (Fig. 6-3B) by the time it reaches the cell body.

Quite surprisingly, in motor neurons there seems to be (for some synapses at least) little or no tendency for peak amplitude of synaptic potentials to decrease between the time a signal arrives on some relatively remote part of the dendritic tree and when it finally gets down to the cell body (Iansek and Redman, 1973). The transfer of electrical charge appears somewhat independent of position, at least for the endings of group IA fibers (large caliber muscle stretch afferents). Synaptic drive (current power) and the geometric electrical properties of the dendrites are such that distal synapses are as effective, or nearly so, as proximal ones. In these neurons the presence of dendritic spines and a booster mechanism (see next section) for strengthening transient and feeble excitations at the tips of branches are two reasons why distal and proximal synapses can have a similar influence.

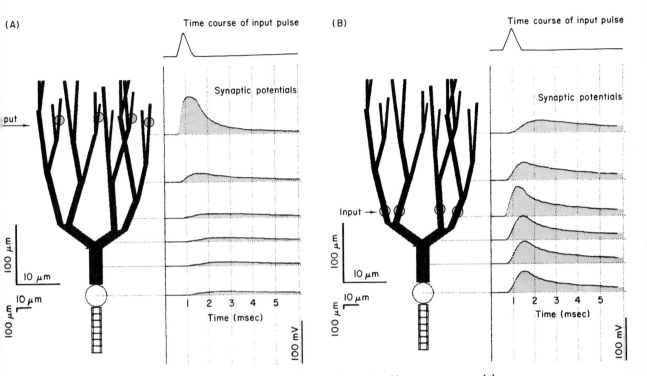

Fig. 6-3. Behavior of synaptic potentials in a Purkinje cell simulated by computer modeling. A symmetrical pulse is applied (top record) which represents the opening and closing gradually of a standard number of synapses on the branches marked by a shaded circle along the upper level of the dendrites (A) or lower level of dendrites (B). The time function and strength of input to one branch is the same in all cases. Distally active synapses generate a potential which decays rapidly and is extremely reduced when it reaches the cell body. Active synapses closer to the cell body are less attenuated. Model parameters are those described in Pellionisz and Llinas (1977) using a 5 MΩ input resistance. (Figure courtesy of Pellionisz and Llinas.)

B. Role of Dendritic Spines in Integration: The Synaptic Equalizer

Most dendritic excitatory synapses in the CNS are on spines (bulbous protrusions of the dendrite with a narrow neck). The diameter of the spine neck in a Purkinje cell is small, about ten times the distance across the synaptic cleft, or 2000 Å compared to 200 Å. Such a constriction gives the neck very high longitudinal resistance, about 20 MΩ (20×10^6 Ω). In contrast, a typical dendritic cable has a low longitudinal resistance, only a few ohms. (Remember, the resistance of a cylinder is *inversely* proportional to its diameter.)

Spines are believed to have two functions: (1) to maintain and protect currents during synaptic transmission from decreases caused by large local variation of input resistance along the length of the dendrite and (2) to convert synapses into a nearly constant current source. Both functions aid the neuron in obtaining a linear summation of all synaptic potentials regardless of their position on the dendrites (Llinas and Hillman, 1969). In keeping with this interpretation, spines tend to become more and more numerous on the more distal ramifications of the dendritic tree. The Purkinje cell of the cerebellum is a good example; its finer dendritic divisions are studded with spines and therefore usually referred to as "spiny branchlets."

Synapses at the tips of dendrites must inject sufficient current to have effects on the cell body. Active synapses imposed between such distal synapses and the soma, however, oppose these effects by decreasing the local resistance of the membrane. Currents can also flow out through an activated low resistance synapse, so that active synapses near each other could drastically reduce the effectiveness of each other. Therefore, we can say that adjacent synapses could "short-circuit" each other, were it not for spines.

It is currently theorized that by isolating synapses on spines, the short-circuit effect is minimized. More of the current from distal active synapses flowing in the cable—the dendritic core—will bypass the high resistance routes back into the necks of active spines in favor of the low resistance path to the soma. Spines thus maximize the effectiveness of remote synapses by offering great obstacles—their necks—to current flow from these synapses out of the channel shared by all synaptic currents flowing to the soma: the dendrites.

Spines also convert synapses into "constant current-injecting devices," such that each synapse can make an approximately equal contribution independent of its position. The high resistance of the spine neck does indeed significantly reduce the current injected into the core of the dendrite at that point, but because the resistance of the cable core is very low, the size of individual synaptic currents is reduced very little once it enters the core.

Therefore, the spine and its neck are a great "equalizer." (An entertaining way to think about this is to recall that once in the Old West a Colt .45 revolver was called the great "equalizer." There, as here, the little guy had just as good a chance as the big guy, and the distance mattered little.) No matter where it is located, if a synapse has a spine it will inject a very similar current into the soma. Spines provide a critically important way of equalizing the effectiveness of synapses over an expanse of dendritic surface that is vast and far-reaching with respect to each synapse (see Fig. 6-4).

Spines may also serve as a means to modify the effectiveness of particular dendritic synapses. A slight difference in the diameter of the neck of a spine could

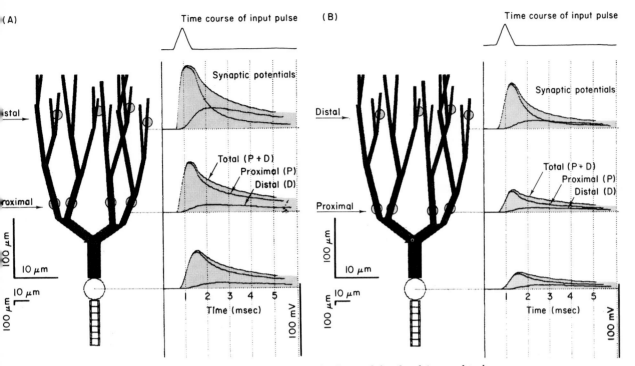

Fig. 6-4. Synaptic inputs at top of dendrite and near the base of the dendrite tend to be equalized when the synapses terminate on a spine with a relatively high resistance neck. Data are generated from a computer model of a Purkinje cell as described in Fig. 6-3. In (A) synapses terminate on a relatively low resistance spine (5 MΩ). The figure shows the potentials generated when the upper level synapses alone (D) or lower level (P) alone are active or when both are active together (T). Synapses active on the inner dendrite account almost completely for the summated potential (T) at the cell body. In (B) all synapses terminate on high resistance spines (25 MΩ). Synaptic activity nearest the cell body (P) is greatly reduced by the imposing spine necks. Now the summated potential at the cell body is a more balanced composite of upper and lower level synaptic action. It should be pointed out that the short circuit effect is not illustrated because in this particular cell when both synaptic sets are activated at once the current from upper level synaptic activity reaches the lower level synaptic sites when their action is nearly over. Thus currents from the outer synapses are spared the short circuit. (Courtesy of Pellionisz and Llinas.)

greatly alter the ease with which a current gets through. Small changes in spine geometry can modify the amount of current injected into the dendritic core. As was noted in Chapter 5, one of the mechanisms underlying long-term neuronal responsiveness or potentiation in the hippocampus may prove to be an increased diameter in the necks of spines. Perhaps, by shrinking or swelling, the neck region could play a critical role in learning or memory.

C. Inhibition: Stopping Is as Important as Starting

Neurons receive inhibitory as well as excitatory signals. Up to now we have said little about these important messages. Inhibitory signals are essential to the operation of the brain. Inhibition cuts into excitation and sculptures patterns of activity from larger blocks of general excitatory activity. Furthermore, inhibition is necessary to stop what has been started. We shall see inhibitory interneurons serving in a feedback capacity to inhibit further firing, just like a brake applied after the accelerator in a motor vehicle. Brake failure is disastrous and so is loss of inhibition. In the CNS when inhibition is removed pharmacologically, the brain readily goes into a seizure, an explosive and often self-injurious display of runaway excitation.

Inhibitory neurons also serve to provide *contrast*—sharp edges or limits to patterns of neuronal activity, as in the clear-cut transitions between shades of what we see in a photograph that has "snap." Old-fashioned long-exposure photographs gave blurry borders because they did not have "snap." Lateral inhibition, as found in the cerebral cortex alongside columns of cells, acts to sharpen up beams of excitation; the same phenomenon is seen in many other neural structures where analytical functions are especially well developed.

Inhibition is, therefore, an essential feature of brain operation: it provides the shading to give the mechanism appropriate responses, fine control and clarity of analysis. It refines excitation and enhances integration.

The most common mode of inhibition in the brain is a decrease in resistance across the neuronal membrane and a hyperpolarization (hypernegativity away from firing levels) probably mediated by an increase in Cl^- ion permeability (Baker, 1976). (In CNS neurons, the equilibrium potential for chloride is probably about -100 mV.) Inhibition "defuses" excitation for two reasons: (1) the same amount of excitation will be less effective because the membrane potential is farther from threshold, and (2) excitatory currents will be shunted out of the dendrite through the areas of reduced resistance (see also Chapter 5, Section III, B, 1). This "one-two punch" can effectively knock out or hammer patterns of excitation into the desired state of control (Fig. 6-5).

A less common mode of inhibition, used by some catecholaminergic systems, is mediated by an *increase* in membrane resistance along with the usual hyperpolarization. Here, inhibition is due to the hyperpolarization itself, which moves the membrane farther from the action potential threshold (see also Chapter 5, Section IV, C).

Most often, inhibitory synapses are placed on the cell body. There, they can have the "last word" on whether to let excitation pass and discharge the neuron. The mathematical study of neurons suggests, however, that distal dendritic inhibition can be more selective and offer finer control (at least in some cases) than inhibition of the soma (Redman, 1976). However, if inhibition is to be generalized and have maximum impact on excitatory inputs to the proximal regions of dendrites, the optimal location for inhibitory input is the soma.

In summary, in the classical projection neuron with passive dendritic conduction, dendrites integrate all excitatory and inhibitory currents over space and time by summation. Currents spread electrotonically in the processes of the neuron and are added up or subtracted, as on an abacus, by the membrane investing the cell body. The threshold for initiating an action potential is lowest at the *axon hillock*, so when the total inward depolarizing current at the axon hillock is strong enough to bring the membrane potential there past threshold, the neuron fires. The

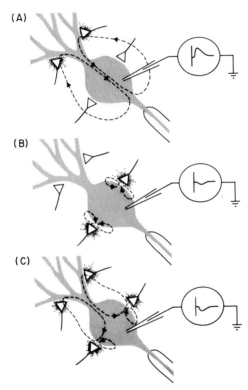

Fig. 6-5. Mechanism of synaptic inhibition. (A) Dendritic excitatory synaptic activity resulting in inward currents and depolarizations. (B) An inhibitory synaptic activity causing a decrease in membrane resistance and a hyperpolarization of the cell membrane. The permeability is increased primarily to Cl^-. Chloride ions are more concentrated outside the cell than inside so Cl^- flows in and makes the interior more negative. An outward flow of K^+ ions may also contribute. (C) Effect of inhibition on excitation. Excitatory synaptic currents leak out through the lower resistance created by inhibition and so dissipate prior to reaching the axon hillock. The hyperpolarization also makes threshold further away so that suprathreshold stimulation is insufficient to fire the cell. Arrows show the direction of positive ion flow.

neuron may receive thousands, perhaps hundreds of thousands, of inputs, but it has only one output line (the axon) and only one kind of output message, a pattern of action potentials.

In a sense, then, all a neuron can do is *fire* or *not fire*. Such a binary choice may seem meager and disappointing as far as the role of individual nerve cells goes, but consider again the space and time aspects of neuronal activity, now with respect to output to other neurons rather than to input of dendritic signals to cell body. Where does that message go? How many other neurons in various places throughout the brain and spinal cord get a copy of that message through branches of that axon? How important is the message? How urgent? These answers lie in the candidate codes—a tremendous range of response from a "blip" now and then, through an uneven "stuttering," to a ceaseless volley of signals (an electrical storm of reported events) (see Chapter 3).

Synaptic currents reflecting the activity patterns of thousands of synapses reach the axon hillock in waves and discharge it. In a busy neuron we can envision synaptic currents at the hillock fluttering above and below threshold. The firing pattern depends on how long depolarization exceeds threshold, as well as on other individualized firing properties of the neuron which differ widely among the various types of cells. Large suprathreshold synaptic potentials will stay above threshold for a longer period of time and thus cause multiple action potentials, since the potential will take longer to decay below threshold. Sustained depolarization of this sort can cause repetitive firing at a particular range of frequencies peculiar to that neuron.

Neurons respond differently. They have "personalities"—some are unusually talkative, others quiet, still others moderately conversational. Some neurons respond to a single stimulus with a single action potential. Others respond with short self-limiting bursts of spikes to a single strong input. Some interneurons fire very rapidly, like machine guns to a touch on the trigger, 800 spikes per second to a brief stimulus! In general, neurons have particular input–output functions or ratios characteristic of the cell class. These characteristics are analogous to the distinctive patterns produced by guns—a pistol, an automatic rifle, a machine gun. The same disturbance, pulling the trigger, gives a single report or repetitive series of bursts.

In the CNS, neurons are always firing to a greater or lesser degree, depending on whether they are discharging spontaneously (as many of them do) or just "resting," waiting to discharge to some stimulus. If an electrophysiologist lowers a microelectrode into the brain of an anesthetized animal, neurons will be found that are discharging, and in some cases the scientist can easily recognize particular cells by their discharge pattern. Purkinje cells in the cerebellar cortex exhibit strong intrinsic activity and are always spontaneously active. Excitation does not initiate their activity; it only speeds the rate up, as inhibition slows it down. You can readily imagine the coding value of such frequency modulation. The cell's function can be increased or decreased. Spinal motor neurons, on the other hand, await activation. When they work, muscles contract and tasks are performed; sometimes, they are better off doing nothing. But in the end, the fine structure of each neuron is tailored to allow that cell to perform its own role in the integration of body activity.

D.   Projection Neurons with Active Dendrites

In some neurons there is another mode of propagation in dendrites in addition to the normal passive spread of current with decay over distance. Dendrites in some cells generate potentials, that are similar to an action potential, and so propagation is *active*. The earliest observation that normal neurons could produce a propagated dendritic potential was with intracellular recording in hippocampal pyramidal cells (Spencer and Kandel, 1961). Small "all-or-none" potentials, called fast prepotentials, were often seen prior to action potentials in the pyramidal cell axon. Evidence was found to suggest that these prepotentials represented activity of distal patches of electrically active membrane, perhaps located at dendritic bifurcations.

Better evidence came later, however, from studies on the cerebellar Purkinje cell. In a rather remarkable experiment, Llinas and Nicholson (1971) penetrated a neuronal process with a fine electrode, recorded an action potential, and then, by passing a small current to fill the process electrophoretically with a dye, proved by subsequent microscopic study that the process was in fact a dendrite.

Now we know that action potentials or spikes are generated in dendrites of other neurons besides those of the pyramidal cells of the hippocampus and Purkinje cells of the cerebellar cortex (see Pellionisz and Llinas, 1977; Stone and Freeman, 1971), but at the present time the abundance of neurons with active dendrites in the CNS is not known. Their presence may be expected, however, where the cell has an elaborate and far-reaching dendritic tree on which remote distal synapses appear to need a booster system of this sort to communicate with the cell body.

Action potentials on Purkinje cell dendrites appear to be Ca^{2+} *spikes*, rather than the Na^+-based spikes typical of axons. Remember, it is only necessary to have a positive equilibrium potential and excitable membrane channels in order to generate an action potential. Calcium has an equilibrium potential of $+80\,mV$. Since this high level of equilibrium potential will ensure a high driving force, once Ca^{2+} ions start to flow across, calcium appears to offer a good choice for giving feeble distant signals enough push to reach the axon hillock and affect events there. In fact, excitable Ca^{2+} channels exist at synaptic boutons, so it is not too surprising that dendritic action potentials use Ca^{2+} currents. In the Purkinje cell these action potentials seem to be initiated and more or less confined to branch points of the dendritic tree.

The most obvious significance of having active membrane in the dendrites is that it permits amplification of the weak and fleeting currents from distant synapses. Even if the dendritic action potentials were abortive and did not progress to the soma, at least the response (as far as it got) would prolong the effective time course of synaptic action (Redman, 1976). If active membrane is located at bifurcations, as the evidence suggests, these regional patches could serve as local integrative centers—dendritic areas of summation which could increase the functional versatility of a neuron manyfold by allowing simultaneous integration at many autonomous locations. Dendritic action potentials, generated at bifurcations separated by appropriate intervening inexcitable membranes, will reach the soma via a sort of pseudosaltatory (jumping or leaping) conduction and greatly and expeditiously influence the probability and rate of axon firing.

Highly branched dendritic trees may pose more of a problem for passive conduction of distal synapses than would be expected for less impressive arborizations. Activation of only one branch might lead to shunting of current from the active branch into inactive ones, and not to the cell body. Any current flowing back into inactive branches would thereby diminish the current available to spread down the parent branch to the soma. Active membrane at nodal or branch points could remove the requirement for uniform excitation at several branches simultaneously for maximal current spread to the soma. In effect, then, active membranes may "plug" an inactive dendritic branch and prevent it from backfilling with current. This "plug" effect appears to be another useful function served by active membrane at dendritic nodal point.

E. Local Circuit Neurons and Local Circuit Functions

1. DENDRO-DENDRITIC SYNAPSES. It has long been known that some nerve cells, notably in the retina and olfactory bulb, lack identifiable axons; these cells are called *amacrine cells*. Any output from them must proceed through the dendrites or soma. In the retina, such cells, disposed horizontally, mediate interactions among receptor cells, while others, disposed vertically, are involved in information transfer between bipolar and ganglion cells. Such interactions are by way of reciprocal dendritic contacts and serial synapses (triads). In the olfactory bulb, a more rapid inhibition of the output neuron (mitral cell) by its tiny neighbors (internal granule cells of the amacrine variety) than would have been expected through feedback loops involving additional neurons and greater synap-

tic delay led to the discovery of two-way dendro-dendritic synapses between the two types of cells (Shepherd, 1974).

Excitation from the mitral cell dendrite is instantly reciprocated by inhibition of that dendrite by its smaller counterpart. Think of a jockey who reins in an exuberant horse moment by moment and not after the animal has run too far too fast and thereby lost the race. The small granule cell (the jockey) inhibits the activity of the large mitral cell (the horse) constantly and immediately by apposed dendrites (instead of with the reins and bit). Such an arrangement represents a refinement, in the way of a bypass, of conventional feedback loops involving other neurons; such loops necessitate more time for limiting output response. Such swift inhibition extends also to adjacent mitral cells via spread of excitation within the granule cell to neighboring mitral cell dendrites. In contrast to classical neurons, the olfactory cells are not polarized and often process information without primary involvement of the soma.

Neurons without axons also appear to serve in local circuit functions. Such circuits provide mechanisms for a "lateral computation" system of fast, *parallel-processing* units. Long-distance circuits in the nervous system, on the other hand, pass along and combine messages in an *in-series* form of processing. The distances involved in local circuits are short enough to permit synaptic interactions to occur in a graded fashion through passive current spread and voltage-dependent Ca^{2+} influx at the synapse. Action potentials need not be involved. Such graded interactions may be highly modifiable and are particularly sensitive to rapid, localized alterations of membrane properties and changes in the extracellular environment.

2.   OTHER LOCAL CIRCUIT INFLUENCES.   Briefly we shall mention local influences mediated by changes in the external milieu of the neuron. The cells of the brain are bathed by an extracellular fluid which fills the extracellular space and which is the immediate environment of the cells. Salts, molecules and hormones rise and fall in this fluid calling out the tide of events of brain and body fluids.

Afferent activity and cell discharge causes changes in the concentration of extracellular K^+ and Ca^{2+} ions. Neuronal activity increases extracellular K^+ levels and can actually decrease extracellular Ca^{2+}. Extracellular K^+ levels, for example, can increase from the normal 3 mM up to 15 mM with only miminal activation of the local circuit. This raised K^+ may alter the excitability state of a neuronal pool.

Nutrients are brought into the brain via the bloodstream, but this interaction between the brain's extracellular fluid and the blood composition is two edged—the brain must get some things and not others. Neurons could not perform reliably unless their overall chemical environment were reasonably independent of whimsical fluctuations of blood compositions. Generally the brain's fluids are regulated and protected from changes in blood composition by the *blood–brain* _barrier_. The blood–brain barrier serves to stabilize the external environment of the neurons. It makes the brain a kind of private room in which the surge in sugars, amino acids, etc., which accompany eating, drinking and changes in body fluids are virtually unnoticed.

However, there are certain key exceptions where changes in body fluids affect local brain activity. Specific brain areas, such as the hypothalamus, are exquisitely sensitive to blood levels of certain molecules such as glucose. Cells in the hypothalamus which are sensitive to glucose activate neuronal circuits which stimulate animals to seek food and eat when blood levels of glucose fall (see Chapter 13). Hormones may also have an influence over the operation of local circuits. Populations of neurons are selectively affected by hormones. Hippocampal neurons, for example, readily accumulate certain steroid hormones which probably in turn alter the functional state of this pool of neurons. Thus, release of specific hormones into the bloodstream can act generally on small pools of neurons. Some of the ways in which the brain is open to the general chemical status of the blood are important in the maintenance of homeostasis and the adaptation of behavior. Changes in fluid composition in contact with the brain can, in special cases, provide important graded signals. We will discuss these signals in more detail in later chapters (see Chapters 13 and 16).

F.   Conclusion and Summary

Neurons are highly sophisticated computational devices. For a single neuron, integration depends on the types of inputs impinging on it, the places where they arrive on the cell (dendrites versus soma), the geometry of the dendrites, the propagation characteristics of those dendrites (passive or active), and the highly individualized relation of the output signal to a specified level of depolarization. Output can be a pattern of action potentials, as in cells with axons, or a graded potential, as in amacrine neurons.

The importance of these graded interactions is that they greatly increase the functional capacity of the nervous system. It is still clear that the bulk of information processing appears through the classic sequence (action potentials, synaptic transmission, integration and action potentials), but local interactions appear to exert a subtle and vital influence and extend the integrative capacity of neurons. It was once thought that the nervous system operated in spite of these modulatory effects, but as more and more are discovered in relationship to specific functions and specific systems, it is clear that the nervous system uses them to gain the maximal capacities of its neurons and its informational processing capacities.

Is integration simply electrical as we have implicity assumed? Or is integration chemical as well? As we have witnessed in the previous chapter on synaptic transmission, each message causes a different set of ionic changes and in certain cases metabolic ones. Transmitters that are inhibitory, for example, bring the same basic message (inhibition) to the surface of the neuron, but they may be construed as lending a different affective state or diffuseness. Their time courses differ and, most significantly, the metabolic consequence of their action is unique. Dopamine alters cAMP levels in the cell; γ-aminobutyric acid, another transmitter, does not. If, then, the consequence is different and if this alters the affective state of the cell (its response to other inputs), then there must be another level of integration underlying the transient electrical one: a type of shifting, abiding pattern of neuronal metabolism. For example, some cells have rhythms and are more or less responsive depending on the part of the cycle in which they are functioning. In the pineal gland we have seen that neurotransmitter metabolism is cyclic as a result of the metabolic influence of its synaptic input. A neuron then is not simply excited, inhibited or modulated. It is affected by what came earlier (or what happens all at once) much like the corporate executive whose decision will sway one way or another depending on what he had for lunch, coffee or scotch. Neurons integrate in relation to their state which is set by certain of its inputs over its prior history.

There appear to be levels of integration: foreground integration and background integration. Foreground integration is up front using electrical signaling, and background integration is setting a metabolic temperament to these excitations. We shall now turn to an analysis of the organization of CNS transmitters.

III.   Chemical Coding of Brain Circuitry

The identification of transmitters for particular neurons and their organization in the CNS is at the crossroads of cellular and behavioral neurosciences. The cellular approach requires knowledge of neurotransmitters in order to understand and analyze mechanisms of synaptic transmission and integration and in order to develop and identify drugs which can selectively manipulate the systems. The behavioral approach, aimed at understanding more global functions, depends on knowledge of organization and characteristics of the subordinate systems.

The emphasis in chemical neuroanatomy is to identify the function of different systems in the integrative activity of the brain. It is now clear that different behavioral and physiological functions are served by discrete brain systems, and the proper performance of certain behaviors depends on the normal operation of these systems. In this section then we will describe the organization of the better known pathways in brain and spinal cord which use different transmitters. We will also briefly describe the role that some of these pathways play in the control of behavior and how knowledge of the transmitters allows, in certain cases, the treatment of previously incurable disorders.

A.   Organization of Neurotransmitter Systems in the CNS

1.   DISTRIBUTION OF NOREPINEPHRINE PATHWAYS.   Great interest in the catecholamines, *norepinephrine* and *dopamine*, was stimulated by clinical observations in the 1950's; the major tranquilizers (reserpine and chlorpromazine) were found to ameliorate certain agitated psychotic states. Patients were calmed by these drugs, but more important, they showed a definite reduction in symptomatology, a lessening of disturbances in thinking and of hallucinatory behavior. These drugs were potent catecholamine antagonists, and thus it was suggested that the agitated psychoses were due to overactivity in noradrenergic and/or dopamine-containing neurons (Schildkraut, 1967). This *catecholamine theory of affective disorders* will be discussed in Chapter 17. To fully appreciate the function of these catecholamines, however, we must look at their widespread distribution within the brain in specific anatomical pathways.

Norepinephrine

The mapping of catecholamine pathways in the CNS is the direct result of a satisfactory method of visualizing them. It was found that upon treatment of tissue sections with formaldehyde (Falck *et al.*, 1962) or glyoxylic acid (Lindvall and Björklund, 1974) catecholamines become fluorescent so that catecholaminergic cells and their processes can be readily visualized in great detail. Histofluorescence methods, plus the use of lesions and direct chemical analysis, have served as the main methods for describing the circuitry of particular neurotransmitter systems (Heller, 1975; Harvey *et al.*, 1963).

As shown in Fig. 6-6, norepinephrine (NE) fibers originate from a relatively few neurons in the pons and medulla, but these fibers project to nearly every principal brain region. Although their innervation is usually very sparse in these target regions (NE synapses are less than 1% of the total of brain terminals), noradrenergic fibers have a profound influence upon behavior.

The noradrenergic cell groups do not correspond to the better known nuclei seen in classically stained preparations of the brain. Consequently, they are

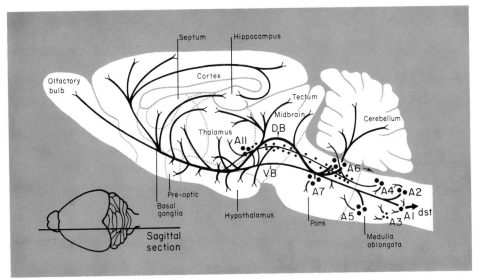

Fig. 6-6. Noradrenergic cell bodies and their projections shown in sagittal plane (see inset). The dots represent location of cell bodies and are identified by the letter A followed by an Arabic number. DB, dorsal bundle; VB, ventral bundle; dst, descending spinal tracts.

designated by capital letters and Arabic numbers: A1–A7 plus A11 (Dahlström and Fuxe, 1964; Björklund and Nobin, 1973; Björklund *et al.*, 1973). The missing combinations A8, A9 and A10 are allocated to dopamine-containing cell bodies (see below), along with three additional groupings: A12, A13 and A14. Groups A1–A4 are located in the medulla oblongata, while A5–A7 lie in the pons. A6, which originates from a deeply pigmented pontine nucleus, the *locus coeruleus* (blue place), is one of the most important groups of NE cells.

Neurons of the locus coeruleus have elaborately branched axons which ramify within the entire brain. Some branches pass to the overlying cerebellum, where they terminate on the fanlike Purkinje cells. Others enter a distinct bundle that runs forward to innervate the forebrain, including the cerebral cortex. As shown in Fig. 6-6 this bundle is an offshoot of a thick cable of axons ascending from other NE cell bodies in the medulla, such as A1 and A2. At the level of the pons, fibers separate to form the *"dorsal bundle"* just mentioned. This bundle innervates the hypothalamus, thalamus (including the geniculate bodies of the auditory and visual pathways), hippocampus and cerebral cortex. In addition, fibers pass to the septum (the partition under the corpus callosum), basal ganglia, amygdala, limbic lobe (including the ancient olfactory cortex surrounding the amygdala) and olfactory bulb. Truly, the locus coeruleus fibers have a very widespread distribution, and, unlike the ascending fibers of the sensory systems we have studied, they can go *directly* to the cerebral cortex without passing through a "relay" nucleus in the thalamus.

Except for this remarkable A6 group, most of the other NE cells in the lower brain stem contribute primarily to the main cable, the *"ventral bundle."* These axons ascend more deeply in the reticular core of the stem, turning downward near the specific lemniscal pathways that carry somesthetic signals, and travel forward directly alongside the hypothalamus. At the level of that neuroendocrine "command console," the fibers of the dorsal and ventral bundles merge and then separate again to pursue their final courses in the forebrain. The ventral bundle also innervates the hypothalamus, as well as the basal regions of the forebrain and parts of the limbic system. Most of these pathways to the forebrain are uncrossed.

The NE cells in the medulla and pons also apparently send axons to the traditional brain stem nuclei amongst which they lie (or of which they form certain parts). Two of the nuclei (A1 and perhaps A2) send axons down to the gray matter of the spinal cord. In short, through this massive system of fibers coursing up and down the neuraxis, the NE cells innervate pretty nearly every major structure in the CNS. It is very reminiscent of the sympathetic nervous system, a far-flung network of neurons, ganglia and fibers that integrates the body's viscera and vasculature in stress responses. Indeed, many look upon the NE system as the sympathetic nervous system of the CNS.

The peripheral sympathetic system (not shown in Fig. 6-6) also sends some of its fibers into the brain at the points where the pineal and pituitary glands are attached, above the thalamus and below the hypothalamus, respectively. It also supplies the neurohypophysis, the lobe of the pituitary that was originally an outgrowth of the embryonic brain.

The above description is just a brief overview of the actual detail that has been gathered on this remarkable system in recent years. This new knowledge has come about through the use of histochemical techniques that detect the presence of catecholamines by their fluorescence under ultraviolet light. Additional methods have been used to verify the novel observations made by histofluorescence. Carefully placed brain lesions in experimental animals have been a valuable aid in verifying the origin of particular pathways. For example, destruction of the locus coeruleus (A6) obliterates the major NE innervation of the cerebellum except for a small region near the front of that structure which appears to originate from one of the other NE cell groups (A4). Recently, a compound called 6-hydroxydopamine has been widely used to investigate the anatomy and function of the NE system. When this compound is injected near catecholamine-containing neurons, their axons and axonal terminals accumulate it and are killed. Apparently, when *6-hydroxydopamine* is metabolized, toxic metabolites are created which cause the self-destruction of the catecholaminergic terminals that imbibed it.

2. DISTRIBUTION OF DOPAMINE PATHWAYS. The dopamine-containing (DA) cell bodies lie primarily in the depths of the midbrain, in front of the noradrenergic elements of the pons and medulla. The major cell groups A8 and A9 lie in a large, deeply pigmented mass of neurons called the *substantia nigra* (black body). The fibers of these DA cells run up to the largest basal ganglia, the caudate nucleus and putamen. These two closely related and massive structures are collectively called the *striatum* due to the striped appearance that fibers of cortical origin impart to them. Accordingly, the output of A8 and A9 forms the very important *nigrostriatal* pathway. These fibers are extremely fine, and in fact their existence was not and still has not been detected with the classical silver methods that are used (in a manner much like the photographic process) to impregnate such features. Yet the slender threads that comprise the nigrostriatal DA pathway contain about three-quarters of all the dopamine in the brain.

$$HO-\text{benzene ring}-CH_2-CH_2-NH_2$$
$$HO-$$

Dopamine

Based on combined histofluorescence and chemical studies, it is estimated that the number of nigrostriatal DA neurons in the rat brain is 3500, and approximately 16% of all axons in striatal slices appear to be dopaminergic. As shown in Fig. 6-7, axons from A8 and A9 ascend deeply in the reticular formation to course

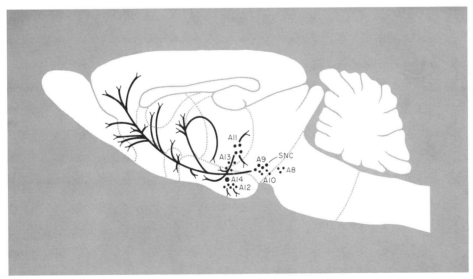

Fig. 6-7. Dopaminergic cell bodies and their projections. The dots represent location of cell bodies and are identified by the letter A followed by an Arabic number. SNC, substantia nigra.

into the forebrain past the hypothalamus as the NE fibers do. Farther up, fibers peel off to enter the caudate and putamen, as well as the globus pallidus (white sphere), through which the motor output of the two striatal components passes en route to thalamus and motor cortex. A topographical orderliness is apparent in the organization of the nigrostriatal pathway: the upper fibers leave the main bundle before the lower ones, and other orderly relationships are noted between the locations of the cells of origin and the points of fiber termination.

This nigrostriatal pathway plays an important role in motor integration. Injury to it, or deficits in its delivery of dopamine to its targets, can result in severe motor disturbances. Normally, if the substantia nigra is stimulated on one side, an

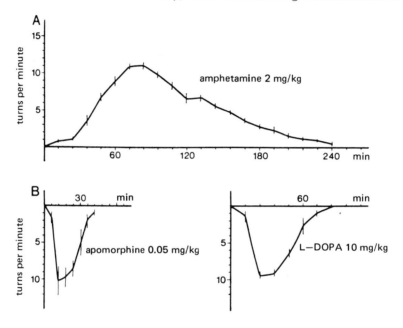

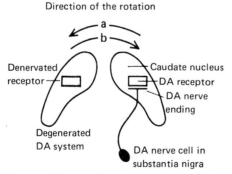

Direction of the rotation

Diagram of the experimental situation-horizontal projection of the nigro striatal DA neuron system

Fig. 6-8. The direction of rotation is toward the least "DA-affected" side. (A) Amphetamine which releases dopamine causes the animal to rotate in direction "a," i.e., toward the lesioned side. (B) Apomorphine or L-dopa, which act primarily on the denervated side as dopamine agonists, cause the animal to rotate toward the opposite side, i.e., direction "b." These agents are more effective on the denervated side because the receptors have become supersensitive as a result of denervation (see Chapter 4). (From Ungerstadt, 1974.)

animal will turn its head to the opposite side. Such a response may be duplicated by unilateral injection of DA directly into the striatum. But if a lesion is placed in the nigrostriatal pathway on one side, the head will be turned to the same side, that of the lesion. The reason for this effect is that DA acts like an inhibitory transmitter. If its effect is removed on one side (by interrupting the path through which it comes, for example), increased striatal activity will result on that side of the brain, with turning of the head to that side. Drugs which affect DA activity also affect turning; the direction of rotation is always toward the least "DA-affected side" (Fig. 6-8). Thus a normal balance in striatal output is necessary for normal motor activity, in regard to other movements as well as those of the head. The head movements are obviously affected because fibers from the putamen component of the striatum lead back down to the nigra, from which another pathway seems to pass to the tectum. The tectum, we recall, is a region in which orientation mechanisms are found; its output is directed (among other places) to the motor neurons that activate the neck muscles. The *rotational model* is significant because it provides a simple way to study synaptic function in a simple quantifiable behavior which is related to a particular transmitter (Ungerstedt, 1974).

The other two groupings of DA neurons are as well defined as the above pathway and illustrate again the more restrictive innervation of the system when compared to its NE counterpart. A10, medial to the nigra, is the source of the *meso-limbic system* (from mesencephalon, or midbrain, to limbic system). It innervates the cortex of frontal and limbic lobes, the septal region that lies between the larger limbic structures and hypothalamus and several regions near the olfactory tract. The remaining cell groups include a *tuberoinfundibular* system, in which cell bodies in the tuberal swelling of the hypothalamus innervate the pituitary stalk at the median eminence around its base. This system is insensitive to the destructive effects of 6-hydroxydopamine; it resembles the neighboring neurosecretory cells in that prolonged activity depletes its terminals of transmitter. Another group of DA neurons, situated above this system, sends fibers into the front part of the hypothalamus. To date, no descending DA axons have been found, in contrast to the numerous ones of the NE system.

3. DISTRIBUTION OF SEROTONERGIC PATHWAYS. The cell bodies that contain serotonin (5-HT) primarily lie scattered along the upper edge of the brain stem midline, from the lower part of the midbrain down into the medulla oblongata (Fig. 6-9). In this region the median of the neuraxis is clearly marked by a vertical stripe of nerve fibers (as if drawn with a pen and straight-edge) in which nerve cell bodies are entangled. This bisecting stripe is called the *raphé* (seam); therefore, the 5-HT cell bodies are in the *raphé nuclei*. These are small, dispersed cell clusters with logical but long Latin names. Like the NE and DA cells, the

5-HT cells themselves are given letter/number combinations, in this instance from B1 to B9.

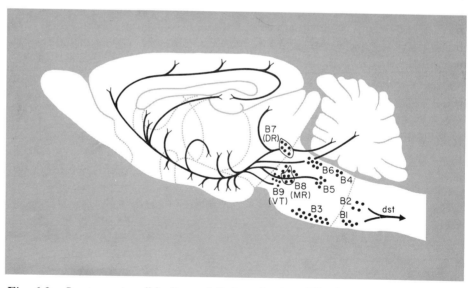

Serotonin

The serotonergic pathways are quite widespread, with terminals in the reticular formation, hypothalamus, preoptic area, septum, hippocampus, cortex, basal ganglia and amygdala (Dahlström and Fuxe, 1964; Fuxe and Jonsson, 1974; Fuxe *et al.*, 1970; Ungerstedt, 1971). The hypothalamic innervation is pronounced just above the crossing of the optic nerves; the suprachiasmatic nucleus there has been implicated in the regulation of biological rhythms. Serotonergic cell bodies also innervate the cerebellum, and fibers from B1, B2 and B3 travel to the spinal cord to end in the gray matter at many levels. Furthermore, some 5-HT axons even terminate in the lining of the brain cavities, or ventricles. There they form bare endings, i.e., no synaptic junctions are made.

The serotonergic system appears to play a critical role in sleep and sleep-related activities. Destruction of the raphé nuclei or depletion of 5-HT stores leads to total insomnia, and subtotal procedures of this type bring about loss of

Fig. 6-9. Serotonergic cell bodies and their projections. The dots represent location of cell bodies and are identified by symbols B1–B9. DR, dorsal raphé nucleus; VT, ventral tegmentum; MR, median raphé nucleus.

6. INTEGRATION: PUTTING IT ALL TOGETHER

slow-wave sleep time proportional to the serotonin loss. Moreover, drugs such as LSD (D-*lysergic acid diethylamide*) act primarily on this system. LSD is a potent inhibitor of serotonin's effect on certain peripheral tissues, such as smooth muscle. This finding has led to the speculation that serotonin might be involved in hallucinatory behavior, and possibly in the hallucinations experienced by psychotic patients. Subsequent research has shown that LSD does, in fact, selectively depress the firing of 5-HT neurons in brain. Furthermore, LSD appears to enhance sensory input, as indeed depletion of serotonin levels in brain also does. In contrast, elevated serotonin levels may decrease one's sensitivity to pain.

Studies of 5-HT content of brain tissue obtained from depressed persons who had committed suicide show significantly lower values than in accident victims. Also, 5-hydroxyindoleacetic acid (the major metabolite of 5-HT) in the cerebrospinal fluid is significantly lower in depressed patients than in hospitalized control individuals. Thus one form of depression seems to be related to decreased activity in the serotonin system.

In general, it appears that 5-HT normally acts in an inhibitory way in a variety of behaviors, while dopamine acts in an excitatory manner. These apparent opposed effects upon behavior, however, do not mean that 5-HT and DA are inhibitory and excitatory synaptic transmitters. On the contrary, for example, the DA released by the nigrostriatal pathway inhibits the firing of neurons in the caudate nucleus. Yet this inhibitory action as a transmitter results in excited motor responses: head turning, rigidity and tremor. There are many suggestions as to the explanation of this paradoxical effect, such as inhibition of neurons that normally inhibit other neurons, thus allowing the latter to escape from normal constraint. But for the most part these mechanisms are not well understood.

4. DISTRIBUTION OF CHOLINERGIC NEURONS. A histochemical method to localize acetylcholine (ACh), like the ones used to hunt for *monoamines* (5-HT, NE and DA), is not available. Instead, the location of cholinergic neurons and their innervation patterns have had to be inferred, chiefly by noting the distribution of their ACh hydrolytic and synthetic enzymes. These are, respectively, acetylcholinesterase (AChE) and choline acetyltransferase (ChAc). If a neuron contains both of these, it can be identified as cholinergic. The presence of ChAc is critical: some neurons contain AChE but not ChAc, so they cannot synthesize ACh and therefore cannot be cholinergic. Consequently, results based on AChE staining alone must be viewed with great caution.

$$H_3C-\overset{\overset{\displaystyle CH_3}{|}}{\underset{\underset{\displaystyle CH_3}{|}}{N^+}}-CH_2-CH_2-O-\overset{\overset{\displaystyle O}{||}}{C}-CH_3$$

Acetylcholine

The most recent mapping of cholinergic brain pathways has made use of immunohistochemistry. Choline acetyltransferase has been purified, and antibodies made to the enzyme. These antibodies recognize ChAc specifically. The tissue can be incubated with them and the distribution of the enzyme shown by staining them in various ways. This promising technique is only in its infancy, however, and so the information gleaned by it is incomplete. Thus while much is known, the map of the cholinergic system is not as well worked out as those for the monoaminergic systems.

Cholinergic neurons appear throughout the nervous system. The best known examples are the motor neurons of the brain stem and spinal cord; both those that supply skeletal muscle and those that synapse upon visceral neurons in various autonomic ganglia are cholinergic. In the brain, one of the best documented cholinergic pathways is the *septohippocampal* pathway which connects the *septum*, a thin partition beneath the corpus callosum with the hippocampus (Fig. 6-10). Septal lesions virtually obliterate hippocampal ChAc activity and high-affinity choline uptake (Lewis *et al.*, 1967; Kuhar *et al.*, 1975). Similarly, lesions lower down in the septal region result in a partial loss of cholinergic properties in the amygdala, hypothalamus and midbrain (Oderfeld-Nowak *et al.*, 1976). Thus several ACh pathways seem to emanate from this portal region of the forebrain. There is also evidence for ACh neurons in the striatum; it is possible that these are the cells normally inhibited by the nigral DA system.

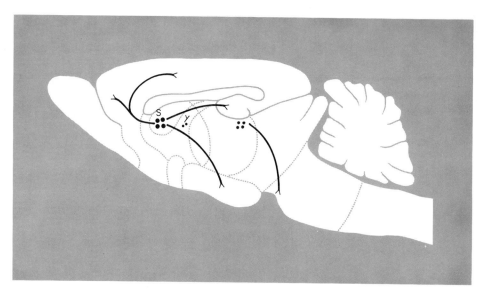

Fig. 6-10. Cholinergic cell bodies and their projections. The dots represent presumed locus of cholinergic cell bodies and brown lines the presumed projections. For details see text. S, septal nucleus.

6. INTEGRATION: PUTTING IT ALL TOGETHER

Cholinergic neurons also seem to be present in the cerebral cortex, although where their axons terminate is not well understood.

Two major ACh pathways ascending to the forebrain from the brain stem reticular formation have been described (not shown in Fig. 6-10). Unfortunately, descriptions of them are based primarily on stains for AChE activity and thus are not as well documented as the connections just described (Lewis and Shute, 1967; Shute and Lewis, 1967). A *dorsal* path is directed toward the tectum and thalamus; it arises in the midbrain core not far from the tectum and innervates the two colliculi, the pretectal region just in front and several thalamic nuclei, including the two geniculate bodies. It is thus aimed at structures which process auditory, visual and somesthetic information. A *ventral* path is clearly limbic in its upward influences; it arises from the substantia nigra and a region in between the two nigral masses and sends fibers to the hypothalamus, the complex overlying subthalamic region and the basal forebrain. These targets are not as easily characterized collectively, but they lie in the midst of visceral and somatic motor machinery. Both these pathways are implicated in arousal mechanisms that are necessary to activate forebrain components for more selective functions. In this regard, it is interesting to note that brain ACh content varies with different functional states, being highest during sleep and lowest during periods of excited activity.

5. DISTRIBUTION OF GLYCINE AND GABA NEURONS. Glycine and *γ-aminobutyric acid* (GABA) are two amino acids which serve as important inhibitory transmitters in the CNS. Glycine acts only in the spinal cord and lower brain stem. In the cord, it seems to be localized in the innumerable small interneurons that inhabit the region of gray matter between the sensory and motor neurons. These intermediate elements inhibit the motor neurons and other cells that lie nearby.

$$\begin{array}{c} COOH \\ | \\ H-C-NH_2 \\ | \\ H \end{array}$$

Glycine

$$H_2C-CH_2-CH_2-COOH$$
$$\;\;|$$
$$NH_2$$

γ-Aminobutyric acid

γ-Aminobutyric acid is the major inhibitory transmitter of the brain (Roberts *et al.*, 1976). In some brain regions it may account for up to one-third of all synaptic terminals. γ-Aminobutyric acid neurons seem to pervade the CNS, and GABA-nergic cells may be the major class of local circuit neurons. The basket cells of the hippocampus and cerebellum, for example, are known to be GABA-nergic; the powerful inhibitory effects of these cells, which invest their target neurons in baskets of fine axonal branches, are well known. They provide sharpening and contrast to the activities of the structures in which they lie by subduing the excitability of neurons adjacent to those that are in critical stages of response. Other local circuit neurons in the midbrain, thalamus and cortex appear to be GABA-nergic, and similar roles for them may be expected; however, only a few projection neurons (that is, ones which send impulses over long distances) use GABA. The cerebellar Purkinje cell is the best known example. This neuron is the final cell through which impulses of the cerebellar cortex flow; it delivers its inhibitory messages to deep cerebellar masses of neurons that excite motor control centers in the brain stem. There also seems to be a GABA-nergic projection from the basal ganglia to the substantia nigra. This pathway thus reciprocates the DA nigrostriatal system (Fig. 6-11), and an interesting clinical correlation of these mutually related influences is now emerging (see Section IV). Only recently has an _immunohistochemical method_ become available to study GABA-nergic pathways. This technique permits visualization of the enzyme glutamic acid decarboxylase (GAD) that is responsible for GABA synthesis.

As one might expect from what has already been seen, GABA-nergic neurons are extremely important in the overall operation of brain circuitry, not merely in local feedback and contrast circuits. Blocking or removing their action usually results in a seizure. A substantial reduction of GABA-nergic activity has been found in brains of patients afflicted with _Huntington's chorea_ (Shoulson and Chase, 1975). This disease is associated with neuronal degeneration in the cerebral cortex and basal ganglia, particularly in the frontal lobe and head of the caudate nucleus. Its cardinal signs are mental deterioration and involuntary movements which usually appear in middle life. The word "chorea" means "dance," and indeed the early, subtle manifestations are brisk, graceful, complex movement "fragments." Ultimately, the condition leads to dementia. It is thought to involve the loss of GABA-nergic (and also some cholinergic) cells in the striatum, thus reducing GABA content in the midbrain targets that striatal fibers reach. A notable one, of course, is the substantia nigra.

Elevated striatal dopamine in Huntington disease indicates that the DA nigrostriatal system has been freed from its normal GABA-nergic inhibition. Huntington chorea has long been regarded as an hereditary, familial disease, and is now known to be a dominant genetic disorder which appears in virtually all ethnic and racial groups with a prevalence rate of about 5 per 100,000 people.

6. GLUTAMATE. With the possible exception of acetylcholine, all the transmitters so far described have been predominantly (if not exclusively) inhibitory. It is generally believed that the major excitatory transmitters are the acidic

amino acids, notably glutamate and aspartate (Davidson, 1976). Research on the organization of glutamate systems has depended solely on biochemical methods. Study of the distribution of these neurons is fraught with difficulty. Glutamate is present in every neuron; it is a major molecule in central neural metabolism. Three techniques are useful: (1) application of glutamate to neurons to see if they are excited by it, together with use of specific glutamate antagonists to see if these block the action of applied glutamate and of the naturally excited pathway; (2) survey of glutamate uptake by axon terminals and analysis of their distribution in the brain by various chemical methods; and (3) search for glutamate release from terminals after stimulation in various brain areas.

$$COOH-CH_2-CH_2-\underset{H}{\overset{NH_2}{C}}-COOH$$

Glutamate

There is now good evidence that glutamate is a transmitter of the pathway from the cerebral cortex to the basal ganglia (see Fig. 6-11). In addition, it may be

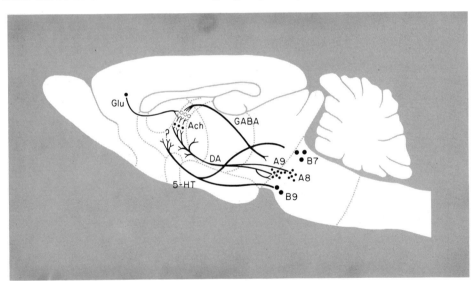

Fig. 6-11. Presumed transmitter interactions. Shown are the serotonergic cell bodies B7 and B9 projecting to the caudate nucleus along the pathway marked 5-HT. The innervation of caudate by these serotonergic fibers is now known, but may be onto the same cells innervated by dopaminergic fibers. The dopaminergic cell bodies A8 and A9 are shown projecting to the caudate nucleus onto cholinergic cell bodies, along the nigrostriatal bundle marked DA. The short cholinergic neurons within the caudate are in turn thought to innervate GABA-nergic neurons shown as open circles in the caudate nucleus. The GABA-nergic neurons in turn are thought to send long projections back to the dopaminergic cell bodies in A9 along a pathway marked GABA. Glutamate-releasing fibers (Glu) project from the cortex to basal ganglia.

the transmitter for the pathway from the temporal lobe cortex to the hippocampus, as well as for various intrinsic hippocampal circuits (Storm-Mathisen, 1977; Cotman and Hamberger, 1978). It also appears to fulfill many of the criteria of a neurotransmitter in the cerebellar cortex (the parallel fibers of which run like telephone lines to the Purkinje cell) (Young *et al.*, 1974; Sandoval and Cotman, 1978) and in the olfactory system (the tract which distributes olfactory impulses to a variety of basal forebrain structures) (Bradford and Richards, 1976; Yamamoto and Matsui, 1976; Harvey *et al.*, 1975). Obviously much more work is needed to identify and localize the various excitatory transmitters that must be present in the ever-active brain.

7.   ENKEPHALINS AND ENDORPHINS.   In 1975 startling reports appeared: the brain contained its own endogenous opiates: peptides called *enkephalins* and *endorphins*. Opium is found only in plants; it is obtained from the milky juice of the unripe seed pod of the poppy. What is the brain doing with such substances?

The first findings of endogenous brain opiates arose out of the free flow of scientific investigation into the causes of addiction. Man has used opium and its derivatives since the time of ancient Greece to alleviate pain and attain euphoria. Addictiveness, however, was only recognized as a severe problem after the drug became an established treatment in clinical medicine. The administration of opiates to wounded soldiers in the Civil War resulted in a significant social problem in the United States. Over the years, this problem has increased in magnitude and prompted research into the basis of addiction.

If opiates act on brain, then the brain must have opiate receptors. A search for them began; it led to the discovery that brain cell membranes contain highly specific receptors for opiates (Goldstein, 1976; Snyder, 1977). Such membranes incubated with radioactive opiates bind them, and this binding can be blocked by antagonists which specifically interfere with opiate action. Known neurotransmitters, however, or endocrine hormones do not compete with opiates. Strange, though, that the brain should have receptors for a plant substance which causes euphoria and ultimately addiction.

As a long shot, John Hughes and Hans Kosterlitz of the University of Aberdeen in Scotland wondered if the brain might have opiate compounds because it normally contains opiate receptors. Again, a search began. They extracted the chemical substances from 500 kg of brain and looked for a material that would act like morphine.

Their discovery is now history. A brain peptide did indeed have opiate-like action. They coined the name "enkephalin" from the Greek word meaning "in the head" to describe it (Hughes, 1975; Hughes *et al.*, 1975).

It was a simple experiment. They used the principal duct from the testis of the guinea pig: the *vas deferens*. This duct is known to have in its wall opiate receptors resembling those in the brain. It is used, therefore, as a biological test structure by which to assay tissue fractions for opiate activity. The vas deferens, immersed in an artificial body fluid, is mounted between two electrodes and anchored to a transducer that is in turn connected to a polygraph. Stimulation of the vas through the electrodes brings about rhythmic contractions which are recorded on the polygraph. As shown in Fig. 6-12, opiates such as normorphine, when applied to the vas, inhibit its subsequent contractions. Thus fractions sus-

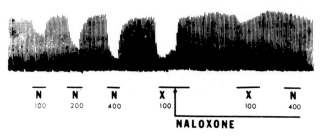

Fig. 6-12. Effect of normorphine (N) and enkephalin (X) on contractions of vas deferens. Naloxone blocks the action of enkephalin. (From Hughes, 1975.)

pected to contain opiate-like molecules can be applied to this sensitive muscular tube and gauged as to their effectiveness in suppressing contractions. The enkephalin markedly inhibited these contractions, but its effect was blocked by an opiate antagonist (*naloxone*). This was a critically important finding. Only when the inhibition of contractility is lessened or blocked altogether by known opiate antagonists can one be sure that the active molecule has opiate action. This precautionary test is essential, since other molecules unrelated to opiate pharmacodynamics will also inhibit contraction.

It is now known that the brain contains many endogenous peptides which have opiate-like activity. One group is called the enkephalins, after the example we saw above. These substances are pentapeptides which possess morphine- or opium-like activity. They show the following sequence of amino acids: H–tyrosine–glycine–glycine–phenylalanine–X–OH. If the amino acid "X" is methionine, the molecule is known as *Met⁵-enkephalin*; if it is leucine, then it is *Leu⁵-enkephalin*. There are only these two enkephalins, and together they correspond to the brain peptide discovered by Hughes and his colleagues at Aberdeen.

The other group of opiate-like molecules are the endorphins. "Endorphin" is a general term used for any endogenous body material that has morphine-like activity. Thus enkephalins are endorphins, but not all endorphins are enkephalins. There are many endorphins; the most common carry the prefixes alpha, beta and gamma. It is now known that the amino acid sequence in these peptides also occurs in a pituitary hormone implicated in fat metabolism, β-lipotropin.

The story behind this discovery is interesting and illustrates the sometimes fortuitous nature of science. The very day after the biochemist John Morris had worked out the amino acid sequence in the enkephalins he attended a seminar on the chemical structure of pituitary hormones. When a lantern slide of the structure of β-lipotropin flashed upon the screen, Morris saw something that looked familiar. He was quick to recognize the sequence of Met[5]-enkephalin and β-endorphin buried right in the middle of the hormonal molecule (Fig. 6-13). Such accidental discoveries are far from unusual. Progress in science often results from a sudden realization of the significance of relationships, of the meaning of things, which come to attention merely by chance.

The regional distribution of enkephalins (Met- and Leu-) and of β-endorphin (a prominent member of that group) in the brain is shown in Table 6-1. They are particularly concentrated in the pituitary. In the case of β-endorphin at least

Table 6-1 Distribution of immunoassayable opioid peptides in brain and pituitary gland[a]

	β-Endorphin (ng/mg tissue)		Enkephalin (mU Enk/mg tissue)	
Pituitary				
Whole	269±20	(11)	72±4	(6)
Adenohypophysis	128±9	(3)	3.7±0.7	(3)
Neurohypophysis and pars intermedia	1500±600	(3)	740±47	(3)
Pineal	4.8±0.8	(10)	19±2	(7)

	β-Endorphin (ng/gm tissue)		Enkephalin (U Enk/gm tissue)	
Brain				
Whole	108±8	(10)	25±2	(6)
Hypothalamus	490±30	(5)	120±7	(6)
Septum	234±34	(3)	85±7	(6)
Midbrain	207±15	(5)	32±1	(6)
Medulla and pons	179±5	(5)	30±4	(6)
Striatum	None	(5)	112±11	(6)
Hippocampus	None	(5)	13±1	(6)
Cortex	None	(5)	15±2	(6)
Cerebellum	None	(5)	5±1	(6)

[a] From Rossier et al. (1977)

some of the cell bodies and elements containing them reside in the gland itself, but others may lie in the overlying hypothalamus or elsewhere. Both kinds of peptides are also present in relatively high amounts in the structures and circuits of the limbic system. Most brain endorphins are encountered in axon terminals,

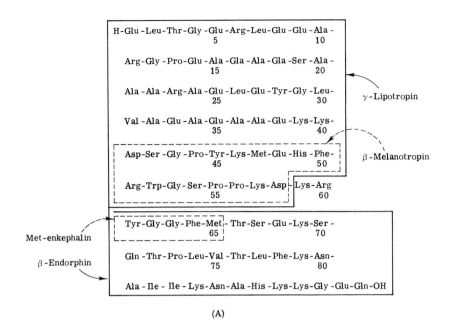

H-Glu -Leu-Thr-Gly -Glu -Arg-Leu-Glu -Glu -Ala -
               5   10

Arg-Gly -Pro-Glu -Ala -Gla -Ala -Gla -Ser -Ala -
              15   20

Ala -Ala -Arg-Ala -Glu -Leu-Glu -Tyr-Gly -Leu-
              25   30

Val -Ala -Glu -Ala -Glu -Ala -Ala -Glu -Lys-Lys-
              35   40

Asp-Ser -Gly -Pro-Tyr-Lys-Met-Glu -His -Phe-
              45   50

Arg-Trp-Gly- Ser-Pro-Pro-Lys-Asp Lys-Arg
              55   60

Tyr-Gly-Gly-Phe-Met - Thr-Ser -Glu -Lys-Ser -
              65   70

Gln -Thr-Pro-Leu-Val -Thr-Leu-Phe-Lys-Asn-
              75   80

Ala -Ile - Ile - Lys-Asn-Ala -His -Lys-Lys-Gly -Glu-Gln-OH

γ-Lipotropin

β-Melanotropin

Met-enkephalin

β-Endorphin

(A)

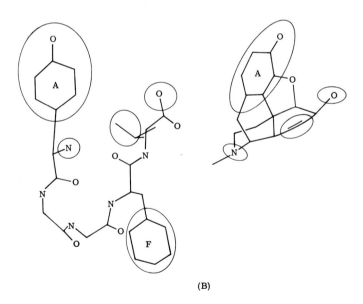

(B)

Fig. 6-13. (A) Sequence of β-lipotropin hormone. The α-, β- and γ-endorphins have amino acid sequences identical to residues 61–76, 61–91 and 61–77, respectively. Met[5]-enkephalin is recognized in sequence 61–65. (B) Three-dimensional structure of Leu[5]-enkephalin (left) compared to morphine (right). There are many similarities between the two molecules. (From Smith and Griffin, 1978, copyright by the American Association for the Advancement of Science.)

and their distribution corresponds in general to that of the opiate receptors discovered before them in brain. Immunohistochemical methods allow the precise localization of endorphin- and enkephalin-containing neurons and the mapping of their fiber distributions throughout the CNS. It is clear that endorphins and

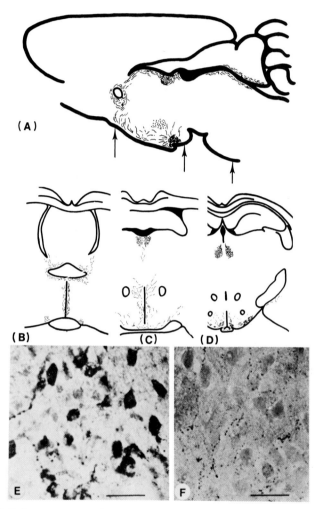

Fig. 6-14. (A) Schematic saggital view of β-endorphin-reactive neurons and fibers in the rat brain. The neuronal perikarya in the basal hypothalamic region (arrows) give rise to fibers that sweep forward to enter the preoptic area and then course within the periaqueductal region of the diencephalon and pons. (B)–(D) Schematic coronal view of β-endorphin neurons and fibers taken at the levels indicated in (A). Note that the reactive fibers tend to lie close to the ventricular surfaces of the diencephalic structures they innervate. (E) Cluster of neurons which stain for the presence of β-endorphin. (F) β-Endorphin fibers within the thalamus. Several long varicose fibers are seen. (From Bloom *et al.*, 1978.)

6. INTEGRATION: PUTTING IT ALL TOGETHER

enkephalins are present in anatomically distinct cells and pathways. β-Endorphin-containing cell bodies are primarily present in the basal hypothalamus. Their organization does not correspond to classical hypothalamic nuclei. Very few, if any, such cells exist in other portions of the rat brain. Fibers from hypothalamic neurons distribute to midline areas throughout the diencephalon and pons (Fig. 6-14). Caudal to the level of the locus coeruleus, β-endorphin fibers are very sparse, and none are present in the medulla and spinal cord. Enkephalin fibers are particularly prominent in the basal ganglia, amygdala and portions of the spinal cord and are clearly distinguished from the organization of β-endorphin fibers (Bloom et al., 1978). Neurons containing β-endorphin in rat brain exist separately from those containing enkephalin.

The endorphins appear to serve many extremely important functions in the CNS, functions of profound interest and importance. They have analgesic properties, and thus may represent naturally occurring, "built-in" anesthetic agents involved in temperature regulation (Holaday et al., 1978), which is not altogether become addicted to endorphins (see Chapter 17). Endorphins also appear to be involved in temperature regulation (Holoday et al., 1978), which is not altogether surprising. Pain and temperature sensibilities have long been known to be related in several ways; they travel over closely apposed pathways and come together both in brain structures and in stressful feelings. Additionally in this regard, there is some evidence that endorphins can influence reward and mood (see Chapter 17). Opiate peptides, such as enkephalins, may play a drive-reducing function. In other words, once a reward is attained opiate peptides may bring the behavior to a satisfying termination (Belluzzi and Stein, 1977; Stein, 1978).

Overall, then endorphins seem to play a number of powerful, if mysterious, roles in regulating our innermost states and feelings. More is likely to come soon in this exciting story, which could have such enormous impact in medicine and upon our lives, but this fascinating field is so new that the first chapter has only just been written, with little time elapsed in which to understand it.

IV. The Functional Role of Transmitters in the Brain

It is through the action of transmitters in specific connections that we reach the next level of integration beyond that of the single nerve cell. Specific neurochemical networks, hard at work, pulse out their patterns to the periphery, drive different responses or create different moods. We have mentioned that noradrenergic systems appear to play a particular role in pleasure and mood. We have also mentioned that the dopaminergic systems in their normal operation seem important for a balanced mental state, as well as for well-regulated movement. It is now recognized that certain alterations of basal ganglia DA activity can lead to schizophrenia, just as certain others can result in movement disorders. We saw that the normal fluctuations of the serotonergic and cholinergic systems participate in the broad (if not global) neural functions of sleep and arousal, respectively, and we noted that GABA-nergic systems keep the brain in a controlled state of excitation by bringing in inhibition, and that disorders of these systems may appear in genetically based diseases. Finally, recently discovered peptides, the endorphins, seem to be involved in pain; somehow, if the system is altered, addiction can result. This list of things we have seen is only partial, but it illustrates some of the many ways in which specific neurotransmitter systems are involved in integrated functions.

The above is not to imply, of course, that each transmitter serves a particular brain function. We can only say that one or another function is tied to a particular transmitter, and that if that substance is absent or present in excessive amounts, some disorder of function may be expected. We must emphasize that these transmitter systems are only parts of larger neuronal systems, and that these parts play interdependent and interrelated roles. Indeed, as we saw, some of these interrelationships are already known: the antagonistic actions of catecholaminergic and serotonergic systems on behavior, the reciprocal and circular influences of dopaminergic and GABA-nergic systems in movement control.

Later we shall discuss our current understanding of the causes and treatment of pain (Chapter 12). Then in Chapter 17 we shall look at the basis and treatment of psychiatric disorders, alcoholism and addiction. For now, however, we shall illustrate how, through basic research, it has been possible to understand and treat the disorder known as Parkinson's disease.

Parkinson's disease is a chronic, progressive degenerative disease of the CNS. It is associated with muscular rigidity, tremor and poverty of movement. The patient has severe difficulty in initiating voluntary motor activity. There is a delay in starting a movement, and if it is to continue it often may occupy the entire attention of the person. Parkinson, the physician who first described the disease in 1817, defined it as ". . . involuntary tumultuous motion, which lessened muscular power, in parts not in action and even when supported; with the propensity to bend the trunk forward, and to pass from a walking to a running pace: the senses and intellects being injured." The patient has extreme difficulty in maintaining a normal or desired amplitude of movement; this feature is the most disabling. For example, a Parkinsonian may start to walk with a normal 18-inch stride, but very rapidly the distance is reduced so that each step covers no more than a few inches. Balance is exceedingly precarious, and patients fall easily. A dramatic example of the same problem is seen in handwriting: it progressively deteriorates during the course of the disease. And as shown in Fig. 6-15, it diminishes in size as the individual writes until it becomes extremely small and illegible.

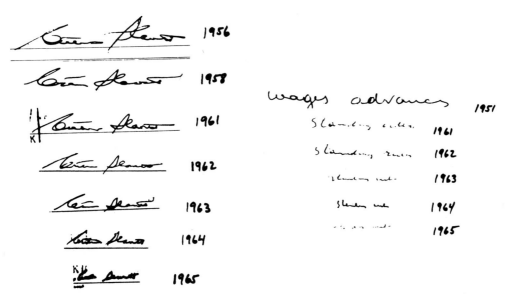

Fig. 6-15. Samples of the signature of two patients with Parkinson's disease. Over the course of a few years their writing became micrographic and illegible. (From Schwab, 1972.)

Parkinsonism is one of the most prevalent nervous disorders. Studies in Great Britain, Sweden and the United States give an incidence of at least 60 in 100,000 to 114 in 100,000. The incidence is higher in older people (Selby, 1968).

The disease has long been known to be associated with pathological changes in certain of the basal ganglia, but these alterations were subtle and not clearly understood. In 1955 the German anatomist Hassler noted that there were fewer nerve cell bodies in the diseased substantia nigra in individuals with Parkinsonism. When it became known a few years later that the basal ganglia had a rich dopaminergic innervation, this discovery prompted an extensive study of dopamine in the human brain, particularly in the brains of patients suffering motor disorders known to involve the basal ganglia. Hornykiewicz, an Austrian neurologist, found that in the brains of Parkinsonians DA was decreased to very low levels in the caudate nucleus, putamen and substantia nigra (Hornykiewicz, 1971, 1974). In addition, the concentration of homovanillic acid, a perfectly stable compound under postmortem conditions, was also subnormal in these three areas. This corollary finding was important, because it ruled out the possibility that the low DA levels in Parkinsonism were due to breakdown of dopamine after death. It appeared then as if the loss of dopaminergic cells in the substantia nigra caused a loss of DA in the other two areas, and that this accounted in part for the Parkinsonian symptomatology.

One of the best examples of the causal relationship between striatal DA deficiency and this symptomatology came from a study of a patient with hemi-

Parkinsonism, where the disease is primarily unilateral. In this person, although striatal DA was subnormal on both sides, the deficiency was much more pronounced on the side opposite to the symptoms (Table 6-2), as expected on the basis of the circuitry, which is crossed. The deficit appears quite specific to DA, since concentrations of serotonin in the striatum on the two sides were similar. Moreover, a deficiency in DA metabolism was not seen in other movement disorders, such as Huntington chorea. These results prompted attempts to therapeutically replenish striatal dopamine in patients with Parkinsonism.

Table 6-2 Dopamine and serotonin in the right and left striatum of a case with hemi-Parkinsonism with symptoms predominantly on the right side of the body[a]

	Dopamine (μg/gm)		Serotonin (μg/gm)	
	Normal	Hemi-Parkinson (right side)	Normal	Hemi-Parkinson (right side)
Caudate nucleus			0.33(6)	
right side	3.28(4)	1.25	—	0.26
left side	3.55(4)	0.59	—	0.26
Putamen			0.32(6)	
right side	3.73(4)	0.93	—	0.26
left side	4.74(4)	0.13	—	0.21

[a] From Hornykiewicz (1971).

It was argued that, since the disease was associated with a DA deficiency in brain, biochemical manipulations which would temporarily replenish DA stores would lessen the motor symptoms. Perhaps it would be possible to give patients additional dopamine or a DA precursor to restore striatal dopamine. Dopamine, however, could not be given since it does not pass the blood–brain barrier. Moreover, administration of an amino acid precursor, tyrosine, would not have been helpful because tyrosine hydroxylase is rate-limiting. On the other hand, L-dopa, the immediate precursor of dopamine, seemed to offer hope of success. Its enzyme, dopa decarboxylase, is not rate-limiting, and L-dopa does pass the blood–brain barrier. Observations on the effect of L-dopa in the brains of laboratory animals showed that it was readily converted to dopamine and that there was a marked accumulation of DA in the basal ganglia.

The first clinical trials with L-dopa in patients with Parkinson's disease were highly successful. The initial description of its dramatic effect on poverty of movement shows why L-dopa therapy has revolutionized the prognosis for many Parkinsonian patients:

6. INTEGRATION: PUTTING IT ALL TOGETHER

The effect of a single intravenous administration of L-DOPA was, in short, a complete abolition or substantial reduction of akinesia. Bedridden patients who were unable to sit up, patients who could not stand up from a sitting position, and patients, who when standing, could not start walking, performed all these activities with ease after L-DOPA. They walked around with normal associated movements and they could even run and jump. The voiceless, aphonic speech, blurred by palilalia and unclear articulation, became forceful and clear again as in a normal person. For short periods of time the patients were able to perform motor activities which could not be prompted by any other known drug to any comparable degree. This DOPA effect reached its peak within 2–3 hours and lasted, in diminishing intensity, for 24 hours (Hornykiewicz, 1974).

Since its inception the therapeutic effect of L-dopa has been firmly established. This story represents at this time the best example of a rationally developed drug treatment for a CNS disorder based on neuroanatomical and neurochemical understanding of the nature of the disease.

Dopamine deficiency, however, is not the only underlying problem in Parkinsonism. Studies in laboratory animals show that a cholinergic/dopaminergic balance is involved in normal motor control. When tested on single cells in the caudate nucleus, ACh is usually excitatory and DA usually inhibitory. Accordingly, it has been suggested that a functional equilibrium exists in the striatum between excitatory ACh and inhibitory DA mechanisms in normal striatal motor control (McGeer et al., 1961; Hornykiewcz, 1971). This hypothesis is in line with the fact that anticholinergic drugs have been used as a partially successful treatment in Parkinsonism. Most of the rigidity and tremor is abated, but the poverty of movement (akinesia) does not respond. The beneficial action of these drugs is probably due to a decrease in the relative hyperactivity of ACh mechanisms in the striatum, freed as those systems seem to be from their normal nigrostriatal DA inhibition. By normalizing the ratio between ACh and DA, these anticholinergic agents work toward balancing the equilibrium.

The use of L-dopa, however, is not without its own problems. A number of adverse side effects such as nausea are experienced by patients under L-dopa therapy. The large amount of L-dopa that has to be administered, however, undoubtedly contributes to the adverse reactions. Less than 5% reaches the brain; the remainder is metabolized to catecholamines in the rest of the body. It was suggested that administration of an inhibitor of dopa decarboxylase that did not itself cross the blood–brain barrier might relieve some of the adverse peripheral reactions. Inhibiting this enzyme, which converts L-dopa to DA, would thus lower body DA levels without affecting DA concentration in the brain. Use of such an inhibitor, carbidopa, allows the concurrent dose of L-dopa to be reduced by about 80%, ameliorating anorexia (loss of appetite), nausea and vomiting while maintaining therapeutic efficiency.

None of the treatments described cure Parkinsonism. In the absence of continued therapy the patient most often regresses, and in some cases L-dopa therapy continued over a prolonged period becomes progessively less effective, and side reactions can develop. Nonetheless, for the first time it is possible to alleviate the disastrous symptoms of the disease.

V. Summary

Integration at the level of the single cell is a microstruggle, a tiny battle of excitation and inhibition that takes place against the modulating background of the slow-acting inputs. We have described how inputs are integrated by single cells and in groups of cells, and how this results in precisely summated outputs and ultimately in specific behavioral responses. We have seen how disturbances in integration, as in the basal ganglia, can bring about disordered function, and how an understanding of the anatomical and neurochemical systems involved leads to a strategy to alleviate or abolish the dysfunction. As we said in the beginning of this chapter, integration occurs at a number of levels. In subsequent chapters we shall study it at the level of systems: the visual, auditory and motor systems.

The scintillating spatiotemporal pattern of signals we have envisioned in the normal brain is highly reliable, and can give precise, predicted outputs time and time again throughout a lifetime. It is built for reliability but at the same time can deliver flexibility. Behaviors are modified during a lifetime, and we, like practically all animals, can learn and remember our experiences. How does the nervous system achieve these dual functions of reliability and flexibility? In succeeding chapters we shall see the highly adaptable qualities of the nervous system: like a society or nation, it is plastic and able to modify its properties as a function of previous experience. It builds itself from its history.

As the story unfolds we shall discover the unique operational and plastic properties of single neurons viewed against the backdrop of their circuitry. We shall learn how a circuit carries out specific functions. We shall witness, as well as we understand the matter at this time, how cellular properties, as parts of larger systems, give us the capacity to see, hear, feel, and move—and to learn and remember.

Key Terms

Active dendrites: Dendrites which are excitable and generate small local "all or none" potentials; such potentials appear to be largely Ca^{2+}-based.

Amacrine cells: Neurons which lack axons; they are in the retina and olfactory bulb.

γ-Aminobutyric acid (GABA): The major inhibitory transmitter in the mammalian brain. It is used by local circuit neurons and other neurons in many brain areas.

Axon hillock: Region of the cell body from which the axon arises. It is often the site where action potentials are initiated. The threshold for initiating an action potential is lowest at the axon hillock.

Blood–brain barrier: A term used to refer to the fact that certain substances in the body have restricted access to areas of the brain.

Ca^{2+} spikes: Action potentials based on regenerative Ca^{2+} currents instead of Na^+ currents. Ca^{2+} spikes appear to exist in active dendrites.

Dendritic spines: Small, narrow-necked, bulbous protrusions of dendrites. Spines appear to maintain and protect conducting dendritic currents from local synaptic activity, and they appear to convert synapses into constant current-injecting devices.

L-Dopa: The precursor which is converted to dopamine by dopa decarboxylase. L-Dopa administration is used to alleviate the symptoms of Parkinson's disease.

Electrotonic conduction: Conduction of localized, graded potentials that are determined by the passive electrical properties of cells. The measure of this passive decay is the space constant.

Endorphin: Any endogenous molecule that has opiate-like activity.

Enkephalins: Pentapeptides which possess opiate-like activity; their sequence is tyrosine–glycine–glycine–phenylalanine–X–OH, where X is either leucine (Leu-enkephalin) or methionine (Met-enkephalin). Enkephalins are a specific type of endorphin.

Histofluorescence method: A histochemical method of analysis used to reveal the presence of dopamine, norepinephrine or serotonin in tissue sections. Each different transmitter fluoresces with a distinct color.

Huntington's chorea: A disease characterized by involuntary movement and mental deterioration. It is believed to be due to a loss of neurons in the cerebral cortex and basal ganglia.

6-Hydroxydopamine: A compound which destroys catecholaminergic neurons.

Immunohistochemical method: A method of analysis which uses an antibody to a substance (such as a neurotransmitter-synthesizing enzyme) to "stain" it in tissue sections. The antibody reacts specifically with the substance (its antigen). The antibody, in turn, is usually identified by a secondary reaction which produces a fluorescent signal or otherwise readily identifiable reaction product.

Locus coeruleus: A region of the pons where one of the most important groups of noradrenergic cell bodies are found. These neurons project widely throughout the brain.

D-Lysergic acid diethylamide (LSD):   A potent antagonist of serotonergic receptors.

Meso-limbic system: A dopaminergic projection which originates in a cell group in the mesencephalon (A10) and projects to the limbic system (frontal and limbic lobes, hypothalamus, septal region and several regions near the olfactory tract).

Monoamine: Any amine, $R-NH_2$, that has one organic substituent (R) attached to the nitrogen group (e.g., dopamine, norepinephrine, serotonin).

Naloxone: A specific receptor antagonist for opiates and opiate-like compounds.

Parkinson's disease: A chronic, progressive disease characterized by muscular rigidity, tremor and poverty of movement. It appears due, in part, to the degeneration of dopaminergic neurons in the substantia nigra.

Passive dendrites: Dendrites which do not generate action potentials; inexcitable dendrites. Currents spread by electrotonic conduction.

Raphé nuclei: A group of nuclei along the midline of the brain stem whose neurons are serotonergic; their projections are widespread.

Rotational model: Dopamine stimulation of the striatum produces rotation to the opposite side when the striatum is asymmetrically stimulated. The direction of rotation is always toward the least stimulated side.

Septum: An area of the brain rich in cholinergic neurons. These neurons project primarily to the hippocampus via the septohippocampal pathway.

Spatiotemporal summation: The process whereby all synaptic potentials impinging on a neuron's dendrites are integrated over time and space.

Substantia nigra: The locus of a major cell group of dopaminergic neurons which form the nigrostriatal pathway and innervate the striatum.

General References

Cooper, J. R., Bloom, F. E., and Roth, R. H. (1978) "The Biochemical Basis of Neuropharmacology." 3rd Ed. Oxford Univ. Press, London and New York.

Schmitt, F. O., Dev, P., and Smith, B. H. (1976). Electrotonic processing of information by brain cells. *Science* **193**, 114–120.

Shepherd, G. M. (1974). "The Synaptic Organization of the Brain," Chapter 6. Oxford Univ. Press, London and New York.

References

Baker, R. (1976). Pharmacological profile of inhibition in the vestibular and ocular nuclei. *In* "Drugs and Central Synaptic Transmission" (P. B. Bradley and B. N. Dhawan, eds.), pp. 227–234. Macmillan, New York.

Bartholini, G., Burkard, W. P., Pletscher, A., and Bates, H. M. (1967). Increase of cerebral catecholamines caused by 3,4-dihydroxyphenylalanine after inhibition of peripheral decarboxylase, *Nature (London)*, **215**, 852–853.

Belluzzi, J. D., and Stein, L. (1977). Enkephalin may mediate euphoria and drive-reduction reward. *Nature (London)*, **226**, 556–558.

Björklund, A., and Nobin, A. (1973). Fluorescence histochemical and microspectrofluorometric mapping of dopamine and noradrenaline cell groups in the rat diencephalon. *Brain Res.* **51**, 193–205.

Björklund, A., Moore, R. Y., Nobin, A., and Stenevi, U. (1973). The organization of tuberohypophyseal and reticulo-infundibular catecholamine neuron systems in the rat brain. *Brain Res.* **51**, 171–191.

Bloom, F., Battenberg, E., Rossier, J., Ling, N., and Guillemin, R. (1978). Neurons containing β-endorphin in rat brain exist separately from those containing enkephalin: Immunocytochemical studies, *Proc. Natl. Acad. Sci. U.S.A.* **75**, 1591–1595.

Bradford, H. F., and Richards, C. D. (1976). Specific release of endogenous glutamate from piriform cortex stimulated *in vitro*. *Brain Res.* **105**, 168–172.

Cotman, C. W., and Hamberger, A. (1978). Glutamate as a CNS neurotransmitter property of release, inactivation and biosynthesis. *In* "Amino Acids as Neurotransmitters" (F. Fonnum, ed.), pp. 379–412. Raven, New York.

Dahlström, A., and Fuxe, K. (1964). Evidence for the existence of monoamine-containing neurons in the central nervous system. I. Demonstration of monoamines in the cell bodies of brain stem neurons. *Acta Physiol. Scand.* **62**, Suppl. 232, 1–55.

Davidson, N. (1976). "Neurotransmitter Amino Acids." Academic Press, New York.

Falck, B., Hillarp, N.-A., Thieme, G., and Torp, A. (1962). Fluorescence of catecholamines and related compounds condensed with formaldehyde. *J. Histochem. Cytochem.* **10**, 348–354.

Fuxe, K., and Jonsson, G. (1974). Further mapping of central 5-hydroxytryptamine neurons: Studies with the neurotoxic dihydroxytryptamines. *Adv. Biochem. Psychopharmacol.* **10**, 1–12.

Fuxe, K., Hökfelt, T., and Ungerstedt, U. (1970). Morphological and functional aspects of central monoamine neurons. *Int. Rev. Neurobiol.* **13**, 93–126.

Goldstein, A. (1976). Opioid peptides (endorphins) in pituitary and brain. *Science* **193**, 1081–1086.

Harvey, J. A., Heller, A., and Moore, R. Y. (1963). The effect of unilateral and bilateral medial forebrain bundle lesions on brain serotonin. *J. Pharmacol. Exp. Ther.* **140**, 103–190.

Harvey, J. A., Scholfield, C. N., Graham, L. T., and Aprison, M. H. (1975). Putative transmitters in denervated olfactory cortex. *J. Neurochem.* **24**, 445–449.

Heller, A. (1975). Central monoaminergic function. *In* "The Nervous System" (R. O. Brady, ed.), Vol. 1, pp. 409–418. Raven, New York.

Holaday, J. W., Wei, E., Loh, H., and Li, C. H. (1978). Endorphins may function in heat adaptation. *Proc. Natl. Acad. Sci. U.S.A.* **75**, 2923–2927.

Hornykiewicz, O. (1971). Neurochemical pathology and pharmacology of brain dopamine and acetylcholine: Rational basis for the current drug treatment of Parkinsonism. *In* "Contemporary Neurology" (F. H. McDowell, ed.), Vol. 8, pp. 33–65. Davis, Philadelphia.

Hornykiewicz, O. (1974). The mechanisms of action of L-DOPA in Parkinson's disease. *Life Sci.* **15**, 1249–1259.

Hughes, J. (1975). Isolation of an endogenous compound from the brain with pharmacological properties similar to morphine. *Brain Res.* **88**, 295–308.

Hughes, J., Smith, T. W., Kosterlitz H. W., Fothergill, L. A., Morgan, B. A., and Morris, H. R. (1975). Identification of two related pentapeptides from the brain with potent opiate agonist activity. *Nature (London)*, **258**, 577–579.

Iansek, R., and Redman, S. J. (1973). The amplitude, time course and charge of unitary excitatory postsynaptic potentials evoked in spinal motoneuron dendrites. *J. Physiol. (London)*, **234**, 665.

Kuhar, M. J., Simon, J. R., and Rommelspacher, H. (1975). Studies of cholinergic neurons. *In* "Current Developments in Psychopharmacology" (W. B. Essman and L. Valzelli, eds.), Vol. 2, pp. 1–27. Spectrum, New York.

Kuno, M. (1971). Quantum aspects of control and ganglionic synaptic transmission in vertebrates. *Physiol. Rev.* **51**, 467–478.

Lewis, P. R., and Shute, C. C. D. (1967). The cholinergic limbic system: Projections to hippocampal information, medial cortex, nuclei of the ascending cholinergic reticular system, and the subfornical organ and supraoptic crest. *Brain* **90**, 521–540.

Lewis, P. R., Shute, C. C. D., and Silver, A. (1967). Confirmation from choline acetylase: Analyses of a massive cholinergic innervation to the rat hippocampus. *J. Physiol. (London)* **191**, 215–224.

Lindvall, O., and Björklund, A. (1974). The organization of the ascending catecholamine neuron systems in the rat brain as revealed by the glyoxylic acid fluorescence method. *Acta. Physiol. Scand., Suppl.* **412**, 1–48.

Llinas, R., and Hillman, D. E. (1969). Physiological and morphological organization of cerebellar circuits and various vertebrates. *In* "Neurobiology of Cerebellar Evolution and Development," pp. 43–73. Am. Med. Assoc., Chicago, Illinois.

Llinas, R., and Nicholson, C. (1971). Electrophysiological properties of dendrites and somata in alligator Purkinje cells. *J. Neurophysiol.* **33**, 332–351.

McGreer, P. L., Boulding, J. E., Gibson, W. C., and Foulkes, R. G. (1961). Drug-induced extrapyramidal reactions. *J. Am. Med. Assoc.* **177**, 665.

Oderfeld-Nowak, B., Narkiewicz, O., Wieraszko, A., and Gradkowska, M. (1976). Acetylcholinesterase and choline acetyltransferase activity in the amygdala of rat brain after septal lesions. *Brain Res.* **106**, 396–402.

Pellionisz, A., and Llinas, R. (1977). A computer model of cerebellar Purkinje cells. *Neuroscience* **2**, 37–48.

Redman, S. J. (1973). The attenuation of passively propagating dendritic potentials in a motoneuron cable model. *J. Physiol. (London)* **234**, 637.

Redman, S. J. (1976). A quantitative approach to integrative function of dendrites. *In* "Neurophysiology II," Vol. 10 International Review of Physiology (R. Porter, ed.), pp. 1–35. Univ. Park Press, Baltimore.

Roberts, E., Chase, T. N., and Tower, D. B., eds. (1976). "GABA in Nervous System Function." Raven, New York.

Rossier, J., Vargo, T. M., Minick, S., Ling, N., Bloom, F. E., and Guillemin, R. (1977). Regional dissociation of β-endorphin and enkephalin contents in rat brain and pituitary. *Proc. Natl. Acad. Sci. U.S.A.* **74**, 5162–5165.

Sandoval, E., and Cotman, C. W. (1978). Evaluation of glutamate as a neurotransmitter of cerebellar parallel fibers. *Neuroscience*, **3**, 199–206.

Schildkraut, J. J. (1967). The catecholamine hypothesis of affective disorders: A review of supporting evidence. *Am. J. Psychiatry* **122**, 509.

Schwab, R. S. (1972). Akinesia paradoxica. *Electroencephalogr. Clin. Neurophysiol. Suppl.* **31**, 87–92.

Selby, G. (1968). Parkinson's disease. *In* "Handbook of Clinical Neurology" (P. J. Vincken and G. W. Bruyn, eds.), Vol. 6, pp. 173–211. Wiley, New York.

Shepherd, G. M. (1974). "The Synaptic Organization of the Brain," Chapter 6. Oxford Univ. Press, London and New York.

Sherrington, C. S. (1947). "Integrative Action of the Nervous System." Yale Univ. Press, New Haven, Connecticut.

Shoulson, I., and Chase, T. N. (1975). Huntington's disease. *Annu. Rev. Med.* **26**, 419–426.

Shute, C. C. D., and Lewis, P. R. (1967). The ascending cholinergic reticular system: Neocortical, olfactory and subcortical projections. *Brain* **90**, 497–520.

Smith, G. D., and Griffin, J. F. (1978). Conformation of [Leu^5]enkephalin from X-ray diffraction: Features important for recognition at opiate receptor. *Science* **199**, 1214–1216.

Snyder, S. H. (1977). Opiate receptors and internal opiates. *Sci. Am.* **236**, 44–56.

Spencer, W. A., and Kandel, E. R. (1961). Electrophysiology of hippocampal neurons IV. Fast prepotentials. *J. Neurophysiol.* **24**, 272–285.

Stein, L. (1979). "Biology of Reinforcement: A Tribute to James Olds." Academic Press, New York (to be published).

Stone, J., and Freeman, J. A. (1971). Synaptic organisation of the pigeon's optic tectum: A Golgi and current source-density analysis. *Brain Res.* **27**, 203–221.

Storm-Mathisen, J. (1977). Localization of transmitter candidates in the brain: The hippocampal formation as a model. *Prog. Neurobiol.* **8**, 119–181.

Ungerstedt, U. (1971). Stereotaxic mapping of the monamine pathways in the rat brain. *Acta Physiol. Scand.*, *Suppl.* **367**, 1–48.

Ungerstadt, U. (1974). Functional dynamics of central monoamine pathways. *In* "The Neurosciences: Third Study Program" (F. O. Schmitt and F. G. Worden, eds.), pp. 695–704. MIT Press, Cambridge, Massachusetts.

Yamamoto, C., and Matsui, S. (1976). Effect of stimulation of excitatory nerve tract on release of glutamic acid from olfactory cortex slices *in vitro*. *J. Neurochem.* **26**, 487–491.

Young, A. B., Oster-Granite, M. L., Herndon, R. M., and Snyder, S. H. (1974). Glutamic acid: Selective depletion by viral induced granule cell loss in hamster cerebellum. *Brain Res.* **73**, 1–13.

7

Elementary Learning and Behavioral Plasticity

Learning is the most important thing that people do. One of the most obvious facts of experience is that we are changed by it. We learn to think, to speak and to relate to our world and to each other. The ability to learn and remember is the essential condition for the development and maintenance of culture. In this

255

chapter, we consider some of the simpler forms of learning and behavioral plasticity; more complex aspects are considered in Chapter 8.

Most, if not all, species of animals with nervous systems appear to have the ability to learn, and, as we have emphasized in several chapters, the nervous system is highly plastic. Much recent research on the neurobiology of behavioral plasticity has been on simple forms of learning in relatively simple animals. Furthermore, attention has been restricted to relatively simple circuits, such as found in the spinal cord. Such research is based on the assumption that the neuronal basis of behavioral plasticity in simpler systems might be similar to that of learning and memory in more complex systems, as found in humans. But we do not know whether different species use the same neuronal mechanism to learn and remember. The nervous systems of mammals are quite different from those of nonmammals. It is obvious, for example, that human memory systems have more storage and retrieval capacity than the snail or the frog. So extraordinary is this capacity, in fact, that it has been estimated that the number of bits of information in memory in a well-educated adult is greater than the number of neurons in the brain. This astonishing fact attests to great complexity in the underlying neural mechanisms. Indeed, the physical complexity of the human brain, or for that matter of any mammalian brain, is a formidable barrier to understanding learning and memory. Nevertheless, the fundamental cellular mechanisms of learning and memory might be the same, or at least similar, in all species, and species differences in memory processes and systems might only reflect differences in the numbers of cells involved and the patterns of their interconnections.

Faced with the great complexity of the mammalian brain, many neuroscientists interested in learning have adopted the "model systems" approach. They have used invertebrates with simpler nervous systems, or isolated subsystems of the vertebrate nervous system, such as the spinal cord, which can be shown to have behavioral plasticity.

The history of science provides many examples of simplified models or subsystems that have led to major advances. In the neurosciences, the squid axon is perhaps the most celebrated model system. This single nerve fiber is very large and very "hardy." It can be removed from the squid and kept alive for a long time in a dish. Indeed, it is so durable that its axoplasm can be squeezed out, like toothpaste from a tube, and replaced with various ionic solutions (see Chapter 4). Further, this axon behaves like a vertebrate unmyelinated nerve fiber. With this simplified model, therefore, basic processes can be analyzed in comparison with mammalian nerve fibers. The two essential features of a model system, then, are simplicity (and hence ease of analysis) and appropriateness. We must be sure that the preparation is not only simple but also a good model of the process in question.

Let us start with a few definitions. *Plasticity* is a general term with a long history. In current usage plasticity can refer to virtually any form of change in the nervous system or behavior, ranging from axon sprouting and modification of dendritic spines, through changing levels of neurotransmitters and their enzymes, to human learning and memory. The term *behavioral plasticity* was introduced by William James in 1890 to refer to any meaningful change in behavior. This term, in the sense intended by James, is useful as an "umbrella" to include habituation, sensitization and all varieties of learning from classic conditioning to complex human learning and cognition. This usage allows us to avoid profitless arguments, such as is habituation "really" learning?

We should distinguish two major forms of elementary behavioral plasticity. In one form, exemplified by *habituation* and *sensitization*, a change is induced in an already existing response to a stimulus. This form is <u>nonassociative</u>: other responses are not involved. In the other form, exemplified by classic conditioning, a new response is brought out. Pavlov's dogs, for example, learned to salivate to a previously neutral sound stimulus. This form is associative: a new stimulus–response relationship is established. The general term often used for this category is associative plasticity or <u>*associative learning*</u>. It can include all forms of learning from basic Pavlovian conditioning to complex human learning. Even this simple dichotomy, however, is not without problems. Thus, the extent to which the neutral stimulus is really "neutral" is still a matter of some debate in the field of behavioral conditioning.

I.   Habituation and Sensitization

If a drop of water falls on the surface of the sea just over the flower-like disc of a sea anemone, the whole animal contracts vigorously. If, then, a second drop falls within a few minutes of the first, there is less contraction, and finally, on the third or fourth drop, the response disappears altogether (Jennings, 1906). Here in this marine polyp with the primitive nerve net is clearly exhibited one of the most pervasive phenomena of the animal kingdom—decrement of response with repeated stimulation. Almost every species studied, from amoeba to man, exhibits some form of response decrement when the stimulus is frequently repeated or constantly applied (Harris, 1943). The ubiquity of the phenomenon plus its obvious survival value suggests that this kind of plasticity must be one of the most fundamental properties of animal behaviour. (Sharpless and Jasper, 1956, p. 655).

Habituation appears to be the most ubiquitous form of behavioral plasticity. All multicellular organisms show it, as do virtually all reflexes (except possibly some monosynaptic ones). Thus, it seems to be an extremely important behavioral mechanism for adaptation and survival.

Habituation is more than a part of survival, however. It is also a most important process in human behavior, as evident in adaptation to adverse but unavoidable stimuli and stresses (Glass and Singer, 1972). It serves to eliminate response patterns which are not useful. Those of us who live in cities scarcely notice the high background noise. We become used to familiar sounds (the ceaseless roar of traffic on the avenues, the constant din of others' conversations, the seemingly ever-present tattoo of a jackhammer), and we hardly notice physical contacts as we walk along the streets (the crowding, the jostling and bumping). Even in our homes, we become habituated to familiar but biologically irrelevant stimuli, the ticking of an alarm clock or a fan on a hot summer day. Animals also show such habituation; a rabbit cares little about a butterfly.

Habituation is currently of great interest in neurosciences and psychology. This interest has its origins in four important studies on habituation: one on the startle response and spinal reflexes in the rat (Prosser and Hunter, 1936), a second on electroencephalographic (EEG) arousal (Sharpless and Jasper, 1956), a third on auditory evoked potentials (Hernández-Peón, 1960), and a fourth in the Soviet Union on many things from human behavior to the mollusc nervous system (Sokolov, 1960, 1963; Pakula and Sokolov, 1973). All these studies emphasized that habituation is an important aspect of behavioral plasticity or learning, that the nervous system itself exhibits habituation and that neurobiological analysis of the underlying mechanisms is feasible. These papers stimulated extensive research on behavioral plasticity. There is now growing agreement on the synaptic mechanisms involved and on our ability to predict and understand even rather complex aspects of behavioral habituation, based on these mechanisms.

So what is habituation? *Habituation* is generally defined as a decrement in response to an initially novel stimulus when it is given repeatedly (Harris, 1943; Humphrey, 1930, 1933). Response decrements to very rapid stimulation (more than 100 per second) are generally excluded, as are decrements resulting from trauma, drugs, etc. The main features of habituation, which precisely and universally characterize it, are given below.

A.   Characteristics of Habituation

There are nine features of habituation which characterize it at the level of behavioral responses (Thompson and Spencer, 1966). They are necessary in order to identify the phenomenon and to define in detail the relationships between stimulus (or training variables) and response. In brief, the parameters are as follows.

1. Repeated stimulation results in a decrease in response (usually a negative exponential).

2. Spontaneous recovery occurs after stimulation is stopped.

3. Repeated series of stimuli cause greater habituation; long term effects occur.

4. Habituation is directly proportional to stimulus frequency.

5. Habituation is inversely proportional to stimulus intensity.

6. Recovery may be prolonged with additional stimulation, even though the response decrement is already at zero.

7. Habituation shows some degree of generalization, i.e., involvement of other stimuli.

8. Presentation of another (usually extra strong) stimulus causes restoration of the response, "dishabituation."

9. The amount of "dishabituation" itself habituates with repetition.

A number of other terms have been used for behavioral habituation as characterized here, *adaptation*, for example. However, adaptation is often used for processes limited to sensory receptors or to central fatigue (in contrast to muscle fatigue, which is based on processes limited to the muscle and neuromuscular junction). Other terms used more or less equivalently with habituation include "stimulus satiation" (Glanzer, 1953) and "reactive inhibition" (Hull, 1943). There is an interesting parallel between habituation and extinction of conditioned responses (Humphrey, 1930). Except for the obvious difference that conditioned responses must first be learned, extinction and habituation are strikingly similar processes.

B. Invertebrate Monosynaptic Models of Habituation

The most complete analysis to date of neural mechanisms underlying habituation and sensitization is the work of Kandel and associates on the invertebrate, *Aplysia* (Fig. 7-1) (for a review see Castellucci and Kandel, 1976a; Kandel, 1977). Using the gill (and siphon) withdrawal reflex, Kandel and associates have been able to move from a behavioral analysis in the intact animal to a quantal analysis of transmitter mechanisms at an identified synapse.

The great advantage of invertebrates lies in the fact that in many cases the nervous system is relatively simple. A diagram of the abdominal ganglion of *Aplysia*, containing the motor neurons for siphon and gill, is shown in Fig. 7-2. Many of the neurons are so large and are so easily recognized from animal to animal that they have been given their own names! The names are not very personal (right one, right two, etc.) but they do allow one to speak about specific neurons. *Aplysia* has a total of about 15,000 neurons, grouped into 9 major ganglia.

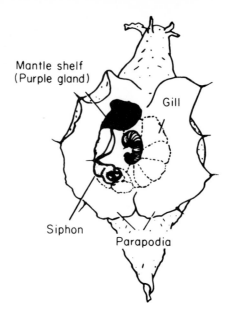

Fig. 7-1. Dorsal view of an *Aplysia*. (From Pinsker *et al.*, 1970, copyright by the American Association for the Advancement of Science.)

The behavioral response of the gill-withdrawal reflex is controlled by the abdominal ganglion, which contains only about 2000 neurons. For behavioral studies, the habituation stimulus is a brief jet of seawater delivered via a Water Pik, a relatively natural tactile stimulus. The response shows clear and systematic habituation to a stimulus repeated every minute or so, shows spontaneous recovery over a period of many minutes and exhibits dishabituation (see Fig. 7-3).

Habituation of the response shows most of the essential parametric characteristics of behavioral habituation (see Section I,A). In addition, and most important, it is also possible to demonstrate that dishabituation is a superimposed sensitization process.

The siphon response is habituated and another response—that of the purple gland—is tested only at the beginning and end of siphon habituation. Neck stimulation, an effective dishabituating stimulus for siphon habituation, is then applied. It causes comparable increases both in the habituated siphon response and in the nonhabituated purple gland test response (Carew *et al.*, 1971). These results are in perfect agreement with related work on spinal flexion reflexes and rat startle response showing the independence of habituation and sensitization.

Fig. 7-2. (A) Dorsal view of the abdominal ganglion illustrating identified cells. The motor neurons for siphon and gill have been darkened. (From Frazier, 1967.) (B) Photograph of an actual ganglion. (From Coggeshall, 1967.)

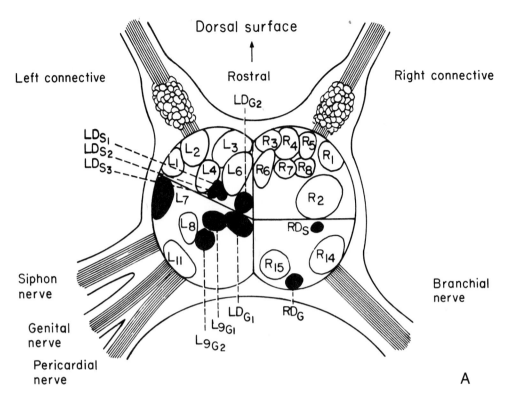

Dorsal surface

Rostral

Left connective

Right connective

LD$_{G2}$

LD$_{S1}$
LD$_{S2}$
LD$_{S3}$

L$_2$ L$_3$ R$_3$ R$_4$ R$_5$

L1   R$_1$

L$_4$ L$_6$ R$_6$ R$_7$ R$_8$

L$_7$ R$_2$

L$_8$ RD$_S$

L$_{11}$ R$_{14}$

R$_{15}$

LD$_{G1}$ RD$_G$

L$_{9G1}$

L$_{9G2}$

Siphon
nerve

Genital
nerve

Pericardial
nerve

Branchial
nerve

A

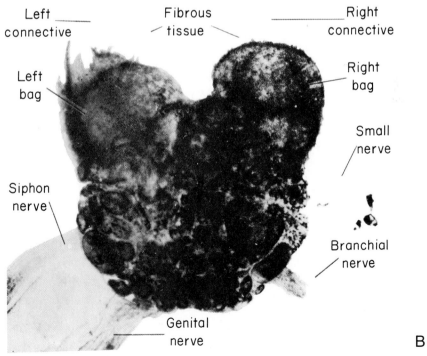

Left
connective

Fibrous
tissue

Right
connective

Left
bag

Right
bag

Small
nerve

Siphon
nerve

Branchial
nerve

Genital
nerve

B

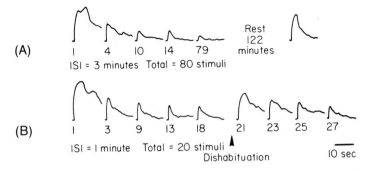

(A)

Rest
122
minutes

1   4   10   14   79

ISI = 3 minutes   Total = 80 stimuli

(B)

1   3   9   13   18   21   23   25   27

ISI = 1 minute   Total = 20 stimuli

Dishabituation

10 sec

Fig. 7-3. Habituation, spontaneous recovery, and dishabituation of the gill-withdrawal reflex. Photocell record from two response habituations in a single preparation. The interval between stimuli (ISI) and total number of habituatory stimuli are indicated. (A) Decrement of the response with repetition of the tactile stimulus. Following a 122-minute rest the response was almost fully recovered. (B) A later experiment from the same preparation. After rehabituation of the response a stimulus consisting of a strong and prolonged tactile stimulus to the neck region was presented at the arrowhead. Successive test responses were facilitated for several minutes. (From Pinsker *et al.*, 1970, copyright by the American Association for the Advancement of Science.)

So now, having demonstrated that behavioral gill withdrawal is a good model of habituation, Kandel and associates analyzed reduced preparations, focusing on a system that included the gill and siphon connected by nerves to the abdominal ganglion. Intracellular recordings could be made both from the motor neurons and the mechanoreceptors during repeated tactile stimulation of the siphon skin.

A necessary step in the analysis is the identification of the motor neurons controlling the behavioral response. Some 13 motor neurons control the response. The afferent side of the reflex is mediated by a cluster of about 24 mechanoreceptors innervating the siphon skin. These have direct *monosynaptic* connections to the motor neurons and indirect polysynaptic connections via excitatory and inhibitory interneurons.

It is first necessary to rule out peripheral factors. Stimulation of the skin at a rate that produces habituation results in no decrement in afferent input (Byrne *et al.*, 1974), and stimulation of motor neurons intracellularly at rates that would yield habituation of the reflex produces no decrement in the motor response. Finally, dishabituation does not alter the properties of the sensory receptors or nerve muscle functions of the reflex. Consequently, both habituation and dishabituation must result from changes in the central nervous system—the abdominal ganglion.

The entire pattern of habituation and dishabituation can, of course, be produced by stimulation of the afferent siphon nerve rather than siphon skin. The complex excitatory synaptic potential produced by such stimulation exhibits habituation and dishabituation of the intracellular responses of a motor neuron. The decrease in the complex excitatory synaptic potential could be due either to changes in properties of the motor neuron, e.g., a change in input resistance, or to a change in the synaptic actions on the motor neuron (or prior to it). Input resistance of the motor neuron measured during habituation and dishabituation does not change, i.e., the general membrane properties of the motor neuron are unaffected.

The monosynaptic connections on motor neurons made by single sensory cells also exhibit habituation (Castellucci *et al.*, 1970; Castellucci and Kandel, 1974) (Fig. 7-4). Thus the locus of the habituation process is at the synaptic terminals of the sensory cells. Excitatory postsynaptic potentials recorded from interneurons activated monosynaptically by these sensory fibers also decrease. Consequently, interneuron processes such as recruitment of central inhibition could be ruled out. Examples of habituation of the monosynaptic excitatory postsynaptic potentials are shown in Fig. 7-4. It is important to determine whether dishabituation (sensitization) occurs in this same monosynaptic pathway from stimulation of the head. It does, as shown in Fig. 7-4. This facilitation does

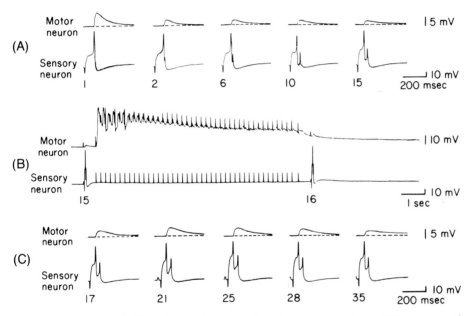

Fig. 7-4. Synaptic habituation and sensitization at monosynaptic excitatory connections between a sensory and motor neuron. In this experiment, a sensory neuron which makes a monosynaptic connection within a motor neuron is stimulated repetitively and the motor neuron's response recorded intracellularly. (A) Habituation. Repetitive stimulation of the sensory nerve once every 10 seconds generates an excitatory synaptic potential in the motor neuron which decrements with the number of stimuli. Stimulus numbers 1, 2, 6, 10 and 15 are shown. (B) Absence of a change in the sensory neuron. A strong stimulus (6 per second train for 4 seconds) is applied to the connection after the fifteenth stimulus. The firing pattern of the sensory neuron is unaffected. (C) Sensitization. Heterosynaptic stimulation to the connective partially restores the amplitude of the synaptic potential. (From Castellucci and Kandel, 1976a.)

not involve an increase in the firing of the sensory neuron stimulated for habituation training. On the basis of these studies a schematic theoretical diagram of the mechanisms of habituation and sensitization in this system can be formulated (see Fig. 7-5).

So far then we have isolated the locus of habituation to the monosynaptic connection between the sensory nerve and the motor neuron (Fig. 7-5), and we have seen that habituation is due to altered synaptic action rather than a change in motor neuron input resistance. The critical question now is to identify the nature of the synaptic change. It must be either a presynaptic or postsynaptic process.

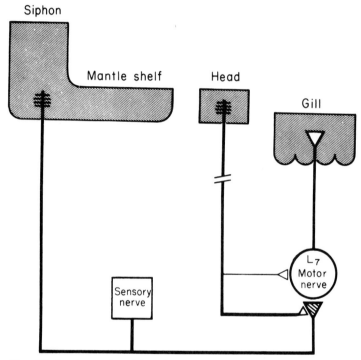

Fig. 7-5. Simplified schematic wiring diagram to indicate the locus of the postulated plastic changes underlying habituation and dishabituation (sensitization) of the gill-withdrawal reflex. Only one sensory neuron and one motor neuron are represented. Habituation is due to a decrement in excitatory transmission at the synapse (hatched area) between the mechanoreceptor neurons and the motor neurons. Dishabituation (sensitization) is due to heterosynaptic facilitation at the same synapse. A hypothetical pathway which synapses on the presynaptic terminals of the sensory fibers and mediates the proposed presynaptic facilitation is indicated. The dishabituatory stimulus also produces an excitatory input to the motor neuron. Dishabituation can be produced by a strong stimulus to most parts of the animal's body surface, although only the head is indicated in the diagram. The exact neural pathway from the head, indicated by the interrupted line, has not yet been worked out. (From Castellucci *et al.,* 1970. Copyright 1970 by the American Association for the Advancement of Science.)

7. ELEMENTARY LEARNING AND BEHAVIORAL PLASTICITY

There might be some type of decrease in transmitter release or some type of decrease in the action of the transmitter on the motor neuron.

In an appropriate monosynaptic system, pre- versus postsynaptic change can be attacked directly by examining the behavior of the *miniature synaptic potentials*. Since transmitter is released in quantal packets, the average amplitude E for an evoked excitatory synaptic potential is given by

$$E = m \times \bar{q}$$

where $\bar{q}$ is the mean size of the postsynaptic potential produced by a single quantum and the value of m is determined by the number of transmitter quanta released presynaptically. The value of $\bar{q}$ is determined from the response of the postsynaptic transmitter receptors. Values for both of these parameters can be estimated experimentally.

The ideal experiment is to record intracellularly from a neuron, in this case the motor neuron, and stimulate a single afferent fiber to that neuron under conditions where the total amount of transmitter released is very small. Under these conditions, the synapse will sometimes fail to transmit, other times will transmit only 1 quantum, other times 2 quanta and so on. The resulting frequency distribution of unitary amplitude, twice unitary amplitude, etc., will be random and form a Poisson distribution. Recall that an action potential increases the.probability that quanta are released, and so when release is low the number of quanta discharged to a single action potential will vary in a random fashion. An analogy is to consider a group of allergic individuals all of whom have identical allergies and sneeze in the same way. If a wind blows a little pollen, just about the threshold amount, into the room perhaps no one will sneeze, or only one, or two and so on.

Now if the decremental process underlying habituation is a decrease in probability of transmitter release, there will be a corresponding increase in the number of failures and a reduced frequency of release in the various categories (1 quantum, 2 quanta, etc.) but no change in the amplitude of the unitary response, the twice unitary response, etc. Alternatively, if there is a postsynaptic decrease in receptor sensitivity, there will be no change in percent failures and a decrease in the actual amplitudes of the excitatory synaptic potentials.

In order to perform quantal analysis, it is necessary to "step down" the release of transmitter. Otherwise too many quanta are released and individual quanta cannot be resolved. Release is suppressed by increasing the Mg^{2+} concentration and decreasing the Ca^{2+} concentration of the bathing solution to the point where failures of transmission occur and unitary, twice unitary, etc., responses can be resolved.

Results of these experiments, shown in Fig. 7-6, are beautifully consistent

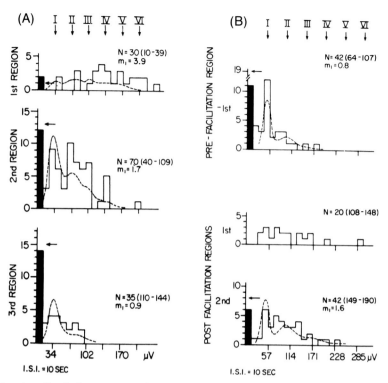

Fig. 7-6. Amplitude histograms of excitatory synaptic potentials and failures evoked by stimulation of sensory neuron during synaptic depression and facilitation. The two values in parentheses next to each histogram refer to the first and last excitatory synaptic potential of a stable region where the amplitude of the synaptic potential changed less than 15%. (A) Synaptic depression: histograms from the successive regions. With repeated stimulation at interstimulus intervals of 10 seconds successive regions show proportionately more failures. That is, the 30 stimuli in the first region produced 2 failures, the next 70 stimuli produced 12 failures and the last 35 stimuli produced 14 failures. The position of the unit peak and the positions of the later peaks do not change, indicating that $\bar{q}$ has not changed while m decreases. (B) Synaptic facilitation: histograms from the region preceding the facilitating stimulation and from two subsequent regions following the stimulus. Prior to facilitation there are many failures. The region following the facilitating stimulus has proportionately fewer failures but the unit peak position of its multiples are not altered, indicating that the estimate of m increased by q does not change. With continued stimulation (second region) the number of failures is still proportionately reduced but the unit peak remains the same. Interstimulus intervals are 10 seconds. In (A) and (B) the dotted lines illustrate theoretical curves based upon the Poisson distribution obtained by assuming a coefficient of variation of 30% for the unit excitatory synaptic potentials. (From Castellucci and Kandel, 1976a.)

with the presynaptic hypothesis (Castellucci and Kandel, 1976b; Kandel, 1976). As habituation develops, the percentage of failures increases, as do the frequencies of low quantal responses, but the amplitudes of the unitary, twice unitary, etc., potential remain unchanged. That is, $\bar{q}$ remains constant but m decreases. In the analogy, the sneeze ($\bar{q}$) remains constant, but the average number/stimulus (m)

decreases. Following a sensitizing stimulus, there is a striking reduction in the percent of failures but no apparent change in the amplitude of the unitary, twice unitary, etc., potentials (see Fig. 7-6). That is $\bar{q}$ again remains consistent but m increases.

In summary, the analysis of habituation and dishabituation of the gill-withdrawal reflex indicates that these behavioral modifications result from plastic changes in the excitatory transmission of previously existing connections. The mechanisms share a common locus, the presynaptic terminals of the sensory neurons projecting on their central targets (see Fig. 7-5). Habituation involves a homosynaptic depression of the terminals due to a repeated activity of the sensory neurons. Dishabituation involves presynaptic facilitation of the synaptic action of the sensory neuron, we postulate, as a result of a pathway that synapses on the sensory neuron terminals. In each case, there is an alteration in transmitter release, and in both cases, receptor sensitivity seems to be unaffected (Castellucci and Kandel, 1976a, pp. 30–32).

A separate form of gill-withdrawal habituation in *Aplysia* can apparently be mediated peripherally. Both habituation and dishabituation in the withdrawal reflex response of a single gill pinnule (a pinnule is the functional element—about 15 pinnules comprise the entire gill) to direct tactile stimulation (drops of water falling upon the pinnule) can be obtained even when all connections with the central nervous system have been severed (Peretz, 1970).

Thus there are indeed two distinct pathways of gill withdrawal response in *Aplysia*, one involving the entire gill and the abdominal ganglion (Kupfermann *et al.*, 1970, 1971) and the other concerning only a single gill pinnule (Peretz, 1970). In the former, identifiable motor neurons make direct synaptic contact with the gill musculature, bypassing all peripheral nerve plexi. Functional central connections through the abdominal ganglion are necessary for mediating the full withdrawal reflex response. The second locus of habituation occurs entirely within the peripheral nerve plexus. Stimulation of the intact peripheral pathway is the necessary and sufficient condition for habituation of the pinnule reflex response. The independence of the two pathways is also supported by the lack of generalization of habituation from one pathway to the other in the semi-intact preparation (Kupfermann *et al.*, 1971).

C. Spinal Reflex Models of Habituation

Reflexes of the spinal mammal (in which the spinal cord has been transected) have been most widely used as a model system for analysis of habituation. The neuronal circuitry of the vertebrate spinal cord is better understood than that of the brain. Spinal reflexes can be studied in animals immobilized and/or anesthetized after spinal section. Further, a spinal reflex, such as the *flexor reflex* elicited by a painful stimulus, appears to be an excellent illustration of simple adaptive behavior—a withdrawal response to avoid injury. In studies of flexor reflex habituation in the hindlimb, the spinal cord is usually cut in the mid-thoracic region. Various hindlimb muscles and nerves are then dissected out for particular types of stimulation and response measurements. The basic procedure involves application of an electrical shock to the skin. If this stimulus is given every few seconds, the limb flexes. This avoidance response typically decreases in strength, i.e., habituates, upon repeated stimulation. If a strong shock is given to some other region of the skin or to another afferent nerve, responses to the original test stimulus will increase in vigor for a time. This enhanced response is called *"dishabituation"* or *sensitization*.

What are the possible mechanisms underlying flexor reflex habituation in the acute spinal cat? The mechanisms have been analyzed in a series of experiments by Spencer and Thompson and colleagues (Thompson and Spencer, 1966; Spencer *et al.*, 1966a,b,c). The flexor reflex is a multisynaptic reflex, involving many connections between stimulus and response (see Fig. 7-7). To determine the basis of habituation it is necessary to consider peripheral versus central

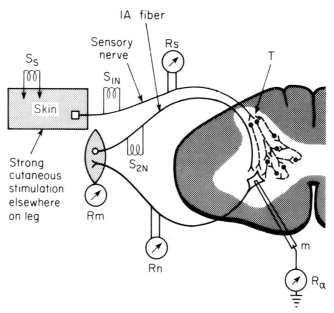

Fig. 7-7. Experimental arrangements used to study habituation and sensitization of the hindlimb flexion reflex in the acute spinal cat. Electrical stimuli can be delivered to skin (S_s) or to afferent nerves (S_{1N}, cutaneous nerve; S_{2N}, muscle nerve). Responses can be recorded from the afferent nerve (R_s), the muscle (R_m), the ventral root (R_n), or the motor neurons ($R\alpha$) with microelectrode (m). (After Thompson, 1967.)

7. ELEMENTARY LEARNING AND BEHAVIORAL PLASTICITY

effects, and to identify where they take place. As scientists, we must be like detectives, seeking important clues and ruling out alternate possibilities.

Is habituation due to a decrement in the stimulus going into the spinal cord? The flexor reflex or the muscle is habituated to repeated skin shock. Figure 7-8 shows habituation and spontaneous recovery of the reflex. During repeated stimulation, there is no decrease in the afferent nerve response monitored at R_s. Therefore, the muscle response habituation cannot be due to any decrease in the incoming nerve activity.

The possibility that flexor reflex habituation is due to muscle fatigue or changes at neuromuscular junctions can be ruled out by recording ventral root (Rn) responses. The same decrease in response occurs as when the motor nerve response is measured. These findings suggest that the processes responsible for habituation are central rather than peripheral. Therefore, spinal reflex habituation must be due to processes occurring within the spinal cord.

Perhaps the most critical data are from intracellular recordings from motor neurons participating in the flexor reflex being habituated (m in Fig. 7-7). Perhaps response habituation is due to a decreased excitability of the motor neurons. It is necessary to test the excitability of the motor neurons. The excitability of the motor neurons can be measured independently of the cutaneous nerve habituation stimuli by stimulation of the large group of IA sensory fibers (S_{2N}) that have

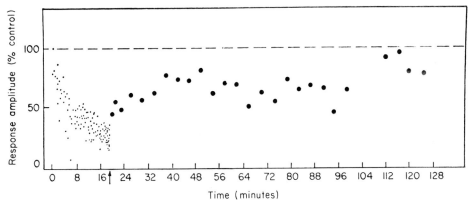

Fig. 7-8. Habituation (zero minutes to arrow) and spontaneous recovery (arrow to 128 minutes) of the hindlimb flexion reflex of the spinal cat in response to repeated skin shocks. (Stimuli were brief trains of shocks, 5 in 50 msec, delivered every 10 seconds during habituation and every 3 minutes during spontaneous recovery, except for a 12-minute period of no stimuli at about 100 minutes.) At slow stimulation rates of 1/minute the response remains at or near 100%. The response measured is tension developed by contraction of the tibialis anterior muscle, expressed as a percentage of mean initial control response amplitude. (From Thompson and Spencer, 1966.)

direct monosynaptic connections on the alpha motor neurons. If the monosynaptic response of the motor neurons recorded intracellularly does not change during the course of habituation, then it follows that the tonic excitability of the motor neurons is unchanged.

As shown in Fig. 7-9, the excitability of spinal motor neurons does not change during habituation to repeated cutaneous nerve stimulation. On these grounds we may conclude that the general excitability of the motor neuron does not change during habituation. This in turn means that the change must occur prior to the motor neurons within the spinal cord.

One earlier theory of habituation is that activity of the postsynaptic neuron acts back on the afferent terminals in a negative feedback manner as a result of

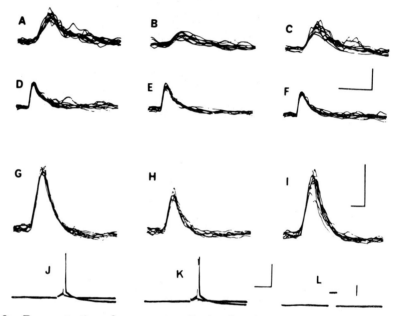

Fig. 7-9. Demonstration of constant amplitude of interpolated monosynaptic potentials and stability of threshold to applied depolarizing currents during period of polysynaptic decrement in deep peroneal motor neurons. (A)–(C) Polysynaptic potentials to single shock stimuli delivered to posterior femoral cutaneous nerve. (A) Control period established by stimulating at 30-second intervals. (B) Period of decrement during stimulation at 1-second intervals. (C) Period of recovery, stimuli at 30-second intervals. (D)–(F) Monosynaptic potentials to stimuli delivered to deep peroneal nerve at 30-second intervals during periods corresponding to those in (A), (B) and (C), respectively. Note constancy of monosynaptic responses during period of polysynaptic potential decrement. (G)–(I) are identical to (A)–(C) but from a different motoneuron in the deep peroneal group. (J) and (K) show responses to depolarizing current pulses of shape shown in (L) during control and decrement periods corresponding to (G) and (H). Note that pulse continues to be of threshold-straddling intensity. Calibrations: (A)–(F) time = 10 msec, voltage = 2 mV; (G)–(I) time = 10 msec, voltage = 10 mV; (J) and (K) time = 5 msec, voltage = 50 mV; (L) vertical bar represents 1×10^{-8} A. (From Spencer et al., 1966c.)

repeated stimulation. In the spinal cord, interneurons synapse directly on a primary afferent terminal and inhibit transmitter release from those terminals (see Fig. 7-7). This feedback action, called presynaptic inhibition, could act on primary afferents and decrease the effective input volley (see, e.g., Hernández-Peón, 1960). To examine this possibility the terminals are stimulated through a microelectrode (T in Fig. 7-7) and the antidromic response recorded in the cutaneous nerve (Groves et al., 1970). This test is very sensitive to the occurrence of presynaptic inhibition (i.e., depolarization) of the terminals. The test shows no change in afferent terminal excitability during habituation or sensitization of the reflex response. Consequently, presynaptic inhibition of the afferent terminals is ruled out as the mechanism of habituation.

The possibility that postsynaptic inhibition acts on the motor neuron at the time of each habituation stimulus can also be ruled out. Some motor neurons show predominant inhibition (inhibitory synaptic potentials) to the habituating stimulus. These also habituate. Many motor neurons show mixed excitatory–inhibitory synaptic potential responses to the polysynaptic habituating stimulus. The possibility that the evoked inhibitory synaptic potential component grows but is masked by the excitatory synaptic potential can be ruled out by manipulating the inhibitory synaptic potential so that "pure" excitatory synaptic potential is recorded. (The polarity of the inhibitory postsynaptic potential (IPSP) is reversed using chloride injection and intracellular hyperpolarization of the motor neuron.) Such "pure" excitatory synaptic potentials show the same habituation. Finally, the possibility that pre- and postsynaptic inhibitory processes are occurring elsewhere in the system (in the interneurons between input fibers and motor neurons indicated by "?" in Fig. 7-7) may be tested with drugs. Strychnine abolishes most known instances of postsynaptic inhibition in the spinal cord and picrotoxin markedly reduces presynaptic inhibition (Eccles, 1964). Administration of these drugs, separately and in combination, has no significant effects on habituation. Consequently, presynaptic and postsynaptic inhibition are not crucially responsible for the response decrements seen during habituation.

In conclusion, in this series of experiments, we have seen that it is possible to rule out conclusively adaptation of skin receptors, decrements in afferent nerve conduction, presynaptic inhibition of cutaneous nerve terminals, muscle fatigue, decrements in motor nerve conduction, and alterations in motor neuron excitability as possible loci of the neuronal process responsible for habituation. All that remains are interneurons. The pharmacological studies argue strongly against pre- and/or postsynaptic inhibition acting at interneurons as possible mechanisms. These findings suggest the habituation is due to synaptic depression localized to presynaptic terminals at interneurons (Spencer et al., 1966c; Thompson and Spencer, 1966). Perhaps the mechanisms at the synapse are similar to those in Aplysia; however, this has not been established.

D. Dishabituation versus Sensitization

Dishabituation is defined as the disruption of previously established habituation of a response by the presentation of another, usually stronger, stimulus. Many, including Pavlov who discovered habituation, believed that dishabituation is simply the removal of habituation. It is now clear this must be revised. For spinal reflexes there is no such process as dishabituation (Thompson and Spencer, 1966). For example, if dishabituation is a specific disruption of the habituation process, then "dishabituation" should not cause an increase in a control response that has not yet been habituated. However, it does (see Fig. 7-10).

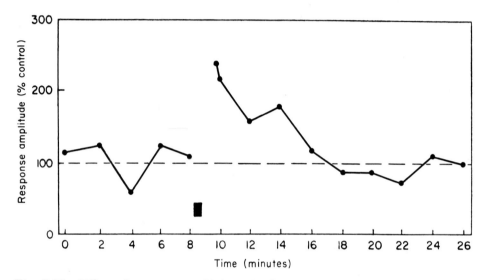

Fig. 7-10. Effect of a strong sensitizing stimulus on a control reflex response. Test stimulus was a brief train of shocks to skin once every 2 minutes and the sensitizing stimulus (solid bar) was a strong shock train delivered elsewhere on the limb for 15 seconds. (From Thompson and Spencer, 1966.)

It is now clear that dishabituation is, in fact, a separate superimposed facilitation or _sensitization_ process. Intracellular data are consistent with this notion. Intracellular recordings from motor neurons during "dishabituation" of an habituated response reveal increased bombardment of the motor neurons by tonic waves of depolarization. The "dishabituation" is clearly a superimposed excitatory synaptic action, a sensitization process.

The studies reviewed above all involved spinal reflexes. In a study of startle responses in intact rats (Groves and Thompson, 1970), dishabituation of the habituated startle response is also an independent superimposed sensitization process. These observations strongly support the view that repeated stimulation results in the development of two separate and/or independent processes in the nervous system, namely, habituation and sensitization.

Studies of spinal interneuron activity accompanying habituation and sensitization of the flexion reflex indicate the existence of two broad classes of plastic interneurons (Groves and Thompson, 1970, 1973). One class shows only response decrement to repeated stimulation, no matter how strong the stimulus or how much sensitization the reflex shows (Fig. 7-11). These are called type "H" (habitua-

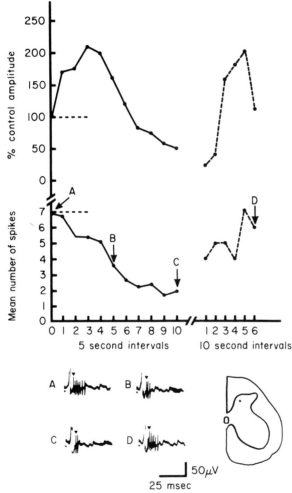

Fig. 7-11. Simultaneous recording of flexor muscle response (upper graph) and activity of spinal interneuron (lower graph) to repeated cutaneous shocks given 2/second during habituation and 1 per 10 seconds during recovery. Examples of neuron responses and location of neuron given below. The neuron shows only habituation even though the muscle shows marked sensitization—it is a type "H" interneuron. (From Thompson and Glanzman, 1976.)

tion) neurons. They are found in the more dorsal layers of the spinal gray matter. The other class shows marked initial increases in responsiveness when moderate or strong stimuli are used. These increases parallel sensitization of the behavioral reflex (see Fig. 7-12). These are called "S" (sensitization) neurons, and they are found in more ventral layers of the spinal gray matter, i.e., closer to the motor neurons. In short, the two categories of interneurons behave as though they reflect the two separate processes of habituation and sensitization.

The spinal flexion reflex is of course polysynaptic, probably involving at least two interneurons, and likely more, in series between afferent fibers and motor neurons. Analysis of such systems is difficult because the interneurons usually cannot be identified unless they are monosynaptically activated by the afferent fibers. The H and S neurons are probably in the reflex path or at least involved in

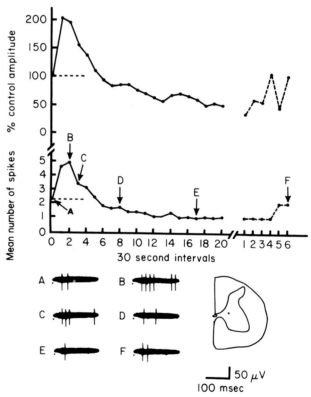

Fig. 7-12. Simultaneous recording of flexor muscle response (upper graph) and activity of spinal interneuron (lower graph) to repeated cutaneous shocks given 2 per second during habituation and 1 per 30 seconds during recovery. Examples of neuron responses and location of neurons are indicated below. The neuron shows marked sensitization followed by habituation and parallels the response of the muscle closely—it is a type "S" interneuron. (From Groves and Thompson, 1973.)

7. **ELEMENTARY LEARNING AND BEHAVIORAL PLASTICITY**

the flexion reflex. This cannot be proven, but it is a reasonable inference—they are the only classes of interneurons that show changes. Many other interneurons respond to the stimuli but show no changes during habituation. The interneurons in the reflex path must show change since the afferent volley is constant and excitation of the motor neurons becomes markedly decreased during habituation.*

E.   Monosynaptic Models of Plasticity

In analyzing mechanisms of synaptic plasticity it is of great advantage to be able to study processes at a monosynaptic pathway where the circuitry is well defined and readily accessible to experimental manipulation. It is also of great interest to study the processes in the brain in order to see how they compare to those in the spinal cord and invertebrates. A new and quite astonishing preparation is the brain slice, particularly the hippocampal *brain slice*.

The *hippocampus* is removed from the brain of a rat or other animal and cut into slices about 400 μm thick in a plane which preserves most intrinsic circuitry (Fig. 7-13). The slices are then transferred into a small chamber filled with artificial media (Ringer's solution) of the same composition as body fluids. The most remarkable finding is that the synaptic potentials and general behavior of the circuitry are identical to that in the intact animal (Dudek *et al*., 1976; Andersen *et al*., 1973, 1977). The advantages of this preparation are great. Looking down on the slice with a microscope experimenters can see before them the rows of neurons so they know exactly where to place the stimulating and recording electrode. Moreover, the preparation is readily manipulated. It is an easy matter to change the ionic composition of the medium and rapidly introduce drugs at known concentrations (White *et al*., 1978a). Hippocampal slices "live" outside the brain for 14 hours or more.

Hippocampal pathways are extraordinarily modifiable and can deliver different responses as a function of stimulus frequencies which are within their normal operating range. The pathway from the cerebral cortex to the granule cells of the hippocampus displays both habituation and potentiation. At low frequencies the response habituates, and at high frequencies it potentiates. Both excitatory synaptic potentials and spike measures of granule cell responses exhibit clear habituation and spontaneous recovery. In brief, this system shows eight of the nine parametric features of habituation (Teyler and Alger, 1976). Stimulus generaliza-

---

* A potentially very promising vertebrate spinal model for analysis of reflex habituation that may provide a solution to the problem of identifying critical interneurons is the plantar cushion reflex (Egger and Wall, 1971; Egger *et al*., 1976).

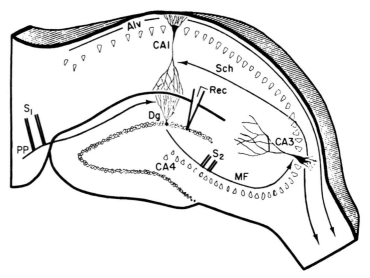

Fig. 7-13. Schematic diagram of a hippocampal slice. A recording micropipette (Rec) is shown positioned in the granule cell layer of the dentate gyrus (Dg). And a bipolar stimulating electrode (S_1) is always placed on the axons of the perforant path (PP) which project to the middle and outer third of the molecular layer of the granule cells. (From Dudek *et al.*, 1976.)

tion (parameter 7, Section I,A) was not tested and would not be expected to occur in a monosynaptic pathway.

This pathway exhibits, as previously noted (Chapter 5), a potent and long lasting low frequency potentiation. Stimulation at a rate of 10 to 15 pulses per second of the perforant path results in potentiation of the granule cell response that can last for minutes to hours, both in the intact hippocampus and in the explant preparation (Alger and Teyler, 1976; Andersen *et al.*, 1973; Bliss and Lømo, 1973; Douglas and Goddard, 1975; White *et al.*, 1978b). Several authors have recently proposed that this form of persistent potentiation induced by relatively "normal" physiological conditions may provide a neuronal substrate for learning and memory (Andersen *et al.*, 1977; Berger and Thompson, 1978; Lynch *et al.*, 1977; White *et al.*, 1978b). Although quantal analysis has not been done in this preparation, the present data are entirely consistent with the notion that habituation is due to a decreased probability of transmitter release from perforant path fiber terminals, whereas long term potentiation appears to be due to post-synaptic excitability changes. One of the advantages of the preparation is that since the transmitters of some hippocampal pathways are known, analysis of the mechansim is greatly facilitated (see Chapter 6).

In summary, this monosynaptic system in the hippocampus shows both habituation and long term potentiation as a function of stimulus frequency over

7. ELEMENTARY LEARNING AND BEHAVIORAL PLASTICITY

what may be considered normal physiological conditions. It is a particularly "plastic" synapse. Curiously, another hippocampal pathway displays potentiation but not habituation. Thus even within a brain area the plasticity characteristics vary extensively. The behavior of the hippocampal pathways is in striking contrast to a skeletal neuromuscular junction, for example, which delivers quite a consistent response over physiological frequencies. In turn, since the hippocampus participates in many adaptive functions, it is expected that its pathways are plastic.

A monosynaptic pathway in the isolated frog spinal cord has also provided a useful model of habituation in the vertebrate central nervous system (Farel et al., 1973; Farel, 1974; Glanzman, 1976; Thompson and Glanzman, 1976). In brief, the spinal cord is removed from the frog and maintained in a perfusion system in vitro. Perhaps most important, this simplified monosynaptic system exhibits retention or "memory" of habituation, a critical parameter distinguishing habituation as a simple form of behavioral plasticity or learning from neuronal refractory phenomena (see parameter 3, Section I,A). The effects of a first series of habituating stimuli persist and are retained by the synapse for a substantial period of time. Further, this retention does not show itself with single test stimuli, but rather as an increased rate and degree of habituation to a subsequent "training" series of stimuli. It is in many ways analogous to the improvement in performance over repeated practice sessions in much more complex learning.

Habituation appears here, as elsewhere, to be a presynaptic mechanism. A direct test using quantal analysis (see the studies by Kandel and associates above) indicates that increasing habituation is accompanied by an increased number of failures of unitary excitatory synaptic potentials recorded intracellularly from the motor neuron (Glanzman, 1976). This result argues for a decrease in probability of transmitter release from the terminals as the mechanisms of habituation in this system.

II. General Theories of Habituation

The first modern formulation of a general "brain systems" theory of habituation is that proposed by Sokolov in 1960. It has proved extremely influential and useful. The theory, often termed the model-comparator theory, is schematized in Fig. 7-14. Sokolov initially developed it to account for results of his studies of habituation of the human orienting response. In essence, he proposed that the cerebral cortex forms a model, i.e., some kind of pattern of neuronal activity, corresponding to a repeated stimulus. The reticular formation of the brain stem, on the other hand, is postulated to serve as a model-comparator and amplifier. If the stimulus

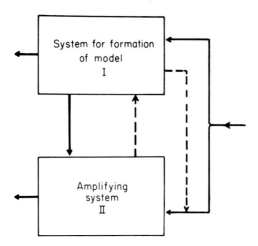

Fig. 7-14. Sokolov's model of habituation involving comparator and amplifier components. A model develops against which are compared new stimuli. If they differ from the habituating stimulus, an increased response will result. (From Sokolov, 1960.)

changes, a new pattern of activity results. The reticular formation makes the comparison and produces an increase in arousal.

Sokolov's theory accounts particularly well for the interesting phenomenon of "dishabituation" to a stimulus suddenly reduced in intensity below the level used in habituation. City dwellers, for example, find the silence of the forest "deafening." It can also account for the so-called missing stimulus effect. If a habituating stimulus is repeated at a constant rate until habituation has occurred and then one stimulus is omitted, responses to the next stimulus will sometimes be increased or "dishabituated." This effect, incidentally, is often difficult to obtain in animals—it has been observed primarily in studies of the human orienting response. Sokolov, however, did not attempt to specify the neural mechanisms that might underlie his general theory. In particular, the nature of the "model formation" process in the cerebral cortex was not considered in terms of possible synaptic processes. Another theory of habituation (Wagner, 1976), similar to Sokolov's but more detailed, assumes that habituation is a kind of "short term" memory (Atkinson and Shiffrin, 1968).

An alternative *"dual-process" theory* of habituation was proposed by Groves and Thompson in 1970. It was based primarily on the idea that dishabituation is not a specific disruption of habituation, but a separate superimposed process of sensitization, as noted for the spinal flexor reflex (see Section I,C). That sensitization is a separate process is shown by its development, when the habituating stimulus is moderate to strong in intensity, *prior* to the onset of habituation in all systems from spinal reflexes to intact human behavior (see Fig. 7-15, and Thompson *et al.*, 1973). Finally, in their studies of spinal interneurons (see Section I,C), only two classes of "plastic" interneurons during reflex habituation were found—some that showed only decreases and others that showed increases followed by variable decreases.

7. **ELEMENTARY LEARNING AND BEHAVIORAL PLASTICITY**

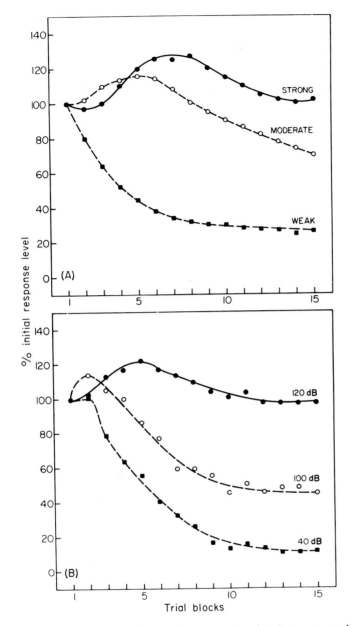

Fig. 7-15. Habituation and sensitization of response amplitude to repeated stimulation as a function of stimulus intensity for two quite different response systems: (A) hindlimb reflex of acute spinal cat to skin shock. (From Groves and Thompson, 1970.) (B) intact human skin potential base level to sound. Note the increase above initial response level with stronger stimulation. (From Thompson *et al.*, 1973.)

These observations led to the notion that a repeated stimulus causes two independent processes in the nervous system—habituation in the reflex pathway and a more generalized sensitization of the "state" of the system. The theory is schematized in Fig. 7-16. Examples of how the two processes can interact to yield actual habituation curves are shown in Fig. 7-17.

Perhaps the most important contribution of the "dual-process" theory is its emphasis on sensitization as a separate and very important process both at behavioral and neural levels. Examples of this were given above in the discussion of various model systems. Sensitization may even serve as a necessary substrate for more complex forms of associative learning (Groves and Thompson, 1970; Castellucci and Kandel, 1976a).

Another important aspect of the dual-process theory is that it assumes only the basic synaptic processes of synaptic depression and facilitation, the two processes shown to underlie habituation and sensitization in the model biological systems already discussed. It is in this sense a purely mechanistic theory. Furthermore, it has been possible to account for and predict a wide range of complex behavioral phenomena of habituation on this basis (see Thompson et al., 1973).

In comparing the two theories it must be noted that they differ primarily in emphasis and extent—Sokolov emphasizes the formation of a stimulus model but does not go on to explain its basis, whereas Groves and Thompson's dual-process

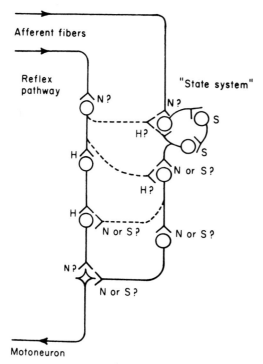

Fig. 7-16. Schematic diagram of possible neuronal substrates of habituation and sensitization. (N indicates nonplastic synapses; H indicates habituation synapses; S indicates sensitizing synapses.) (From Groves and Thompson, 1970.)

7. ELEMENTARY LEARNING AND BEHAVIORAL PLASTICITY

theory emphasizes the independence of habituation and sensitization, and proceeds to define the nature of the underlying synaptic processes. In the dual-process theory, what occurs is simply synaptic depression in the stimulus–response pathway. If this occurrence is equated with the "stimulus model formation process" in Sokolov's theory, the two theories are then not as different as they may seem at first. In any event, the major function of a general theory is to provide a framework for subsequent research. Both theories have served this purpose well.

III. Cellular Mechanisms of Habituation and Sensitization

A. Habituation

In all studies where it has been possible to look at habituation in monosynaptic pathways, the mechanism is *synaptic depression*. Depression at neuromuscular junctions is frequency dependent and is thus believed due to transmitter depletion (see Chapter 5). However, in central synapses, whatever the mechanism is that underlies synaptic depression and mediates habituation, it is not depletion. In both *Aplysia* (Castellucci and Kandel, 1976a) and in frog spinal cord (Farel, 1974) a set of habituated synapses can be sensitized by a "dishabituating" stimulus and suddenly transmit an increased rate. This immediate upsurge of activity shows that transmitter stores have not been depleted. Consequently, at the cellular level, habituation is due to a decreased probability of transmitter release from presynaptic terminals and is not simply a result of transmitter depletion.

B. Sensitization

There are at least two possible cellular mechanisms for "dishabituation" or sensitization—presynaptic excitation and postsynaptic excitation. It is important to emphasize that there is no neurophysiological evidence that dishabituation ever disrupts habituation per se; it is always a superimposed facilitation (excitation). In *Aplysia*, dishabituation of the gill-withdrawal reflex is due to presynaptic excitation, superimposed on the depressed activity of habituated terminals (Fig. 7-5) (Castellucci and Kandel, 1976a,b). In the spinal flexor reflex, on the other

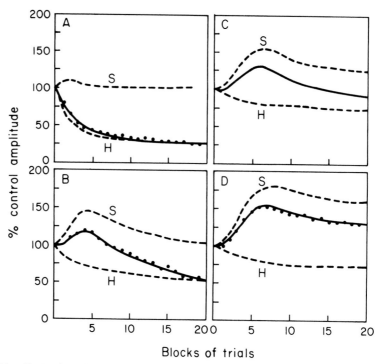

Fig. 7-17. Basic idea of the dual-process theory of habituation. Processes of sensitization (S) and habituation (H) (dashed lines) occur to varying extents as a function of stimulus and training conditions and interact to produce final behavioral outcome. (Solid lines and dots are actual behavioral results for flexor reflex.) (From Groves and Thompson, 1970.)

hand, dishabituation is at least partially due to increased postsynaptic excitation, tonically exerted.

C. Endoneural Habituation

Sokolov has explored at the cellular level a most interesting form of habituatory response which does not appear to involve synaptic processes at all (Pakula and Sokolov, 1973). Repeated intracellular stimulation at low rates of certain neurons in the snail results in a decreased response of the cells with no accompanying change in membrane excitability. These cells may in fact be "latent" pacemakers. If so, repeated stimulation might interact with intracellular pacemaker mechanisms to alter cellular responsiveness. Hence the term "endoneural": whatever the process is, it seems to be inside the cell. The extent to which such a process may be involved in habituation of behavioral responses remains to be determined.

IV. Future Directions

A number of questions regarding habituation remain to be answered. What is the subcellular mechanism responsible for decreased probability of transmitter release? What is the relation between short term and long term habituation, particularly in terms of underlying synaptic processes? And to what extent do these subcellular and cellular mechanisms of habituation and sensitization in simple model systems hold true for more complex biological systems and humans? Finally, what are the relations, if any, between all these mechanisms and more complex forms of behavioral plasticity such as associative learning?

V. Associative Learning

The more complex forms of learning involve associations. As a result of experience we bring stimuli together and learn to respond in distinct ways. The associations may be internal or external as Fig. 7-18 illustrates. In pairing stimuli we learn the relationships between them and we remember them, and thereby become products of our experiences.

The early roots of knowledge on associative learning lie in the pioneering work of the Russian physiologist Ivan Pavlov (1927). In the course of experiments on digestion in dogs he noted that certain secretions occur in the absence of food. For one thing he observed how specific oral stimuli promoted the flow of saliva and other digestive fluids, such as gastric juice. He also saw, as had others before him, that when an experimenter entered the room or when the food was presented the dogs began to salivate—to produce what were first called "psychic secretions." They appeared to be "mind triggered" instead of initiated by the food itself by way of receptors. Pavlov was very well read; he recognized the importance of defining the ways in which stimuli determine behavioral responses. So he set up several experiments. In the first, he showed the dog the color red (to suggest meat) as the conditioning stimulus. Then he used stimuli appropriate to the surface receptors activated to food getting and eating, but eventually he decided to try a neutral stimulus like a light or a buzzer; he would follow that with food to the mouth. Soon the dog learned that a light or buzzer was followed by food, and the dog became conditioned; i.e., the animal would salivate simply to the neutral or conditioning stimulus. Subsequent to these early experiments many workers have used such Pavlovian, or classical conditioning procedures to study learning.

In *classical conditioning* the *conditioning stimulus* (light, tone, etc.) and the unconditional stimulus are under the precise control of the experimenter. *Unconditional stimuli* are those that by the innate structure of the organism

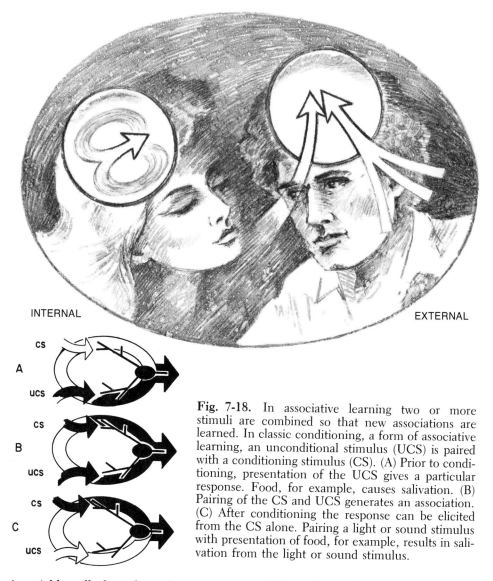

INTERNAL

EXTERNAL

Fig. 7-18. In associative learning two or more stimuli are combined so that new associations are learned. In classic conditioning, a form of associative learning, an unconditional stimulus (UCS) is paired with a conditioning stimulus (CS). (A) Prior to conditioning, presentation of the UCS gives a particular response. Food, for example, causes salivation. (B) Pairing of the CS and UCS generates an association. (C) After conditioning the response can be elicited from the CS alone. Pairing a light or sound stimulus with presentation of food, for example, results in salivation from the light or sound stimulus.

invariably will elicit the reflex or response independent of its learning history. Recently, classical conditioning procedures have been used in simple systems to explore the neural mechanisms of associative learning.

Possible cellular mechanisms for even the simplest forms of associative learning remain unknown, and good models are hard to find. The ant and octopus are both known to learn very well, but they also have very complicated nervous systems and therefore are not as suitable as model systems as they might appear to be.

7. **ELEMENTARY LEARNING AND BEHAVIORAL PLASTICITY**

The classical conditioning of the spinal flexor reflex appears to be a most promising model. Whether such conditioning could be obtained was the topic of heated debate some years ago, after its initial description (Shurrager and Culler, 1938; Patterson, 1976). However, in recent years several laboratories have independently duplicated the phenomenon (Fitzgerald and Thompson, 1967; Patterson *et al.*, 1973; Buerger and Dawson, 1968; Durkovic, 1975). One standard preparation utilizes a spinally transected cat, anesthetized and then pharmacologically immobilized. The conditioning stimulus (CS) is a shock at threshold level to a cutaneous nerve (superficial peroneal) and the unconditional stimulus (UCS) is a strong shock to the foot of the same limb. The response is the reflex volley recorded from the deep peroneal motor nerve. In brief, paired stimulus training results in a significant increase in motor nerve response to the CS. Appropriate unpaired control training does not produce an increase (see Fig. 7-19).

In establishing the suitability of such models of associative learning, we must demonstrate that they exhibit the behavioral characteristics of classical conditioning. This is much more difficult to do than for habituation, a simpler form of plasticity. In classical conditioning optimal conditioning occurs when the CS terminates shortly before the onset of the UCS. Conditioning does not occur when the UCS stimulus precedes the CS.

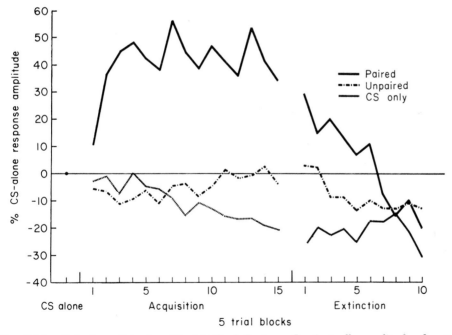

Fig. 7-19. Spinal conditioning. The hindlimb flexion reflex (actually amplitude of motor nerve volley) was conditioned in acute paralyzed spinal cats. Unpaired (CS and UCS not paired in time) and CS-only controls did not show learning. (From Patterson *et al.*, 1973.)

Spinal conditioning does show the same interstimulus interval effect as classical conditioning (best conditioning occurs when the CS precedes the UCS by about 200–400 msec), and does not show backward conditioning (when the UCS precedes the CS). Also spinal conditioning, like classical conditioning, is more effective when trials are massed than when they are spaced (see Patterson, 1976). These important demonstrations argue strongly that spinal conditioning can serve as a legitimate model of classical conditioning, and, for a variety of reasons, the mechanism of plasticity in this model must occur in interneurons. In summary, the stage appears to be set for analysis of neural mechanisms in this promising experimental paradigm.

A simple model which has all the requirements of a typical Pavlovian behavior is the conditioning of the third eyelid or *nictitating membrane response* in the rabbit (Gormezano *et al.*, 1962). A tone can serve as the CS and a light puff of air on the cornea as the UCS. The rabbit learns to blink when it hears the tone. This reproducible response develops in a few hours of training, displays very little spontaneous activity and thus can be quantified precisely in a single session. The challenge, and it is a formidable one, is to identify the circuitry controlling the response and to find out where and how it is changed.

In the initial experiments neuronal activity was examined in the hippocampus, because this structure has been implicated in learning. The activity of groups of hippocampal neurons was recorded during conditioning (Berger *et al.*, 1976). Very little activity occurs after the CS or the UCS in controls given unpaired presentations of these stimuli. However, subjects which received standard conditioning show an increase in activity to the UCS after a few pairings of tone and air puff. The acquired neuronal response to the UCS "moves forward" in time as conditioning progresses, eventually occurring with the tone, prior to air puff onset. These changes occur in the early stages of conditioning, prior to the development of a stable conditioned nictitating membrane response. When the conditioned response does occur, the neuronal response invariably precedes it by a brief and relatively constant interval (25–35 msec). In short, the neuronal effect is "time-locked" to the nictitating membrane response.

The most striking aspect of this study, however, is that the hippocampal response has a wave form over time very similar to the wave form of the nictitating membrane response (see Fig. 7-20). In other words, the hippocampal neurons seem to "model" the sequence of muscle movements involved in the eyelid behavior, in terms of electrical wave form properties. It is clear, however, that the hippocampal neuronal activity is not simply "motor commands" for the nictitating membrane, because the neuronal effects do not accompany spontaneous or reflexly elicited blinking of the third eyelid prior to conditioning.

It seems remarkable that the neuronal activity of a structure such as the hippocampus, which is not necessary for motor performances of complex learned

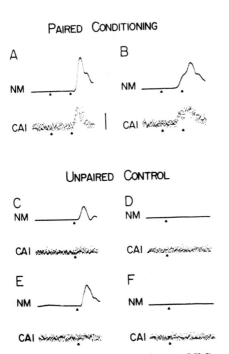

PAIRED CONDITIONING

UNPAIRED CONTROL

Fig. 7-20. Upper traces: Average nictitating membrane (NM) response for one block of eight trials. Lower traces: hippocampal unit poststimulus histogram for one block of eight trials. (A) First block of eight paired conditioning trials, day 1. (B) Last block of eight paired conditioning trials, day 1, after conditioning has occurred. First cursor indicates tone onset; second cursor indicates air puff onset. (C) First block of eight unpaired UCS-alone trials, day 1. (E) Last block of eight unpaired UCS-alone trials, day 2. Cursor indicates air puff onset. (D) First block of eight unpaired CS-alone trials, day 1. (F) Last block of eight unpaired CS-alone trials, day 2. Cursor indicates tone onset. Total trace length is 750 msec. Height of vertical bar to right of CA1 unit poststimulus histogram in (A) is equivalent to 13 neural spike events. (From Berger *et al.*, 1976, copyright by the American Association for the Advancement of Science.)

tasks already acquired, should so closely follow the muscular activity involved in a simple reflex movement such as the nictitating membrane response. It seems from these data that the hippocampus could form temporary "templates" of recently associated stimuli and responses. The simplicity of the nictitating membrane response may have made it possible to detect the template in this case. Many brain structures which receive fibers from and connect to the hippocampus must also be involved in the development of learning (Berger and Thompson, 1978), but it is also clear that certain brain structures are not involved. The deep auditory nuclei which receive the CS (the tone) and the motor nuclei controlling the nictitating membrane are not implicated in learning.

Studies using invertebrate model systems have been only partially successful in identifying the neural events of conditioning. One ingenious preparation that appeared to offer promise was the headless cockroach and its learning of leg position, as studied by Horridge. This preparation is illustrated in Fig. 7-21. Learning in this model involves positioning a limb so as to avoid a shock, a form of instrumental avoidance conditioning. The preparation receives a shock whenever the limb is lowered to the point where contact with a water surface is made. The yoked control receives a shock at the same time regardless of its position. The result is that the experimental limb ends up avoiding contact as compared to the control in subsequent testing. However, two problems have developed with this model. First, similar learning effects can be obtained in preparations where the ganglion is destroyed, leaving only the peripheral nerves and muscles of the leg (Eisenstein and Cohen, 1965). There is still a difference—the preparation without a ganglion does not retain its "learning" as well as that in which the ganglion is intact. The other problem is more general. Use of the yoked control can introduce systematic nonlearning effects (Church, 1964). Recently Church and Lerner (1976) reanalyzed the data of Einsenstein and Cohen in terms of a mathematical (probablistic) model of the yoked procedure which assumes that no learning or associative processes are operating, only performance variables. Computer simulation of the model predicted exactly the outcome of their experimental ganglion-intact learning.

Hoyle (1965) has developed a most interesting analogue of the Horridge paradigm at the cellular level, recording intracellularly from both muscle and motor neuron in the headless locust. In brief, changes in the frequency of motor discharge are followed by nerve stimulation in a contingent manner. If nerve stimulation occurs after decreases in motor discharge, the mean rate of such discharge increases substantially ("up-learning"). If nerve stimulation occurs after

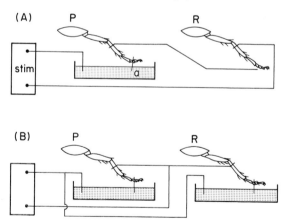

Fig. 7-21. Experimental arrangement for the study of "conditioning" in the cockroach prothoracic ganglion. (A) Training phase. The P leg is shocked whenever it touches the water (a) and the R leg is shocked whenever the P leg is shocked. (B) Testing phase. Each leg is now shocked when it touches the water independently of the other. (From Horridge, 1962.)

7. ELEMENTARY LEARNING AND BEHAVIORAL PLASTICITY

increases in motor discharge, the mean rate decreases ("down-learning"). Noncontingent nerve stimulation does not yield such changes. Hoyle has recently presented most interesting evidence, suggesting that the mechanism may lie in alterations of the ionic properties of the motor neuron membrane at nonsynaptic sites, i.e., not involving changes in synaptic actions (Woollacott and Hoyle, 1977). Such alterations might be the performance variables given by Church and Lerner (see above) for the Horridge headless cockroach model.

The development of additional biological models of associative learning in which mechanisms can be analyzed is a challenge for future research. It is possible that useful invertebrate preparations will be found. For example, Gelperin (1975) reported rapid food aversion learning by the terrestrial mollusk, *Limax*. Additional possibilities have been suggested by other workers.

At some point, simplified models of complex learning will reach fundamental limits, for the very reason that apes cannot learn to speak. The hope is that basic processes of learning, such as classical conditioning and avoidance learning, can, at the very least, be established in preparations where analysis is possible.

VI. Summary

The behavior of most, if not all, animals is plastic. Research on behavioral plasticity aims to provide an understanding of the basic neural processes underlying these changes in response produced by experience. Experiments have focused upon invertebrates, or upon parts of invertebrate or vertebrate nervous systems which display plasticity. Such models are used because of their simplicity. In every case we must judge whether the model of the process or phenomenon of interest is a good one.

Much research has dealt with habituation, that decrease in response resulting from repeated stimulation. The neural systems underlying habituation of limb flexion in spinally transected rats and cats have been extensively investigated. Habituation turns out to be due not to changes in sensory receptors or sensory nerves, motor neuron excitability or muscle fatigue, but to changes in interneurons. Studies of interneuron activity indicate that there are two types of interneurons, those whose activity decreases to repeated stimulation and those whose activity increases, and dishabituation appears to be not a disruption of habituation but a superimposed sensitization by means of neuronal excitation.

Studies of habituation in *Aplysia* indicate that habituation is due to a decrease in the probability of transmitter release from the presynaptic terminals of sensory neurons. Dishabituation is produced by facilitation (through excitation) of synaptic terminals. Similar findings have been obtained in studies of interneurons (including cells of the hippocampus) and of a monosynaptic pathway in the isolated frog spinal cord.

Theories of habituation have attempted to account for the fact that such habituation can be produced by a change in stimulation. One theory proposes that with stimulation, a neural model (a pattern of neuronal activity) is formed, and arousal occurs when sensory input does not match the model. This theory seems most appropriate for complex stimulus processing. A "dual-process" theory proposes that repeated stimulation leads to habituation in reflex pathways and generalized sensitization of the neural "state." In the latter theory the habituation to the stimulus consists only of synaptic depression in the stimulus–response pathway.

The cellular mechanisms underlying simple associative learning are not known. Learning can be obtained in "spinal" frogs and rats. Studies of classical conditioning in spinal animals or in the rabbit's nictitating membrane response suggest that the behavioral changes are due to alterations in interneurons, including those higher interneurons of the hippocampus, not to changes in sensory and motor nerve cells.

Future research must be directed toward the mechanisms responsible for the changes in neuronal activity occurring in habituation and associative learning in these model systems. Ultimately, investigators must address the question of the relevance of these relatively simple phenomena to more complex forms of learning.

Key Terms

Associative learning: A type of learning whereby a new response is brought out as a result of associations between stimuli. It includes all forms of learning from basic Pavlovian conditioning to complex human learning.

Classical conditioning: An experimental paradigm developed by Pavlov in which an originally neutral stimulus, the conditioned stimulus (such as light or tone), is paired with an unconditioned stimulus (such as food). This unconditioned stimulus evokes a particular innate response, such as salivation. After pairing, the neutral, or conditioned stimulus, evokes a response similar to that of the unconditioned stimulus.

Dishabituation: The disruption of a previously established habituation of a response by the presentation of another, usually stronger, stimulus; sometimes called sensitization.

"Dual-process" theory: A theory of habituation which states that a repetitive stimulus causes two independent processes in the nervous system: habituation in the reflex pathway and a more generalized sensitization (increase in sensitivity) of the "state" of the system.

Flexor reflex: The reflexive withdrawal of a limb (its flexion) when the skin receives a painful stimulus.

Habituation: A decrease in an already existing response to an initially novel stimulus when it is given repeatedly. Habituation is the simplest form of learning; it is non-associative.

Monosynaptic pathway: A single-synapse pathway.

Nictitating membrane: A thin membrane found in the eye of many animals, just beneath the lower lid, and capable of being drawn across the eyeball; it is a third eyelid. Classical conditioning of the nictitating membrane has been used to study the neuronal mechanisms of learning. The animal learns to blink in response to a conditioned stimulus (a tone, for example) when it is repeatedly paired with an air puff on the cornea (the unconditioned stimulus).

Nonassociative learning: The simplest form of learning whereby a change is produced in an already existing response to a repetitive stimulus. Associations between stimuli are not involved (habituation and sensitization are examples).

Sensitization: Any increase in sensitivity to a stimulus, repetitive or otherwise.

General References

Hoyle, G. (1979). Mechanisms of simple motor learning trends. *NeuroSciences* **2**, 153–155.

Kandel, E. R. (1976). "Cellular Basis of Behavior," Freeman, San Francisco, California.

Kandel, E. R. (1977). Neuronal plasticity and the modification of behavior. *In* "Handbook of Physiology" (E. R. Kandel, ed.). Sect. 1, Vol. 1, Part 2, pp. 1137–1182. Am. Physiol. Soc., Bethesda, Maryland.

Thompson, R. F. (1976). The search for the engram. *Am. Psychol.* **31**, 209–227.

Thompson, R. F., and Glanzman, D. G. (1976). Neural and behavioral mechanisms of habituation and sensitization. *In* "Habituation: Perspectives from Child Development, Animal Behavior and Neurophysiology" (T. J. Tighe and R. N. Leaton, eds.), pp. 49–93. Lawrence Erlbaum Associates, Hillsdale, New Jersey.

Thompson, R. F., and Spencer, W. A. (1966). Habituation: A model phenomenon for the study of neuronal substrates of behavior. *Psychol. Rev.* **73**, 16–43.

References

Alger, B. E., and Teyler, T. J. (1976). Long-term and short-term plasticity in the CA1, CA3, and dentate regions of the rat hippocampal slice. *Brain Res.* **110**, 463–480.

Andersen, P., Teyler, T. J., and Wester, K. (1973). Long-lasting change of synaptic transmission in a specialized cortical pathway. *Acta Physiol. Scand., Suppl.* **396**, A30, 34.

Andersen, P., Sundberg, S. H., Sveen, O., and Wigström, H. (1977). Specific long lasting potentiation of synaptic transmission in hippocampal slices. *Nature (London)* **266**, 736–737.

Atkinson, R. C., and Shiffrin, R. M. (1968). Human memory: A proposed system and its control processes. *In* "The Psychology of Learning and Motivation" (K. W. Spence and J. T. Spence, eds.), Vol. 2, pp. 89–195. Academic Press, New York.

Berger, T. W., and Thompson, R. F. (1978). Neuronal plasticity in the limbic system during classical conditioning of the rabbit nictitating membrane response. I. The hippocampus. *Brain Res.* **145**, 323–346.

Berger, T. W., Alger, B., and Thompson, R. F. (1976). Neuronal substrate of classical conditioning in the hippocampus. *Science* **192**, 483–485.

Bliss, T. V. P., and Lømo, T. (1973). Long-lasting potentiation of synaptic transmission in the dentate area of the anaesthetized rabbit following stimulation of the perforant path. *J. Physiol. (London)* **232**, 331–356.

Buerger, A. A., and Dawson, A. M. (1968). Spinal kittens: Long-term increases in electromyograms due to a conditioning routine, *Physiol. Behav.* **3**, 99–103.

Byrne, J., Castellucci, V., and Kandel, E. R. (1974). Receptive fields and response properties of mechanoreceptor neurons innervating siphon skin and mantle shelf in *Aplysia*. *J. Neurophysiol.* **37**, 1041–1064.

Carew, T. J., Castellucci, V. F., and Kandel, E. R. (1971). An analysis of dishabituation and sensitization of the gill-withdrawal reflex in *Aplysia*. *Int. J. Neurosci.* **2**, 79–98.

Castellucci, V., and Kandel, E. R. (1974). A quantal analysis of the synaptic depression underlying habituation of the gill-withdrawal reflex in *Aplysia*. *Proc. Natl. Acad. Sci. U.S.A.* **71**, 5004–5008.

Castellucci, V., and Kandel, E. R. (1976a). An invertebrate system for the cellular study of habituation and sensitization. *In* "Habituation: Perspectives from Child Development, Animal Behavior, and Neurophysiology" (T. J. Tighe and R. N. Leaton, eds.), pp. 1–47. Lawrence Erlbaum Associates, Hillsdale, New Jersey.

Castellucci, V., and Kandel, E. R. (1976b). Presynaptic facilitation as a mechanism for behavioral sensitization in *Aplysia*. *Science* **194**, 1176–1178.

Castellucci, V., Pinsker, H., Kupfermann, I., and Kandel, E. R. (1970). Neuronal mechanisms of habituation and dishabituation of the gill-withdrawal reflex in *Aplysia*. *Science* **167**, 1745–1748.

Church, R. M. (1964). Systematic effect of random error in the yoked control design. *Psychol. Bull.* **62**, 122–131.

Church, R. M., and Lerner, N. D. (1976). Does the headless roach learn to avoid? *Physiol. Psychol.* **4**, 439–442.

Coggeshall, R. E. (1967). A light and electron microscope study of the abdominal ganglion of *Aplysia californica*. *J. Neurophysiol.* **30**, 1263–1287.

Douglas, R. M., and Goddard, G. V. (1975). Long-term potentiation of the perforant path-granule cell synapse in the rat hippocampus. *Brain Res.* **86**, 205–215.

Dudek, F. E., Deadwyler, S. A., Cotman, C. W., and Lynch, G. (1976). Intracellular responses from granule cell layer in slices of rat hippocampus: Perforant path synapse. *J. Neurophysiol.* **39**, 384–393.

Durkovic, R. G. (1975). Classical conditioning, sensitization and habituation in the spinal cat. *Physiol. Behav.* **14**, 297–304.

Eccles, J. C. (1964). "The Physiology of Synapses," Academic Press, New York.

Egger, M. D., and Wall, P. D. (1971). The plantar cushion reflex circuit: An oligosynaptic cutaneous reflex. *J. Physiol. (London)* **216**, 483–501.

Egger, M. D., Bishop, J. W., and Cone, C. H. (1976). Sensitization and habituation of the plantar cushion reflex in cats. *Brain Res.* **103**, 215–228.

Eisenstein, E. M., and Cohen, M. J. (1965). Learning in an isolated prothoracic insect ganglion. *Anim. Behav.* **13**, 104–108.

Farel, P. B. (1974). Dual processes control response habituation across a single synapse. *Brain Res.* **72**, 323–327.

Farel, P. B., Glanzman, D. L., and Thompson, R. F. (1973). Habituation of a monosynaptic response in vertebrate central nervous system: Lateral column-motoneuron pathway in isolated frog spinal cord. *J. Neurophysiol.* **36**, 1117–1130.

Fitzgerald, L. A., and Thompson, R. F. (1967). Classical conditioning of the hindlimb flexion reflex in the acute spinal cat. *Psychonom. Sci.* **8**, 213–214.

Frazier, W. T., Kandel, E. R., Kupfermann, I., Waziri, R., and Coggeshall, R. E. (1967). Morphological and functional properties of identified neurons in the abdominal ganglion of *Aplysia californica*. *J. Neurophysiol.* **30**, 1288–1351.

Gelperin, A. (1975). Rapid food-aversion learning by a terrestrial mollusk. *Science* **189**, 567–570.

Glanzer, M. (1953). Stimulus satiation: An explanation of spontaneous alternation and related phenomena. *Psychol. Rev.* **60**, 257–268.

Glanzman, D. L. (1976). Synaptic mechanisms of habituation. Doctoral Dissertation, University of California, Irvine.

Glass, D. C., and Singer, J. E. (1972). "Urban Stress." Academic Press, New York.

Gormezano, I., Schneiderman, N., Deaux, E. B., and Fuentes, I. (1962). Nictitating membrane: Classical conditioning and extinction in the albino rabbit. *Science* **138**, 33–34.

Groves, P. M., and Thompson, R. F. (1970). Habituation: A dual-process theory. *Psychol. Rev.* **77**, 419–450.

Groves, P. M., and Thompson, R. F. (1973). Dual-process theory of habituation: Neural mechanisms. *In* "Habituation" (H. V. S. Peeke and M. J. Herz, eds.), Vol. 2, pp. 175–205. Academic Press, New York.

Groves, P. M., Glanzman, D. L., Patterson, M. M., and Thompson, R. F. (1970). Excitability of cutaneous afferent terminals during habituation and sensitization in acute spinal cat. *Brain Res.* **18**, 388–392.

Harris, J. D. (1943). Habituatory response decrement in the intact organism. *Psychol. Bull.* **40**, 385–422.

Hernández-Peón, R. (1960). Neurophysiological correlates of habituation and other manifestations of plastic inhibition. *Electroencephalogr. Clin. Neurophysiol., Suppl.* **13**, 101–114.

Horridge, G. A. (1962). Learning of leg position by the ventral nerve cord in headless insects. *Proc. R. Soc. London* **157**, 33–52.

Hoyle, G. (1965). Neurophysiological studies on "learning" in headless insects. *In* "The Physiology of the Insect Central Nervous System" (J. E. Treherne and J. W. L. Beament, eds.), pp. 203–232. Academic Press, New York.

Hull, C. L. (1943). "Principles of Behavior." Appleton, New York.

Humphrey, G. (1930). LeChatelier's rule and the problem of habituation and dehabituation in *Helix albolabris*. *Psychol. Forsch.* **13**, 113–117.

Humphrey, G. (1933). "The Nature of Learning." Harcourt, New York.

James, W. (1890). "The Principles of Psychology." Holt, New York.

Jennings, H. S. (1906). "Behavior of the Lower Organisms." Columbia Univ. Press, New York.

Kandel, E. R. (1976). "Cellular Basis of Behavior." Freeman, San Francisco, California.

Kandel, E. R. (1977). Neuronal plasticity and the modification of behavior. *In* "Handbook of Physiology" (E. R. Kandel, ed.), Sect. 1, Vol. 1, Part 2, pp. 1137–1182. Am. Physiol. Soc., Bethesda, Maryland.

Kupfermann, I., Castellucci, V., Pinsker, H., and Kandel, E. (1970). Neuronal correlates of habituation and dishabituation of the gill-withdrawal reflex in *Aplysia*. *Science* **167**, 1743–1745.

Kupfermann, I., Pinsker, H., Castellucci, V., and Kandel, E. R. (1971). Central and peripheral control of gill movements in *Aplysia*. *Science* **174**, 1252–1256.

Lynch, G. S., Dunwiddie, T., and Gribkoff, V. (1977). Heterosynaptic depression: A postsynaptic correlate of long-term potentiation. *Nature (London)* **266**, 737–739.

Pakula, A., and Sokolov, E. N. (1973). Habituation in *Gastropoda*: Behavioral interneuronal and endoneuronal aspects. *In* "Habituation" (H. V. S. Peeke and M. J. Herz, eds.), Vol. 2, pp. 35–107. Academic Press, New York.

Patterson, M. M. (1976). Mechanisms of classical conditioning and fixation in spinal mammals. *In* "Advances in Psychobiology" (A. H. Riesen and R. F. Thompson, eds.), Vol. 3, pp. 381–436. Wiley, New York.

Patterson, M. M., Cegavske, C. F., and Thompson, R. F. (1973). Effects of a classical conditioning paradigm on hind-limb flexor nerve response in immobilized spinal cats. *J. Comp. Physiol. Psychol.* **84,** 88–97.

Pavlov, I. (1927). "Conditioned Reflexes." Oxford Univ. Press, London and New York.

Peretz, B. (1970). Habituation and dishabituation in the absence of a central nervous system. *Science* **169,** 379–381.

Pinsker, H., Kupfermann, I., Castellucci, V., and Kandel, E. R. (1970). Habituation and dishabituation of the gill withdrawal reflex in *Aplysia. Science* **167,** 1740–1742.

Prosser, C. L., and Hunter, W. S. (1936). The extinction of startle responses and spinal reflexes in the white rat. *Am. J. Physiol.* **117,** 609–618.

Sharpless, S., and Jasper, H. (1956). Habituation of the arousal reaction. *Brain* **79,** 655–680.

Shurrager, P. S., and Culler, E. A. (1938). Phenomena allied to conditioning in the spinal dog. *Am. J. Physiol.* **123,** 186–187.

Sokolov, E. N. (1960). Neuronal models and the orienting reflex. *In* "The Central Nervous System and Behavior" (M. A. B. Brazier, ed.), pp. 187–276. Josiah Macy, Jr. Found., New York.

Sokolov, E. N. (1963). Higher nervous functions: The orienting reflex. *Annu. Rev. Physiol.* **25,** 545–580.

Spencer, W. A., Thompson, R. F., and Neilson, D. R., Jr. (1966a). Response decrement of the flexion reflex in the acute spinal cat and transient restoration by strong stimuli. *J. Neurophysiol.* **29,** 221–239.

Spencer, W. A., Thompson, R. F., and Neilson, D. R., Jr. (1966b). Alterations in responsiveness of ascending and reflex pathways activated by iterated cutaneous afferent volleys. *J. Neurophysiol.* **29,** 240–252.

Spencer, W. A., Thompson, R. F., and Neilson, D. R., Jr. (1966c). Decrement of ventral root electrotonus and intracellularly recorded PSPs produced by iterated cutaneous afferent volleys. *J. Neurophysiol.* **29,** 253–274.

Teyler, T. J., and Alger, B. E. (1976). Monosynaptic habituation in the vertebrate forebrain: The dentate gyrus examined *in vitro. Brain Res.* **115,** 413–425.

Thompson, R. F. (1967). "Foundations of Physiological Psychology." Harper, New York.

Thompson, R. F., and Glanzman, D. G. (1976). Neural and behavioral mechanisms of habituation and sensitization. *In* "Habituation: Perspectives from Child Development, Animal Behavior, and Neurophysiology" (T. J. Tighe and R. N. Leaton, eds.), pp. 49–93. Lawrence Erlbaum Associates, Hillsdale, New Jersey.

Thompson, R. F., and Spencer, W. A. (1966). Habituation: A model phenomenon for the study of neuronal substrates of behavior. *Psychol. Rev.* **73,** 16–43.

Thompson, R. F., Groves, P. M., Teyler, T. J., and Roemer, R. A. (1973). A dual-process theory of habituation: Theory and behavior. *In* "Habituation" (H. V. S. Peeke and M. J. Herz, eds.), Vol. 1, pp. 239–271. Academic Press, New York.

Wagner, A. R. (1976). Priming in STM: An information-processing mechanism for self-generated or retrieval-generated depression in performance. *In* "Habituation: Perspectives from Child Development, Animal Behavior and Neurophysiology" (T. J. Tighe and R. N. Leaton, eds.), pp. 95–128. Lawrence Erlbaum Associates, Hillsdale, New Jersey.

White, W. F., Nadler, J. V., and Cotman, C. W. (1978a). A perfusion chamber for the study of CNS physiology and pharmacology *in vitro. Brain Res.* **152,** 591–596.

White, W. F., Nadler, J. V., and Cotman, C. W. (1978b). Pre- and postsynaptic loci for short and long term plasticity. *Fed. Proc., Fed. Am. Proc. Exp. Biol.* **37,** 524.

Woollacott, M., and Hoyle, G. (1977). Neural events underlying learning in insects: changes in pacemaker. *Proc. R. Soc. London, B. Ser.* **195,** 395–415.

8

Complex Learning and Memory

Learning and memory involve a complex set of processes by which experiences alter the nervous system in ways such that the changes endure and effect subsequent experience and behavior. The problem of understanding the neuronal basis of learning and memory is not a simple one of determining the neuronal residue of experience. In order to understand memory we will ultimately need to know many things, including how experiences are selected for storage, how they are stored, how they are integrated with other memories, how they are retrieved and how they lead to changes in behavior. Neuronal plasticity is only one aspect of learning and memory.

The complexity of the problem may be illustrated by considering what is involved in using an unfamiliar telephone number. The information is obtained by looking the number up in a directory. Note that one may see many numbers (i.e., the numbers are present in the visual field) but only one set is selected for use. The memory can be *indicated* by speaking, dialing, pushing buttons or in other ways, such as writing or simply identifying the sequence of numbers as the correct number. The memory can be discriminated from all other sequences of numbers including other telephone numbers you are capable of recalling. The memory is formed rapidly, it is usually transient, but, with rehearsal or repetition, can become long-lasting.

This is but one example of memory. We learn and remember isolated experiences, complex events, and skills. It is important to note that memory does not consist of the particular responses made during the course of learning experience. We can acquire information simply through sensory experiences (watching, reading, listening, etc.) and we learn to perform skills such as language in which responses can and do occur in different and novel sequences.

It is obvious that simple models of neuronal plasticity which assume that memories are formed as a consequence of repetitive activation of the same neuronal elements in precise sequence will not provide a complete explanation of memory for either the relatively simple learning of a telephone number or the learning of the more complex skill of language. Understanding of the detailed processes by which information is selected, stored and sequenced is well beyond the current state of knowledge, but ultimately such understanding is essential for a complete understanding of the neurobiological bases of memory.

I. Approaches to the Neurobiological Bases of Memory

If learning occurs, as logic seems to require, because of changes produced in the nervous system, it should be possible to discover what the changes are and where they occur. Three basic approaches have been used in an attempt to understand the neuronal basis of memory. The most commonly used technique is that of making brain lesions in different brain regions following training to see whether damage to specific neural structures produces loss of retention of a learned response. A second approach involves examining changes in brain anatomy, chemistry, and physiology that are correlated with learning. A third approach involves the use of a variety of experimental techniques to modulate the retention of recently acquired memories.

II. Effects of Brain Lesions on Retention

Research using brain lesions to discover the locus or loci of memory traces or *"engrams"* has been vigorously carried out for decades (Lashley, 1950). Lesions in many brain regions are known to impair both acquisition and retention. For example, in an extensive and systematic series of studies Thompson and Thorne (1973) trained rats in a visual pattern discrimination task and examined the effects of discrete lesions to numerous brain regions on retention of the learned response. As was expected, impairment was produced by lesions of the visual cortex. In addition, marked impairment was produced by lesions of the posterior thalamus, a region not considered to be important for visual function.

The problem with such studies is that the findings are difficult to interpret. One would like to be able to conclude that the lesion impaired retention because it destroyed a portion of the brain tissue containing the memory trace. However, it is difficult to dissociate the effects of the lesion on memory from the effects on other processes influencing behavior, including perception, motivation, arousal and locomotor activity (Isaacson, 1976). Further, if a lesion does not affect retention, it cannot be concluded that the damaged region has no role in memory in normal animals. Lesion studies can only indicate how behavior is altered by the lesion. They do not readily reveal the function of the damaged tissue. The problem is further complicated by the evidence that lesions do not simply remove tissue. It is clear from evidence reviewed in Chapter 6 that the brain can become reorganized following a lesion. Axons from undamaged cells can sprout and innervate synaptic regions vacated by the brain lesions. Because of these logical, methodological, and neurobiological problems, lesion studies by themselves are not likely to provide an understanding of the neural basis of memory.

III. Neurobiological Correlates of Memory

When animals are trained, numerous physiological changes are produced. Much recent research has investigated such changes in an attempt to determine whether the changes are involved in the neural mechanisms that underlie retention of a response. Before turning to the findings let us first briefly consider the complexity of the problem. First, if a neural correlate is involved in processes underlying the retention of a learned response, the correlate must be present after training and remain as long as retention of the response can be demonstrated. However, the search for such correlates must not be restricted by the assumption that all learning results in long-term or permanent changes in the nervous system. There is no reason to assume that all consequences of experience are permanent. Many experiences are of little significance and need not be stored permanently. However, enduring brain changes should be produced by experiences that are particularly meaningful or frequently repeated. Obviously we need to understand the conditions under which memories are transient as well as those that produce long-lasting memory if we are to find neural correlates of learning which are causally involved in retention. Second, learning probably occurs most if not all of the time. When we train animals we do not necessarily change them from a "non-learning" to a "learning" state. Rather we merely control what is learned by controlling the stimulation received and the responses made. Thus, neural changes recorded are correlates found with specific experimental training conditions. Whether such correlates are the same as those that occur when animals observe the world or when you read this chapter remains to be determined. Third, learning and memory are not directly observed. They are inferred from changes in behavior. Behavior can change for a variety of reasons, such as changes due to fatigue, arousal and motivation. Great ingenuity and care is needed in conducting behavioral studies in order to be able to assure that the changes in behavior are due to learning and retention and not to other influences. These complexities will be illustrated by some of the experimental findings in this area.

IV. Neurophysiological Correlates of Learning

The majority of studies on correlates of learning have involved the examination of patterns of electrical brain activity as animals are trained. Electrical activity is of interest primarily because electrophysiological instruments are capable of responding to the rapid shifts (on the order of milliseconds) in activation and degree of activation exhibited by neural systems. Three types of electrophysiological measures commonly used in studies of memory are shown in Fig. 8-1.

V. EEG Studies of Learning

The first studies of electrophysiological correlates of learning examined changes in patterns of _electroencephalographic (EEG) activity_ produced by training. It is

8. COMPLEX LEARNING AND MEMORY

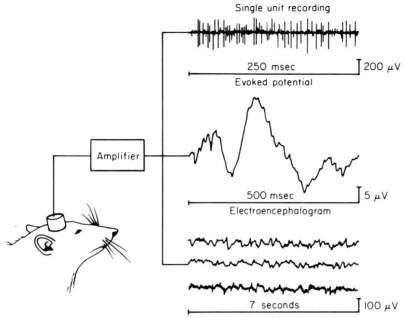

Fig. 8-1. A number of kinds of electrical measurements can be recorded from the brain of an animal. Among them are single unit activity which is the record of the firing patterns of individual nerve cells. Single unit recordings can be made either from very fine electrodes that penetrate a cell or from electrodes placed in close proximity to several neurons. An evoked potential is the electrophysiological response to a discrete stimulus delivered to the animal. Last, is shown the electroencephalogram (EEG), which is an ongoing record of activity recorded from the brain region.

generally agreed that EEG waves are algebraic summations of excitatory and inhibitory postsynaptic potentials (EPSP's and IPSP's). The EEG represents spontaneous oscillatory potentials generated by cell neurons within the range of the recording electrode. Thus, the EEG provides a measure of the activity of a large population of cells. The number of cells in the population varies with the size of the recording electrode, since the greater the diameter of the electrode, the lower the resistance. An *evoked potential* can be thought of as an EEG wave that is time-locked to a specific stimulus.

EEG waves vary in frequency from synchronized high-voltage low-frequency waves of 1–14 Hz to *desynchronized* low-voltage high-frequency (14–80 Hz) waves. Synchronous cortical EEG activity is associated with quiet sleep, while desynchronized EEG activity is associated with alertness and active or REM sleep (see Chapter 14).

The question asked in studies of EEG correlates of learning is whether there are changes in the EEG pattern that are associated specifically with the acquisition of the response. In the 1950's many studies investigated EEG activity during

V. EEG STUDIES OF LEARNING 299

instrumental conditioning. In these studies animals were trained to respond to a conditioned stimulus (CS) by making some conditioned response, such as pushing a lever at the onset of a light in order to receive food. Prior to the pairing of the light with the food the light elicited a brain response comparable to that of similar irrelevant stimuli. However, as the light flash grew more meaningful as a consequence of the association with food, it elicited a change in the EEG response. This response consisted primarily of EEG desynchronization.

The primary difficulty with these studies, of course, is that EEG desynchronization, even though it is signal-specific (i.e., elicited consistently only by a novel CS or one that the animal has learned is meaningful), could well be a correlate of signal-specific _arousal_, rather than of learning. The EEG arousal may occur because the animal has learned the significance of the stimuli, and not because the EEG changes are involved in the processes underlying learning (Thompson et al., 1972).

Numerous experiments examined changes in the _hippocampal theta rhythm_ (4–7 Hz) during learning. In cats, theta rhythm is elicited during training. Moreover, the theta rhythm becomes more stable as the cats master the task. Many brain regions other than hippocampus show similar theta rhythms and changes during acquisition (Adey, 1970). Other studies suggest that theta rhythm is more specifically related to learning than is cortical desynchronization. In one study (Grastyan et al., 1959) theta rhythm was only prominent in the early trials of training, and disappeared once the animal mastered the task, even though cortical desynchronization continued. Further, the theta rhythm was only present when the animal paid specific attention to a meaningful stimulus, as is shown in Fig. 8-2. These kinds of findings suggest that theta rhythms are more selectively related to meaningful, novel or complex stimuli than is cortical EEG desynchronization.

There is other evidence that theta activity is a correlate of acquisition. In one recent study, EEG activity was recorded for 30 minutes after rats were trained on a simple task. The amount of cortically recorded theta rhythm from individual rats was highly correlated with the retention performance which the animals subsequently exhibited on a later retention test (Landfield and McGaugh, 1972). The theta rhythm can be relatively specifically driven by stimulating the septal nuclei regions of theta-range frequencies (e.g., 5–8 Hz) without producing many other aspects of arousal. In recent studies, the theta rhythm of rats was driven in this way following training. In comparison to implanted controls, or to animals in whom the theta rhythm was blocked by high frequency septal stimulation, the animals with driven theta exhibited superior retention performance. Since this procedure represents a relatively specific experimental manipulation of an EEG pattern, with little involvement of many other components of the arousal complex, these findings suggest that theta rhythms may be signs of processes involved in the formation of memory (Landfield, 1976, 1977; Wetzel *et al.*, 1977).

VI. Unit Studies of Learning

Millions, perhaps billions, of neurons are activated by even the simplest stimulus, such as a light flash. The essential measure in studies of <u>unit activity</u> during learning is generally a change with training in amount or rate of single or multiple cell firing in a given brain region following presentation of a stimulus. Nearly all cortical cells measured by investigators generally change their ongoing activity in response to presentation of a stimulus. The latency (delay between the stimulus and the response of a cell) may vary greatly among cells of different areas, with the response of visual cortical cells occurring first, for example, to a light flash, whereas the response of cells of the auditory cortex may occur earliest to a click. Nevertheless, cells in many cortical and subcortical areas respond with some latency to even the simplest stimulus and, moreover, most cells within a responsive region will be either excited or inhibited by the stimulus. Thus, a great number of brain cells are involved in processing even the simplest information. The activity of a single cell provides little insight into the *pattern* of information being processed or stored by millions of cells. However, the study of a single cell can provide some understanding of the *common* aspects of the behavior of cells of its type during a particular stimulus or learning situation. The study of single or multiple unit activity then provides detailed information about the behavior of components of an aggregate during activation of a brain region.

Many studies have examined the effects of different kinds of training procedures on the firing patterns of neurons. For example, a series of experiments studied the patterns of responses of single neurons in the prefrontal cortex of monkeys as the animals performed a delayed response task (Fuster, 1973). The neuronal activity was recorded from chronically implanted microelectrodes. In these experiments, as shown in Fig. 8-3, the monkeys were extensively trained to perform the delayed response task. On each trial the monkeys had to observe which of two containers contained a bit of food. Then a screen was lowered to block the animals' view of the food and was raised 18 seconds later. After they were trained, unit responses were recorded throughout the delay and the subject's accuracy of choice was observed. As can be seen in Fig. 8-3, several patterns of unit activity were observed. In some cells, unit activity increased during the delay, whereas in others unit activity decreased. Still other cells showed various patterns of increase and decrease in firing rates during the delay. Comparable patterns were not

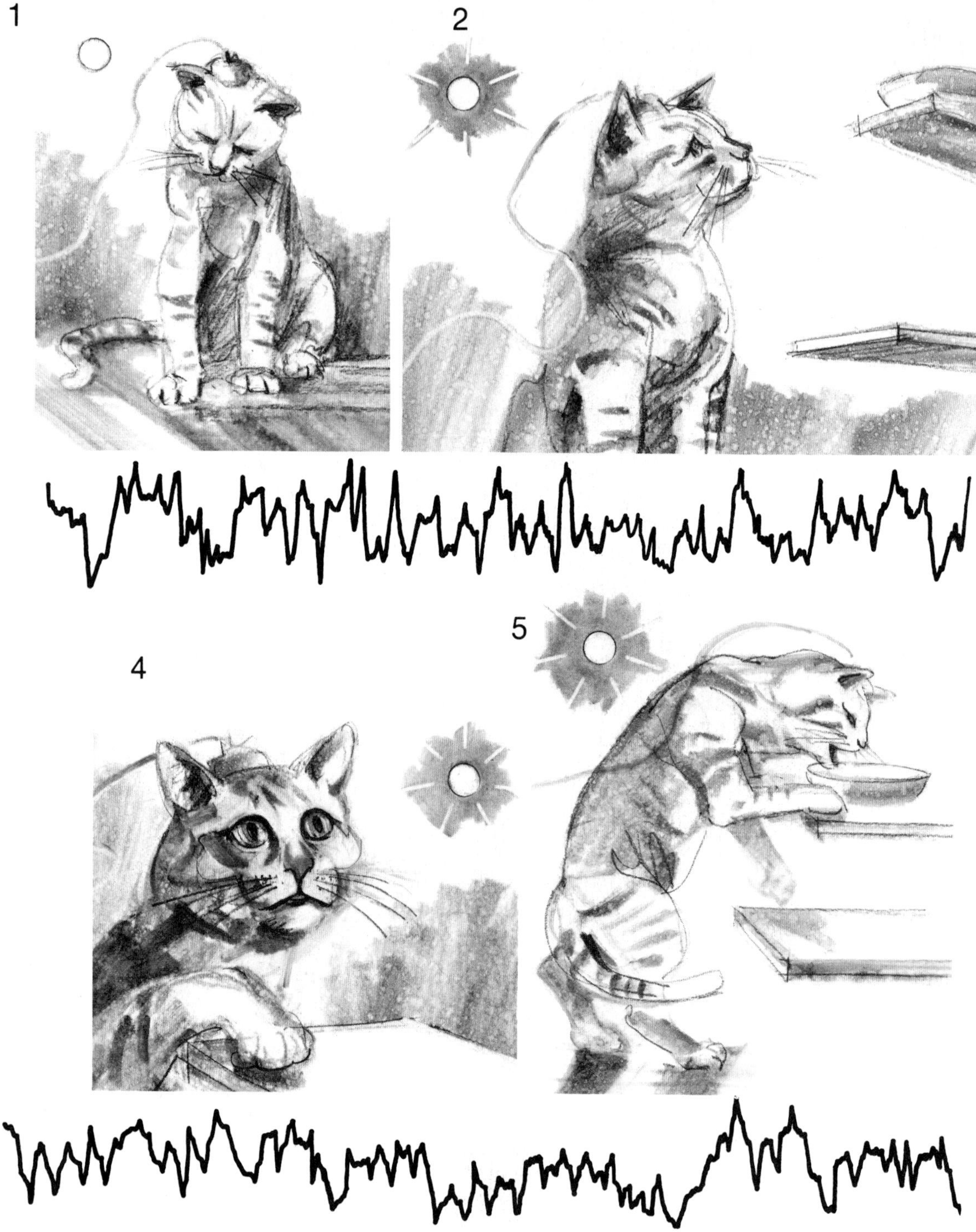
1
2
4
5

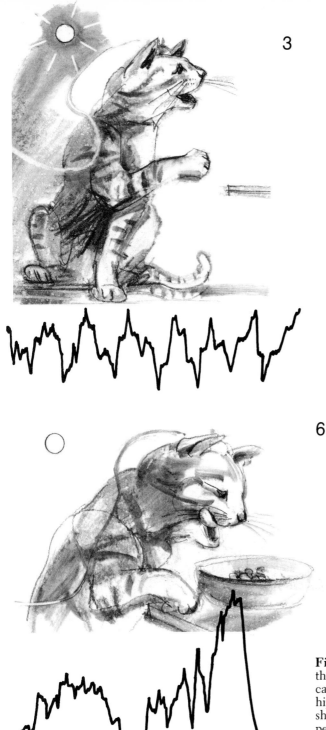

3

6

Fig. 8-2. When the light, the conditioned stimulus that signals the appearance of food, is presented, it causes the appearance of rhythmic theta activity in the hippocampus correlated with an orienting response shown below panels 2 and 3. The theta activity disappears as the cat obtains the food. (Data from Grastyán *et al.*, 1959.)

303

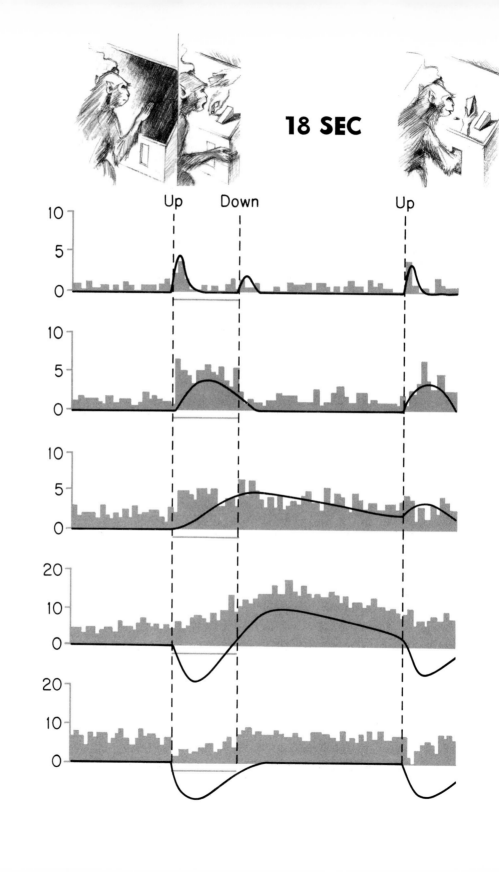

18 SEC

observed in animals tested without prior delayed-response training. These results suggest that the cells in this region of the brain are involved in processes that play some critical role in short-term memory. This interpretation is consistent with findings that delayed-response performance is impaired if this brain region is depressed by cooling.

A number of recent studies have shown that animals can be trained to alter rates of unit activity through the use of rewards. For example, one recent study reported that the rate of firing of cells in cat visual cortex following the presentation of a visual stimulus could be increased if cats were rewarded (with brain stimulation) on trials in which the cells responded with increases in firing rates (Shinkman *et al.*, 1974). Since the cats were paralyzed during the experiment, the changes could not have been caused by changes in sensory stimulation or feedback from motor responses. However, the changes might have been caused by alterations in levels of arousal and thus caused indirectly by changes occurring elsewhere in the brain. Consequently, without additional information concerning the specificity of the changes, studies of this kind can only serve to show that changes in cellular activity can be instrumentally conditioned. It is not clear from such studies that the cells whose activity is recorded are involved in the mechanisms underlying learning.

One clear advantage of unit studies is that the precise time point of a firing rate increase is somewhat easier to determine than is the time point of a change in EEG pattern (because the EEG change must persist longer to be unequivocal). Thus, unit studies are more suited for the study of latency differences in responses of various brain areas to a CS. Moreover, since unit changes are also somewhat easier to differentiate from background than are small EEG changes in many brain structures, the investigation of the time course of development of these changes in various brain areas is facilitated by microelectrode studies of unit activity.

Olds and his colleagues (1972) adopted an interesting and unique strategy. It is extremely difficult to determine whether an observed correlate is causally related to the changes in learning and memory. The pattern of a neuron's firing may change merely because the neuron under study is stimulated by neurons that are changed by training. As Olds put it, "How can we, from an enormous number

---

Fig. 8-3. Joaquin Fuster (1973) studied the activity of single units in the prefrontal cortex of the monkey during delayed response conditioning. In this task the monkey was shown the location of food, but then he had to wait for 18 seconds, with a screen between him and the food, before he could get it. During this delay period, the monkey had to remember under which object the food had been placed. A number of different types of cells were encountered during this research that may be associated with short-term memory. The histograms show the activity of individual cells while the heavy lines show the basic patterns of firing. Movements of the screen are shown above the dashed lines. (Data from Fuster, 1973.)

of changes fed back upon changes in a confusing web of neuron behavior cycles and neuron–neuron epicycles, sort out the critical changes which come first, and being at the sites of the learning cause the others?" (Olds, 1973). It might be that the critical measure is the latency of a neuron's response to a new stimulus. If a unit changes its rate of firing during training and if the latency of the response of the unit is very short, then it is likely that the unit is directly rather than indirectly involved in the learning process. That is, it is suggested that the brain regions where changes are found might be regions containing the neural changes underlying the acquisition of the conditioned response. Experiments to investigate this possibility studied, in many brain regions, the latencies of cells (multiple units) whose patterns of activity are changed during a simple learning task. In these studies rats were trained simply to orient toward a pellet dispenser at the onset of a tone. A tone (CS+) signaled the presentation of a food pellet, and a second tone (CS−), which did not signal food was interspersed with the CS+ tones. In certain restricted regions of the brain, signal-specific increases of the unit response occurred at latencies of less than 20 msec. Many of the regions sampled in this study did not show short latency changes. These findings appear to point to some regions of the brain in which cellular activity may be causally related to the behavioral change. The fact that the cells' responses precede the behavior makes it possible for the cells' activity to be causally related to the learning. If the cells are involved, what is their role? Are they part of a neural circuit that is the neural memory? Or are the cells important because of other influences, such as possibly modulating cells with longer response latencies? For the present, the changes in unit activity must be regarded as correlates of learning. It remains to be determined whether the neural changes are critically involved in the learned behavior.

In studies such as these, in which changes in the nervous system are to be interpreted as reflecting associative changes, i.e., alterations in the meaning of the stimulation, it is essential that other factors that might influence the amplitude or pattern of the evoked neural activity be held constant. This is a complicated but important problem in studies of learning, since factors such as changes in the intensity of the stimulus at the receptor as well as the animal's state of excitability might produce changes that could be regarded as being due to memory processes.

A series of recent experiments recorded multiple unit activity from several brain regions during the classical conditioning of a pupillary dilation response in paralyzed cats (Oleson et al., 1975). Under these conditions the sensory stimulation could be kept constant and, thus, ruled out as a cause of the changes in neural activity. Using the pupillary response as a measure of learning, the findings indicated that systematic changes in evoked multiple unit activity occurred during training. The animals showed evidence of conditioning, discriminating between two auditory signals, and reversal learning. Evoked multiple unit activity in the

306

auditory cortex, somatic cortex, and even the cochlear nucleus showed essentially similar results.

However, the role of such changes is not at all clear, since the acquisition of neural changes sometimes followed rather than preceded the behavioral changes. These findings serve to emphasize the need for careful examination of the relationship between development of behavioral changes and the development of changes in neuronal activity. This type of information can of course only be obtained when the behavioral and neural responses are observed in the same subjects.

Other recent studies recorded multiple-unit activity from the brains of rabbits trained in an _active avoidance task_ (Gabriel et al., 1975). The rabbits were required to move (in a wheel) in response to the CS+ in order to avoid shock, and to remain motionless in the presence of the CS−. Once this discrimination was mastered, they had to master the reverse discrimination. That is, the CS+ and CS− tones were interchanged. The results showed development and reversal of short latency (5–40 msec) signal-specific unit responses in the medial geniculate nucleus (MGN) during differential conditioning and reversal of the discriminative avoidance response. Of particular interest in this study was the fact that the signal-specific unit response shifted back and forth rather abruptly, favoring the old CS+, then the "new" CS+, during the early sessions of reversal training. However, the signal-specific unit activity of MGN was very often independent of the learned behavioral response in the early stage of reversal training; in some subjects the behavioral conditioned response showed reversal several sessions prior to reversal of the neuronal activity.

The activity units in different brain regions may shift with the course of the conditioning. For example, signal-specific, multiple-unit activity response was recorded in the rabbit limbic cortex during avoidance conditioning. The limbic neuronal activity was present in the intermediate stages of discrimination training when the behavioral discrimination was beginning to develop. However, the limbic cortex showed only a marginal signal-specific effect in the final stages of acquisition when the behavioral discrimination was well established. Instead, the anteroventral nucleus of the thalamus, a region with reciprocal fiber connections to the limbic cortex, showed a large signal-specific unit effect at the end of discrimination training. These findings suggest that the cortex was perhaps more involved in mediating the early stages of behavioral learning, whereas the thalamus may have been involved in the well-learned behavior.

A very likely, and simpler, alternative to this interpretation, however, is that the degree of nonspecific cortical arousal (which increased the unit response) decreased as the animal acquired the task, while the thalamic response continued to develop. Very similar decreases in the anatomical extent of EEG desynchronization of cortical regions were also seen with overtraining in early EEG studies.

VII. Evoked Potentials

One of the major purposes of studies of changes in the activity of neurons as a consequence of training is the hope of finding cells that are directly involved in the learning. Thus, as we have noted, the electrophysiological studies of unit activity are frequently conducted in an attempt to locate cells that are parts of neural circuits which provide the basis of a memory trace. The basic assumption of this approach is that memories are based on neural circuits. Although this assumption is appealing and therefore widely accepted, it is not beyond question. In fact, the "switchboard" view of learning—that is the view that learning is based on the formation of specific connections between nerve cells—is not well supported by existing evidence. For example, as was discussed above, lesion studies have not shown that specific memories are lost when brain tissue is destroyed. Sometimes even very large lesions fail to cause retention losses. Furthermore, when an animal is trained, changes in firing patterns can be recorded in a large proportion of cells (from 10 to 70% in various studies). This suggests that each cell is affected by many experiences. Given this degree of complexity, how are specific memory circuits formed? John (1972) suggests that specific circuits are not formed and that information is represented by a common mode of activity in units located in many regions of the brain. The important feature of firing is the coherence of firing patterns in ensembles of neurons. The coherence can be measured in patterns of evoked potentials or as statistical averages of unit discharges. The findings of a series of studies indicate that training produces highly specific changes in the wave shapes of evoked potentials recorded from several brain regions. Furthermore, the response of a trained animal to a stimulus is predicted by the shape of the evoked potential, which is elicited by the stimulus (John, 1967, 1972).

In these studies, food and water-deprived cats were trained to perform two responses, e.g., bar pressing for water and hurdle jumping to avoid shock. The subjects were required to make both responses within the same experimental session, and different stimuli were used to signal each response. The stimuli were trains of simple, repetitive stimuli (tones, light flashes) which differed in terms of the frequency of repetition. For example, in a particular experiment, a cat might be required on some trials to press a bar for water at the onset of a 3 per second flashing light, and on other trials in the same session to jump a hurdle to avoid shock signaled to a 10 per second click. In some experiments, the stimuli were of the same modality, differing only in repetition frequency. Moreover, in some of these studies, both responses led to the same reinforcer (e.g., water), whereas in other experiments the responses led to different reinforcers (e.g., water and shock avoidance), as in the example given above. During performance, evoked potentials (EP's) to each stimulus within the train of repetitive stimuli were recorded from various regions of the brain.

The wave form of late components of the EP's elicited by each flash within a train of 3 per second light flashes (which signaled water) were distinctly different from the EP's elicited by light flashes given at 10 per second (which signaled foot shock). Further, the unique wave shapes of the EP's elicited by the signals "predicted" with great accuracy which of the two alternative responses the subject was about to perform. This was true even for trials on which the subjects made errors. Thus, if the 10 per second train signaled hurdle jump, but the cat erroneously performed a bar press, the EP wave shapes to the 10 per second signal were not the usual ones, but instead were those ordinarily associated with the 3 per second signal and a bar press! Further, if the cat was presented with a 6.5 Hz signal (midway between the 10 per second and 3 per second signals), the EP's were similar to the EP's to the 3 per second signal if the 3 per second response was performed, and they were similar to the 10 per second EP's if the 10 per second response was performed. Thus, the EP wave form predicted how the animal "interpreted" a signal that was intermediate between the two original signals.

On some occasions during early training wave shapes appropriate to both responses appeared, and frequently there was a switching back and forth from one wave shape to the other during the initial training trials. However, wave shapes appropriate to the behavior-about-to-happen consistently occurred in the later training trials, just prior to the occurrence of that behavior. Interestingly, the same EP could be recorded from many of the brain areas. These results are consistent with the view (Lashley, 1950) that memory for a given behavior is widely distributed in the brain.

In other experiments cats were trained to push a lever on the left to a 3 per second signal, and a lever on the right to a 10 per second signal, with the signals being of the same modality and the reward being similar. Even under these circumstances, differences in EP wave forms differentiated the two learned responses. These experiments attempted to control for the possibility that the wave forms might reflect different patterns of generalized systems activation, rather than different patterns of specific learned information. Nevertheless, the possibility of different wave forms being influenced by different motor areas involved in turning right or left still remains. Although it seems nearly impossible to rule out such general effects, these data continue to suggest that learned information may be at least partially coded in changes within large neuronal aggregates.

On the basis of findings such as these, John suggests that information about an experience is represented by coherent activity in ensembles of cells and that the information will be activated or "read-out" when a stimulus (even a novel one) activates the representative system, ". . . in such a way as to cause release of a common mode of activity like that stored during the learning experience" (John, 1972).

These theoretical arguments and experimental findings provide difficulty for theories that assume that memories are based on the formation of specific circuits. However, the alternative theory raises a number of questions. In particular, what is the basis of the alteration in the coherence of firing in ensembles? Are the changes in the evoked potentials due to stable changes at specific synaptic sites of specific cells? Are the ensembles merely more complex circuits? How do the ensembles activate specific units that control behavior? These questions must be addressed in subsequent development of the cellular "ensemble" hypothesis.

VIII. Neurochemical Correlates of Training

The electrophysiological changes produced by training are, of course, merely signs that neural activity has changed. If it is assumed that a change in neuronal activity results from a change in the particular cells whose discharges are recorded, the question is, what is the basis of the change? What cellular changes cause the cells to alter their rates of firing? Activation of a neuron by training very likely triggers chemical changes that in some way alter the cells' probability of firing. Such changes might, in turn, produce an increase in transmitter substances in presynaptic terminals or alter the receptive properties of postsynaptic sites on dendrites. Such changes might presumably require the synthesis of ribonucleic acid (RNA) and protein. It might even be that training causes the synthesis of specific species of RNA and protein.

During the past two decades, a large number of studies have investigated the effects of training on the synthesis of RNA and protein. While many of the findings and interpretations are controversial, the overall evidence does support the general view that training stimulates RNA and protein synthesis. In these experiments animals, usually rats or mice, are trained on a task. Control animals are given some kind of stimulation but are not given specific training. The animals are then sacrificed and the brains are analyzed for changes in RNA or protein. Studies focusing on RNA have measured changes in the ratios of bases in the RNA as well as the incorporation of radioactive precursors into RNA. For example, in the studies by Hydén and Egyhazi (1962), rats were trained to climb a sloping wire for a food reward, then the RNA in cells in the vestibular nucleus of the trained rats was compared with that of control rats subjected to stimulation produced by rotation. The results suggested that the training increased RNA and altered the composition of RNA in the cell nucleus.

In a series of experiments, Glassman and his colleagues (see Glassman, 1974) investigated the effects of active avoidance training on the incorporation of radioactively labeled uridine into RNA. Mice were trained to jump to a small platform in order to avoid a foot shock. "Yoked" controls received the conditioned stimulus (light and buzzer) and the unconditioned stimulus (foot shock) but were not allowed to learn to avoid the shock. The findings suggested that the avoidance training increased the incorporation of the uridine into RNA, particularly in the hippocampus and diencephalon. Similar results have been obtained by other investigators. For example, in rats, training on a visual discrimination task increased the incorporation of radioactive precursors into RNA. The effect was particularly pronounced in the cells of the hippocampus and visual cortex (Matthies *et al.*, 1973).

These results suggest that active avoidance training increases RNA in neurons in specific regions of the brain. However, both the biochemical and the behavioral findings of these experiments are difficult to interpret. In many of the incorporation studies, it is not clear that the changes measured reflect increased synthesis of RNA. Other evidence indicates that, in mice, training on an active avoidance response decreases the amount of radioactivity measured in uridine monophosphates (UMP) (Entingh *et al.*, 1974). Since UMP radioactivity has in many studies been used as the correction factor for measuring the incorporation of labeled uridine into RNA, the conclusion that training increases RNA synthesis is seriously questioned by these findings. It is clear nonetheless that the avoidance training procedures affect brain biochemistry. At the behavioral level, it is important to consider whether the neurochemical changes are associated with the formation of memory or whether they reflect changes caused by sensory stimulation, arousal stress, or performance of the response. Since the yoked controls also experience the lights, hunger and shock stimuli they presumably learn something. Why then should their brains differ from those of the animals that were trained to avoid the shock? The problem of the appropriate control for training is a very difficult matter.

In a series of experiments, Horn and his colleagues (1973) have attempted to clarify both the biochemical and behavioral questions concerning the effects of training on RNA synthesis. In their studies newborn chicks were subjected to imprinting procedures. A flashing yellow light was presented for 60 minutes. This training produces a strong and sustained approach response. The training also produces an increase in incorporation of labeled precursors into what is presumed to be RNA (and protein). However, what aspects of the imprinting procedure produce the chemical changes? In order to attempt to answer this question, split-brain chicks were produced by surgically severing the supraoptic commissure. The chicks were then exposed to the flashing light while one eye was covered with a patch, so that one side of the brain received the imprinting information but both sides of the brain were influenced by other factors such as arousal and stress. The chicks' brains were then analyzed for incorporation of labeled uracil into acid-insoluble substances presumed to be RNA. The incorporation in the trained side of the brain was higher than in the untrained side. The effect was obtained only in the forebrain "roof." Other brain regions were not affected. Other experiments showed that in chicks with intact brains, monocular imprinting does not differentially affect incorporation in the two halves of the brain. Furthermore, incorporation is much less enhanced by stimulation with the flashing light if the chicks are given extensive imprinting training on the previous day such that they have already "learned." Overall these findings suggest that the changes in incorporation are related to the learning that occurs during the imprinting session and are not caused simply by arousal, stress, or sensory stimulation. It may be that there are alternative interpretations that have not been tested. The effects may be due, for example, to some nonmemorial consequences of the flashing light. But these findings strongly suggest that the chemical changes may be critically involved in learning.

Numerous studies have also reported that training increases the incorporation of labeled amino acids into protein. For example, protein synthesis is increased by visual discrimination learning (Matthies et al., 1973) and imprinting (Horn et al., 1973). Recent studies indicate that, in goldfish, training produces specific changes in the pattern of brain protein synthesis (Shashoua, 1976). In these experiments a small styrofoam float was attached to the ventral midline of the fish. Initially the fish were suspended upside down. However, they learned to adjust to the float and swim normally within a few hours as is shown in Fig. 8-4. The response was retained for over 1 week. Changes in protein synthesis were studied by injecting the animals with the amino acid ^{3}H- or ^{14}C-valine immediately after the animals were trained and then analyzing the radioactivity in protein of different fractions of brain tissue. The training increased valine incorporation only in a cytoplasmic fraction and not in a nuclear or synaptosomal fraction. Further, changes were obtained in only some types of protein. Animals that did not learn showed no changes in brain protein. Thus, the effects appeared not to be due to stress or exercise. It could be that such changes are due to arousal associated with the learning or to changes occurring as a consequence of the learning (e.g., decreased stress). Further research is needed to determine whether the changes are specifically related to the acquisition of the response.

Perhaps the most dramatic as well as controversial experiments in studies of the neurobiology of memory are those investigating the possibility that memory might be transferred from one individual to another by injecting extracts taken from the brain. Clear evidence of memory transfer by means of chemical extracts would provide the possibility of discovering the chemical nature of changes underlying memory. This possibility has stimulated a number of memory-transfer experiments in recent years. In the earliest experiments evidence of memory transfer was obtained in studies in which trained planaria were fed to naive planaria (McConnell, 1962). However, comparable results were then obtained by feeding planaria

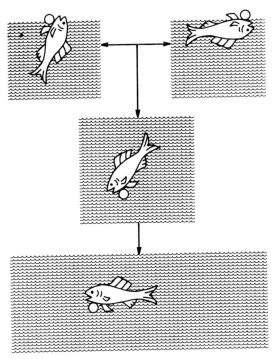

Fig. 8-4. A small polystyrene foam float was attached to the chin of each goldfish after injection of a radioactive label into the brain. The goldfish then had to learn to swim in a new way to compensate for the float. This training experience produced specific changes in brain protein synthesis. (Redrawn from Shashoua, 1968.)

tissue obtained from planaria that were stimulated but not given training (Hartry *et al.*, 1964). Thus the basis of the effect is not clear.

Most memory transfer studies have used rats, mice, or goldfish (Byrne, 1970; Ungar, 1970). In general the findings are extremely conflicting, and as a consequence no firm conclusions can be drawn. Research has not as yet specified either optimal or reliable procedures for producing a transfer effect. Further, it is not at all clear what type of molecule might be responsible for producing the effect (McGaugh, 1967). Should such experiments be reproducible, it should be possible to determine the basis of the effects. At the present time, the memory transfer effect must be regarded as not yet convincingly demonstrated.

Most of the research in this area has investigated the possible role of the synthesis of macromolecules. There is, however, other evidence that brain chemistry is altered by experience. Environmental stimulation can alter the activity of enzymes involved in the regulation of cholinergic transmitters (Rosenzweig *et al.*, 1972). Furthermore, there is evidence that training alters the turnover of brain norepinephine (Lewy and Seiden, 1972). Obviously, much research is needed to provide an understanding of the specific chemical changes involved in memory storage.

IX. Experimental Modulation of Memory Storage Processes

It is clear that the electrical and chemical activity of the brain is altered by experience. However, additional research is needed as to whether the neurobiological correlates of training discussed in Section VIII provide measures of changes that underlie the memory. Another approach to the study of the neural basis of learning and memory involves the study of the effects on memory of treatments that alter brain activity at the time that the changes underlying learning are presumed to occur. When learning occurs it seems unlikely that permanent neural changes occur instantaneously. Some changes must, of course, occur very rapidly, since we know that we routinely remember and use information acquired within milliseconds or seconds. Such memory is essential for integrating sequential experience, such as language and music, and for integrating motor responses. However, there is extensive evidence that the long term retention of recently acquired information can be altered by many different types of treatments administered after the learning experience. In general, the degree of the effect of the treatment on retention is greatest if the treatment is administered shortly after learning. These findings suggest that the treatments act in some way (or ways) to modulate the processes involved in establishing or "consolidating" the neural changes underlying long term memory. Much recent research on *memory consolidation* has been based on the hope that understanding the ways in which the nervous system is influenced by treatments affecting retention will provide clues to the neural processes underlying learning (Glickman, 1961; McGaugh and Herz, 1972).

X. Retrograde Amnesia

When the "consolidation hypothesis" was first proposed by Mueller and Pilzecker in 1900 it provided an explanation for the well-known phenomenon of *retrograde amnesia* seen following head injury (McDougall, 1901). Human patients who suffer head injury may have a permanent loss of memory for experiences that occurred seconds, hours, or sometimes days *prior to* the injury. In general, the length of the period of retrograde amnesia varies with the severity of the injury. If

8. COMPLEX LEARNING AND MEMORY

the patient has only a short period of "posttraumatic amnesia," that is, if the patient quickly recovers consciousness after the injury, the period of retrograde amnesia is usually short. If the injury produces unconsciousness and confusion for days or weeks, then a long period of retrograde amnesia results. Clinical evidence summarized by one study of retrograde amnesia produced by head injury is shown in Fig. 8-5 (Russell and Nathan, 1946). In the patients studied (50 per group) retrograde amnesia of greater than 1 minute was found in 14% of patients with brief (less than 1 hour) posttraumatic amnesia and 28 to 76% of patients with longer posttraumatic amnesia.

Shortly after the introduction of _electroconvulsive shock_ (ECS) as a treatment for mental disorders (Cerletti and Bini, 1938), it was found that the treatments sometimes produced retrograde amnesia. Some of the memory loss is only temporary and due to inability to retrieve information. However, under some conditions the effects appear to be permanent (Fink _et al._, 1974). We will return to this problem in Section XXI.

These clinical studies stimulated extensive experiments investigating the effects of ECS on the behavior of laboratory animals. In now classic studies, Duncan (1949) and Gerard (1949) found that ECS produced retrograde amnesia in rats and hamsters. In the past several decades subsequent research has attempted to determine why ECS and other brain treatments alter animals' memory for experiences occurring prior to the treatments. The most generally accepted

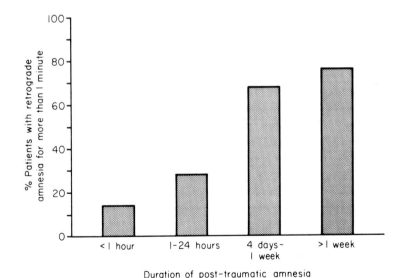

Fig. 8-5. Head injury produces both retrograde amnesia and posttraumatic amnesia. The percentage of cases, in which retrograde amnesia of greater than 1 minute is seen, increases dramatically as the duration of posttraumatic amnesia increases. (Data from Russell and Nathan, 1946.)

view is that the treatments alter retention by influencing processes involved in memory consolidation. However, such treatments may also affect retrieval of memory as well as alter factors that influence the performance of learned responses (McGaugh and Herz, 1972; Lewis, 1969).

XI. Effects of Direct Electrical Stimulation of the Brain

Following Duncan's and Gerard's studies, numerous studies confirmed and extended the finding that ECS produces retrograde amnesia (Thompson, 1958; Glickman, 1961). In these studies, diagrammed in Fig. 8-6, the animals (usually mice or rats) are first trained on some simple task. Then they are given a treatment either immediately after the training or after an interval of time. At a later time, usually at least 1 day or longer after the training, the animals are tested

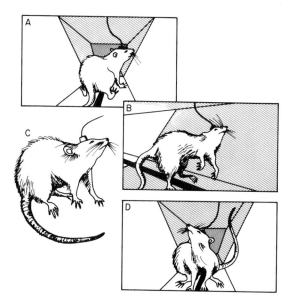

Fig. 8-6. In the experimental study of memory storage processes, animals are often trained in an inhibitory avoidance task. In this procedure, the rat is placed in the lighted portion of an alley (A). When the rat steps into the darkened portion of the runway, it receives a short foot shock (B) followed by a treatment, such as stimulation of a particular brain region (C). Some time later, usually at least 1 day, the rat is tested for retention. If the animal refrains from entering the darkened area, where it had been shocked, then it is assumed that the animal remembers the training. If, however, the rat reenters the dark side, then the treatment is said to have produced retrograde amnesia for the training experience. In this case, it appears that the animal remembers because it is staying in the lighted side and away from the place where it had been shocked (D).

to see whether they remember the training experience. In general, the treatments are most effective, that is, cause greatest memory losses, if they are administered immediately after training. As is shown in Fig. 8-7, degree of modulation of retention observed decreases as the time interval between training and posttraining treatment is increased. In the early research on the problem, the ECS was administered by passing electrical current through animals' heads by means of electrodes attached to their ears. Recent research has investigated the effects of direct electrical stimulation of the brain.

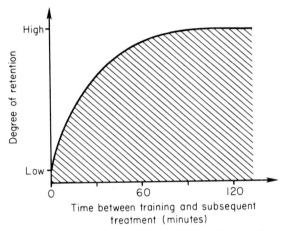

Fig. 8-7. A typical retrograde amnesia gradient obtained in studies of memory disruption. As the interval between the time of training and administration of the amestic treatment increases, the degree of retention increases. As the experimental conditions are changed, the slope of the gradient also changes. (From McGaugh, 1973.)

Electroconvulsive shock treatments elicit brain seizures and bodily convulsions. However, neither the convulsions nor the brain seizures play any critical role in producing the amnesic effects (McGaugh, 1974). If the current is applied directly to the surface of the brain cortex in rats, the length of the gradient of retrograde amnesia varies directly with the intensity of the electrical current (Zornetzer, 1974). Different gradients can be obtained with different experimental treatments. For example, in one study different cortical regions were stimulated with currents of varying intensity at an interval varying from 1 second to several hours after the rats were trained on an *inhibitory avoidance task* (see Fig. 8-6). On the training trial, the rats were punished with a mild foot shock as they stepped from one compartment to another compartment of a straight alley. They were then given cortical stimulation of various intensities. The following day the rats were tested for retention of the experience. The results of this experiment are shown in Fig. 8-8. With lower intensities (2 to 4 mA) of cortical stimulation, retention was affected only if the current was applied within seconds after the

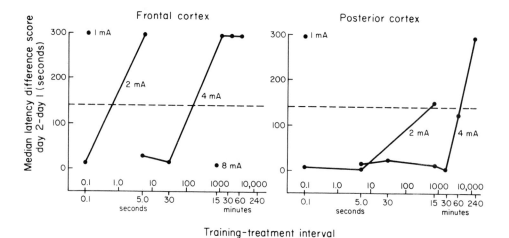

Fig. 8-8. Median difference scores (entrance latency on day 2 minus day 1) showing amount of retention of an inhibitory avoidance task. All median latencies less than 140 seconds (dashed line) are significantly lower than latencies for animals receiving footshock only (median = 300 seconds). The length of the retrograde amnesia gradients ranged from 5 seconds to 240 minutes depending on the location of the electrodes and the intensity of the stimulation. (From Gold *et al.*, 1973b.)

training. With a higher intensity (8 mA), amnesia was produced even if the treatments were administered at an interval of 1 hour following training (Gold *et al.*, 1973a). Even longer gradients of retrograde amnesia can be produced with ECS by varying the intensity and duration of the treatment and by administering several treatments after the training (Mah and Albert, 1973). These findings are comparable to those of studies of the effects of the convulsant drug, flurothyl, on memory in chicks. The *gradient of amnesia* varies with the dose and duration of the treatment (Cherkin, 1969). Memory storage processes appear to remain susceptible to modulating influences of brain stimulation for at least several hours following training. It is clear that no single treatment condition can provide a measure of "storage time." Retrograde amnesia gradients are products of the specific experimental conditions under which they are obtained.

When electrical stimulation is delivered either by means of peripheral electrodes or directly to the brain cortex, memory effects are usually produced when the current also elicits brain seizure activity. Currents that elicit seizures also have other effects, such as inhibition of brain protein synthesis (Cotman *et al.*, 1971; Dunn *et al.*, 1974). However, electrical stimulation applied to some subcortical brain regions produces alteration in memory even if the stimulating current is well below the seizure threshold. Amnesic effects have been obtained with low-intensity (subseizure) stimulation of several structures including the caudate nucleus, substantia nigra, hippocampus, mesencephalic reticular formation (MRF), and the amygdala (McGaugh and Gold, 1976; Kesner and Wilburn, 1974).

Such findings have been interpreted by some investigators as suggesting that the electrical stimulation interferes with neural processing of information which is occurring in the region stimulated. For example, in rats, recent memory is disrupted by stimulation of the mesencephalic reticular formation, and the formation of long term memory is impaired by posttraining stimulation of the hippocampus. On the basis of these findings, it has been suggested that the two neural structures have different functions in short and long term memory (Kesner, 1973). There are, of course, other possible interpretations of these results. The memory effects might be produced because stimulation of these two structures produces quite different effects in other regions of the brain. Or it might be that stimulation produces the same effects in the two regions, but that the two regions have different thresholds for response to the stimulation.

The important contribution of subcortical brain stimulation studies is that they indicate that memory can be altered by low-intensity electrical stimulation applied to relatively specific brain regions. For example, the findings of a series of studies indicate that amygdala stimulation produces retrograde amnesia. Studies using unilateral stimulation indicate that the degree of amnesia produced varies with the locus of the electrode within the amygdala, as shown in Fig. 8-9 (Gold *et al.*, 1974; McGaugh and Gold, 1976). However, this finding does not mean that memory processing occurs in this brain region. It seems more likely that activation of this region leads to widespread changes that have a modulating influence on memory storage processes. In view of evidence (discussed in Section XV) that pituitary hormones may affect memory storage it could be that brain stimulation modulates memory through the release of pituitary hormones, or the brain stimulation might cause the release of transmitters at the terminals of the neurons stimulated. If the stimulated structures project throughout the brain as with the monoamine systems discussed in Chapter 6, then numerous brain regions could be affected by stimulation of a restricted brain region (see Kety, 1972).

XII. Facilitating Effects of Brain Stimulation

The interpretation that brain stimulation modulates memory storage processes is also supported by evidence that retention can be enhanced by posttraining stimulation of several brain regions. Facilitating effects are produced only if the stimulation is administered shortly after training. For example, in an elegant series of experiments, Bloch and his colleagues (Bloch, 1970) gave rats electrical stimulation of the mesencephalic reticular formation immediately after training sessions. Rate of learning was enhanced by the stimulation. Further, they found that the amnesia produced by postsession administration of the depressant drug fluothane

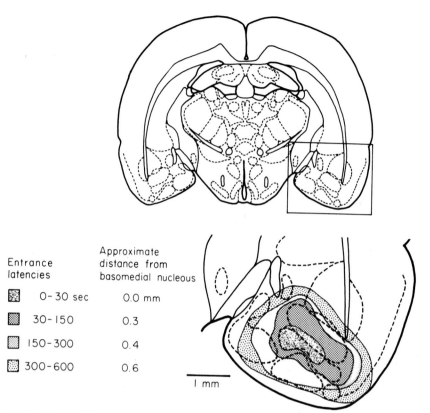

Entrance latencies

		Approximate distance from basomedial nucleous
▨	0-30 sec	0.0 mm
▨	30-150	0.3
▨	150-300	0.4
▨	300-600	0.6

1 mm

Fig. 8-9. Electrical stimulation in, or very near, the basomedial nucleus (BM) of the amygdala produced the greatest disruption of memory. As the site of stimulation was moved further from the basomedial nucleus, latencies increased, indicating better retention. (Data from McGaugh and Gold, 1976.)

could be prevented if the electrical stimulation of the reticular formation were given in the interval between the termination of the training and the administration of the fluothane.

Experiments have confirmed Bloch's other finding that learning is enhanced by postsession electrical brain stimulation. In one study (Denti *et al.*, 1970), rats received reticular stimulation immediately after each training trial on a one-way active avoidance task. The learning of the group given postsession stimulation was superior to that of animals which had electrodes implanted but which did not receive stimulation, but the learning of the stimulated animals was inferior to that of control rats which did not have electrodes implanted. Thus the posttrial stimulation appeared to partially compensate for a lesion-produced impairment of learning. However, facilitation of learning by posttrial electrical stimulation of the reticular formation can also be obtained in studies in which the lesion produced by the implantation of the electrode does not impair learning. Comparable results have been obtained with posttraining hippocampal stimulation (Landfield *et al.*, 1973; Destrade *et al.*, 1973).

Several studies have shown that memory can be impaired or enhanced by posttrial electrical stimulation of the amygdala. The same type of stimulation can produce either impairment of memory or facilitation of memory, depending on the experimental conditions. As is shown in Fig. 8-10, animals given posttraining amygdala stimulation show poor retention following training on an inhibitory avoidance task in comparison with either unimplanted controls or controls bearing amygdala electrodes if a relatively high level of foot shock is used during training (Fig. 8-10A). However, if a low-level foot shock is used during training, the implanted animals have poor retention. Further, with low-level foot shock, posttrial stimulation of the amygdala facilitates retention. These findings indicate that brain stimulation does not simply disrupt or enhance retention. The modulating influences of stimulation vary with the state of the animal produced by the experimental conditions (Gold *et al.*, 1973b, 1975; Gold and McGaugh, 1975).

It is clear that brain stimulation can modulate retention. The fact that the

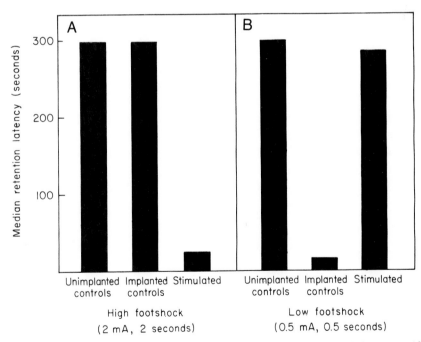

Fig. 8-10. Stimulation of the amygdala was given immediately after inhibitory avoidance training. The implanted controls showed a retention deficit for training with low foot shock (B), but not with the high foot shock (A). When compared with their control groups, amygdala stimulation facilitated retention of training with low foot shock (B), but impaired it with high foot shock (A). (From Gold *et al.*, 1975.)

effects are time dependent provides strong support for the view that the stimulation alters memory storage processes. It is also clear that there is considerable anatomic specificity in the stimulation effects. However, brain stimulation experiments have not located "memory neurons" or even "memory structures." They have located structures that, when stimulated, produce modulating influences on memory storage. With more information of this kind it should eventually be possible to determine which of the effects of brain stimulation are critical for producing the modulating influence on memory.

XIII. Effects of CNS Stimulants on Memory

A variety of drugs, including CNS stimulants such as strychnine, picrotoxin, pentylenetetrazol, bemegride, and amphetamines, enhance retention when they are administered to animals either shortly before or shortly after training (McGaugh, 1968, 1973). Enhancing effects of stimulants have been obtained in many tasks and with several species of animals. Furthermore, as is the case with brain stimulation, the degree of modulation of retention decreases as the time between the training and the drug injection is increased.

Figure 8-11 summarizes findings of several studies of the effects of strychnine, pentylenetetrazol, and amphetamine on learning by mice of a visual discrimination response. Each day the mice received a drug injection either before or after they were given training on the task. The degree of enhancement of learning with each drug varied with the dose used and the time of drug administration. These findings suggest that the drugs alter retention by modulating memory storage processes. The basis of the modulating influences is not yet understood. Some clues are provided by recent studies of alterations in hormones and neurotransmitters as is discussed in Sections XV–XVII.

XIV. Effects of Inhibition of RNA and Protein Synthesis

Numerous studies have investigated the possible roles of RNA and protein synthesis in memory storage by administering antibiotic drugs that interfere with RNA and protein synthesis (Agranoff, 1967; Barondes and Cohen, 1968). There is substantial evidence that drugs such as puromycin, cycloheximide, acetoxycycloheximide and anisomycin disrupt retention in rats, mice and goldfish if the drugs are administered shortly before or after training. A diagrammatic summary of studies of puromycin's effects on learning and memory in goldfish is shown in

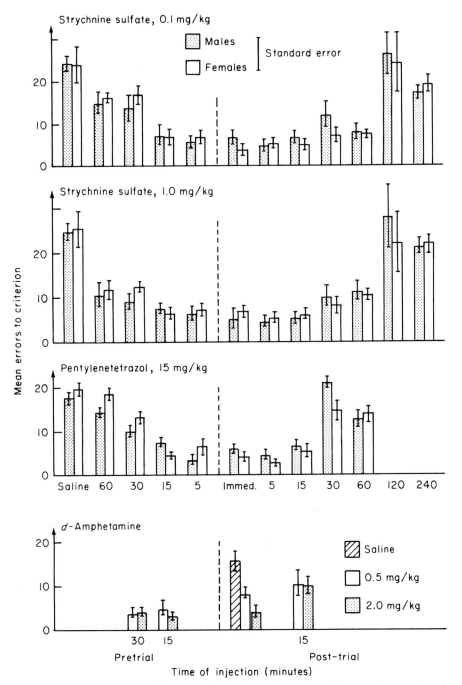

Fig. 8-11. Mice were trained in a visual discrimination task and were given various drug treatments at different times before or after training. Those mice that received the drug treatments close to the time of training took fewer trials to learn the task. (From McGaugh and Herz, 1972.)

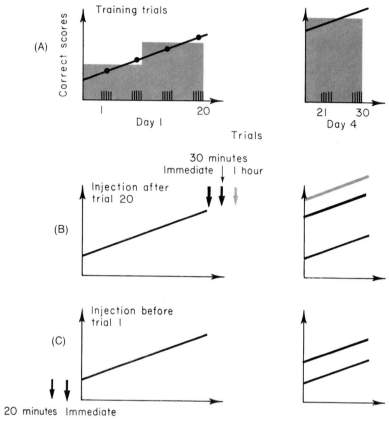

Fig. 8-12. (A) Fish were given 20 training trials, in blocks of 5, on day 1 and were tested for retention on day 4. (B) Puromycin injected immediately after trial 20 reduced performance on day 4 to the level of naive animals. Puromycin injected 30 minutes after training resulted in an intermediate level of retention, while puromycin injected 1 hour after training had no effect on retention. (C) Puromycin injected immediately before trial 1 had no reliable effect on acquisition but blocked retention measured on day 4. Puromycin injected 20 minutes before the first acquisition trial left acquisition unimpaired but blocked some facilitation. (From McGaugh and Herz, 1972, as adapted from Agranoff *et al.*, 1966.)

Fig. 8-12 (Agranoff *et al.*, 1966). In general, retention impairment is produced by inhibition of protein synthesis only if protein synthesis is inhibited by greater than 90%. Under some conditions the degree of impairment is related to the duration of protein synthesis inhibition. In one study (Flood *et al.*, 1975b) mice received a series of injections of anisomycin in order to prolong the duration of inhibition of protein synthesis following training (see Fig. 8-13). One injection was given before training and another 2 hours after training. These injections produced an inhibition of protein synthesis lasting approximately 4 hours but little amnesia (10% of animals). Animals given a third injection 4 hours after training had prolonged

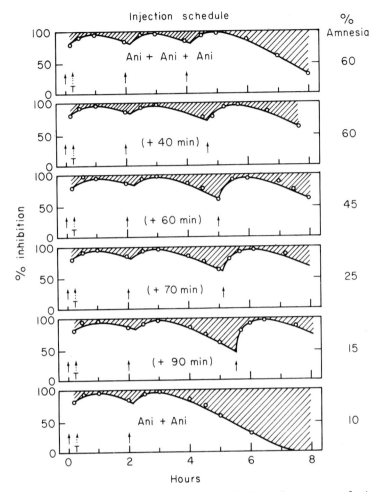

Fig. 8-13. The effect of inhibition of protein synthesis on the percent of mice showing amnesia for training in an inhibitory avoidance task. Three injections of the protein synthesis inhibitor anisomycin (Ani) produced significantly greater amnesia than just two successive Ani injections. These findings can be interpreted to indicate that protein synthesis related to memory formation was occurring 4 to 6 hours after training. (From Flood *et al.*, 1975b.)

inhibition of protein synthesis and increased amnesia (60%). The third injection did not markedly affect retention if administered 5½ hours after training. The protein synthesis occurring between the second and third injection appeared to block the effects of the later injection.

The impairing effects of anisomycin on retention in mice can be attenuated by stimulant drugs, such as strychnine, pentylenetetrazol and amphetamine, given shortly after training. The amnesic effects are potentiated by CNS depressants. This is particularly interesting since the stimulants and depressants do not significantly affect protein synthesis. Thus, the drugs appear to act by influencing other processes which can override the impairing influences of inhibition of brain protein synthesis. The important point is that consolidation can occur with markedly reduced brain protein synthesis (greater than 90% inhibition) if the CNS is stimulated. These findings pose interesting questions concerning the role of protein synthesis in memory storage.

Recent evidence also indicates that memory is impaired by reversible inhibition of RNA synthesis (Thut *et al.*, 1973; Kobiler and Allweis, 1974). Under some conditions the memory losses produced by inhibitors of RNA and protein synthesis are temporary, whereas under others the losses appear to be permanent. These findings suggest that the treatments may affect the retrieval as well as the storage of memory processes. However, the fact that the degree of retention loss depends upon the training-treatment interval indicates that the effects are not due to nonspecific influences such as illness.

These experiments are also difficult to interpret in terms of the mechanism responsible for the amnesia. The findings that inhibitors of RNA and protein synthesis impair retention are of course consistent with the findings reviewed above suggesting that training stimulates RNA and protein synthesis. However, it could be that these drugs influence learning because of other influences on neuronal functioning. It could be that memory storage is disrupted by any treatment that disrupts cellular metabolic processes. Further studies are needed to determine the biochemical bases of the effects of these drugs on memory.

XV. Endogenous Modulators of Memory Storage

In recent years, several endogenous substances have been suggested as possibly playing a modulating role in memory storage. Kety (1972) has suggested that catecholamines, particularly norepinephrine, released in affective states might have the effect of promoting memory storage. De Wied and his associates (de Wied, 1974) have shown that ACTH and peptide fragments of ACTH alter retention. Numerous recent studies have examined the effects of adrenocorticotropic hormone (ACTH) and ACTH analogues, particularly the 4 to 10 peptide sequence of the ACTH molecule. ACTH or $ACTH_{4-10}$ both retard the extinction of learned avoidance responses. The fact that the 4 to 10 peptide has effects that are similar to ACTH is interesting because $ACTH_{4-10}$ does not affect the adrenal cortex. This suggests that ACTH may influence retention by directly influencing brain processes. Flood *et al.* (1976) examined the effects of $ACTH_{4-10}$ on retention of active and inhibitory responses in mice. Two forms of the peptide were used: in one the *l* form of the amino acid phenylalanine was the seventh amino acid in the sequence, while in the other the *d* isomer of phenylalanine was in the seventh position. Other evidence (Bohus and de Wied, 1966) has suggested that the *l* form of $ACTH_{4-10}$ is the portion that affects behavior. In support of this view Flood *et al.* (1976) found that retention was enhanced by posttraining administration of $ACTH_{4-10}$ with *l*-phenylalanine and impaired by the *d* form. However, the *d* form blocked the enhancement produced by the *l* form and potentiated the amnesia produced by anisomycin.

Hormones of the posterior pituitary may also play some role in modulating memory. Van Wimersma Greidanus *et al.* (1975) reported that rats with a genetic defect in the ability to synthesize vasopressin are unable to learn an inhibitory avoidance response. However, the animals of this strain (Brattleboro) were able to learn the response if vasopressin was administered immediately after training. Furthermore, the learning of normal animals was impaired by intraventricular injections of vasopressin antibodies (van Wimersma Greidanus *et al.*, 1975).

The findings of these recent studies strongly suggest that pituitary hormones have regulatory influences in memory storage in addition to their other well-known endocrine influences.

Other recent studies have shown that administration of pituitary and adrenal hormones as well as treatments which alter catecholamine metabolism can produce both retrograde amnesia and facilitation of memory storage. Several experiments have examined the effects of posttrial subcutaneous administration of several hormones, including epinephrine, norepinephrine, and ACTH, on the retention by rats of an inhibitory avoidance response (Gold and van Buskirk, 1975, 1976; Gold *et al.*, 1977). In these studies, rats were given a single trial on an inhibitory avoidance task and a retention test 24 hours later. The results are shown in Fig. 8-14A and B. Moderate doses of these hormones were found to enhance retention if the hormone was administered within a few minutes after training. A high dose of ACTH impaired retention. Hormones administered 2 hours after training did not affect subsequent retention. These findings provide clear evidence that memory storage processes are influenced by hormones administered after training and thus provide support for the view that hormones may be directly involved in the modulation of memory storage. It is not clear, however, how peripherally administered hormones modulate central neural processes, since there is much evidence suggesting that these hormones do not pass the blood–brain barrier. It is possible that small amounts might pass the barrier, particularly in the region of the hypothalamus. It is also possible that the peripheral injections may cause the release of ACTH or directly influence the CNS by altering circulatory activity. Thus, while it is not clear exactly how peripherally administered hormones affect brain activity, it is clear that they do produce alterations in brain functioning. It remains to be determined whether all

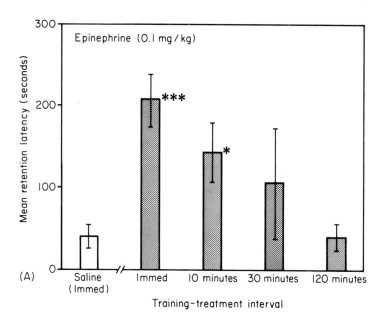

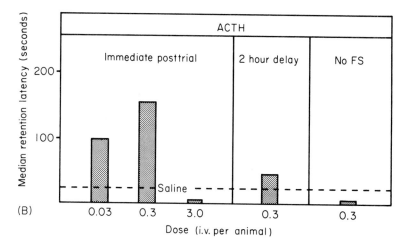

Fig. 8-14. (A) Retention latencies for animals that received either saline or epinephrine immediately after training, or epinephrine at various times after training. The effectiveness of epinephrine in facilitating retention decreased as the training-treatment interval increased. (From Gold and van Buskirk, 1975.) (B) The effects on memory of ACTH injections given after inhibitory avoidance training. The effect of immediate posttraining injections varied with dose as an inverted-U function. Animals receiving the two lowest doses of ACTH had significantly enhanced performance, while 3.0 I.U. of ACTH impaired retention. Delayed injections had no effect on later retention performance. (From Gold and McGaugh, 1977.)

of these hormones have directly acting central effects or whether they have peripheral effects that have a common action centrally.

Other peptides found in the brain may influence memory storage processes. One set of substances, known collectively as the endorphins (see Chapter 6), has recently been the subject of intensive investigation in many research laboratories. Recall that the term endorphin means endogenous morphine-like substance and that this class of molecules also includes the enkephalins. Endorphins bind to opiate receptors in the brain and other parts of the body, and stimulate cells in ways similar to morphine or heroin. Although the endorphins are capable of producing analgesia, many researchers feel that their primary function may be the modulation of some aspects of behavior (de Wied et al., 1978) and not control of pain.

There is now evidence that those neural systems influenced by opiates and naturally occurring opioids may modulate memory mechanisms. For example, an injection of morphine given after training impairs memory in rats, while injections of naloxone, a substance that blocks opiate receptors, enhances memory. This effect appears mediated specifically by opiate receptors because morphine blocks the memory enhancing effect of naloxone when they are given together (Jensen et al., 1978; Messing et al., 1979). In addition, naloxone will produce memory facilitation when injected directly into the amygdala (Gallagher and Kapp, 1978). These data and others indicate that endorphins play an important role in memory mechanisms. However, the precise way in which opioid systems in the brain and body act to influence memory processes is largely unknown.

There is much recent evidence suggesting that retention is influenced by posttraining alteration in brain catecholamines. For example, amphetamine enhances retention when administered shortly after training (McGaugh, 1973). However, it has not yet been shown that this effect is due to an action on central catecholamines. Somewhat more direct evidence has been provided by studies using drugs which block catecholamine biosynthesis. For example, the enhancing effects of posttraining injections of amphetamines are blocked by α-methyl-p-tyrosine (α-MPT), a compound that interferes with the synthesis of dopamine, the precursor of norepinephrine. Further, the impairing effects of posttraining administration of α-MPT were attenuated by administering L-dopa—the precursor of dopamine (Fulginiti and Orsingher, 1971; Fulginiti et al., 1976). In addition, recent research indicates that retention is impaired by posttrial administration of diethyldithiocarbamate (DDC), an inhibitor of dopamine β-hydroxylase, the enzyme that converts dopamine to norepinephrine (Randt et al., 1971; McGaugh et al., 1975). The results of one study using mice are shown in Fig. 8-15. These results are consistent with the interpretation that the retention impairment is due to a decrease in norepinephrine. However, the findings must be interpreted cautiously

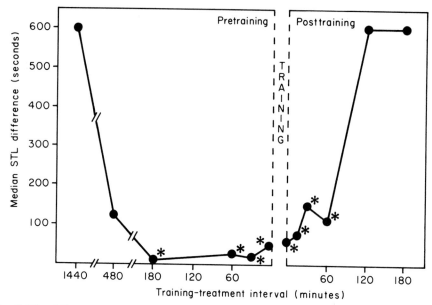

Fig. 8-15. Mice were injected with 900 mg/kg diethyldithiocarbamate (DDC) either before or after inhibitory avoidance training and retention was measured as the difference between the latency to step through (STL) on training day and the time to step through on test day. DDC administered as long as 180 minutes before training, or 60 minutes after training, significantly impaired retention. (Redrawn from Haycock *et al.*, 1977.)

because DDC chelates heavy metals and undoubtedly affects other brain systems involving metal-requiring enzymes.

Another approach to the problem is that of administering catecholamines directly to the brain to see whether such treatment will affect retention. There is some evidence that, in mice, memory can be facilitated by posttrial intraventricular administration of catecholamines. Somewhat clearer evidence of a role for catecholamines in memory has been provided by recent studies in which animals were given DDC before training and intraventricular injections of norepinephrine after training. A study using these procedures (Stein *et al.*, 1975) found that the memory deficit produced by DDC was significantly attenuated by norepinephrine (10 mg) if the intraventricular injection was given immediately after training. Administration of norepinephrine 2 hours or more after the training did not affect retention. Subsequent studies have confirmed these findings. In these experiments, rats were injected with DDC (680 mg/kg) 30 minutes before receiving a training trial on an inhibitory avoidance task. Immediately after the training trial, norepinephrine was injected into the lateral ventricle by means of an implanted cannula. As Fig. 8-16 shows, learning was impaired in the DDC-treated animals. However, a dose of 0.1 μg of norepinephrine attenuated the retention

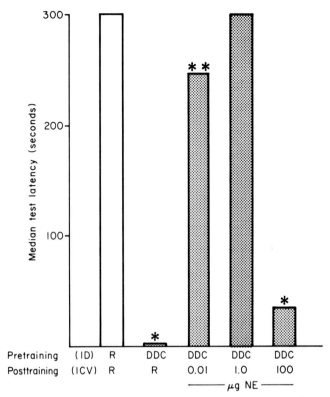

Fig. 8-16. Diethyldithiocarbamate (DDC), an inhibitor of norepinephrine (NE) biosynthesis was peripherally administered (IP) to rats 0.5 hour before training or immediately after training. Ringers saline (R), or various doses of NE, was injected into the lateral ventricles (ICV). The 0.01 μg dose of NE significantly attenuated the DDC amnesia (**), while those animals that received no Ringers saline or 100 μg NE after training showed significant amnesia (*). Although the 1.0 μg dose of NE produced a substantial elevation in median test latency, this difference was not significant. (Redrawn from Meligeni *et al.*, 1978.)

deficit produced by the DDC (Meligeni *et al.*, 1975). These findings provide additional support for the view (Kety, 1970, 1972) that central norepinephrine plays a role in memory storage. Obviously, additional studies are needed to determine whether substances other than norepinephrine might also attenuate DDC-induced retention deficits. Diethyldithiocarbamate-induced retention deficits can also be attenuated by peripheral subcutaneous injections of norepinephrine (Meligeni *et al.*, 1975). This effect is difficult to interpret in terms of a direct action of norepinephrine on the brain. The peripheral effects might act indirectly, for example, through influences on the pituitary gland or on the circulatory system.

Other recent attempts to investigate the role of catecholamines in memory have involved the use of brain lesions. Most of the norepinephrine-containing terminals in the cerebral cortex appear to arise from cell bodies of the locus coeruleus, which is located in the midbrain. Lesions of this structure produce a decrease in cortical norepinephrine. There is some evidence to suggest that locus coeruleus lesions produce deficits in learning (Anlezark *et al.*, 1973). However, this effect has not been confirmed (Amaral and Foss, 1975). Zornetzer and Gold (1975) reported that animals with a unilateral locus coeruleus lesion have an increased susceptibility to ECS-induced amnesia. In normal (i.e., un-lesioned) mice, ECS produced amnesia for inhibitory avoidance training only if the treatment was administered shortly after the training. However, in mice with locus coeruleus lesions, an ECS treatment produced a retention deficit even if the treatment was administered several days after the training. The lesion (which was made immediately after training) did not, by itself, affect retention.

XVI. Peripheral Catecholamines

Recent research findings have suggested that the memory-enhancing effects of amphetamine may be mediated by peripheral systems, and that catecholamines in parts of the body other than the brain may play an important role in modulating memory storage processes. Peripherally administered injections of amphetamine cause memory facilitation, whereas amphetamine given directly into the ventricles of the brain does not have an effect on memory at all.

Moreover, an amphetamine derivative, 4-OH-amphetamine, which does not readily enter the brain, facilitates memory when given to rats after training to the same extent as does amphetamine, which readily enters the brain (Martinez *et al.*, 1979). Thus, it seems that the site of action of amphetamine on memory facilitation may not necessarily be in the brain. Amphetamines may be working on the sympathetic nervous system or other peripheral catecholaminergic systems. In support of this hypothesis, removal of the adrenal medulla combined with peripheral sympathectomy abolishes the memory-enhancing effect of *both* amphetamine and 4-OH-amphetamine.

These studies taken together indicate that peripheral catecholaminergic systems are of great importance in the modulation of memory storage processes. It is possible that these findings may explain why peripheral administration of epinephrine and norepinephrine attenuates the degree of amnesia produced by DDC (see Section XV). Thus, the peripheral body state appears to interact with the brain states to determine the efficiency of memory storage.

XVII. Sleep and Memory Modulation

Effects comparable to those produced by locus coeruleus lesions have also been obtained by depriving mice of the stage of sleep referred to as *active sleep* or REM sleep (see Chapter 14). In one study mice were trained on an inhibitory avoidance task and then deprived of active sleep for two days. An ECS treatment produced amnesia when administered immediately after the termination of the sleep deprivation, which was 48 hours after the training. In mice not deprived of sleep the ECS produced amnesia only if administered shortly after training.

Evidence from other studies has provided additional support for the view that active sleep may influence memory storage processes (Bloch *et al.*, 1977). In these studies, rats were trained daily on a simple task. During the early stages of training, active sleep increased after each training session. Further, the amount of active sleep occurring after training decreased after the animals had learned the task but increased again if they were then taught a new task. The learning of the task was retarded by depriving animals of active sleep for several hours immediately after each training session. If the animals received posttraining electrical stimulation of the mesencephalic reticular formation there was no increase in active sleep following the training. Such stimulation enhances retention in normal animals. It is not yet clear just what aspects of sleep deprivation are responsible for the influence on retention. It might be that hormones released during active sleep normally serve as memory storage modulators. There is some evidence that the learning deficit produced by active sleep deprivation is related to a decrease in catecholamines. Hartmann and Stern (1972) reported that L-dopa (a precursor of dopamine and norepinephrine) attenuates the impairing effects of sleep deprivation on retention.

XVIII. Brain Pathology and Memory

A number of conditions that affect brain functioning in humans produce defects in memory storage. A review of some of the features of memory pathology in human patients will illustrate the complexity of the problems as well as some implications of these disorders for our understanding of the neurobiological bases of memory.

Disturbances of memory can occur in conjunction with alterations in mood or in association with the global changes in brain function that accompany aging. Such conditions can affect perceptual and motor skills and a wide range of cognitive abilities, along with memory capacity. Amnesia can also occur as a relatively pure disorder, in apparent isolation from other deficits in cognitive abilities. The analysis of such amnesias has provided a large body of information about the structure and organization of normal memory and its neurobiological substrate. Amnesias of this type have multiple causes, but share many common features.

XIX.   The Amnesic Syndrome: An Introduction

The best studied case of a human memory disorder is that of the patient H.M. who, at the age of 16, developed epileptic seizures which increased in severity until by the age of 27 they could no longer be controlled by anticonvulsive medication. Consequently, in 1953 surgery consisting of radical bilateral excision of the mediotemporal region including the anterior two-thirds of the hippocampus, the parahippocampal gyrus, uncus, and amygdala was performed (Fig. 8-17) (Scoville and Milner, 1957; Milner, 1972). A similar surgical procedure had been performed several times previously on severely psychotic patients without apparent adverse effect. Following surgery, H.M. exhibited no alteration in personality, an above average intellectual capacity (I.Q. 117), and an intact immediate memory as demonstrated by a normal facility for conversation. By contrast, he exhibited, after the surgery, a marked impairment in the ability to learn new material. His main problem is that once his attention is diverted the immediately preceding experiences are forgotten. He has considerable awareness of his memory defect. "Every day is alone in itself. . . . You see, at this moment, everything looks clear to me, but what happened just before? That's what worries me. . . . It's like waking from a dream. I just don't remember" (Milner, 1970).

Extensive testing has further clarified this remarkably pure *amnesic syndrome*. H.M. was unable to reduce his errors in a 28-choice-point, visual stylus maze during 215 trials. Normal subjects reached a criterion of three consecutive errorless runs in about 20 trials. Another test involved an extension of the familiar digit span procedure. Subjects attempt progressively longer lists of digits. When an error is made, the same list is presented repeatedly until it is done correctly. Under these conditions, normal subjects can extend their digit span up to 20 digits, requiring fewer than 15 trials to succeed at any list length. H.M. was unable to extend his digit span of six by a single digit even after 25 repetitions of the same seven-digit list (Drachman and Arbit, 1966). Despite this severe global amnesia for most kinds of material, H.M. showed evidence of acquiring motor skills and other tasks that might be termed "proprioceptive" or "perceptuomotor" (Corkin, 1968). Thus, H.M. learned a mirror drawing task at the normal rate over a 3-day period. It is very interesting to note that while he demonstrated good performance on this task, he denied that he had any memory of it.

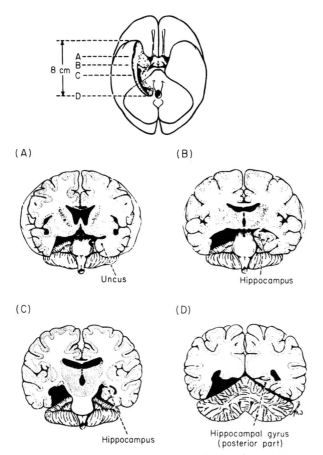

(A)   (B)

Uncus   Hippocampus

(C)   (D)

Hippocampus   Hippocampal gyrus
(posterior part)

Fig. 8-17. Diagrams showing cross-sections of the human brain. The estimated area that was removed from H.M.'s brain is diagrammed. The operation was a bilateral single-stage procedure, but here, for illustrative purposes, one side is shown intact. (From Milner, 1972.)

Global amnesia can result from a variety of other conditions, including head trauma, diencephalic tumor, *Korsakoff psychosis*, electroconvulsive therapy, focal brain wounds, certain viral infections (e.g., *Herpes simplex* encephalitis) and toxemias, and some degenerative diseases (e.g., Alzheimer's disease). Although these amnesias are seldom as severe or as clearly circumscribed as in the patient H.M., several well-studied cases suggest that the general pattern of dysfunction described for H.M. has considerable generality (Starr and Phillips, 1970; Zangwill, 1966).

For example, the patient N.A. was stabbed in basal brain near the midline in 1960. Since that time he has had a marked loss of memory for events that have occurred since the time of his accident. However, he has no other detectable intellectual deficit. Like H.M., N.A. also exhibits insight into his condition "The recording record doesn't let me know whether it's on the good side or the bad side. . . . Sometimes I can remember and sometimes I can't. . . ." (L. R. Squire, unpublished observations; Teuber *et al.*, 1968).

XX. Retrograde Amnesia in Human Patients

The long term memories of patients H.M. and N.A. have recently been tested by objective questionnaire techniques. These techniques ask about persons or events that can be associated with specific past time periods. Thus, one test asks subjects to name photographs of famous persons, and another asks for details about past public events. Memory for events that occurred after the onset of amnesia is markedly impaired (for H.M., after 1953; for N.A., after 1960). Memory for events prior to the injury and surgery is normal. The results of these objective tests are consistent with the impression from informal conversations that these patients have good recall of their early lives. H.M. reportedly has a retrograde amnesia for events that occurred 1 to 3 years before his surgery. N.A. seems to have a patchy retrograde amnesia covering about 6 months prior to his accident.

Results with objective remote memory tests indicate that retrograde amnesia can be extensive in a variety of circumstances. Korsakoff psychosis, electroconvulsive therapy, or diencephalic tumor can cause loss of memory for events that occurred many decades before the onset of amnesia. Remote memory defects thus seem to occur with acute amnesia as caused by electroconvulsive therapy or unusually severe head trauma or with severe conditions, such as Korsakoff psychosis or third ventricle tumors, that can be associated with loss of initiative and some cognitive dysfunction in addition to amnesia (Sanders and Warrington, 1971; Squire, 1975; Ignelzi and Squire, 1976).

As we have emphasized, a large body of animal studies and studies of patients exhibiting brief retrograde amnesia indicate that retrograde amnesia tends to be temporally graded such that the severity of amnesia is inversely proportional to the age of the memory at the time of the treatment or injury. Are extensive memory losses for remote memory also retrograde? This issue cannot be settled easily by informal interviews, since sampling artifacts could easily lead to an impression of a temporal gradient of retrograde amnesia. That is, when an interview covers a period of many months or years, questions about the remote or distant past tend to sample a greater time interval and to be more general than questions about the recent past. One is likely to be asked more questions about what happened yesterday than about what happened on one day 5 years ago.

The temporal organization of remote memory loss has recently been investigated with a new questionnaire technique designed to permit the equivalent sampling of past periods (Squire and Slater, 1975). Subjects were asked to recognize the names of television programs that were broadcast for only one season. Various control procedures suggested that the programs for each time period had been exposed to general audiences about equally, and that the material was learned close to the time that the program was on the air. Normal subjects performed best on questions about programs that were broadcast recently and more poorly on questions about programs that were broadcast many years ago. Following a series of five electroconvulsive shock treatments, depressed psychiatric patients exhibited a selective impairment for material learned 1 to 3 years before treatment but no impairment for material learned 4 to 16 years before treatment (Fig. 8-18) (Squire *et al.*, 1975). The lost memories were recovered within 2 weeks after the last treatment. These results provide strong evidence that remote memories are temporally organized and that the resistance of memory to disruption can gradually increase over a period of years. Similar results have been reported using a public events questionnaire with Korsakoff patients (Seltzer and Benson, 1974).

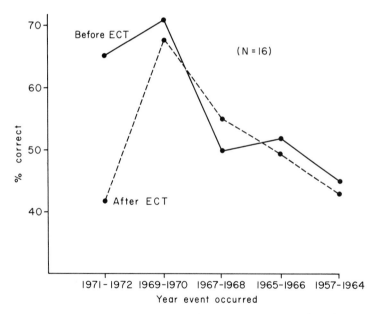

Fig. 8-18. A test of remote memory designed to minimize sampling bias was administered to psychiatric patients who were to receive series of bilateral electroconvulsive therapy (ECT) treatments. The test was given before the first treatment and 1 hour after the fifth treatment. The ECT selectively impaired performance on questions covering the period of 1971–1972. Test was conducted in 1974. (From Squire *et al.*, 1975.)

These findings make several points about the biology of memory. First, since resistance can develop gradually over a period of years, the development of resistance must depend on gradual changes in neural mechanisms underlying "long term" memory. Second, and paradoxically, there must be two distinct consequences of the passage of time after learning. Material in memory becomes resistant to disruption and also becomes gradually more difficult to recall. The neural substrate of memory apparently changes so that resistance to disruption develops as forgetting occurs.

XXI. Neuropathology

Given the multiple causes of amnesias, it is perhaps surprising that the brain regions involved are so delimited. The critical structures appear to be the hippocampal formation and certain midline diencephalic structures. The hippocampus appears to be particularly susceptible to anoxia and cerebral ischemia as well as to the neuropathological changes associated with some diseases (e.g., encephalitis and Alzheimer's disease). Bilateral damage to this structure is sufficient to produce global amnesia.

Extensive documentation of the neuropathology of Korsakoff's disease indicates that the mammillary bodies, dorsal medial nucleus of the thalamus, and the terminal reaches of the fornix are the critical structures associated with amnesia (Victor *et al.*, 1971). These structures appear to be particularly sensitive to the thiamine deficiency that accompanies chronic alcoholism. Other evidence comes from the severe amnesic syndromes associated with intracranial tumors in this region. Tumors pressing bilaterally on the mammillary bodies or tumors that compress the floor and walls of the third ventricle can cause global amnesia (Williams and Pennybacker, 1954; Ignelzi and Squire, 1976).

In instances of unilateral dysfunction, the amnesic syndrome is less severe and follows the familiar asymmetry of hemispheric function with respect to language. This point is best illustrated in the series of epileptic patients sustaining left or right temporal excisions who have been studied by Milner (1974) and her colleagues. Patients with left temporal excisions exhibit a material-specific deficit in the retention of verbal material, or material that can be verbally labeled, but do not exhibit a deficit in the retention of nonverbal material (e.g., faces, spatial relationships, and abstract drawings). Patients with right temporal excisions exhibit the opposite pattern of deficit. The severity of the memory deficit following left or right temporal removal is related to the extent of hippocampal excision (Milner, 1974).

XXII. The Psychological Defect in Amnesia

Since the analysis of amnesia can provide details of normal human information processing and provide clues as to how this processing can go awry, it is of interest to try to specify precisely the nature of amnesia at the psychological level. Probably the most straightforward explanation of the amnesic syndrome is that new information is not adequately consolidated. According to this view, material in short term memory does not reach long term memory. However, it is possible that the amnesia is due, at least in part, to a difference in retrieving information. Specifically, it has been proposed that amnesia may occur because at the time of retrieval many memories are available and interfere with each other for recall (Warrington and Weiskrantz, 1970). Two important facts about amnesia seem consistent with such a theory. First, when amnesics try to recall word lists they frequently recall words from previously learned lists, clearly indicating that some learning has occurred after all. Second, the performance of amnesics is greatly enhanced by providing cues at the time of retest. For example, one group of amnesics exhibited no deficit in retention when they were provided the initial three letters of previously learned words, but were markedly impaired when they had to read each word and indicate whether or not they had seen it previously. These findings with cues mean that amnesics can store some amount of information and weaken explanations suggesting that amnesia is due to a complete failure of the storage process.

A study of the amnesic patient N.A. suggests, however, that prompting does not exert a unique effect on the memory of amnesic patients. Normal subjects can be helped by prompts to an even greater extent. As shown in Fig. 8-19, N.A. recalled fewer details than control subjects about public events that occurred in 1970 to 1975. To test the value of promptings, the 154 details that could be recalled by N.A. and the control group (N = 7) were read to each subject one at a time. As they were read, subjects indicated which details they specifically remembered to be true and which ones they did not remember. The results (Fig. 8-19) indicate that cueing substantially improved recall for both N.A. and for the control group. Considerably more details were recognized by the control group than by N.A. Other tests indicated that these results were not due to differences in response bias.

Taken together, the results of prompting studies agree that amnesic patients have available much more information than they can produce by free recall. In the same way, normal subjects have available much more information than they can produce by free recall. The effects of promptings can be explained by supposing that amnesics store less new information than normals so that they cannot be helped as much by promptings as normals can. The evidence is

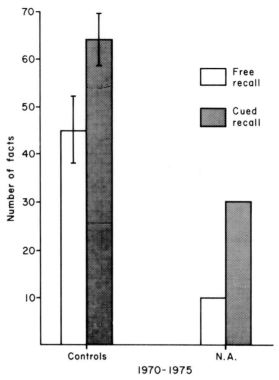

Fig. 8-19. Free recall of details about 26 news events that occurred in 1970–1975 and recognition of these details (cued recall) by N.A. and by normal controls. (From Squire and Slater, 1976.)

therefore consistent with the hypothesis that amnesia reflects reduced capacity to store information in an enduring form.

XXIII. The Organization of Memory in the Brain

The study of amnesia and its neuropathology leads to several general conclusions about the neurology of memory. In the first place, it is obvious that neither the hippocampal region nor the diencephalic midline can be the locus of the structural alterations subserving long term memory, since most old memories are not affected. The hippocampal formation and certain diencephalic structures therefore appear to constitute an essential anatomical substrate for the formation of enduring memories that are stored elsewhere. Since severe anterograde amnesia can occur even though older memory is mostly normal (cases H.M. and N.A.), new learning capacity and remote memory capacity must to some extent depend

8. COMPLEX LEARNING AND MEMORY

on different mechanisms. The neural mechanisms involved in recording information for subsequent long term use must be different from the mechanisms involved in recalling experiences from remote memory.

The facts of retrograde amnesia provide further information about how memory changes with time. A disruption soon after learning can produce permanent loss of memory (brief retrograde amnesia). In the case of brief retrograde amnesia, the disruption apparently erases or rapidly dissipates the storage process that has just been initiated. The storage process continues to change and at some interval after learning, perhaps minutes or hours, it apparently reaches a threshold, since disruption after this interval causes only transient amnesia. In this case, the storage process has become somewhat resistant so that memory can recover when the after effects of the disruption have dissipated. The storage process undergoes still further changes that can continue for years beyond this point, and at a later time disruption may not cause even a temporary loss of memory.

At the present time, the available information about amnesia is largely descriptive, and it is difficult to choose definitively between competing theories. Nevertheless, enough is now known about the amnesic syndrome to establish several general principles about the global structural organization of memory. The facts now available provide many constraints for neurobiological theories of memory.

XXIV. Summary

Learning and memory involve processes by which experiences produce enduring changes that affect behavior. Memory does not consist simply of responses made during learning. We readily learn and perform skills such as language in which responses occur in novel sequence.

Brain lesions can impair learning and retention. However, such studies are difficult to interpret since they only reveal how behavior is altered by the lesion. Lesion studies have not revealed the anatomical locus of memory. Many neurobiological changes are produced by training. Studies of electrical brain activity indicate that training alters EEG activity, hippocampal theta activity, firing patterns of single cells, and shapes of evoked potentials. However, it has not as yet been determined that these correlates of learning are involved in the mechanisms underlying learning and memory. The electrophysiological changes produced by training are signs that neural activity has been altered. Training of laboratory animals also produces neurochemical changes. Findings of several studies suggest that RNA and protein synthesis is increased by training. Further, in goldfish, training appears to alter the pattern of brain protein synthesis. Experiments have investigated the possibility that memory might be transferred from one involvement to another by means of brain extracts. The findings of such studies are highly conflicting. Memory "transfer" by means of brain extracts has not yet been convincingly demonstrated.

Numerous studies have shown that memory can be altered (either enhanced or impaired) by treatments that alter brain activity. In general the treatments are most effective if administered shortly before training or shortly after training. The treatments appear to affect memory by altering the processes involved in the storing or consolidation of recent experiences. Treatments found to be effective in influencing memory include electrical stimulation, stimulant drugs, drugs affecting RNA and protein synthesis, drugs affecting neurotransmitters, and hormones. These findings suggest that normal variations in memory storage may be due to modulating influences of neurotransmitters and hormones.

Studies of memory pathology in humans indicate that memory processes are altered by brain damage. Patients with an amnesic syndrome seem to have a selective loss in the ability to learn new information. Patients given a series of electroconvulsive therapy treatments may have temporary retrograde amnesia for information learned up to several years before the treatment. These findings suggest that memory storage processes may continue to change with time long after an experience.

Overall, research findings indicate that the nervous system is altered in many ways by experiences. Understanding the specific ways that neurobiological changes alter behavior remains an exciting task for future research.

Key Terms

Active avoidance task: A general type of learning task that requires that an animal make a response in order to postpone or prevent punishment.

Active sleep: A phase of sleep characterized by rapid eye movements (REM) and almost complete relaxation of skeletal muscles. The electroencephalogram appears desynchronized and similar to that seen while the subject is awake. Most dreaming occurs during this sleep phase, sometimes called REM sleep.

Amnesia syndrome: A behavioral disorder characterized by impaired memory; there is usually no other detectable intellectual deficit.

Arousal: The excitation or energizing of behavior of an animal or person by either internal or external stimuli.

Desynchronized electroencephalogram: An electroencephalogram characterized by high frequency, low amplitude wave forms.

8. COMPLEX LEARNING AND MEMORY

Electroconvulsive shock (ECS): A brief electrical current applied to the brain that causes convulsions (seizures). When used for therapeutic purposes it is called electroshock therapy.

Electroencephalogram (EEG): The spontaneous electrical activity of the brain as recorded from electrodes placed on the scalp. The electroencephalograph is a machine that amplifies the brain's electrical activity and displays it as waves on chart paper.

Engram: A term for the memory trace or the physical representation of memory in the brain.

Evoked potential: Any transient change in the electrical activity of the brain that is elicited by a discrete stimulus.

Global amnesia: A generalized forgetting of experiences independent of their nature.

Gradient of amnesia: The relationship between memory loss and the time of an amnesia-producing treatment; the degree of memory loss typically declines as the time between training and the amnestic treatment increases.

Inhibitory avoidance task: A behavioral task which requires that animals learn *not* to make a preferred response in order to prevent punishment; often called passive avoidance.

Korsakoff psychosis: Severe mental disturbance, often occurring as a result of alcoholism, that produces severe amnesia. Patients typically have difficulty learning new information as well as recalling past events.

Macromolecule: Any large molecule (e.g., proteins, DNA, RNA).

Memory consolidation: The process which results in the permanent storage of memories; consolidation requires time, but the amount of time that consolidation takes depends on the task.

Retrograde amnesia: A loss of memory for experiences that occurred prior to an injury or experimental treatment.

Theta rhythm: A 4–7 Hz rhythm in electroencephalograms; it is characteristic of the electroencephalographic activity in the hippocampus and appears to be related to some memory storage processes.

Unit activity: The firing pattern of the action potentials of neurons. Single units (one neuron); multiple units (several neurons).

General References

Beach, F. A., Hebb, D. O., Morgan, C. T., and Nissen, H. W., eds. (1960). "The Neuropsychology of Lashley." McGraw-Hill, New York.

Deutsch, J. A., ed. (1973). "The Physiological Basis of Memory." Academic Press, New York.

Gross, C. G., and Ziegler, H. P., eds. (1969). "Readings in Physiological Psychology: Learning and Memory." Harper, New York.

McGaugh, J. L., and Herz, M. J. (1972). "Memory Consolidation." Albion Publ. Co., San Francisco, California.

Rosenzweig, M. R., and Bennett, E. L., eds. (1976). "Neural Mechanisms of Learning and Memory." MIT Press, Cambridge, Massachusetts.

Teyler, T., ed. (1978). "Brain and Learning." Albion Publ. Co., San Francisco, California.

References

Adey, W. R. (1970). Spontaneous electrical brain rhythms accompanying learned responses. In "The Neurosciences: Second Study Program" (F. O. Schmitt, ed.), pp. 225–243. Rockefeller Univ. Press, New York.

Agranoff, B. W. (1967). Agents that block memory. In "The Neurosciences: A Study Program" (G. C. Quarton, T. Melnechuk, and F. O. Schmitt, eds.), pp. 756–764. MIT Press, Cambridge, Massachusetts.

Agranoff, B. W., Davis, R. E., and Brink, J. J. (1966). Chemical studies on memory fixation in the goldfish. Brain Res. 1, 303–309.

Amaral, D. G., and Foss, J. A. (1975). Locus coeruleus lesions and learning. Science 188, 377.

Anlezark, G. M., Crow, T. J., and Greenway, A. P. (1973). Impaired learning and decreased cortical norepinephrine after bilateral locus coeruleus lesions. Science 181, 682–684.

Barondes, A., and Cohen, H. D. (1968). Memory impairment after subcutaneous injection of acetyoxycycloheximide. Science 160, 556–557.

Bloch, V. (1970). Facts and hypotheses concerning memory consolidation. Brain Res. 24, 561–575.

Bloch, V., Hennevin, E., and Leconte, P. (1977). Interaction between post-trial reticular stimulation and subsequent paradoxical sleep in memory consolidation processes. In "Neurobiology of Sleep and Memory" (R. R. Drucker-Colín and J. L. McGaugh, eds.), pp. 255–272. Academic Press, New York.

Bohus, B., and de Wied, D. (1966). Inhibitory and facilitatory effect of two related peptides on extinction of avoidance behavior. Science 153, 318–320.

Byrne, W. L. ed. (1970). "Molecular Approaches to Learning and Memory." Academic Press, New York.

Cerletti, U., and Bini, L. (1938). Electric shock treatment. Boll. Accad. Med. Roma 64, 36.

Cherkin, A. (1969). Kinetics of memory consolidation: Role of amnesic treatment parameters. Proc. Natl. Acad. Sci. U.S.A. 63, 1094–1101.

Corkin, S. (1968). Acquisition of motor skill after bilateral medial temporal-lobe excision. Neuropsychologia 6, 255–265.

Cotman, C., Banker, G., Zornetzer, S., and McGaugh, J. L. (1971). Electroshock effects on brain protein synthesis: Relation to brain seizures and retrograde amnesia. Science 173, 454–456.

Denti, A., McGaugh, J. L., Landfield, P., and Shinkman, P. (1970). Facilitation of learning with posttrial stimulation of the reticular formation. Physiol. Behav. 5, 659–662.

Destrade, C., Soumireu-Mourat, B., and Cardo, B. (1973). Effects of posttrial hippocampal stimulation on acquisition of operant behavior in the mouse. Behav. Bio. 8, 713–724.

de Wied, D. (1974). Pituitary–adrenal system hormones and behavior. In "The Neurosciences Third Study Program" (F. O. Schmitt and F. G. Worden, eds.), pp. 653–666. MIT Press, Cambridge, Massachusetts.

de Wied, D., Bohus, B., Van Ree, J. M., and Urban, I. (1978). Behavioral and electrophysiological effects of peptides related to lipotropin (B-LPH). J. Pharmacol. Exp. Therapeut. 204, 570.

Drachman, D. A., and Arbit, J. (1966). Memory and the hippocampal complex. II. Is memory a multiple process? Arch. Neurol. 15, 52–61.

Duncan, C. P. (1949). The retroactive effect of electroshock on learning. J. Comp. Physiol. Psychol. 42, 32–44.

Dunn, A., Giuditta, A., Wilson, J. E., and Glassman, E. (1974). The effect of electroshock on brain

RNA and protein synthesis and its possible relationship to behavioral effects. *In* "Psychobiology of Convulsive Therapy" (M. Fink *et al.*, pp. 185–197. Holt, New York.

Entingh, D., Damstra-Entingh, T., Dunn, A., Wilson, J. E., and Glassman, E. (1974). *Brain Res.* **70**, 131–138.

Fink, M., Kety, S. S., McGaugh, J. L., and Williams, T. A., eds. (1974). "Psychobiology of Convulsive Therapy," Holt, New York.

Flood, J. F., Bennett, E. L., Orme, A. E., and Rosenzweig, M. R. (1975a). Effects of protein synthesis inhibition on memory for active avoidance training. *Physiol. Behav.* **14**, 177–184.

Flood, J. F., Bennett, E. L., Orme, A. E., and Rosenzweig, M. R. (1975b). The relation of memory formation to controlled amounts of brain protein synthesis. *Physiol. Behav.* **15**, 97–102.

Flood, J. F., Jarvik, M. E., Bennett, E. L., and Orme, A. E. (1976). Effects of ACTH peptide fragments on memory formation. *Pharmacol. Biochem. Behav.* **5**, Suppl. 1, 41–51.

Fulginiti, S., and Orsingher, O. A. (1971). Effects of learning, amphetamine and nicotine on the level and synthesis of brain noradrenaline in rats. *Arch. Int. Pharmacodyn. Ther.* **190**, 291–298.

Fulginiti, S., Molina, V. A., and Orsingher, O. A. (1976). Inhibition of catecholamine biosynthesis and memory processes. *Psychopharmacology* **51**, 65–69.

Fuster, J. M. (1973). Unit activity in prefrontal cortex during delayed-response performance: Neuronal correlates of transient memory. *J. Neurophysiol.* **36**, 61–78.

Gabriel, M., Saltwick, S. E., and Miller, J. D. (1975). Conditioning and reversal of short-latency multiple-unit responses in the rabbit medial geniculate nucleus. *Science* **189**, 1108–1109.

Gallagher, M., and Kapp, B. S. (1978). Opiate administration into the amygdala: Effects on memory processes. *Neurosci. Abstr. (Soc. Neurosci.)* **4**, 258.

Gerard, R. W. (1949). Physiology and psychiatry. *Am. J. Psychiatry* **106**, 161–173.

Glassman, E. (1974). Macromolecules and behavior: A commentary. *In* "The Neurosciences: Third Study Program" (F. O. Schmitt and F. G. Worden, eds.), pp. 667–677. MIT Press, Cambridge, Massachusetts.

Glickman, S. E. (1961). Preservative neural processes and consolidation of the memory trace. *Psychol. Bull.* **58**, 218–233.

Gold, P. E., and McGaugh, J. L. (1975). A single-trace, two-process view of memory storage processes. *In* "Short-Term Memory" (D. Deutsch and J. A. Deutsch, eds.), pp. 355–378. Academic Press, New York.

Gold, P. E., and McGaugh, J. L. (1977). Hormones and memory. *In* "Neuropeptide Influences on the Brain and Behavior" (L. H. Miller, C. A. Sandman, and A. J. Kastin, eds.), pp. 127–143. Raven, New York.

Gold, P. E., and van Buskirk, R. B. (1975). Facilitation of time-dependent memory processes with posttrial epinephrine injections. *Behav. Biol.* **13**, 145–153.

Gold, P. E., and van Buskirk, R. B. (1976). Effects of posttrial hormone injections of memory processes. *Horm. Behav.* **7**, 509–517.

Gold, P. E., Bueno, O. F., and McGaugh, J. L. (1973a). Training and task-related differences in retrograde amnesia thresholds determined by direct electrical stimulation of the cortex in rats. *Physiol. Behav.* **11**, 57–63.

Gold, P. E., Macri, J., and McGaugh, J. L. (1973b). Retrograde amnesia gradients: Effects of direct cortical stimulation. *Science* **179**, 1343–1345.

Gold, P. E., Hankins, L., Edwards, R. M., Chester, J., and McGaugh, J. L. (1975). Memory interference and facilitation with posttrial amygdala stimulation: Effect on memory varies with foot shock level. *Brain Res.* **86**, 509–513.

Gold, P. E., van Buskirk, R., and Haycock, J. W. (1977). Effects of posttraining epinephrine injections on retention of avoidance training in mice. *Behav. Biol.* **20**, 197–204.

Grastyán, E., Lissák, K., Madarász, I., and Donhoffer, H. (1959). Hippocampal electrical activity during the development of conditioned reflexes. *Electroencephalagr. Clin. Neurophysiol.* **11**, 409–430.

Hartmann, E., and Stern, W. C. (1972). Desynchronized sleep deprivation: Learning deficit and its reversal by increased catecholamines. *Physiol. Behav.* **8**, 585–587.

Hartry, A. L., Keith-Lee, P., and Morton, W. D. (1964). Planaria: Memory transfer through cannibalism re-examined. *Science* **146**, 274–275.

Haycock, J. W., van Buskirk, R., and McGaugh, J. L. (1977). Effects of catecholaminergic drugs upon memory storage processes in mice. *Behav. Biol.* **20**, 281–310.

Horn, G., Rose, S. P. R., and Bateson, P. P. G. (1973). Experience and plasticity in the central nervous system. *Science* **181**, 506–514.

Hyden, H., and Egyhazi, E. (1962). Nuclear RNA changes in nerve cells during learning experiment in rats. *Proc. Natl. Acad. Sci. U.S.A.* **48**, 1366–1372.

Ignelzi, R., and Squire, L. R. (1976). Recovery from anterograde and retrograde amnesia following percutaneous drainage of a cystic craniopharyngioma. *J. Neurol., Neurosurg. Psychiatry* **39**, 1231–1235.

Isaacson, R. L. (1976). Experimental brain lesions and memory. *In* "Neural Mechanisms of Learning and Memory" (M. R. Rosenzweig and E. L. Bennett, eds.), pp. 521–543. MIT Press, Cambridge, Massachusetts.

John, E. R. (1967). "Mechanisms of Memory." Academic Press, New York.

John, E. R. (1972). Statistical versus switchboard theories of memory. *Science* **177**, 850–864.

Kesner, R. P. (1973). A neural system analysis of memory storage and retrieval. *Psychol. Bull.* **80**, 177–203.

Kesner, R. P., and Wilburn, M. W. (1974). A review of electrical stimulation of the brain in the context of learning and retention. *Behav. Biol.* **10**, 259–293.

Kety, S. S. (1970). The biogenic amines in the central nervous system: There possible roles in arousal, emotion, and learning. *In* "The Neurosciences: Second Study Program" (F. O. Schmitt, ed.), pp. 324–336. Rockefeller Univ. Press, New York.

Kety, S. S. (1972). Brain catecholamines, affective states, and memory. *In* "The Chemistry of Mood, Motivation, and Memory" (J. L. McGaugh, ed.), pp. 65–80. Plenum, New York.

Kobiler, D., and Allweis, C. (1974). The prevention of long term memory formation by 2,6-diaminopurine. *Pharmacol. Biochem. Behav.* **2**, 9–17.

Landfield, P. W. (1976). Synchronous EEG rhythms: Their nature and their possible functions in memory, information transmission and behavior. *In* "Molecular and Functional Neurobiology" (W. H. Gispen, ed.), pp. 389–424. Elsevier, Amsterdam.

Jensen, R. A., Martinez, Jr., J. L., Messing, R. B., Spiehler, V. R., Vasquez, B. J., Soumireu-Mourat, B., Liang, K. C., and McGaugh, J. L. (1978). Morphine and naloxone alter memory in rats. *Neurosci. Abstr. (Soc. Neurosci.)* **4**, 260.

Landfield, P. W. (1977). Different effects of posttrial driving or blocking of the theta rhythm on avoidance learning in rats. *Physiol. Behav.* **18**, 439–445.

Landfield, P. W., and McGaugh, J. L. (1972). Effects of electroconvulsive shock and brain stimulation on EEG cortical theta rhythms in rats. *Behav. Biol.* **7**, 271–278.

Landfield, P. W., Tusa, R., and McGaugh, J. L. (1973). Effects of posttrial hippocampal stimulation on memory storage and EEG activity. *Behav. Biol.* **8**, 485–505.

Lashley, K. S. (1950). In search of the engram. *Symp. Soc. Exp. Biol.* **4**, 454–482.

Lewis, D. J. (1969). Sources of experimental amnesia. *Psychol. Rev.* **76**, 461–472.

Lewy, A. J., and Seiden, L. S. (1972). Operant behavior changes norepinephrine metabolism in rat brain. *Science* **175**, 454–455.

McConnell, J. V. (1962). Memory transfer through cannibalism in planarians. *J. Neuropsychiatry* **3**, 42–48.

McDougall, W. (1901). Facilitative and disruptive effects of strychnine sulphate on maze learning. *Psych. Rep.* **8**, 99–104.

McGaugh, J. L. (1967). Analysis of memory transfer and enhancement. *Proc. Am. Philos. Soc.* **111**, 347–351.

McGaugh, J. L. (1968). Drug facilitation of memory and learning. *In* "Psychopharmacology: A Review of Progress" (D. H. Efron, ed.), PHS. Publ. No. 1836, pp. 891–904. US Gov. Printing Office, Washington, D.C.

McGaugh, J. L. (1973). Drug facilitation of learning and memory. *Annu. Rev. Pharmacol.* **13**, 229–241.

McGaugh, J. L. (1974). Electroconvulsive shock: Effects on learning and memory in animals. *In* "Psychobiology of Convulsive Therapy" (M. Fink *et al.*, eds.), pp. 279–283. Holt, New York.

McGaugh, J. L., and Gold, P. E. (1976). Modulation of memory by electrical stimulation of the brain. *In* "Neural Mechanisms of Learning and Memory" (M. R. Rosenzweig and E. L. Bennett, eds.), pp. 549–560. MIT Press, Cambridge, Massachusetts.

McGaugh, J. L., and Herz, M. J. (1972). "Memory Consolidation." Albion Publ. Co., San Francisco, California.

McGaugh, J. L., Gold, P. E., van Buskirk, R. B., and Haycock, J. W. (1975). Modulating influences of hormones and catecholamines on memory storage processes. *Prog. Brain Res.* **42**, 151–162.

Mah, C. J., and Albert, D. J. (1973). Electroconvulsive shock-induced retrograde amnesia: An analysis of the variation in the length of the amnesia gradient. *Behav. Biol.* **9**, 517–540.

Matthies, H., Lossner, B., Ott, T., Phole, W., and Rauca, C. (1973). The intraneuronal regulation of neural connectivity. *Proc. Int. Congr. Pharmacol.* 5th, 1972 Vol. 4, pp. 29–38.

Meligeni, J. A., Ledergerber, S. A., and McGaugh, J. L. (1975). Reversal of diethyldithiocarbamate induced amnesia by norepinephrine. *Neurosci. Abstr. (Soc. Neurosci.)* **1**, 514.

Meligeni, J. A., Ledergerber, S. A., and McGaugh, J. L. (1978). Norepinephrine attenuation of amnesia produced by diethyldithiocarbamate. *Brain Res.* **149**, 155–164.

Messing, R. B., Jensen, R. A., Martinez, Jr., J. L., Spiehler, V. R., Vasquez, B. J., Soumireu-Mourat, B., Liang, K. C. and McGaugh, J. L. (1978). Naloxone enhancement and morphine impairment of memory. Submitted for publication.

Milner, B. (1970). Memory and the medial temporal regions of the brain. *In* "Biology of Memory" (K. H. Pribram and D. E. Broadbent, eds.), pp. 29–50. Academic Press, New York.

Milner, B. (1972). Disorders of learning and memory after temporal lobe lesions in man. *Clin. Neurosurg.* **29**, 421–446.

Milner, B. (1974). Hemispheric specialization: Scope and limits. *In* "The Neurosciences: Third Study Program" (F. O. Schmitt and F. G. Worden, eds.), pp. 75–89. MIT Press, Cambridge, Massachusetts.

Mueller, G. E., and Pilzecker, A. (1900). Experimentelle Beitrage zur Lehre vom Gedachtniss. *Z. Psychol.* **1**, 1–288.

Olds, J. (1973). Brain mechanisms of reinforcement learning. *In* "Pleasure, Reward, Preference: Their Nature, Determinants, and Role in Behavior" (L. D. E. Berlyne and K. B. Masden, eds.), Academic Press, pp. 35–63.

Olds, J., Disterhoft, J. F., Segal, M., Lornblith, C., and Hirsch, R. (1972). Learning centers of rat brain mapped by measuring latencies of conditioned unit responses. *J. Neurophysiol.* **35**, 202–219.

Oleson, T. D., Ashe, J. H., and Weinberger, N. M. (1975). Modification of auditory and somatosensory activity during pupillary conditioning in the paralyzed cat. *J. Neurophysiol.* **38**, 1114–1139.

Randt, C. T., Quartermain, D., Goldstein, M., and Anagnosti, B. (1971). Norepinephrine biosynthesis inhibition: Effects on memory in mice. *Science* **172**, 498–499.

Rosenzweig, M. R., Bennett, E. L., and Diamond, M. C. (1972). Brain changes in response to experience. *Sci. Am.* **226**, 22–39.

Russell, W. R., and Nathan, P. W. (1946). Traumatic amnesia. *Brain* **69**, 280–300.

Sanders, H. I., and Warrington, E. K. (1971). Memory for remote events in amnesic patients. *Brain* **94**, 661–668.

Scoville, W. B., and Milner, B. (1957). Loss of recent memory after bilateral hippocampal lesions. *J. Neurol., Neurosurg. Psychiatry* **20**, 11–21.

Seltzer, B., and Benson, D. F. (1974). The temporal pattern of retrograde amnesia in Korsakoff's disease. *Neurology* **24**, 527–530.

Shashoua, V. E. (1968). RNA changes in goldfish brain during learning. *Nature (London)* **217**, 238–240.

Shashoua, V. E. (1967). Identification of specific changes in the pattern of brain protein synthesis after training. *Science* **193**, 1264–1266.

Shinkman, P. G., Bruce, C. J., and Pfingst, B. E. (1974). Operant conditioning of single-unit response patterns in visual cortex. *Science* **184**, 1194–1196.

Squire, L. R. (1975). A stable impairment in remote memory following electroconvulsive therapy. *Neuropsychologia* **13**, 51–58.

Squire, L. R., and Slater, P. C. (1975). Forgetting in very long-term memory as assessed by an improved questionnaire technique. *J. Exp. Psychol., Hum. Learn. Memory* **104**, 50–54.

Squire, L. R., and Slater, P. C. (1976). Remote memory in chronic anterograde amnesia. *Behav. Biol.* **20**, 398–403.

Squire, L. R., Slater, P. C., and Chace, P. M. (1975). Retrograde amnesia: Temporal gradient in very long-term memory following electroconvulsive therapy. *Science* **187**, 77–79.

Starr, A., and Phillips, L. (1970). Verbal and motor memory in the amnestic syndrome. *Neuropsychologia* **8**, 75–88.

Stein, L., Belluzzi, J. D., and Wise, C. D. (1975). Memory enhancement by central administration of norepinephrine. *Brain Res.* **84**, 329–335.

Teuber, H.-L., Milner, B., and Vaughan, H. G. (1968). Persistent anterograde amnesia after stab wound of the basal brain. *Neuropsychologia* **6**, 267–282.

Thompson, R. (1958). The effects of intracranial stimulation on memory in cats. *J. Comp. Physiol. Psychol.* **51**, 421–426.

Thompson, R., and Thorne, B. M. (1973). Brainstem reticular formation lesions: Amnestic effects on learned habituation in the rat. *Physiol. Psychol.* **1**, 61–70.

Thompson, R. F., Patterson, M. M., and Teyler, T. J. (1972). Neurophysiology of learning. *Annu. Rev. Psychol.* **23**, 73–104.

Thut, P. D., Hruska, R. E., Kelter, A., Mizne, J., and Lindell, T. J. (1973). The effect of α-amanitin on passive and active avoidance acquisition in mice. *Psychopharmacologia* **30**, 355–368.

Ungar, G. (1970). Chemical transfer of learned information. *In* "Molecular Approaches to Learning and Memory" (W. L. Byrne, ed.), pp. 179–187. Academic Press, New York.

van Wimersma Greidanus, Tj. B., Bohus, B., and de Wied, D. (1975). The role of vasopressin in memory processes. *Prog. Brain Res.* **42**, 135–141.

van Wimersma Greidanus, Tj. B., Dogterom, J., and de Wied, D. (1975). Intraventricular administration of anti-vasopressin serum inhibits memory consolidation in rats. *Life Sci.* **16**, 637–644.

Victor, H., Adams, R. D., and Collins, G. H. (1971). "The Wernicke Korsakoff Syndrome" (A clinical and pathological study of 245 patients, 82 with post-mortem examinations). Davis, Philadelphia, Pennsylvania.

Warrington, E. K., and Weiskrantz, L. (1974). The effect of prior learning on subsequent retention in amnesic patients. *Neuropsychologia* **12**, 419–428.

Wetzel, W., Ott, T., and Matthies, H. (1977). Post-training hippocampal rhythmic slow activity ("theta") elicited by septal stimulation improves memory consolidation in rats. *Behav. Biol.* **21**, 32–40.

Williams, M., and Pennybacker, J. (1954). Memory disturbances in third ventrical tumours. *J. Neurol., Neurosurg. Psychiatry* **17**, 115–123.

Zangwill, O. L. (1966). The amnesic syndrome. *In* "Amnesia" (C. W. M. Whitty and O. L. Zangwill, eds.), pp. 77–91. Butterworth, London.

Zornetzer, S. R. (1974). Retrograde amnesia and brain seizures in rodents: Electrophysiological and neuroanatomical analyses. *In* "The Psychobiology of Convulsive Therapy" (M. D. Fink *et al.*, eds.), pp. 99–128. Holt, New York.

Zornetzer, S. F., and Gold, M. S. (1975). Effects of locus coeruleus lesions on the susceptibility of labile memory to disruption. *Neurosci. Abst. (Soc. Neurosci.)* **1**, 821.

8. COMPLEX LEARNING AND MEMORY

9

Hearing, Tasting and Smelling, and Feeling

I.   Introduction

Our sensory systems provide us with the ability to hear, feel, taste, smell and see. Through these systems we monitor the world about us. In this chapter we shall focus our discussion on the auditory system but shall also discuss the basic properties of the somesthetic, olfactory and gustatory systems. In Chapter 10 we shall describe in detail the operation of the visual system.

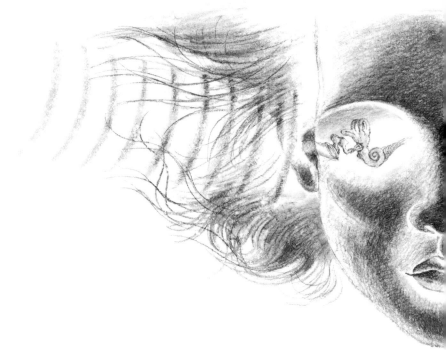

II. Auditory System

Sounds are so much an integral part of our daily lives that we seldom think about them. Without them, however, our lives would be like one continuous silent movie. Conversations with others would lack the subtlety of tone change; music and other spoken art forms—embellishments of man's culture that enrich his environment—would be lost to us. We want to know about sounds. We study them, interpret them and offer prompt, and hopefully, appropriate reactions.

Our ability to perceive sounds and translate them into the language of the brain is the task of the brain's auditory system. It is no simple task, as we are able to discriminate about 400,000 sounds and call into action perhaps as many responses. The simple phonics of a word may be translated into an idea, be committed to memory for future action or produce movement in a part of our body, for example. Hearing is linked closely with speech and provides the basis for man's exceptional ability to communicate. With hearing, instruction is received rapidly and the feeling and thought of others can be perceived readily.

The auditory system not only discriminates sound frequencies and intensities, but it also locates sounds in space. Auditory senses may be highly trained and refined, as in musicians and the blind. Blind people develop their auditory senses to an extraordinary degree—sensing sounds unnoticed by others and

350   **9. HEARING, TASTING AND SMELLING, AND FEELING**

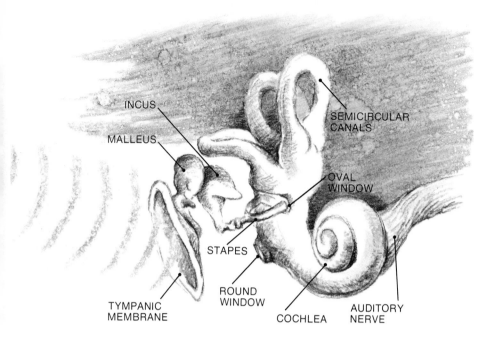

INCUS

SEMICIRCULAR
CANALS

MALLEUS

OVAL
WINDOW

STAPES

ROUND
WINDOW

TYMPANIC
MEMBRANE

COCHLEA

AUDITORY
NERVE

THE AUDITORY SYSTEM

Fig. 9-1. Location and general structure of the receptor system for hearing. A channel from the outer ear leads to the eardrum, or tympanic membrane. The eardrum and ossicles are collectively called the middle ear. The coiled-like structure, the cochlea, is contacted by one of the ossicles (the stapes). The auditory nerve (VIII nerve) projects to the brain.

deriving conclusions beyond expectation. For example, Erasmus Darwin (grandfather of Charles Darwin) wrote, "the late blind Justice Fielding walked for the first time into my room where he once visited me and after speaking a few words said, 'This room is about 22 feet long, 18 wide and 12 high', all of which he guessed with great accuracy." (Stevens *et al.*, 1965).

The auditory system is a masterpiece of engineering. It begins with an incredibly miniaturized receptor system which converts sound into electrical impulses (Fig. 9-1). The receptor system is only about 1 in.³ in overall size. No commercial product can match the size, sensitivity and versatility of the auditory system. Construction of an equivalent receptor system alone from stereo components, for example, would require a wide range frequency analyzer, an amplifier and a device to convert mechanical signals into coded electrical pulses free of distortion. We have no idea, of course, how to construct an equivalent of the auditory regions of the brain.

In Section II,A we shall describe the basic operation of the auditory system and the characteristics of sound perception. We shall then use this information to discuss applications of basic findings toward the analysis and treatment of hearing disorders in people.

A. Basic Organization of the Auditory System

The auditory system is a complex multilayered processing unit which begins with the ear and cochlea (Fig. 9-2). There sounds are transformed into electrical impulses which travel in the auditory nerve to the brain. The auditory nerve projects to the cochlear nuclei in the hindbrain or medulla which in turn connect to the superior olivary nuclei. Signals from the *superior olivary nuclei* pass to two main brain centers, the inferior colliculus in the midbrain and *medial geniculate* body in the thalamus. The main pathway to the auditory cortex is via the medial geniculate. At each station signals are processed and distributed not only to the auditory system but to other systems as well.

A surprising amount of processing takes place directly at the cochlea. The cochlea analyzes the sounds for frequency and intensity and sends coded messages on these parameters into the brain. Brain centers are concerned with the analysis of other aspects of sound. Sound localization in space, for example, is largely delegated to hindbrain and midbrain auditory centers. The role of the auditory cortex is rather mysterious at present. Its loss causes insignificant deficits in hearing and, although it seems involved in certain aspects of sound localization, this also does not appear to be its major task. The auditory cortex is concerned with the decoding of complex acoustic signals used in communication. In a sense the auditory cortex decides about the significance of sounds and when they should have access to the motor system.

In Chapter 2 we noted that processing in the auditory system is carried out publicly with great divergence of information. Unfortunately, as with most public operations, they are complex and not well understood. Consequently a detailed description of integration through the auditory centers of the brain will not be undertaken. However, we shall examine the way the brain integrates signals in the visual and motor systems where the basic processes are better understood. The same principles apply over and over again throughout the brain, and so we will reserve the story for the visual system where it can be told best.

In this chapter we shall focus our discussion on the receptor processes at the cochlea. This has a number of advantages. For one thing, it is very well understood. For another, it provides an excellent illustration of the way a receptor translates a stimulus into brain language. Indeed processing at the cochlea is a prime example of an important concept in sensory systems: much of the initial processing occurs right at the receptor. In fact, as we shall demonstrate, the limits

9. HEARING, TASTING AND SMELLING, AND FEELING

and qualities of the transduction process largely determine our perception of sounds. In order to understand the operation of the receptor processes, we need to understand the physical properties of sound.

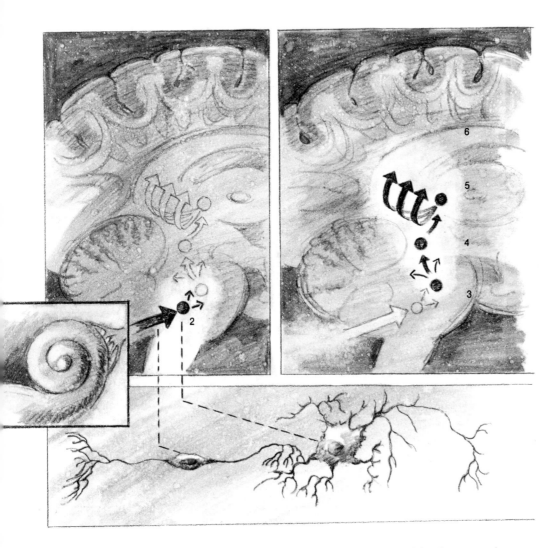

Fig. 9-2. General layout of the auditory system. Sounds are collected by the ear and transduced by the cochlea (1) into action potentials. Primary sensory neurons whose cell bodies are located in the spiral ganglia carry the news to secondary sensory neurons in the cochlear nuclei (2). The cochlear nuclei pass on the information primarily to the superior olivary nuclei (3) which in turn connect to the inferior colliculus (4) then to the medial geniculate (5) and finally to the auditory cortex (6).

1. NATURE OF SOUND. What is sound? Sound consists of pressure variations in the air. All sounds must begin with a mechanical disturbance. An instrument makes sound by causing pressure waves to travel through the surrounding medium. For example, when a tuning fork is tapped, pressure waves are generated by the oscillations of the tuning fork that travel through the surrounding air. The force applied to the air particles causes them to accelerate first in one direction and then the other. Molecules bumping into each other create a compression; molecules bouncing apart create a rarefaction. Sounds are compressions and rarefactions traveling through the air in the form of pressure waves.

The physical properties of this pressure wave determine the nature of the sound. The interval of time elapsing between two successive peak compression phases is called the "period" of the pressure wave. The reciprocal of the period is the frequency of the pressure wave, i.e., the number of complete cycles that occurs per second. Thus, _frequency_ is specified in cycles per second, designated as _hertz_ or Hz, and the period is specified in units of time. For example, if a tuning fork moves from its initial position to its extreme in one direction, then to the extreme in the other direction and returns to its starting position in 1 millisecond (msec), the period of the pressure wave generated by the movement of the tuning fork is 1 msec and the frequency is 1000 cycles per second or 1000 Hz. One thousand cycles of the pressure wave would be generated each second in the surrounding air. Table 9-1 gives a few examples of the sound frequencies people and animals use to communicate. We hear sounds over the frequency range of 15 to 20,000 Hz. Our greatest sensitivity is to sounds between 1000 and 4000 Hz, which is within the range of much of our everyday experiences. Speech sounds, for example, are usually in the range of 200–800 Hz.

Table 9-1 Examples of the frequencies used in communication[a]

Species	Behavior	Principal frequency range (Hz)
Man	Conversation	200–800
	Lowest note of a bass singer	100
	Upper range of a soprano	1000
Dog[a]	Growling	452
	Barking	452–904
Cat[a]	Meowing	760–1520
	Purring	200–400
Pig[a]	Grunting	269–320
Elephant[a]	Trumpeting	640
Whale	—	256,000

[a] From Tembrock (1963).

9. HEARING, TASTING AND SMELLING, AND FEELING

A wave also has an amplitude which specifies the greatness of its pressure variation. The larger the amplitude of the wave at a particular frequency, the louder it sounds. Scientists have worked out a means to define sound intensity in relative terms. Sound *intensity* is measured in <u>*decibels*</u> (deci for tenths and bel for Alexander Graham Bell). The *decibel* (dB) is defined as the log of the ratio of two sound pressure amplitudes

$$\text{number of dB} = 10 \log P_1/P_0$$

where P_1 is the pressure of the louder sound. An increase of 10 dB occurs when P_1 is 10 times greater than P_0, whatever value P_0 may be. Since decibels are the ratio of two sound intensities, it is meaningless unless the comparison sound is known. The reference sound pressure, P_0, is taken to be 0.0002 dynes/cm², approximately the human threshold at 1000 Hz. We can get a better feel for the magnitude of this threshold value when we relate this pressure change to atmospheric pressure. Atmospheric pressure (1 atm) is about 10^6 dynes/cm². Accordingly, a human can detect pressure variations in a sound wave as small as 2 parts in 10^{10} (or 10 billion)! The loudest sound the ear can tolerate has a pressure variation of about 0.004 atm. A normal conversation is about 60 dB which is 10^6 times more intense than the sound threshold level. The ambient sound level in a quiet room is about 40 dB, whereas a rock band is about 130 dB. At 4000 Hz (the sound of a whistling tea kettle), we can discriminate a 40 dB signal from a 40.5 dB signal.

2. RECEPTOR PROCESSES. Inside the ear is a microtransduction device made from membranes and bones (see Fig. 9-1). Briefly previewing the process, the outer ear collects sounds and channels them through the ear canal where they make the eardrum vibrate. These vibrations are picked up by a set of levers made of three small bones (the ossicles) and relayed to the oval window of the cochlea. Vibrations of this window set up waves in the thin watery fluid of the cochlea. Receptors (hair cells) are responsible for the main event—transducing mechanical to electrical energy. They detect, by movement of minute hairs bristling from their free surfaces, the vibrations of the fluid. When they bend they generate an electrical potential whose magnitude is coded as action potentials in the auditory nerve.

3. CHANNELING OF SOUND TO THE EARDRUM. The ear (often specialized as in the fennec fox, see Fig. 9-3) collects sound which passes down a canal to the *eardrum* or the *tympanic membrane*. The canal acts as a resonator (as a pipe organ) so that sound vibrations at the eardrum have a higher pressure than at the external ear. Between 2000 and 5500 Hz, for example, the sound is amplified twofold in this canal. It is the tympanic membrane that captures sound waves and converts them into mechanical vibrations. This membrane is thin and taut and

vibrates when sound pressure waves hit it, just as the diaphragm of a telephone mouthpiece vibrates when you talk into it.

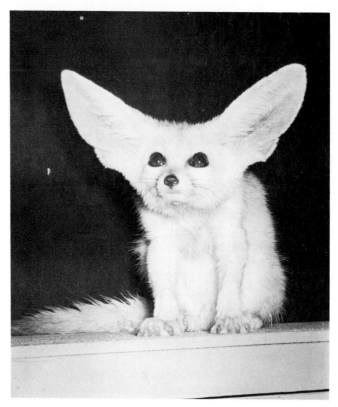

Fig. 9-3. Fennec fox. (Courtesy of the Zoological Society of San Diego, Inc.)

4. TRANSMISSION OF SOUND FROM EARDRUM TO THE COCHLEA. The rear of the eardrum is connected to a set of bones (malleus, incus, and stapes) collectively called the *ossicular system* (Fig. 9-4). These bones form a set of lever arms and work together to amplify mechanical movements and transfer them to the entrance of the cochlea, called the *oval window*. The handle of the *malleus* is attached to the very center of the eardrum. The malleus in turn connects to the *incus*, which connects to the *stapes*. These bones are the smallest in the body— the stapes is about the size of a grain of rice. The ossicular system is constructed so that the inner end of the lever moves through a shorter distance than the outer end. The sound pressure is amplified about two times.

5. IMPEDANCE MATCHING BY THE OSSICULAR SYSTEM. The purpose of the ossicular system is to achieve the transfer of air pressure waves to the liquid of the cochlea without loss. A simple air–water interface reflects 99.9% of the sound

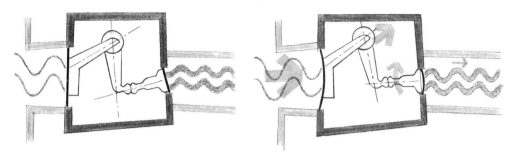

Fig. 9-4. The ossicular system. The diagram shows the transfer of sound energy through the middle ear. Sound waves, shown as wavy lines, displace the eardrum causing the ossicles to move and hammer on the oval window of the cochlea.

back into the air so an interface device is needed. Since fluid has greater inertia than air, more pressure is needed to cause the same degree of vibration in a fluid. In man, the eardrum is about 22 times larger in area than the stapes contacting the oval window of the cochlea (70 mm² compared to 3.2 mm²). The reduction in size applies approximately 22 times more pressure at the oval window of the cochlea than is applied to the surface of the eardrum. This, plus the lever arm amplification, provides *impedance matching* so that sound waves above 500 Hz are transferred at 99.9% transmission efficiency from the ear to the cochlea. That is real efficiency!

Thus, three distinctive processes combine to magnify weak air vibrations. The resonance of the ear canal doubles the vibrations, the mechanical advantage of the ossicles again double it, and the reductive arrangement of the eardrum and oval window provides another 22-fold increase. Overall, then, a sound pressure wave may be amplified 88 times before it sets up a wave in the cochlear fluid.

6.   OPERATION OF THE COCHLEA.   At the cochlea, pressure waves are converted to electrical impulses. The *cochlea* is a coiled tube (shown unrolled in Fig. 9-5) which consists of two main compartments (scala media and scala tympani) separated by a thin membrane, the *basilar membrane*. The entire cochlea is filled with fluid.

We owe our modern understanding of the operation of the cochlea to a communications engineer, George von Békésy (1960), who was awarded the Nobel prize for his work. Békésy wondered how much better the quality of the human ear is than any telephone system. So he watched the events inside the cochlea. He excised the cochlea and bored a tiny hole into it exposing a part of the basilar membrane. This procedure was incredibly delicate. To achieve it, he fashioned some of his own microtools such as scissors with blades a few thousandths of an inch long! The cochlear fluid was withdrawn and replaced with a saline solution of coal and powdered aluminum. By reflecting flashes of intense light off the suspen-

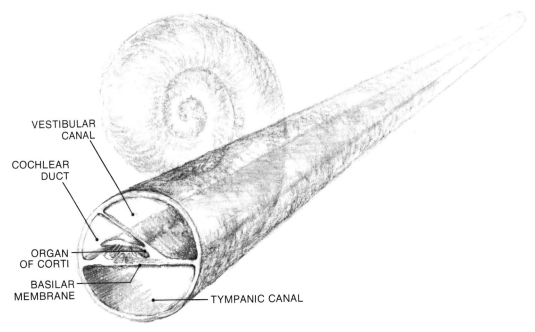

VESTIBULAR
CANAL

COCHLEAR
DUCT

ORGAN
OF CORTI

BASILAR
MEMBRANE

TYMPANIC CANAL

sion, Békésy directly watched the events within the cochlea. He found that sound creates an undulation—a *traveling wave*—along the basilar membrane. As illustrated in Fig. 9-6, the action of the basilar membrane is like a wave rolling back and forth dissipating on each side of a main peak. The basilar membrane is very thin and easily moved. Its movements are similar to the whip action of a rope secured at both ends.

The threshold value for the amplitude of vibration of the basilar membrane is remarkable. A movement somewhat less than the diameter of a hydrogen atom (0.02 Å or 2×10^{-10}cm) can produce an auditory sensation (Rhode, 1971). This is so minute that the random motion of air molecules can be detected under ideal listening conditions. In ordinary conversations the basilar membrane is displaced about 2 Å. Maximum displacements of the membrane approximate the amplitude of motion of air molecules.

Up to this point we have described how vibrations of the stapes on the oval window set up traveling waves in the cochlea and resonate the basilar membrane. How is the frequency of the sound waves analyzed?

The cochlea as a frequency analyzer.   As early as the late 1800s a prominent physician, physicist and physiologist, Hermann Ludwig Ferdinand von Helmholz, proposed that each sound wave of a distinct frequency induced vibrations of a particular part of the basilar membrane. He postulated quite correctly that the cochlea is constructed so that high frequency waves are focused near the

358   9. HEARING, TASTING AND SMELLING, AND FEELING

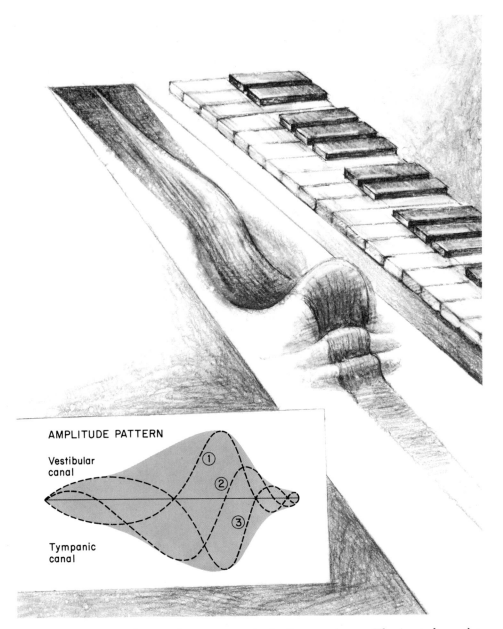

Fig. 9-6. Diagram of a traveling wave on the basilar membrane. The inset shows the basilar membrane position at three successive time periods (1,2,3). The basilar membrane vibrates between the vestibular and tympanic canals. At each frequency the traveling wave forms a maxima at a different part of the basilar membrane. As the keyboard symbolizes, sounds of particular frequencies are precisely and serially ordered on the basilar membrane. High frequency tones generate traveling waves near the base and low frequency ones near the apex.

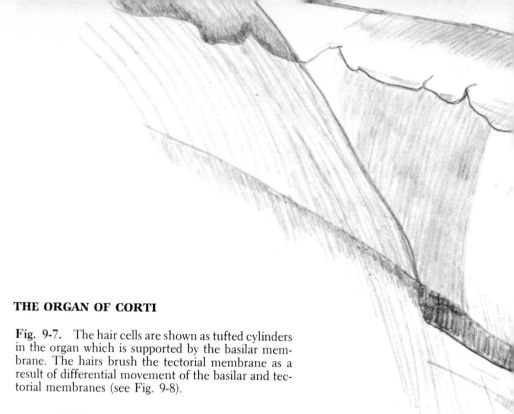

THE ORGAN OF CORTI

Fig. 9-7. The hair cells are shown as tufted cylinders in the organ which is supported by the basilar membrane. The hairs brush the tectorial membrane as a result of differential movement of the basilar and tectorial membranes (see Fig. 9-8).

stapes (the _base_), while low frequency waves oscillate maximally nearer the _apex_ of the cochlea.

The features of the cochlea which provide frequency localization are a result of the resonance qualities of the cochlea. The factors are complex, but they are primarily the result of the conical shape of the cochlea and the differential stiffness of the basilar membrane at each end. Sound vibrations enter the oval window and pass through the basilar membrane causing a bulge in the _round window_. High frequency sounds resonate at the base because the vibrations are rapid and do not have time to pass all the way to the apex and back again to the round window; they damp out a short distance from the stapes. Low frequency waves have longer periods so that these localize near the apex of the cochlea. Also, the membrane is stiffer at the base. This stiffer quality at the base favors high frequency vibrations, whereas the looser quality at the apex favors low frequency vibrations, much as a thin glass vibrates to high frequency sounds and heavier glass to low frequency sounds.

Thus particular frequencies perturb particular parts of the basilar membrane. This eventually activates particular fibers of the VIII nerve, and their activity signifies a particular frequency of sound to the brain. This type of coding is an example of the _place theory_ of coding (see Chapter 4). When a particular fiber responds, it informs the brain of the location along the basilar membrane of the active hair cells.

9. HEARING, TASTING AND SMELLING, AND FEELING

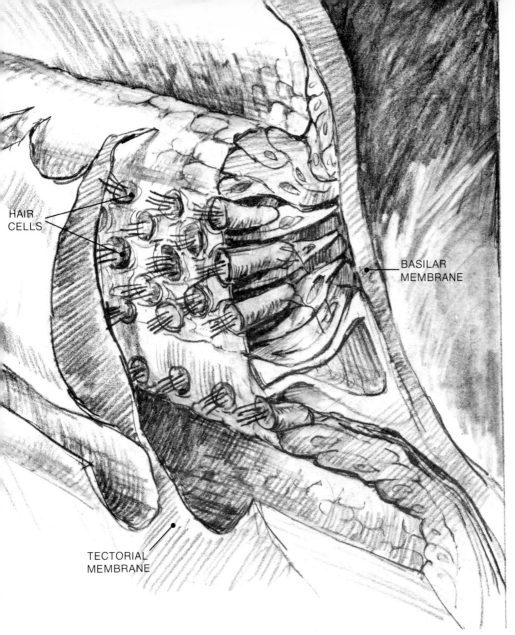

HAIR CELLS

BASILAR MEMBRANE

TECTORIAL MEMBRANE

7. TRANSDUCTION FROM MECHANICAL TO ELECTRICAL SIGNALS. On the surface of the basilar membrane is the *organ of Corti* which contains a series of mechanically sensitive cells, the *hair cells* (Fig. 9-7). It is within the organ of Corti that the actual transduction of mechanical events into neural events occurs. The organ of Corti is supported by the basilar membrane and extends continuously throughout the length of the membrane. Hair cells are arranged in well-defined rows. Each hair cell has approximately 120 *hairs* or stereocilia embedded in the tectorial membrane. The transduction process occurs because the hairs of the

hair cells bend or are displaced as a result of the basilar membrane movements.

The basilar membrane vibrates between the vestibular canal and the tympanic canal according to the frequency and intensity of the stapes movement. This causes the hairs of the hair cells to bend radially in one direction and then the other. The movement of the hairs occurs because there is a relative movement of the tectorial and basilar membranes owing to the fact that the tectorial and basilar membranes are "hinged" at different points (Fig. 9-8). The movement of the hairs from this shearing action of the membranes somehow stimulates the hair cell and results in the excitation of the afferent terminals contacting the base of the cell. The actual mechanisms for the transformation of the mechanical movements to electrical pulses are unknown at present. The primary sensory neurons, those sentinels of the nervous system, relay the news from the hair cells to the *cochlear nuclei* in the brain.

8.   THE PROBLEM OF CODING FOR SOUND FREQUENCY AND INTENSITY.   Auditory nerve fibers have the capacity to code sound stimuli by both temporal and spatial parameters. In describing the operation of the cochlea, we emphasized that the auditory system can code for sound frequency by *place coding* (see Chapter 4). Particular frequencies resonate particular sections of the basilar mem-

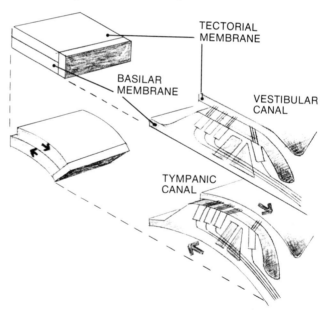

Fig. 9-8.   Diagram of a section of the organ of Corti to show the mechanical movements which stimulate the hair cells. In the top two schematics, the tectorial membrane (upper plane) and the basilar membrane (lower plane) supporting the hair cells are in register. As shown in the bottom two schematics, when a sound wave bends the basilar membrane it causes the two membranes to move differentially, shearing the hairs and stimulating the hair cells.

9. HEARING, TASTING AND SMELLING, AND FEELING

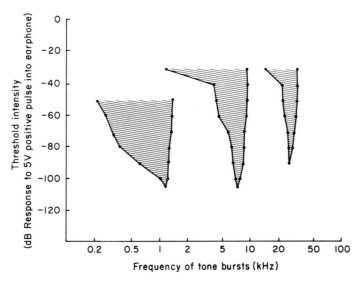

Fig. 9-9. Representative "tuning curves," for three different auditory nerve fibers. Each curve is obtained by setting intensity of tone bursts and measuring frequency range for which spike responses are obtained. The hatched areas within the V-shaped curves show the effective stimulus parameters. Abscissa of lowest point of each curve is defined as characteristic frequency. (Data from Kiang *et al.*, 1962.)

brane and activate select auditory nerve fibers. Auditory nerve fibers have highly selective tuning curves. A *tuning curve* shows the range of frequencies to which an auditory neuron responds at different intensities of sound. The tuning curve is V-shaped showing that a fiber will respond to some minimum intensity of sound only over a narrow range of frequencies (see Fig. 9-9). This suggests that a fiber is tuned to respond to some particular frequency called its "best" frequency.

Auditory fibers terminate in the brain in a well-organized *tonotopic map*. Thus, for example, a particular part of an auditory area is selective to particular frequencies. This tonotopic organization is preserved to a high degree throughout the auditory pathway. It is particularly well displayed in the auditory cortex (see Fig. 9-10).

The discharge patterns of auditory fibers tend to have a constant relationship to the sound stimulus. As shown in Fig. 9-11, action potentials cluster about discrete intervals which usually are phase-locked to the frequency of the sound. This is an example of *phase coding* (a type of temporal code, see Chapter 4) and is specifically referred to as phase-lock coding in the auditory system because the firing of the auditory nerve is locked to the stimulus frequency (Rose *et al.*, 1967). The response of individual cells, however, is not simply a frequency interval in which the cell discharges on every cycle. An action potential may or may not

II. AUDITORY SYSTEM 363

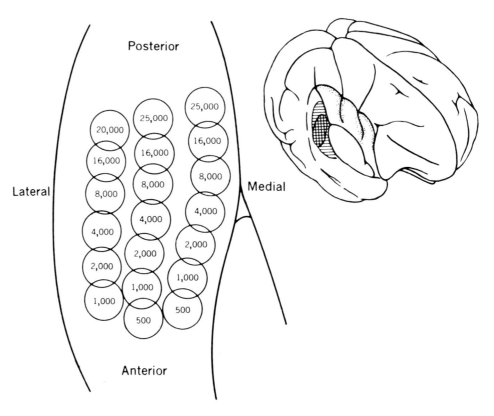

Fig. 9-10. Tonotopic organization of the auditory cortex in the monkey. (*Right*) The location of the auditory cortex. (*Left*) Enlarged drawing showing the representation of frequency within the auditory cortex. (From Mountcastle, 1974.)

occur within each cycle, but when it does it is at a consistent point in time during the cycle. The behavior of individual cells is probabilistic.

What is the extent to which place and temporal codes are used? Phase-lock coding will not occur at frequencies above about 4000 Hz. Thus, for all higher frequencies place coding is the best candidate code for sound frequency. Temporal coding is also probably used at low frequencies below 4000 Hz. A phenomenon called *periodicity pitch* underscores the importance of temporal codes in the detection of sound frequency. In periodicity pitch a high frequency sound, for example, 5000 Hz, is interrupted periodically at a low frequency. Place coding theory would predict that the tone should be recognized as 5000 Hz irregardless of the low frequency intervals because the 5000 Hz portion of the basilar membrane is active. It turns out, though, that the tone is perceived as being at the interruption frequency. Thus the temporal aspects of cell discharge are more important than the place of origin of the fibers for this particular pitch sensation. Temporal

9. HEARING, TASTING AND SMELLING, AND FEELING

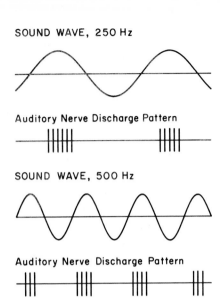

SOUND WAVE, 250 Hz

Auditory Nerve Discharge Pattern

SOUND WAVE, 500 Hz

Auditory Nerve Discharge Pattern

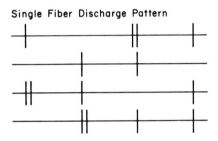

Single Fiber Discharge Pattern

Fig. 9-11. Illustration of temporal coding in the auditory neurons. The discharge pattern is phase-locked to the frequency of the sound wave. The phase-locked pattern at 250 Hz has a larger interval then that at 500 Hz. The afferent discharge pattern in the auditory nerve is made up of the probabilistic firing of single fibers (see lower panel).

coding is implicated in the judgement of the interval of a periodic stimuli below 3000 Hz. Also discrimination of pulses with no fundamental frequency may employ a temporal code. Finally, as will be described in Section II,C, judgments based on timing are especially important in localizing sound.

The general rule is that for high frequencies a place code must be used, while for low or middle range frequencies both place and temporal codes provide information on frequencies. Sound intensity, which also must be coded, is signaled by the discharge rate of cells and the number of cells firing. Sound intensity appears to be coded by a simple frequency code based on the number of action potentials per unit time (see Fig. 9-12).

In summary the receptor system functions as follows. Sounds are collected in a canal in the outer ear and set up vibrations of the ear drum (or tympanic membrane). These vibrations are passed through the middle ear via the ossicular system to the inner ear and the cochlea. The ossicular system consists of three tiny bones which amplify the vibrations of the eardrum and transmit them to the

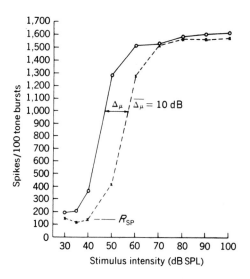

Fig. 9-12. Graph of the rate of cell discharge for a primary afferent unit as a function of sound intensity (solid line). Tone bursts (40 msec) were given at the units best frequency. The dashed line illustrates the effect of efferent stimulation. The same sound stimulus was preceded by 32 shocks of the crossed olivocochlear bundle at 400/second. Tone burst began at 10 msec after the last shock. Intensity scale gives peak-to-peak sound pressure level (SPL). R_{SP}, rate of spontaneous unit activity; $\Delta\mu$, shift of intensity function by efferent stimulation. (From Wiederhold, 1970.)

cochlea. The cochlea, a delicate spiral-shaped structure, converts the sounds to nerve impulses. It is filled with a watery fluid and has a thin membrane, the basilar membrane, stretched from wall to wall along its length. Tiny mechanoreceptor cells, hair cells, are in contact with the basilar membrane. Sound waves cause movements of the cochlear fluid, which cause the basilar membrane to resonate. These membrane movements deflect hair cells and when so disturbed they generate potentials. Axons of primary sensory neurons carry the news via the auditory nerve to auditory centers in the brain. The signals are place and temporally coded.

9. EFFERENT CONTROL OF AUDITION. Besides ascending tracts, the auditory pathway includes descending or *efferent* tracts. Two of these project into the cochlea, the crossed and uncrossed olivocochlear fibers. In the cat there are about 600 such efferent fibers which innervate the hair cells.

Electrical stimulation of the crossed olivocochlear bundle has the effect of decreasing the impulse activity of primary afferent fibers. As shown in Fig. 9-12, the intensity function shifts to the right so that for a given sound intensity above 40 dB the firing rate is decreased the equivalent of a 10 dB reduction in sound intensity. Above 70 dB the primary afferent response saturates and efferent stimulation has no effect.

The function of the crossed olivocochlear bundle may be to raise the threshold of auditory nerve fibers so that they are insensitive to background noise but still responsive to sounds of moderate or high intensity (Dewson, 1967). That is, the system may act to improve the extraction of signal in noise at the cochlea. In one study, moderately intense clicks were masked by the addition of high-rate low-intensity clicks so that the intense clicks could be barely discriminated over

9. HEARING, TASTING AND SMELLING, AND FEELING

the background. When the olivocochlear bundle was stimulated, the intense clicks were unmasked and more readily discriminated (Niedler and Niedler, 1970). Thus efferent activation reduces the background signal in the manner shown in Fig. 9-12, but has relatively little affect on the moderately intense clicks. Behavioral data in support of a role of efferents in improving signal to noise ratios came from a study of rhesus monkeys before and after surgical section of the crossed olivocochlear bundles. The discrimination of vowel sounds of moderate intensity in the presence of background noise was poorer in animals following section of the bundles (Dewson, 1968). Clearly efferent fibers can play an important role in audition. As will be discussed in Section V, efferent fibers can also serve as an aid for protecting the middle ear from excessively loud sounds.

B.   The Perception of Sounds: Pitch and Loudness

What is the relationship between the sensation of a sound and its physical properties? The discipline that studies the response of sense organs to physical stimuli is called _psychophysics_. Psychophysicists try to define and understand the precise rules by which sensations change with stimuli. This science is not limited to hearing but includes all senses—sight, touch, smell, etc. It is the science of peoples' and animals' reactions to the stimuli of pitch and loudness, brightness and hue, taste, smell and touch.

How does pitch vary with frequency? The _pitch_ of a sound is defined as the subjective sensation to sounds of different frequencies. Pitch is a quality measure. It would seem at first glance that over the range of audible sounds doubling the frequency would double the pitch. But the mind has its own influence. In 1937, psychophysicists at Harvard began a series of experiments showing that the relationship is not one to one.

A simple experiment was done to reveal the relationship. An adjustable electronic piano with 20 keys and 20 knobs was built so that turning a knob varied the tone produced by the corresponding key (Fig. 9-13). Five keys were selected from the piano. The _lowest key_ was tuned to a particular frequency, for example, 200 Hz, and the highest to 6500 Hz. Subjects were asked to tune three other keys so as to produce four equal intervals. Intensity was maintained constant. All ten subjects were readily able to do so and each produced a scale in close agreement with the others (Table 9-2).

This procedure was repeated over the other frequency ranges and a comprehensive scale of subjective units was obtained. In generating a scale it is sufficient to have a zero point and then define a unit size. The limit of lower sensation was found to be about 40 Hz so this was called 0. The sensation at a frequency of 1000 Hz (and an intensity of 60 dB) was defined as 1000 and the units

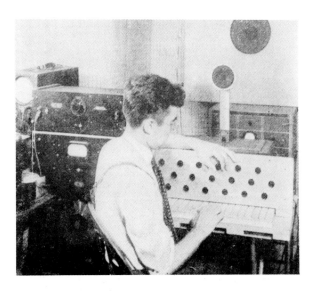

Fig. 9-13. Apparatus used to examine the relation of pitch to frequency (From Stevens and Volkmann, 1940. Copyright by Karl M. Dallenbach, by permission of University of Illinois Press.)

Table 9-2 Frequencies selected by ten subjects asked to fractionate sounds 200–6500 Hz at an intensity of 60 dB into four increments of equal pitch[a]

Frequency division selected, mean (Hz)		867	2022	3393
Percent average deviation among subjects		±6.4	±9.6	±6.6
Frequency increments (Hz)	667 (200–867)	1155 (867–2022)	1371 (2022–3393)	2567 (3393–6500)

[a] In order to carry this out, three intermediate frequencies must be selected. Note that the frequency increments are not arithmetically equal but that they become larger at higher frequencies. (From Stevens and Volkman, 1940.)

were given the name _mels_ (after melody). Thus by definition a sound with a frequency of 1000 Hz and an intensity of 60 dB has a pitch of 1000 mels. The relationship between frequency and pitch shown plotted in Fig. 9-14 is nearly logarithmic. This relationship confirmed the feeling often expressed by musicians that the higher musical octaves sound "larger" than the lower ones.

How good are we at detecting changes in frequency? Sensitivity can be measured by successively presenting pairs of tones to an observer and asking him to decide whether they have the same pitch. At 1000 Hz we can discriminate between two tones when they differ by only 3 Hz. The _just noticeable difference_ (jnd) varies with the frequency. The integral of jnds over frequency results in a curve which virtually coincides with the mel scale (Fig. 9-14). Thus, we can conclude that frequency jnds have equal subjective magnitudes. It was found that 1 jnd is larger than 1 mel (1 jnd equals 4.5 mels).

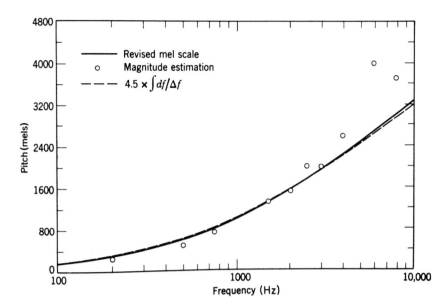

Fig. 9-14. Pitch as a function of sound frequency (solid line) for a loudness level of 60 dB using the mel scale. The dashed line gives the integration of jnds (just noticeable differences) as a function of frequency. The curves virtually coincide showing that frequency jnds have equal psychological magnitudes. (From Zwislocki, 1965.)

The similarity between pitch and the frequency jnd is striking and suggests they have a common basis. The key factor is the distribution of neurons along the basilar membrane. The hair cells are innervated by about 30,000 primary sensory neurons which have their cell bodies in the spiral ganglion (see Fig. 9-1). The density of neurons decreases toward the apex of the cochlea in such a way that intervals of equal sensation represent divisions of an equal number of neurons along the membrane: each unit change on the mel scale corresponds to the movement of the vibration pattern along the membrane by 12 neurons. One mel cannot be detected, since it is less than 1 jnd. The frequency jnd represents the activation of a mere 54 neurons (12 × 4.5), a distance of only about 0.05 mm along the basilar membrane! It is remarkable the CNS can register significant differences with so few cells.

The relationship between neuron distribution, pitch and the jnd is very significant. It means that these psychophysical properties are a result of inherent physical properties of the system, rather than entirely a result of learning or some other psychological construct.

Now that we have examined frequency, let us examine the other physical attribute of sound. How does _loudness_ change with sound intensity? In 1860 a physicist and philosopher, Gustav Theodor Fechner, published one of the most influential books in modern science—Elements of Psychophysics. This book gave birth to the science of psychophysics and has influenced research and thought on this problem for generations. It stimulated a major effort to study human subjects in the laboratory and led to new insights into our lives. The findings of such studies have been used by accoustical engineers for improved communication systems, by architects for buildings and by commercial artists for display, to name just a few applications.

Fechner proposed that the sensation of a stimulus is related to the stimulus by a simple mathematical law: sensation grows as the logarithm of the stimulus. This simple, yet bold, statement aroused many psychologists and inspired others. For a century afterward Fechner's law was a cornerstone of psychological theory.

A simple and direct means of experimentally scaling the magnitude of sensations is called *magnitude estimation*. An observer is presented with two tones and asked to tell how much louder one is than the other. After a series of different sensations are scored by a number of volunteers, the data is analyzed and the relationship determined.

The results of magnitude estimation showed that loudness increases as the cube root of intensity. That is,

$$J = kI^{0.3}$$

where J is the judgment of loudness in sones, k is a constant and I is the intensity of the sound in decibels. One *sone* (from the Latin word, sound) is defined as the loudness of a 1000 Hz tone at an intensity of 40 dB.

The general form of the equation above—known as the power law—gave stable values of sensation magnitudes not only for sound but also for all other sensory systems! Each system has its own exponent. For example, it is 0.33 for the visual sense of brightness and 3.5 for the apparent strength of an electric current applied to the fingers. These power relationships are most remarkable and are a fundamental feature of transduction–perception processes. Unfortunately, however, their exact physiological basis is unknown for any system, but the correlation continues to entice many. The answers will no doubt finally come from further basic research on the functional properties of each system.

The loudness of a sound depends not only on its intensity but also on other tones present at the same time. Obviously, a quiet sound against a loud background is inaudible. Sounds mask other sounds.

Masking affects the perception of sounds in everyday life. It even affects the perception of music. Intense low frequency instruments mask the sounds of weak higher frequency instruments. Musicians take this into account and use it to produce the desired overall effect. Masking is a significant factor when listening to a recorded piece in the home. When a record is played at home, the intensity is usually less than when recorded. Consequently, the masking patterns are changed, and the piece is not heard as in the original performance.

Masking has been studied experimentally by presenting two tones (a masker and test tone) to an observer. In a typical experiment, the masker tone is set at some fixed intensity and frequency. The test tone is set at some fixed frequency and the intensity varied until the test tone is just audible in the presence of the masker. This procedure is repeated for different values of the frequency of the test tone and a masking curve is generated. A typical result is shown in Fig. 9-15. This curve shows exactly how intense the test tone must be at different frequencies in order to detect it in the presence of the masker (1200 Hz) given at different intensities. The data shows that the masker has relatively little effect on tones below its own frequency (1200 Hz), but that tones above this frequency are more difficult to hear in the presence of the masker.

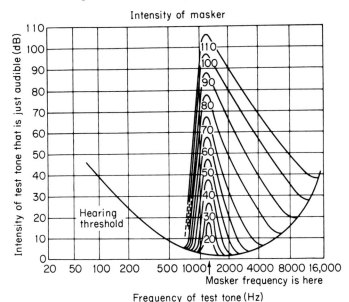

Fig. 9-15. Masking effect of a sound of 1200 Hz on the intensity of test tones that are just audible. The family of curves shows the effect on threshold when the intensity of the masker is increased from 20 to 110 dB. The 1200 Hz tone has little effect on threshold tones of lower frequency than the masker but obscures higher frequency tones particularly at high sound intensities. (From Zwicker and Scharf, 1965. Copyright by the American Psychological Association. Reprinted by permission.)

The masking of tones above the masking frequency is a direct result of the vibration patterns of the basilar membrane. High frequency sounds are quite strictly localized, whereas low frequency sounds tend to produce activity over much of the membrane. Thus, when a tone is weak and only slightly higher in frequency than the masker, no part of the activity pattern can make itself felt above the pattern of the masker.

C. The Perception of Auditory Space

The intensity and frequency of sounds is only a part of our perception of sound. As important is our ability to locate sounds in space. We need to determine where sounds come from in order to behave normally. How are sounds located in space? One way, used in the 1800s, is shown in Fig. 9-16.

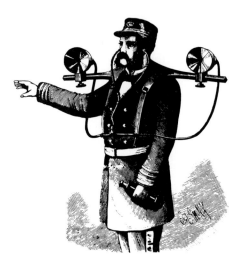

Fig. 9-16. A device used in the late 1800's by ship captains to increase their binaural capabilities and determine with precision the direction of a whistle in the thickest fog. Sounds are located in space because the time relationships and intensity of sounds are different in each ear when the sound is not straight ahead. The device aids in sound localization because the two ear trumpets are more widely spaced and collect more sound than human ears. (From Culver Pictures.)

In 1934 two scientists at Harvard performed an experiment which clearly showed our capacity to locate sounds in space. One person sat in a swivel chair from which extended a 12 ft boom with a loudspeaker at its outer end. Tones ranging up to 10,000 Hz were emitted from the speaker and the observer who was blindfolded was asked to locate the tones as the boom swung through a circle. It was found that low frequency tones (less than 1000 Hz) and high frequency tones (greater than 4000 Hz) could be accurately localized. Errors were most common between 2000 and 4000 Hz.

The nervous system uses information on the exact time and intensity differences at which tones arrive at the two ears to locate sound sources. When sound is straight ahead, it reaches both ears at the same time and intensity so it is perceived as straight ahead. If the head is turned only 3°, a difference is detected. Sounds arrive first at the ear closest to the sources. They also arrive there with the greatest intensity, since the distant ear is partly shielded by the head (Fig. 9-17).

It can be calculated that a sound 3° to the right arrives at the right ear 30 μsec (or 300 millionths of a second) before it arrives at the left. It seems incredible that such a slight difference in time can be discriminated. The reason is that for sounds of relatively long duration the slight delay produces a significant *phase difference* in the signal between the two ears (Fig. 9-18). This is sufficient to allow

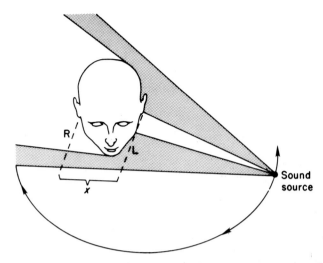

Fig. 9-17. The cues used to locate sound in space are the time and intensity at which sounds reach the two ears. The right ear receives sound slightly after the left because sound travels the extra distance (x). Also the sound intensity reaching the right ear is reduced because the head partly shields the sound. As the tone moves each placement provides unique time–intensity information. The nervous system uses this information to compute the location of the sound.

discrimination of sounds only a few degrees off center at low frequencies. However, it is not sufficient at high frequencies, since the time delay between ears is longer than that required for the sound to complete a cycle. High frequency sounds can complete multiple cycles at certain angles, and there is no way to discriminate whether there has been a single cycle or multiple cycles (Fig. 9-18).

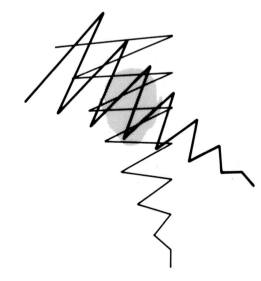

Fig. 9-18. Phase differences are not unique to each angle at high frequencies. The wave can complete more than one cycle in the time necessary to travel between the ears. Each wave is at a crest and trough when it reaches the ears so that the ears receive identical information even though the sound source is located at different positions. At high frequencies sound localization also depends on information on sound intensity.

Thus the sound could originate from any number of places. Another clue is needed. At high frequencies, sound intensity differences between the two ears are used primarily in locating sound sources.

Thus at low frequencies sounds are localized by time or phase differences, whereas at high frequencies intensity differences are also used. The switch occurs in the frequency range of about 2000 Hz. In this range the two mechanisms overlap completely so the error rate is greatest in locating a source.

The brain collects the appropriate information from each ear and computes the location of the sound. It is believed that one key interaction takes place at a small nucleus in the brain stem called the superior olivary nucleus. Here impulses from each ear converge (Fig. 9-19). One theory states that excitatory signals from one ear interact with inhibitory ones from the other ear. A difference signal is generated, characteristic of the particular sound source. This signal is then passed onto higher centers where an appropriate "sense" of the source of sound is created.

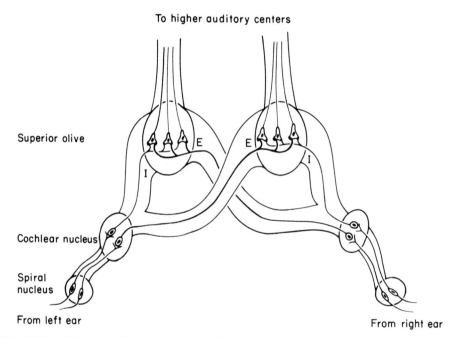

Fig. 9-19. Schematic illustrating a possible mechanism for the localization of sound. E, excitatory signals; I, inhibitory signals. (From van Bergeijk, 1962.)

Such differential cues in the output of the superior olive are passed to higher centers such as the inferior colliculus. According to one theory, the spatial field for sound is mapped onto a spatially distributed population of neurons. That is, sound space is encoded in brain space as a three-dimensional neural map. The

9. HEARING, TASTING AND SMELLING, AND FEELING

data are particularly striking for the owl brain (Knudsen and Konishi, 1978). Auditory units were recorded in a functionally specialized region of the midbrain which is homologous to the mammalian inferior colliculus. With the owl's head in a fixed position, an auditory stimulus was moved around in three-dimensional space while the firing patterns of single cells were examined. It was found that a cell responded only when a sound was at a particular location in space, and the responses shifted location sequentially as the sound source was continuously moved in elevation. By moving the electrode and sound source about systematically, a map of the area was made. It was found that the responsive units in the brain were organized as a three-dimensional space map of auditory space (Fig. 9-20). The cells responded equally well to clicks, bursts or just noise, and sound intensity was unimportant. Moreover, this map depended on the relative input from both ears, since blocking sound to one ear changed the map. Thus the units were clearly organized according to the *location* of the sound source.

We can then conclude that as a result of the integrative activity of auditory circuitry, it appears that certain cells know where a sound is located in the environment. Presumably they pass this information on to other brain areas so that a "sense" of auditory space is created. At present the mechanisms which underlie this perception process are a complete mystery.

The integrative mechanisms for the localization of sound in space are interesting in their own right because they are an example of a time–space transform in the CNS. The auditory system is so wired that it can convert a differential time signal into a spatial neural map. This contrasts to the type of transform for most other sensory processes. In the somatosensory system, for example, place on the body surface is registered as place in the brain. Recall that in Chapter 2 we noted that position of a tactile stimulus on the body is registered as a sensory homunculus in the sensory cortex.

Binaural interactions enrich our sound experiences. Stereophonic recording is an excellent example of how binaural interactions provide richness and authenticity to sounds. Stereophonic sound reproductions create the illusion of a live performance because they give aural spaciousness and richness to sounds, making them freer of masking than monaural reproductions. There is an interesting story which nicely illustrates how real a listening experience can be because of our binaural capacities.

On May 7, 1941 at a meeting of the Acoustical Society of America, Bell Telephone Laboratories demonstrated the first stereophonic playback system (Stevens *et al.*, 1965). The Rochester Symphony Orchestra was featured. Behind the musicians stood three loudspeakers, part of the playback system. Just as the concert was about to begin, the curtain fell. Behind the curtain the orchestra played through the first movement of a symphony. Then a stereophonic recording of the second movement went out over the speakers. The system played

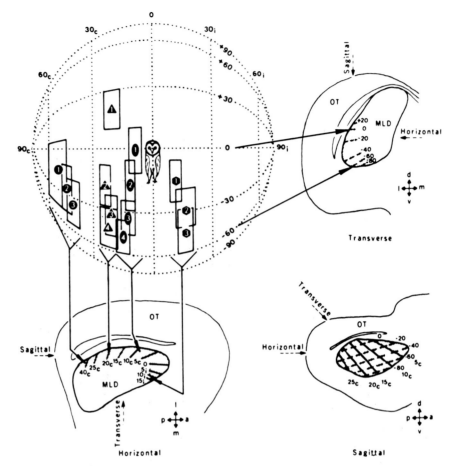

Fig. 9-20. Organization of auditory space in the mesencephalus lateralis dorsalis nucleus (MLD) of the owl. The diagram in the upper left depicts the world of auditory space surrounding the owl. On the right and below the globe are transverse, horizontal and saggital sections of the owl brain. The arrows show meridians in auditory space where a sound activates brain cells at particular places in the nucleus. Isoelevation contours are represented by dashed lines in the transverse and saggital sections; isoazimuth contours are shown as solid lines in the horizontal and saggital sections. OT, optic tectum (From Knudsen and Konishi, 1978. Copyright by the American Association for the Advancement of Science.)

frequencies from 26 to 14,000 Hz and reproduced sounds at intensities up to 120 dB. After the symphony, a representative of the Bell team revealed that half the music was live and half recorded and, to test the quality of the playback system, the audience was to judge which part was live and which was recorded. Half the audience voted one way and half the other—the system was a success. It is clear that given the same music, room and orchestra, music can be recorded and replayed with very close fidelity to the original. Our binaural capacities bless us with the richness of sounds.

The nature of information processing at higher centers and its conversion into an appropriate motor output is not well understood at the present time. Moreover, auditory signals are most frequently considered along with others. The computation is exquisitely sophisticated. Imagine for a moment you are walking along a busy street. You hear a bang. What's that—danger or just an insignificant noise? In a split second you turn and look. Your brain compares and considers all visual and auditory reports, recalls similar past experiences and delivers a decision on the sound's meaning. You may just continue on your way or you may do something differently, but you will probably remember the experience, at least for a time.

In other situations sound information may not be dealt with at a conscious level. Sounds reach our ears but are simply discarded, suppressed by higher order commands of the brain as we concentrate on more significant matters. Not hearing can be just as essential as hearing.

D. Disorders of Hearing

Hearing may be taken for granted until it is lost or until we have difficulty with it. What are the types of problems which arise? What are the diseases that afflict the auditory system and what can be done to correct them? One of the purposes of gaining an understanding of the basic operation of the auditory system, or any sensory system for that matter, is to provide the information necessary to treat disorders of the system. The auditory provides a suitable system to illustrate the active interplay between basic research and clinical medicine. We shall, therefore, describe in moderate detail some of the disorders of hearing and how they are diagnosed and treated. We shall also describe some of the natural defenses that the receptor system has against insult.

Extremely loud sound is dangerous to the ear. Prolonged exposure to sounds of 160 dB or greater, for example, usually causes total deafness. The pressure created is so great it ruptures the eardrum or damages the hair cells.

For moderately loud sounds, the ear has built-in protection devices which we have experienced at one time or another. Several hours of exposure to very loud music or a jack hammer, for example, produce temporary hearing deficits which are a result of our protection mechanism at work. Repeated exposures to such sounds, however, causes permanent hair cell loss.

The movement of the ossicular chain, and therefore the amount of energy transferred to the cochlea, is modulated continuously by the action of the *middle ear muscles*. The middle ear muscles are controlled by efferents from the brain. Contraction of the middle ear muscles, called the *middle ear reflex*, can be evoked by intense stimulation of either ear. The middle ear muscles act to stiffen the middle ear transmission system (eardrum and ossicles) moving the resonance to a higher frequency. This decreases transmission for lower frequencies. Since the amplitude of motion is greatest for lower frequencies, the middle ear reflex is an effective protective mechanism. The effect of the middle ear reflex may be very large, producing an attenuation of cochlear excitation by as much as 20 dB at 1000 Hz. As the latency of the attenuation is on the order of 40 to 160 msec from the beginning of the sound, however, its effect is useful only for damping relatively sustained loud signals and would not be effective, for example, in the case of a gun shot.

It is likely, however, that the middle ear muscles serve in capacities other than as a protection mechanism. It has been found that the middle ear muscles are directly activated during vocalization. This suggests a further and perhaps more important role. These muscles may serve to minimize sensitivity to sounds that we ourselves produce (Carmel and Starr, 1963). The role of the middle ear muscles in audition is another instance illustrating the important concept of efferent modulation of sensory input.

Another safety mechanism protects the ear against excessive pressure changes. Increased pressure, created by the descent of an airplane or racing down a mountain road at 50 mph, for example, pushes on the eardrum and can break it unless the pressure of the air space behind the drum is equalized. The *eustachian tube*—named after its discoverer, Bartolommeo Eustachio—connects the air-filled passage behind the ear drum with the mouth cavity and serves as a passage to equalizing pressure. Sudden pressures changes are felt in the ears until swallowing or yawning opens the eustachian tubes sufficiently to equalize the air pressure. Colds and allergies often plug the tube and hinder our ability to correct for air pressure changes.

E. Alterations in Hearing from Lesions of Auditory Structures in Humans

Studies of the neuroanatomical and neurophysiological bases of audition provide insights into the mechanisms underlying clinical disorders of hearing. Table 9-3 is an outline of the site of pathology, the prominent perceptual deficits, and the methods used to document the various causes of such deficits.

The patient provides important clues when describing the hearing loss that guide the clinician in finding the site of pathology, its mechanism, and the opportunities for therapeutic success. Accurate diagnosis requires the skillful interpretation of a case history, a physical examination and laboratory tests, and the following brief outline should not be used as a guide for self-diagnosis.

Is the hearing loss an isolated complaint or are there accompanying problems

Table 9-3 Hearing loss: pathology, prominent perceptual deficits and method used to document deficit

Site	Sensation	Techniques
Middle Ear	Decreased hearing	Audiogram: air and bone Tympanogram
Cochlear hair cells	Decreased hearing "tinnitus"	Audiogram: air and bone Cochlear microphonic SiSi loudness balance (if hearing loss unilateral)
VIII nerve fibers	Decreased speech comprehension	Speech comprehension Tone decay Békésy audiometry Middle ear muscle contractions VIII nerve potentials Auditory brain stem potentials
Brain stem	Decreased detection of speech signals Localization disorders "tinnitus"	Speech comprehension Filtered speech Tone decay Békésy audiometry VIII nerve potentials Middle ear muscle contractions Auditory brainstem potentials
Cortex	Aphasia if dominant lobe Hallucinations both simple and complex	Dichotic hearing tasks Tests of language

such as double vision, weakness or clumsiness that point to a central nervous system disease? Has the hearing loss occurred in association with exposure to adverse metabolic or environmental factors such as treatment with certain antibiotics that may destroy hair cells or as in an occupation in which the patient is exposed to unusually loud sounds that damage hair cells?

Is the patient an irritable infant with a recent history of upper respiratory infection, suggesting a fluid collection in the middle ear cavity? Does the patient have an accompanying episodic disorder of dizziness suggesting a degenerative process affecting the cochlear and vestibular receptors?

The clinician from both his knowledge of the neuroanatomical and physiological basis of hearing and his experience in "listening" to patients describing their disorders achieves a classification of the probable cause of the hearing impairment. It is interesting that there is a limited variety of subjective descriptions of hearing impairments, and the astute clinician soon learns to correctly classify these disorders.

1. MIDDLE EAR. A decrease in the mobility of the middle ear ossicles or eardrum will occur when the middle ear is infected (*otitis media*) or if the joints between the ossicles become hardened with age (*otosclerosis*). These disorders will impair the perception particularly of low frequency sounds (<2000 Hz). Pressure disorders within the middle ear cavity that result when the eustachian tube is functioning improperly affect hearing over a wide range of frequencies. Such disorders change the stiffness of the eardrum so it cannot vibrate correctly.

The tests used to define peripheral hearing disorders include the following: (1) The *audiogram* in which the intensity of a pure tone acoustic signal is adjusted to be just detectable. Clinical audiometers are calibrated for such "normal" hearing and deviations from the normal curve are expressed in dB of hearing loss. Figure 9-21 contains a typical audiogram for a middle ear deficit producing a conductive hearing loss. Note the major loss occurs below 2 kHz when the sounds are presented via the "air" route using calibrated earphones and that the deficit is corrected if the pure tones are presented by "*bone conduction*" using a vibrating source applied to the mastoid. Bone vibration bypasses the ossicular chain and causes the basilar membrane to be set into vibration revealing that the middle ear is the basis for the hearing loss. (2) The *tympanogram* utilizes changes in the mobility of the eardrum (tympanic membrane) to define the continuity of middle ear mechanisms. The mobility is measured in an air-tight system using plugs to seal the ear canal and recording the compliance of the eardrum and middle ear system as a function of induced pressure changes. The measure will be affected by disorders of the middle ear, eardrum or ossicles but not by cochlear or central lesions of the auditory system. In many cases diagnosis is even simpler. The physician need only look into the ear and see if the eardrum looks abnormal. Infection causes a characteristic redness and, in some cases, an outward bulging of the eardrum.

The treatment of disorders of middle ear function is the most successful form of therapy for hearing loss. Antibiotics most often will stop an infection and hearing returns to normal. Fluid collection in the middle ear can be relieved by a small incision in the eardrum with removal of fluid and placement of an aeration tube in the eardrum. Fluid collections due to the common cold are often treated with an antihistamine so that the eustachian tube is cleared and the middle ear can drain. The hearing loss of otosclerosis can be improved if the immobile stapes (the innermost bone) and its footplate are removed and one end of a small wire is connected to the incus (the middle bone), while the other rests at the oval window of the cochlea. Additionally, a hole in the eardrum can be grafted, ossicular arrangement modified, and donor grafts used.

CASE #1

32 y.o. female with unilateral conductive hearing

loss of moderate degree 2° to left otosclerosis

Otolaryngology
Audiology Service

Date ___10/15/76___

AUDIOLOGICAL EVALUATION

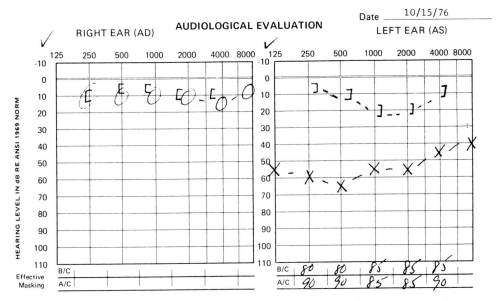

Fig. 9-21. Audiogram. The patient's response to air conducted sounds to the right ear is shown by open circles O and to the left ear by X. The response to bone conducted sounds to the right ear is noted by the C symbol and to the left ear by the J symbol. The right ear was normal. Bone conducted sounds to the left ear could be heard but air conducted sounds could not.

In middle ear disorders that are uncorrected by surgery a hearing aid that selectively amplifies the intensity of the auditory signals is a great benefit. The technology of the hearing aid devices has improved remarkably over the past few years allowing improved function, miniaturization and acceptable cosmetic appearance. Figure 9-22 shows one of the first attempts at a hearing aid.

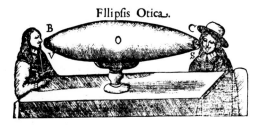

Fllipfis Otica.

Fig. 9-22. Athanasius Kircher (1601–1608) famed inventor tried to help the hard of hearing by designing this "conversation tube." The speaker's voice is amplified in an elliptical tube. Kircher's work was the first to touch this important subject. (Copper engraving, 1673, courtesy of The Bettmann Archive.)

II. AUDITORY SYSTEM

2.   COCHLEAR RECEPTOR.   Disorders of hearing from lesions at this level are related to the site of cochlear dysfunction. For instance, lesions localized at the basal end of the cochlea will affect the high frequency threshold, whereas those that affect the cochlea more diffusely will affect hearing over the entire spectrum.

a.   Meniere's disease.   This disease is thought to be due to increased pressure in the scala media, one of the two main fluid compartments in the cochlea. Initially hearing is impaired primarily at low frequencies (<2 kHz), but eventually the entire spectrum suffers. This loss is also seen using bone-conducted acoustic stimulation. Patients complain of *tinnitus*, which is a spontaneous "ringing" or "buzzing" sound in the affected ear that may even have a quality resembling a pure tone.

b.   Presbycusis.   This is a disorder of high frequency hearing that is associated with aging. The threshold of hearing is raised. There is a loss of hair cells particularly in the basilar portions of the cochlea. A peculiar aspect of this disorder is that individuals experience an uncomfortable "loudness" when intensity is increased. This phenomenon, called "recruitment," accounts for a common experience in conversing with such individuals: raising one's voice to ensure reception may only result in the irascible reprimand, "Don't shout." The hearing impaired ear appears to function like that of a normal ear with increasing increments of stimulus intensity; in some instances it can even become more sensitive than the normal ear. The loudness balance test was devised to demonstrate just this phenomenon for unilateral cochlear pathology. A set of gradually increasing intensity tones are presented to the normal ear and the patient asked to set the signal intensity in the affected ear for equal loudness. Figure 9-23 compares a normal loudness balance measure with one characteristic of a unilateral cochlear impairment.

c.   Ototoxic drugs.   Drugs, particularly certain antibiotics, have as one of their unfortunate side effects a selective destruction of hair cells. The hearing loss from this form of pathology affects the basal end of the cochlea more severely than the apex.

The knowledge gained from electrophysiological studies in animals while recording receptor motion (the cochlear microphonic) and nerve action potentials can be utilized as an objective measure of cochlear function in humans. The recording electrode cannot, of course, be placed inside the cochlea but, under local anesthesia and with the use of a special microscope, it can be placed on the bony cochlea following a small incision in the eardrum. The application of computer techniques for "averaging" low amplitude electrical signals from background electrical events (EEG, EKG) has now allowed the recording of these same receptor potentials from electrodes *remote* from the cochlea as on the eardrum and even on the mastoid, a bone behind the ear. Thus, it is now possible

CASE # 2

40 y.o. male with unilateral sensory hearing loss

of moderate severe degree 2° to right skull fx

Date ___7/18/76___

AUDIOLOGICAL EVALUATION

RIGHT EAR (AD)

LEFT EAR (AS)

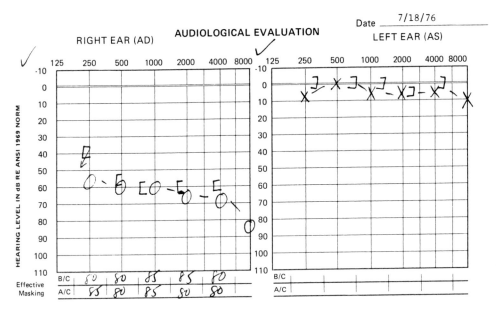

Fig. 9-23. Audiogram. The left ear in this patient was normal, but the patient was unable to hear either bone or air-conducted sound in the right ear. See Fig. 9-16 for symbol key.

to study routinely the peripheral auditory system of man and objectively define cochlear abnormalities and correlate results with the altered sound "perception."

Hair cells unfortunately do not regenerate once they are destroyed. The therapy of cochlear disorders is directed to defining the etiology of the affliction and removing the individual from the source if possible. The discovery that loud sounds can damage hair cells has prompted industry to introduce preventive measures. Sound level meters are used to measure the sound intensity and to define its spectral composition; ear plugs and ear muffs can provide some degree of sound attenuation. The recognition that the effects of intense sound are cumulative has changed the work habits of individuals who must be exposed to loud sound sources.

What hope is there for individuals who have lost their hair cells but who still have functioning VIII nerve fibers? Implantable stimulators are being developed for electrically activating VIII nerve fibers. The electrodes are inserted into the cochlea so as to come into proximity with the VIII nerve fibers. A transducer

II. AUDITORY SYSTEM

converts sounds into electrical impulses to activate the nerve. The pitch is coded by the pulse repetition rates. So far only a few patients have been implanted with these devices and evaluated. At their present state of development, these devices are considered an aid to lip reading. Evidently the stimulus perceived is much like a rhythmic tapping called periodicity pitch (see Section II,A,8). Nevertheless, the patients are enthusiastic about the device because it allows them some awareness of sound, however distorted.

3. VIII NERVE FIBERS. The auditory nerve can be affected by tumors that arise either from abnormal Schwann cells of the adjacent vestibular nerve, or from adjacent tissues such as the meninges or bone. One striking clinical observation is that these patients may not be aware of any hearing impairment. In fact routine audiograms show that the *threshold* of hearing may be normal. However, there is often an impaired ability to understand words presented to the affected ear (speech comprehension test). This result provides an explanation for the fact that some of these patients seek medical attention because of their sudden awareness of an inability to use the telephone with one ear. The *tone decay test* can be remarkably altered in the affected ear. In this test a pure tone is set to be 30 dB above the patient's threshold and the task is to define how long the maintained signal can be perceived. Normally an awareness of the tone will persist for at least 30 seconds. In patients with VIII nerve lesions the sensation of the tone will be lost more rapidly. The tone decay test is actually a measure of adaptation and is commonly abnormal in lesions of the VIII nerve.

The best way to treat tumors of the VIII nerve is to detect them and remove them. If the tumor is very small the patient may be fortunate and not suffer a permanent hearing loss. However, in the vast majority of cases, the removal of the tumor is associated with damage to the nerve and loss of hearing. If it is not removed it will spread, it may damage the facial nerve which is adjacent to the VIII nerve and perhaps eventually affect functions of the brain stem that can lead to even more serious neurological disability.

4. BRAIN STEM. Neurological disorders that affect the brain stem usually involve some portion of the ascending auditory pathway, but complaints of hearing impairment are not prominent in these patients. This pathway is bilateral and diffuse, and the rather extensive lesions necessary to significantly impair the system would be incompatible with life. On the other hand the patient's other symptoms such as visual disorders, vertigo, paresis, or numbness may be so prominent that subtle changes in hearing are unnoticed.

The detection of speech signals embedded in masking noise is difficult for patients with brain stem lesions, suggesting a failure of brain stem binaural mechanisms. The localization of sounds, which depends on binaural time or intensity differences, would also be expected to be impaired.

9. HEARING, TASTING AND SMELLING, AND FEELING

Fortunately, the application of research derived from experiments in animals can now be applied to the localization of brain stem lesions in man. A transient acoustic signal, like a click, evokes a sequence of potentials in each nucleus and tract of the auditory pathway beginning in VIII nerve and culminating in auditory cortex 8–12 msec later. These potentials are of large size (up to 1 mV) if recorded directly from auditory structures, but their amplitude decays rapidly as the recording electrode becomes distant. The use of computer averaging techniques now allows the detection of these attenuated brain stem potentials from an electrode on the scalp. A sequence of seven vertex positive waves in the first 10 msec following a click signal can be detected from an electrode on the scalp of human subjects (Fig. 9-24). The amplitudes of the potentials are less than 1 μV and

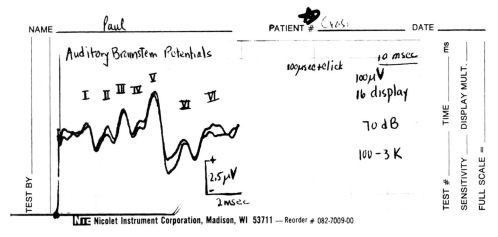

Fig. 9-24. Auditory brain stem potentials.

require the averaging of approximately 2000 click signals for their successful detection out of background EEG activity. Each of the waves appears to be generated principally by a local portion of the auditory pathway. It has been suggested that wave I represents VIII nerve activity, wave II represents cochlear nucleus, wave III represents superior olive and trapezoid body, wave IV and V represent the inferior colliculus, and waves VI and VII the portions of auditory pathway rostral to the midbrain. The test has proved of use for defining the presence and locus of brain stem lesions in humans due to tumors, vascular disease, demyelination and infection. The test is of particular importance in defining the hearing status in young children or in mentally retarded individuals. The early knowledge of a hearing impairment may allow effective therapeutic measures such as a hearing aid or appropriate remedial therapy employing lip reading or sign language.

Brain stem lesions also will affect reflex middle ear muscle contractions by interrupting either the direct or crossed auditory connections to the motor (V and VII) cranial nerves innervating the two middle ear muscles (tensor tympani and stapedius, respectively). The comparison of measurement of middle ear impedance to ipsilateral and contralateral acoustic input can define reflex alterations which may aid in localizing central brain stem lesions.

5. CORTEX. Lesions of cortex in man are very disabling and cause an impairment of the power to use words. The lesion must involve the "dominant" hemisphere (the left hemisphere in 95% of people) in the region of the third prefrontal convolution, temporal lobe, or parietal lobe. The individual may have particular difficulty in understanding language (receptive *aphasia*), talking (expressive aphasia), naming objects (nominal aphasia), or repeating acoustic input (conductive aphasia), and all these functions may be affected to varying degree. It is not completely clear whether mechanisms of aphasia are auditory or semantic in nature. Certainly a disorder of auditory function must account for (1) the prominent generation of phonemic errors in the vocalization of aphasic patients, (2) the failure to detect self-generated errors in contrast to the recognition of speech errors generated by other speakers, (3) the loss of the rhythm of speech in some patients, and (4) the failure to "understand" speech sounds contrasted to the comprehension using other modalities, i.e., mimicry.

The experiments utilizing dichotic processing of acoustic information in humans has revealed special qualities of the left hemisphere for detecting semantic input presented to the right ear and special qualities of the right hemisphere for detecting musical input presented to the left ear. This functional asymmetry of the cerebral hemisphere may be correlated with certain anatomical asymmetries of the temporal lobe that have been defined in postmortem material in man. Research using electrophysiological analysis of electrical activity derived from scalp electrodes may help document these special acoustic processes of the cerebral hemisphere.

III. Somesthetic System

Just as our auditory system is specialized for sound we have a somesthetic system specialized for bodily sensations, an olfactory system for smell, a gustatory system for taste, a visual system for sight, and a vestibular system for monitoring postural stability. We have already discussed the main features of the somesthetic system in Chapter 2 and we shall treat certain aspects of it in other chapters. Thus we shall only briefly describe highlights here in order to place this system in the perspective of other sensory systems.

We need to know what is happening on the skin, in the fabric of connective tissue, in our muscles, joints, tendons, in the heart, lungs, and vital organs. Specialized receptors exist in all these tissues in varying densities to gather information on body state. In fact, they exist everywhere within the body except the brain tissue itself. Several different types of sensory receptors are illustrated in Fig. 9-25.

In the skin, for example, modified surface "sense" cells encapsulate the peripheral axon terminal. At the _Pacinian corpuscle_ (Fig. 9-25C), the classical skin (cutaneous) receptor, pressure applied to the skin distorts the encapsulated terminals causing them to send a coded battery of action potentials to the CNS for analysis. Distortion of the corpuscle causes it to depolarize and produce what is called a "_generator potential_." When such localized, graded differences in voltage across the axon membrane are strong enough, they produce action potentials in a nearby trigger zone of the sensory nerve fiber. The amplitude of this distortion is thus transduced into the amplitude of the generator potential. This in turn is abstracted to a frequency-coded train of nerve impulses.

Receptors are present and ready to detect and collect the flow of energy around and through the organism. Many specialized receptors sense appropriate stimuli. In our skeletal muscles, for example, stretch receptors monitor the pull on muscles, the Golgi tendon organ monitors the tension at joints. Some receptors (nociceptors) respond to painful stimuli or concomitant products of injury either preferentially or following sufficient stimulus intensity. The task of the somesthetic system is to process these and other signals from receptors and distribute them, as appropriate, to other systems.

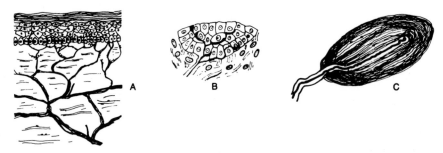

Fig. 9-25. Several types of sensory endings. (A) Free nerve endings. These are present everywhere in the body. In the skin they terminate with arborizations between the epithelial cells. (B) Merkel's disc. A branched nerve fiber which ends in a concave flattened, disc-like formation in close contact with a special epithelial cell. Merkel's discs are scarce in hairy skin but relatively common in the skin of lips, external genitalia and elsewhere. (C) Pacinian corpuscle. These are large encapsulated nerve endings (often 1–4 mm in length). The nerve fiber is enclosed by a large number of cytoplasmic lamellae. In the skin Pacinian corpuscles are abundant at the tips of fingers and toes, the palms of the hands and soles of the feet. Similar corpuscles are found in ligaments and internal organs. (From Brodal, 1969.)

Signals from receptors enter the spinal cord (via the dorsal roots) or the brain (via certain cranial nerves). Recall that body sensations are reported over two contrasting pathways: lemniscal and reticular (see Chapter 2). In general, *lemniscal pathways* are direct, rapid and reliable. Signals enter the spinal cord, synapse in the medulla (dorsal column nuclei), pass to a nucleus of the thalamus (ventrobasal complex) which, in turn, projects to the primary sensory cortex. The majority of primary sensory neurons in this pathway fire in response to movement of hairs or pressure applied to the skin. *Reticular pathways*, on the other hand, exert greater, longer and more generalized influences. They are multisynaptic, branching en route to the thalamus and sensory and other cortical areas, especially at the reticular formation of the brain stem. Receptors of this pathway are sensitive to a crude form of touch and more importantly, to pain and temperature.

In the primary sensory cortex, the body is represented as the *sensory homunculus*, that distorted, largely upside-down (and altogether repugnant) image of half of a body. Thus, distinct parts of cortex receive reports from distinct body areas. Such mapping generates an image of the body in cortical space and orderly relationships are maintained.

Mountcastle, one of the pioneers in the neurophysiological exploration of the somatosensory cortex, discovered one of the key principles of cortical organization, the *cortical column* (Mountcastle, 1978). The cortical column is the basic unit of operation of the cortex. It is a vertically arrayed group of cells, heavily interconnected along the vertical axis of the cortex with a sparse horizontal connectivity. The cortical column is an input–output processing device consisting of a few square millimeters of cortex which receives and transmits signals from other cortical or subcortical areas. The inputs and outputs of cortical columns may differ widely, but as the column is presently envisioned its fundamental design is similar throughout the entire cerebral cortex.

We shall discuss the organization and function of the cortical column in more detail in Chapter 10 on the visual system. We shall also see other aspects of the somesthetic system in later chapters. In Chapter 11 (Moving) we shall describe the role of muscle receptors in the control of movement and posture, in Chapter 12 we shall discuss perception of pain and in Chapter 18 we shall describe other cortical areas closely related to somatic sensations.

IV.   Gustatory and Olfactory Systems

The stimuli for both taste and olfaction are chemical; olfactory compounds must be volatile while those for taste must be water soluble. These two senses often work together. Try tasting while holding your nose, for example, or recall the difficulty of tasting when your sinuses are congested. An onion might be mistaken for an apple! The overlap of these two senses compounds the difficulty of controlling and defining the stimuli. This has made progress in understanding the operations of each system difficult. Most information centers upon the nature and properties of receptors.

There are essentially four *basic tastes* from which others are derived: salty, sour, bitter and sweet. Certain of these qualities are produced by distinct chemical properties. Saltiness is due to the presence of metallic cations (Na^+, K^+, Li^+) with a halogen or other anion (Cl^-, Br^-, NO_3^-, etc.). As salts get larger they begin to taste bitter (e.g., sodium acetate). Sour tastes are due to their acidity. However, this relationship is complex since the degree of sourness does not relate to their hydrogen ion concentration, the chemical basis of acidity. Alkaloid compounds (e.g., quinine) generally produce a bitter taste although unrelated compounds may also as well. Sweet molecules tend to be large, nonionizing, organic molecules with molecular structures that make them hydrogen ion donors. In some manner not yet understood it appears as if removal of hydrogen ions from receptor sites stimulates a sensation of sweetness (Dzendolet, 1968).

The organs of taste, the *taste buds*, are located on the tongue. The tongue contains numerous small infoldings called *papillae*. Several taste buds (approximately 200 for the larger taste buds) are embedded in and protrude from each papilla. Each papilla is sensitive primarily to only one of the four basic tastes. Sweet and salty tastes are detected most readily at the tip of the tongue, sour ones at the sides and bitter ones at the base. Each taste bud consists of 10–15 individual receptor cells (Fig. 9-26). A small extension, called a microvillus, protrudes from the receptor cell toward the surface of the papillae. Individual receptor cells are constantly dying and being replaced. A receptor cell has an average lifetime of 4 to 5 days. Perhaps this decreases even further after a hot, spicy Mexican meal? The receptor cells of the taste buds (and hair cells in the cochlear and vestibular apparatus) are modified epithelial cells called neuroepithelial cells.

Fibers in the facial nerve (VII) and glossopharyngeal nerve (IX) innervate the taste buds. These nerves enter the brain stem where they synapse in the nucleus of the solitary tract. Fibers from this nucleus project along with the medial lemniscus to the thalamic nuclei. Thus, the gustatory system is closely associated with the somesthetic lemniscal system. Sensation of taste appears processed, in part at least, by the primary somatosensory cortex.

Smells, odors . . . how are they processed? Odors do not fall into simple classes such as we have just seen for taste. It is difficult indeed to find a precise, physical property to coincide with a person's description of an odor. Even the same smell can mean different things to different people. What would you guess the basic odors to be? Classifications are based on historic and social, as well as scientific, grounds. Early this century Henning proposed that there are six pri-

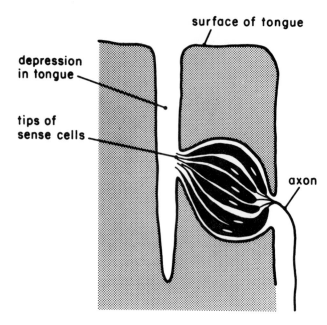

Fig. 9-26. A taste bud. The tips of the sense cells protrude through pores to the surface of the papillae where they are stimulated by various solutions which contact them. (Adapted from Woodworth, 1940.)

mary odors: foul, flavory, fruity, burnt, spicy and resinous. Recent work identifies seven (see Table 9-4), and according to a prominent theory, the *stereochemical theory of odor* (Amoore *et al.*, 1964), an odor is determined, to a large degree, by the structural shape of the volatile molecules. Musky odors, for example, are related to disc-like molecules, camphoraceous to spherical ones, etc.

Table 9-4   **The seven primary odors with chemical and more familiar examples**[a,b]

Primary odor	Chemical example	Familiar substance
Camphoraceous	Camphor	Moth repellent
Musky	Pentadecanolactone	Angelica root oil
Floral	Phenylethylmethyl ethyl carbinol	Roses
Pepperminty	Menthone	Mint candy
Ethereal	Ethylene dichloride	Dry-cleaning fluid
Pungent	Formic acid	Vinegar
Putrid	Butyl mercaptan	Bad egg

[a] From Amoore *et al.* (1964).
[b] Each of the primary odors is detected by a different receptor in the nose. Most odors are composed of several of these primaries combined in various proportions.

9. HEARING, TASTING AND SMELLING, AND FEELING

Olfactory receptor cells are embedded in the olfactory epithelium of the nose. It is a yellowish-brown patch of specialized epithelium located in the upper, posterior part of the nasal cavity. The slender receptor cells are scattered among supporting epithelial cells and are bipolar neurons. They have a unique un-branched dendrite at one end that reaches to the surface of the epithelium and expands into a bulbous terminal provided with cilia; at the other end there is an unmyelinated axon that passes to the olfactory bulb in the olfactory nerve. The transduction process at the receptor is unknown and seemingly insurmountable puzzles exist. A camphor molecule, for example, is over 1000 times the size of a cilium.

Olfactory receptor neurons undergo a continuous turnover every few days throughout life which is accompanied by a continuous renewal of their synaptic endings in the olfactory bulb (Graziadei and Graziadei, 1978). As illustrated in Fig. 9-27 precursor cells (st) divide and differentiate into mature neurons (n)

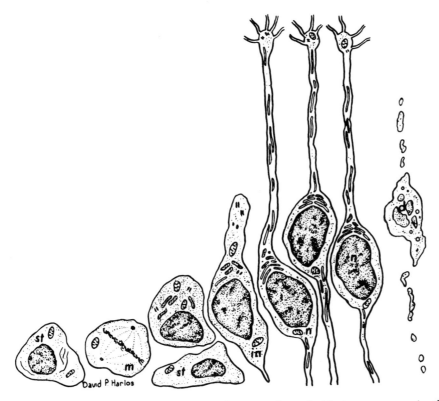

Fig. 9-27. Stages in the differentiation and maturation of olfactory neurons in the olfactory mucosa of adult rodents. The cell marked (n) is a mature receptor neuron; cell (st) is a precursor cell and that marked (d) is degenerating. (From Graziadei and Graziadei, 1978.)

which send an axon into the olfactory bulb and a sensory process to the surface of the epithelium. After a number of days these neurons degenerate and break into debri (d) which is then removed by glial cells.

The primary sensory neurons synapse in the olfactory bulb, that elegantly laminated edifice of neurons found in the front of the brain. The synaptic transactions of the olfactory bulb are reasonably well understood (see Shepherd, 1974). As mentioned in Chapter 3, the olfactory bulb is one of the areas in the CNS where dendrodendritic synaptic transmission exists. Unlike all other sensory systems, information does not project to a sensory relay in the thalamus. Instead, output fibers from the olfactory bulb pass into a variety of structures related to the limbic system including the amygdala and entorhinal cortex. Recall that the limbic system is concerned with emotion (see Chapter 2). Thus it is no surprise that of all the senses, smells are the most closely tied to emotions and emotional behaviors.

The sense of smell in man is not essential to life, but many animals depend on it for their survival. Animals, as well as insects, use odors to mark territories, attract mates, signal sexual receptivity and seek food. For example, ants leave a chemical trail when returning from a food source so that other members of the colony may locate it. Gerbils have a specialized secretory gland on their abdomens which they use to deposit a chemical to mark their territories. Such chemicals, which are secreted by one member of a species and which serve as messengers to others to produce a particular reaction or response, are called *pheromones*. It has been reported that vaginal secretions of rhesus monkeys during certain times of their estrous cycle contain chemicals that are sexual stimulants for males (Michael *et al.*, 1976). However, this finding is controversial since it has not been replicated by others (Goldfoot *et al.*, 1976a). The journal *Hormones and Behavior* published an interesting dialogue on the controversy (see Michael *et al.*, 1976; Keverne, 1976b; Goldfoot *et al.*, 1976b). Some have argued that people secrete pheromones. Perfumes are certainly attractants . . .

V. Summary

Sound is pressure waves in the air, rarefactions and compressions. Our ears capture these microvibrations of the air and analyze them for their frequency and intensity. From this we can perceive a rich spectrum of sounds which we interpret in terms of pitch and loudness. The outer ear, eardrum and ossicles capture nearly all the mechanical energy of sounds and pass it to the cochlea where it is analyzed. Each frequency affects only particular parts of the basilar membrane. High frequency sounds resonate near the base of the cochlea (where the stapes contacts the oval window); low frequency sounds resonate nearer the apex.

Bristles of the hair cells constantly monitor movements of the basilar membrane and when disturbed generate electrical potentials. These are picked up by primary sensory neurons and rushed to the brain for further analysis.

We hear some frequencies better than others. Our ability to just notice the difference between sound frequencies is a direct consequence of the organization of hair cells along the basilar membrane. The frequency just noticeable difference represents the activation of only 54 neurons or a separation of approximately 0.05 mm along the basilar membrane. Loudness, for reasons as yet unknown, increases as the cube root of intensity. We must constantly discriminate specific sounds from a whole spectrum of noise. Most certainly, our ability to hear sounds of different intensities depends on whether or not other sounds are present. Sounds mask other sounds. Sounds of a lower frequency than background noise are easier to hear than those of higher frequencies. This perceptual quality is a direct result of the physical properties of the receptor. High frequency sounds influence only a small portion of the basilar membrane and can easily become masked.

Sound localization requires both ears. At low frequencies the auditory system uses time differences to localize the sound source, whereas at high frequencies time differences and intensity differences are important.

The ear has certain self-protective measures to keep it from becoming damaged due to excessive sound or pressure. In response to excessive sound, the middle ear reflex makes the eardrum and ossicles less responsive. The eustachian tube equalizes pressure inside the ear to that outside.

Pathologies affect all levels of the auditory system. In peripheral hearing disorders, the middle ear can become infected or the ossicles can become hardened. Diagnosis is relatively easy and, in extreme cases, when recovery is poor, a hearing aid can restore normal hearing. The cochlea can be damaged by disease, aging and certain antibotics. Diagnosis is aided by neurophysiological methods which allow direct measures of the performance of the cochlea (the cochlea microphonic) and the activity of the VIII nerve. Hair cells do not regenerate, and so their loss is most serious. The auditory nerve, brain stem and cortex are affected by tumors, stroke or direct insult. The problem can be diagnosed by observing the patients' behavior and monitoring the electrical activity of the auditory system.

The somesthetic system is responsible for processing information on body state. Specialized receptors are present everywhere except the brain itself to collect this information. Pacinian corpuscles, for example, produce a generator potential in response to pressure, which is abstracted to a frequency-coded train of action potentials. Signals enter the spinal cord and cranial nerves. Bodily sensations reported over spinal routes travel in either lemniscal or reticular pathways. Sensory input to the primary sensory cortex is topographically organized creating an image of half of a body called a sensory homunculus. Cortical columns are the fundamental processing units in the sensory cortex as well as other cortical areas.

The gustatory system processes oral stimuli which give us the sensation of taste. Taste buds located in papillae of the tongue respond to salty, sour, bitter or sweet stimuli. The chemical characteristics of these stimuli are distinguishable by taste bud receptor cells. Odors are classified as camphoraceous, musky, floral, pepperminty, ethereal, pungent or putrid. It appears as if the shape of the molecules determine their odor according to the stereochemical theory of odor. Both primary olfactory neurons and gustatory receptors are lost and replaced throughout life. Primary sensory olfactory neurons project to the olfactory bulb and from there into the brain. These olfactory projections are unlike all other sensory systems in that they do not project primarily to a thalamic nucleus. Instead, they are closely linked to the limbic system. Chemical signals, called pheromones, may play a role in social behaviors of many animals. In real life olfactory and gustatory systems are particularly interrelated and often work together.

Key Terms

Aphasia: A loss of language ability.

Audiogram: A test used to discover peripheral hearing disorders. A patient reports his ability to hear air-conducted sounds of different frequencies.

Basic tastes: Salty, sour, bitter and sweet.

Basic odors: According to the stereochemical theory of odor, they are camphorous, musky, floral, pepperminty, ethereal, pungent, and putrid.

Basilar membrane: A membrane extending the length of the cochlea on which the organ of Corti is supported. The basilar membrane decreases in width and stiffness from base (nearest the oval window) to apex of the cochlea. High frequency sounds resonate the membrane nearest its base; low frequency ones nearest its apex.

Bone conducted acoustic potentials: If a vibrating source is placed on the bone near the ear, bone vibrations bypass the ossicular chain and cause the basilar membrane to vibrate directly.

Cochlea: A coiled snail-like bone of the inner ear that contains the receptor system for hearing.

Cochlear nucleus: An auditory nucleus of the medulla which receives input from the auditory nerve; it projects primarily to the superior olivary nucleus.

Cortical column: A vertically arrayed aggregate of neurons heavily interconnected along the vertical axis and working as a functional unit in cortical transactions. Neurons in a cortical column share common properties. The cortex is constructed in principle from millions of these fundamental units, each with its own different inputs and outputs.

Decibels: The measure of sound intensity. The number of decibels is equal to $10 \log P_i/P_0$, where P_i is the pressure of the louder sound.

Eardrum (Tympanic membrane): A thin membrane between outer and middle ear. Its vibrations move the ossicles.

Eustachian tube: A tube which connects the air-filled passage behind the eardrum with the mouth cavity. It serves to equalize pressure between the inner ear and external environment.

Generator potential: A graded potential change produced in sensory receptors in proportion to the magnitude of their mechanical distortion which, if large enough, leads to an action potential in the sensory nerve.

Hair cells: The receptor cells of the cochlea.

Hertz: The international unit of frequency. One hertz equals one cycle per second.

Impedance matching: The efficiency by which sound waves are transmitted from the tympanic membrane to the oval window. Matching is achieved as a result of the reduction in the area from the eardrum to the stapes and the lever arm amplification of the ossicles.

Jnd: The just-noticeable difference for detecting changes in sound frequency.

Lemniscal pathways: A series of pathways over which certain bodily sensations are conveyed (e.g., light touch, movement of hairs). Lemniscal pathways are, in general, direct and rapid.

Loudness: The subjective measure of sound intensity. Loudness increases in proportion to the cube root of intensity. Loudness is measured in sones.

Magnitude estimation: An experimental means of scaling the magnitude of sensations. The subject evaluates sounds and reports their relative loudness.

Masking: The phenomenon whereby one sound can obscure another. A masker tone has relatively more effect on tones above its frequency than below it.

Medial geniculate: An auditory nucleus of the thalamus which projects to the cortex and receives input from the inferior colliculus.

Mel: The unit used to describe pitch.

Meniere's disease: A hearing disorder caused by increased pressure in one of the fluid compartments of the cochlea.

Middle ear reflex: Reflexive contraction of the middle ear muscles caused by sounds, particularly intense ones.

Organ of Corti: A part of the cochlea where the hair cells are located. It is the organ of hearing.

Ossicles: A term used to describe the group of the three small bones of the middle ear (the malleus, incus and stapes).

Otitis media: A disease resulting in a loss of hearing which is caused by a decrease in the mobility of the middle ear ossicles or eardrum when the middle ear becomes infected.

Otosclerosis: A disease resulting in a loss of hearing due to a hardening of the joints between the ossicles.

Ototoxic drugs: Drugs which are toxic to the auditory system.

Oval window: A small membrane-covered opening where the stapes is connected to the cochlea. Vibrations of the stapes on the oval window are transferred to the fluid-filled cochlea.

Pacinian corpuscle: A specialized sensory receptor of the skin which responds to mechanical distortion. This distortion produces a generator potential.

Papillae: Small, nipple-like projections of the tongue.

Periodicity pitch: A phenomenon illustrating the importance of the temporal coding of auditory signals. A high frequency sound interrupted by one of low frequency is perceived as being of the interruption frequency.

Pheromone: A volatile chemical which is secreted by one member of a species and serves as messenger to another member to produce a particular response.

Pitch: The subjective sensation to sounds of different frequencies.

Place theory of hearing: A theory which states that the place along the basilar membrane activated by a sound determines the pitch of the sound perceived.

Presbycusis: A disorder of high frequency hearing that is associated with aging.

Psychophysics: A discipline that studies the responses of sense organs to physical stimuli.

Reticular pathways: Pathways over which certain bodily sensations are conveyed (e.g., crude forms of touch, pain and temperature). Reticular pathways are more diffuse than lemniscal pathways.

Round window: A small, round membrane-covered opening near the oval window which serves to relieve the instantaneous changes in pressure inside the cochlea as a result of sound stimulation.

Sensory homunculus: A term used to describe the topographical representation of the body's image on the cerebral cortex.

Sound frequency: The number of complete cycles per second of a sound pressure wave. The unit of measure is the hertz.

Stereochemical theory of odor: A theory which states that the basic odors are determined primarily by the structural shape of the volatile molecules.

Superior olivary nuclei: Auditory nuclei of the medulla which receive input from the cochlear nuclei and project primarily to the inferior colliculus.

Taste buds: The organs of taste located on the tongue. Many protrude from each of the papillae of the tongue.

Tinnitus: A spontaneous ringing or buzzing sound in the ear which is not caused by external sounds.

Tonotopic map: A term used to describe the orderly organization of frequencies within auditory areas of the brain.

9. HEARING, TASTING AND SMELLING, AND FEELING

Traveling wave: An undulation of the basilar membrane set up by a sound wave.

Tuning curve: A plot of sound frequency versus intensity for auditory nerve fibers; it shows the frequency selectivity of particular fibers.

Tympanic membrane: See Eardrum.

Tympanogram: A test used to detect peripheral hearing disorders. It tests the continuity of middle ear mechanisms.

General References

Dallos, P. (1973). "The Auditory Periphery: Biophysics and Physiology." Academic Press, New York.

Goldstein, M. H., Jr. (1974). The auditory periphery. In "Medical Physiology (V. B. Mountcastle, ed.) 13th ed., Vol. 1, pp. 382–411. Mosby, St. Louis, Missouri.

Jeans, Sir J. (1961). "Science and Music." Cambridge Univ. Press, London and New York.

Lindsay, P. H., and Norman, D. A. (1973). "An Introduction to Psychology." Academic Press, New York.

Mountcastle, V. B. (1974). Central neural mechanisms in hearing. In "Medical Physiology" (V. B. Mountcastle, ed.) 13th ed., Vol. 1, pp. 412–439. Mosby, St. Louis, Missouri.

Stevens, S. S., Warshofsky, F., and the Editors of "Life" (1965). "Sound and Hearing." Time, Inc., New York.

Tobias, J. V. (1970). "Foundations of Modern Auditory Theory," Vol. 1, Academic Press, New York.

Tobias, J. V. (1972). "Foundations of Modern Auditory Theory." Vol. 2 Academic Press, New York.

von Helmholtz, H. (1954). "On the Sensations of Tone." Dover, New York.

Whitfield, I. C. (1967). "The Auditory Pathway." Arnold, London.

Willis, W. D., and Grossman, R. G. (1973). "Medical Neurobiology." Mosby, St. Louis, Missouri.

References

Ades, H. (1959). Central auditory mechanisms. In "Neurophysiology Section: Handbook of Physiology" (H. W. Magsun, ed.), pp. 585–613. Williams & Wilkins, Baltimore.

Amoore, J. E., Johnston, J. W., and Rubin, M. (1964). The stereochemical theory of odor. Sci. Am. 210, 4249.

Brodal, A. (1969). The somatic afferent pathways. In Neurological Anatomy in Relation to Clinical Medicine," 2d ed., p. 34. Oxford Univ. Press, New York.

Carmel, P. W., and Starr, A. (1963). Acoustic and non-acoustic factors modifying middle-ear muscle activity in waking cats. J. Neurophysiol. 29. 598–616.

Dewson, J. H., III (1967). Efferent olivocochlear bundle: Some relationships to noise masking and to stimulus attenuation. J. Neurophysiol. 30, 817–832.

Dewson, J. H., III (1968). Efferent olivocochlear bundle: Some relationships to stimulus discrimination in noise, J. Neurophysiol. 31, 122–130.

Dzendolet, E. A. (1968) A structure common to sweet-evoking compounds. Percep. Psychophys. 3, 6568.

Goldfoot, D. A., M. A. Kravetz, Goy, R. W., and Freeman, S. K. (1976a). Lack of effect of vaginal lavages and aliphatic acids on ejaculatory responses in Rhesus monkeys: Behavioral and chemical analyses. Horm. Behav. 7, 1–27.

Goldfoot, D. A., Goy, R. W., Kravetz, M. A., and Freeman, S. K. (1976b). Letters to the Editor: Reply to Michael et al. (1976). Horm. Behav. 7, 373–378.

Graziadei, P. P. C., and Graziadei, G. A. M. (1978). The olfactory system: A model for the study of neurogenesis and axon regeneration in mammals. *In* Neuronal Plasticity (C. W. Cotman, ed.), pp. 131–154. Raven, New York.

Keverne, E. B. (1976a). Sexual receptivity and attractiveness in the female rhesus monkey. *Adv. Study Behav.* 7, 155–200.

Keverne, E. B. (1976b). Reply to Goldfoot *et al.* (1976a). *Horm. Behav.* 7, 369–372.

Kiang, N. Y-S., Watanabe, T., Thomas, E. D., and Clark, L. F. (1962). Stimulus coding in the cat's auditory nerve. *Ann. Otol., Rhinol., & Laryngol.* 71, 1009–1026.

Knudsen, E. I., and Konishi, M. (1978). A neural map of auditory space in the owl. *Science* 200, 795–797.

Michael, R. P., Bonsall, R. W., and Zumpe, D. (1976). Letters to the editor: Reply to Goldfoot *et al.* (1976a). *Horm. Behav.* 7, 365–367.

Mountcastle, V. B. (1974). Central neural mechanisms in hearing. *In* "Medical Physiology" (V. B. Mountcastle, ed.), 13th ed., Vol. 1, pp. 412–439. Mosby, St. Louis, Missouri.

Mountcastle, V. B. (1978). An organising principle for cerebral function: the unit module and the distributed system. *In* "The Mindful Brain" (G. M. Edelman and V. B. Mountcastle, eds.), pp. 1–50. MIT Press, Cambridge, Massachusetts.

Neff, W. D. (1961). Neural mechanisms of auditory discrimination. *In* "Sensory Communication" (W. A. Rosenblith, ed.), pp. 259–278. MIT Press, Cambridge, Massachusetts.

Nieder, P. C., and Nieder, I. (1970). Crossed olivocochlear bundle: Electric stimulation enhances masked neural responses to loud clicks. *Brain Res.* 21, 135–137.

Rhode, W. S. (1971). Observations of the vibration of the basilar membrane in squirrel monkeys using the Mössbauer technique. *J. Acoust. Soc. Am.* 49, 1218–1231.

Rose, J. E., Brugge, J. F., Anderson, D. J., and Hind, J. E. (1967). Phase-locked response to low-frequency tones in single auditory nerve fibers of the squirrel monkey. *J. Neurophysiol.* 30, 769–793.

Shepherd, G. M. (1974). "The Synaptic Organization of the Brain: An Introduction. Oxford Univ. Press, London and New York.

Stevens, S. S., and Volkmann, J. (1940). The relation of pitch to frequency: A revised scale. *Am. J. Psychol.* 53, 329–353.

Stevens, S. S., Warshofsky, F., and the Editors of "Life" (1965). "Sound and Hearing." Time, Inc., New York.

Tembrock, G. (1963). Acoustic behavior of mammals. *In* "Acoustic Behavior of Animals" (R. G. Bushnel, ed.), pp. 751–786. Am. Elsevier, New York.

van Bergeijk, W. A. (1962). Variation on a theme of Békésy: A model of binaural interaction. *J. Acoust. Soc. Am.* 34, 1431–1437.

von Békésy, G. (1960). "Experiments in Hearing." McGraw-Hill, New York.

Wiederhold, M. L. (1970). Variations in the effects of electrical stimulation of the crossed olivocochlear bundle on cat single auditory-nerve fiber responses to tone bursts. *J. Acoust. Soc. Am.* 48, 966–977.

Woodworth, R. S. (1940). "Psychology," 4th Ed. Holt, New York.

Zwicker, E., and Scharf, B. (1965). Model of loudness summation. *Psychol. Rev.* 72, 3–26.

Zwislocki, J. (1965). Analysis of some auditory characteristics. *In* "Handbook of Mathematical Psychology" (R. D. Luce, R. R. Bush, and E. Galanter, eds.) Vol. 3, p. 47. Wiley, New York.

9. HEARING, TASTING AND SMELLING, AND FEELING

10

Seeing

I. Introduction

How is the world that we see converted into the language of the brain so that we can understand and act in reference to it? This is the task of the visual system.

Suppose that we are watching a person walking down the street. In this common event we take in a tremendous amount of information. We identify many of that person's qualities, such as appearance, color of clothes, direction of movement, and we do it all in three dimensions. As we watch, we gauge the person's size, sex, and possibly recognize something about the nature of his or her movements. We can even project that individual's course and, with a moment's consideration, even estimate how long it might take to reach a particular destination. We relate what we see to what we already know. We are able to make statements about the world we see because we can relate it to an enormous data base that we already possess. "I know that person and that outfit is just like the one. . . ."

The visual system abstracts and then reconstitutes visual stimuli for us. The image of a person or object is broken down into a series of lines and contrasts, each with a given orientation and value. The letter L is a good example of a simple visual stimulus. It consists of contrasting edges with a given shape and proportion. Elementary forms of visual processing, such as of the letter L, are reasonably well understood.

In this chapter we will discover how simple visual processing is thought to work. Visual processing starts at the eye. An image is projected onto a large number of receptor cells, reduced to a series of *on* and *off responses* and relayed to the brain. There stimuli are reconstituted into more and more general responses so that eventually the integrative power of the brain comes forth with sufficient information to create the reality of an object. We shall describe the remarkable capacities of the visual system to analyze and reassemble visual stimuli.

In this chapter, we shall also discuss factors which influence the development of the visual system. Is the processing of visual information genetically encoded and built into the system from birth, or is it developed from early visual experience? In other words, is a particular type of stimulus and the way that we perceive it ingrained into the brain by early experience, or is it inherited and quite independent of experience? This question of the relative importance of heredity versus early experience is a fascinating one, and studies on the development of the visual system are providing new and key insights. The debate is a lively and highly informative one.

A.   Perception

How does an image give rise to the perception of an object? This question is not easily answered. Some physiologists emphasize our tendency to organize and group stimuli into simple units. Look at Fig. 10-1 for a few moments. Even in something as simple as this equally spaced array of dots, there is a tendency for us to see rows and squares. There are, of course, no rows and no squares in this

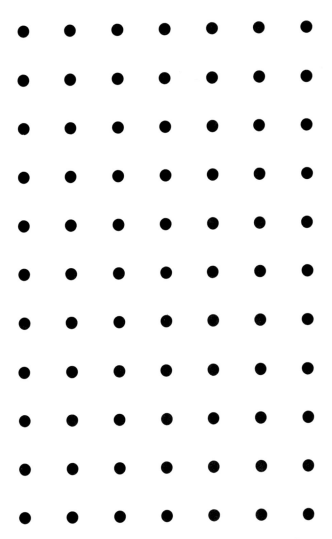

Fig. 10-1. This array of equally spaced dots is seen as continually changing patterns of rows and squares. We see something of the active organizing power of the visual system while looking at this figure. (From Gregory, 1972.)

figure, but we tend to see them anyway. We create them. When we look at this figure, we experience something of the organizing power of the visual system. Our visual system has a powerful capacity to abstract and analyze what we see in terms of what we know. In fact, a few simple lines are all that is necessary to create a meaningful representation of an object. The brain does the rest. A cartoon figure is a good example of this point, since few cartoons are really complete images. Figure 10-2 is a cartoon. What is it? It is not just a set of meaningless lines.

I. INTRODUCTION

401

It is a washerwoman beside her bucket. When we realize this, all of a sudden those strange looking lines take on a new meaning and become a scene that appears almost solid. Once the organizing power of the brain is called into action, a set of lines can become an object, a set of objects a scene, and a set of scenes our whole world.

The abstracting power of the visual system is really most astonishing—a miracle of sorts. Our senses did not give us a picture of the washerwoman, we made the picture. Our senses provide the evidence for checking our hypotheses about the nature of whatever we are looking at. In looking at Fig. 10-2, you may have tried all sorts of different hypotheses about the picture. In fact, an object may be thought of as "a hypothesis suggested and tested by sensory data" (Gregory, 1972). When a hypothesis is wrong, then we err; when it is right, we behave in a logical and intended manner. In large part we guide our behavior on the basis of successful perceptions of our visual world.

We can start in our quest to understand the operation of the visual system by beginning at the eye. Then we shall journey along the neural circuitry, following the coded visual information through the brain, until we reach the visual cortex where some truly amazing computations occur. Frankly, we do not have all the answers, but much is understood about the operation of the visual system and a relatively detailed survey of this, our primary sense, will be most rewarding.

Figure 10-3, which we saw already in Chapter 2, reviews the basic circuitry of the visual system and provides a preview of our trip through the visual system. In Fig. 10-3A light enters the eye and is captured and converted into graded electrical potentials, integrated and passed out of the eye as a coded sequence of action potentials. In Fig. 10-3B signals are passed directly to the _lateral geniculate nucleus_. The lateral geniculate is primarily a relay and organizing center for visual information. In Fig. 10-3C the processed signals are relayed to the _visual cortex_ where feature analysis transpires.

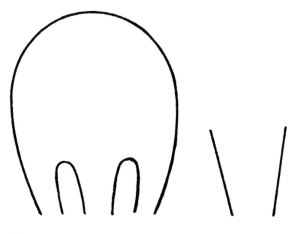

Fig. 10-2. A joke figure: What is When you see it as an object, merely meaningless lines, it will s denly appear almost solid—an obj not a pattern. (From Gregory, 197

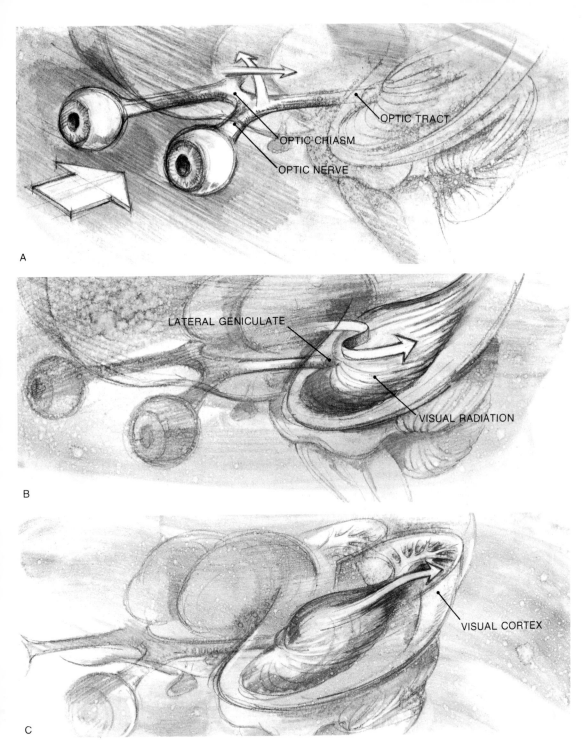

Fig. 10-3. The visual system.

B. Focusing the Image

The role of the eye is to capture an image of objects that we see and to translate that light energy into electrical energy; the eye also performs some computations on the image.

The basic structure of the eye is shown in Fig. 10-4. The neural part of the eye is called the _retina_. It is a filmy layer composed of several layers of cells located at the far side of the eyeball from the place where light enters. The retina receives light and transmits visual information about the light to other parts of the brain. The retina is only about 0.02 inches thick, and it looks like a pink net; in fact, the name retina is derived from the Latin word _rete_ meaning net. The rest of the eye serves only to provide a clear, focused image on the retina, and to move the eye in its socket so that the object that we are most interested in viewing at any moment

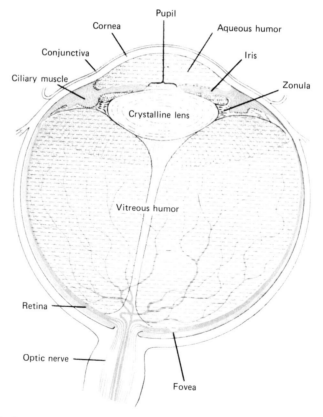

Fig. 10-4. The human eye. The most important optical instrument. Here lies the focusing lens, projecting a minute inverted image to an incredibly dense mosaic of light-sensitive receptors which convert the patterns of light energy into a language the brain can read— chains of electrical impulses. (From Gregory, 1972.)

is projected onto a part of the retina called the fovea. The _fovea_ contains a dense concentration of photoreceptors and is the area of sharpest vision. It has a limited field of view—about 4-in.² at 8 ft.

Light passing into the eye must be focused on the retina. The structures of the eye that permit an image to be formed are analogous to the parts of a camera (Fig. 10-5). The outermost structure of the eye, the _eyelid_, is like a combination dust cover and lens paper. It protects the eye and cleans off dirt and other irritants. Next, there is the _cornea_, the clear front part of the eye, which functions like the first lens in a camera. Most of the optical power of the eye is contained in the curved front surface of the cornea. There, the process of bending the light rays that come from a distant object begins. On the front surface of the lens in back of a small chamber, is a muscle called the _iris_. The iris works in principle like the f-stop or aperture diaphragm of a camera. It controls the amount of light

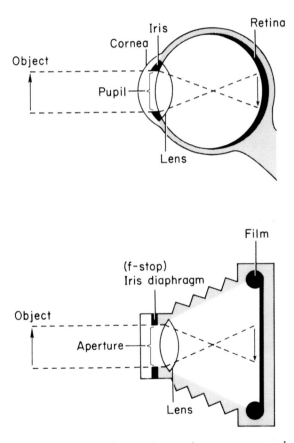

Fig. 10-5. The eye and its parts and operation are in many ways analagous to a camera. (Redrawn from Wald, 1950. Copyright by the American Association for the Advancement of Science.)

I. INTRODUCTION

entering the eye and, when it is contracted to a small opening, increases the *depth of field* (the range of depths that will be in sharp focus). The same principle is used by nearsighted people when they squint to see distant objects more clearly.

In the center of the lens is a round region called the *pupil*. Light enters that

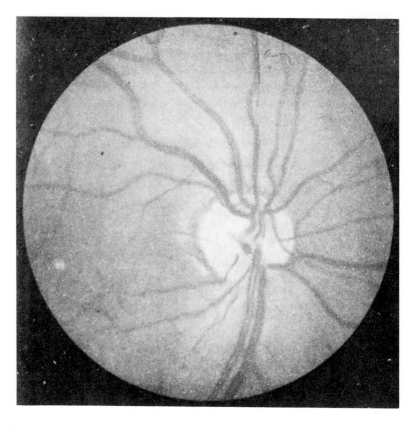

Fig. 10-6. How eyes would look if we could see into them. This photograph is taken with an ophthalmoscope. It shows the spots over the fovea, the retinal blood vessels through which we see the world, and the blind region where the vessels and nerve leave the eyeball. (From Gregory, 1972.)

portion of the pupil that is not covered by the iris. It is a "hole" that looks solid (Fig. 10-6). Light rays entering the pupil are bent further when they reach the large double-convex *lens*. The lens is responsible for the adjustment of focus. In part, focusing in the eye is accomplished as it is in a camera, by slight movements of the lens backward for the distant objects, and forward for close objects. Unlike a camera's lens, however, the lens of the eye achieves most of its focusing power by actually changing its shape, becoming more sharply curved for near objects and relaxing to a flatter shape for distant objects (Fig. 10-7).

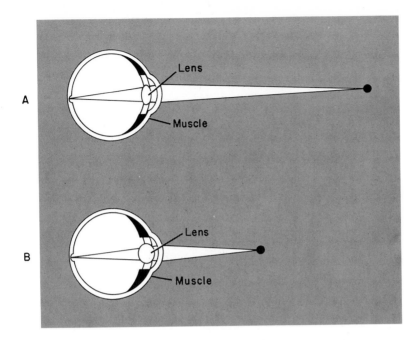

Fig. 10-7. Focusing the eye. For viewing distant objects the eye's lens is flattened because the incoming light rays are nearly parallel and need only a small degree of refraction to be focused (A). On the other hand, light from close objects needs to be refracted a great deal more because the rays are divergent and are still widening as they approach the eye. Therefore, the lens becomes more rounded causing the rays to be bent to a greater degree and come into focus on the retina (B).

II. Common Optical Problems

Many of our visual problems are not defects of the nervous system, but rather defects of the optical parts of the eye. The most common of these result in poor focus of the image and can be corrected by lenses. Although we have only recently understood how the eye focuses images, lenses to correct visual problems have been in use since the thirteenth century.

When the eye is working well, an object in the plane of fixation is brought into sharp focus on the retina by the lens and cornea, a process called *accommodation* (see Fig. 10-8). In *myopia* (nearsightedness), the eye either has too much optical power, or else the posterior chamber is too long. In either case, rays from a distant object are focused on a point in front of the retina and are blurred when they reach the retina. Myopia is corrected by placing a diverging lens in front of the eye to enable focusing on near objects. *Astigmatism* is unequal optical power in two orthogonal axes; interestingly, it occurs almost exclusively on axes near horizontal or vertical rather than on the diagonals. Astigmatism is also simply

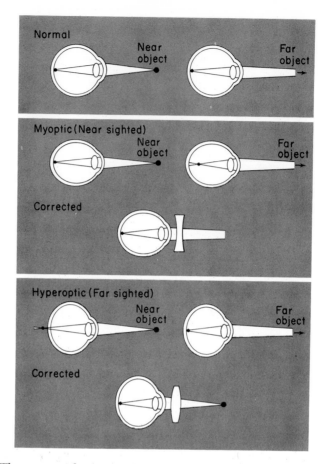

Fig. 10-8. The process of accommodation. In the normal eye an object can be brought into sharp focus on the retina by the lens and the cornea. In myopia (nearsightedness) the light rays from near objects are bent properly but the rays from distant objects are bent too sharply and, therefore, focus in front of the retina. Thus the image is blurred when it reaches the retina. Myopia is corrected by placing a diverging lens in front of the eye for focusing far objects. Hyperopia (farsightedness) is the opposite problem. The light rays from near objects are not bent enough so the image is not in clear focus until after it has passed through the retina. Therefore, the image focused on the retina is blurred. The problem is corrected by placing a converging lens in front of the eye for focusing near objects.

corrected by placing a compensating lens, in this case cylindrical, in front of the eye. Aging often affects focus. As the years pass, the lens becomes less pliable and loses some of its ability to adjust. This loss of the ability to focus or accommodate over a wide range of distances is called *presbyopia* and is a very common optical problem in older people. Although it is optically simple and seems to be due merely to increased rigidity of the lens with age, it is not easy to correct, because spectacle lenses cannot be made that will change their optical power in a few tenths of a second at will. Presbyopia usually cannot be corrected entirely, but bifocals (lenses that have two regions of different optical power) usually provide a satisfactory compromise: one looks through one region of the spectacles to focus on near objects, and through another region of less optical power to see distant objects.

Other optical problems such as *cataracts* and *corneal opacities* may sometimes be corrected by surgery. Cataracts result from the clouding of the eye's lens. Sometimes it is possible to remove the lens or to cut holes in it; this permits the patient to see when wearing very thick spectacle lenses, without which vision remains very badly out of focus. In recent years, it has become possible in some cases to replace a cloudy lens with an artificial lens, which is a considerable improvement over earlier procedures. Corneal opacities sometimes heal with treatment, and in some cases corneal transplants are carried out, although not without risk and difficulty.

Glaucoma is not an optical problem, but a complex condition of damage to the retina which results from a sustained elevation in hydraulic pressure of the aqueous and vitreous humors (the spaces of the eye, see Fig. 10-4). It can be treated and arrested in its early stages by drugs or surgery to reduce the intraocular pressure. Sight is permanently lost if the high pressure is not corrected.

III. The Transduction Process: Light into Electrical Impulses

The eye harnesses light energy and translates it into electrochemical energy at the retina. The retina consists of a few layers of specialized nerve cells (Fig. 10-9 and 10-10). Curiously, the cells that actually receive light energy are located at the very back of the retina, and to get to them the light must first travel through all the outer cells and nerve fibers that make up the retina. There are two types of *receptor cells*, rods and cones (Granit, 1959). *Cones* are the fatter cells and report on color; *rods* are thinner, more sensitive to light and do not report on color. In primates the cones are concentrated in the fovea and, in part, it is this dense concentration of cones that causes the high degree of visual acuity of that area. The rods, on the other hand, are specialized for the reception of dim light, as at night, and they are concentrated in the periphery of the retina outside the fovea (Pirenne, 1967).

Receptor cells connect to the *bipolar cells*. The bipolar cells connect to the *ganglion cells*, which are the only cells that transmit information out of the retina. The general straight-through pathway into and out of the retina is as

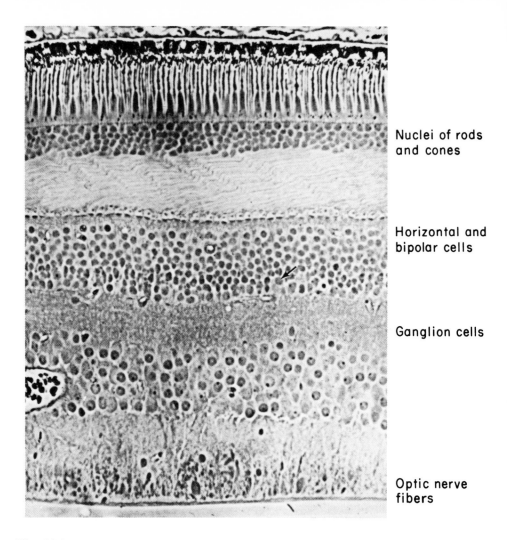

Nuclei of rods and cones

Horizontal and bipolar cells

Ganglion cells

Optic nerve fibers

Fig. 10-9. Organization of the various cell types in the human retina. The cells are arranged in discrete lamina with the rods and cones found in the very back of the retina. Thus light must pass through the other cells before it can activate these receptor cells. Signals from the receptor cells pass to the bipolar cells, then to the ganglion whose axons join together, pass out of the eye and become the optic nerve. Horizontal cells participate in image sharpening and integration. (From Boycott and Dowling, 1969.)

follows: receptor cells to bipolar cells to ganglion cells. Other cell types also exist in the retina, such as the horizontal cells which serve to increase the integrative power of this microtransducing device. Ganglion cell axons travel in fascicles over the surface of the retina to the optic disc, enter the brain and become the optic

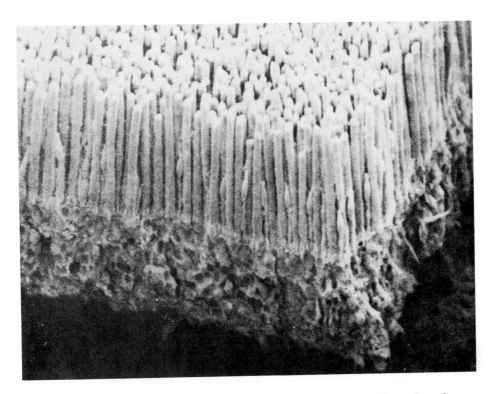

Fig. 10-10. Scanning electron micrograph of the bullfrog retina. The rods and cones appear (as their names imply) as tiny rods or cones. A scanning electron micrograph provides a three-dimensional image of the structure as it actually exists in the tissue. The piece of tissue, usually fixed, is removed from the animal, showered with a fine mist of platinum or gold, placed in a scanning electron microscope and photographed. (From Steinberg, 1973).

nerve. The blind spot can be seen in Fig. 10-6; there and only there is the retina "blind."

Even before the signals enter the brain an amazing amount of analysis takes place right at the retina. Simple and complex forms are analyzed and converted into a neural language that, in some animals at least, is amazingly sophisticated. In the frog, for example, the retina nearly knows the form of a fly is a fly! Similarly, in the human the retina performs a remarkable amount of image analysis.

The general processes transpiring at the retina are outlined in Fig. 10-11, which takes us through the events at the retina as light energy is transduced into electrical energy, and the electrical signals are processed and eventually relayed to the brain via the optic nerve.

III. THE TRANSDUCTION PROCESS   **411**

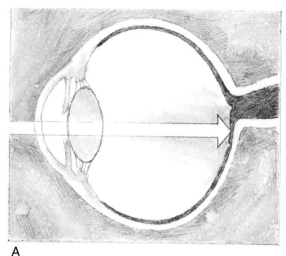

A

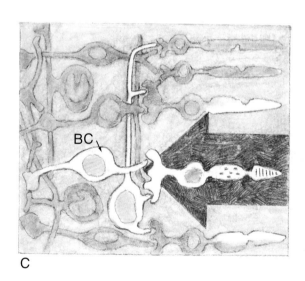

BC

C

THE RETINA

412

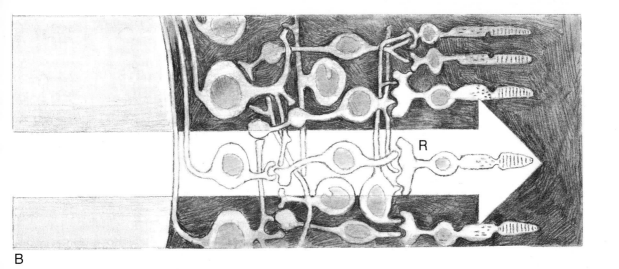

B

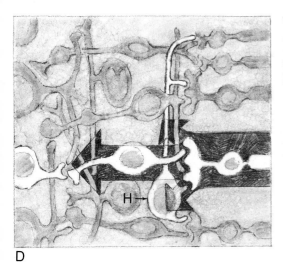

D

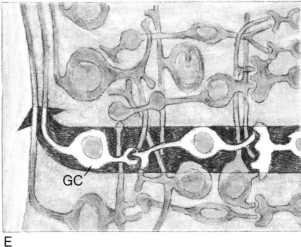

E

Fig. 10-11. (A) Light enters the eye. It passes through the cornea and pupil and is focused by the lens. Light passes through the large chambers and contacts the retina, the neural part of the eye where light is transduced into electrical signals. (B) The receptor cells (the rods and cones) are located at the back of the retina. Light passes through the other cells to signal these receptor cells (R). Rods and cones are the only retinal cells which are directly sensitive to light. (C) Receptor cells make synaptic contact with bipolar cells (BC) (so-named because of their shape). (D) The horizontal cells (H) have an inhibitory action. They inhibit adjacent receptor cell activity and in this way sharpen the signal by inhibiting nearby activity. The bipolar cells activate the ganglion cells. (E) The ganglion cells (GC) send their axons into the optic nerve and carry the message to the lateral geniculate nucleus.

413

A. Receptor Cells

How is light transduced into electrical energy? Rods and cones contain a special light-sensitive pigment called *rhodopsin* which consists of a protein and a chromophore of vitamin A aldehyde called *retinene*. Rhodopsin is located in the membranes of a series of disks (the outer segment) that are stacked at one end of the rod (Fig. 10-12). When individual photons of light enter the rod and hit the rhodopsin molecule, the dramatic conversion begins. *Retinal* absorbs a photon of light; this causes a cis–trans isomerization of the retinal structure (retinal

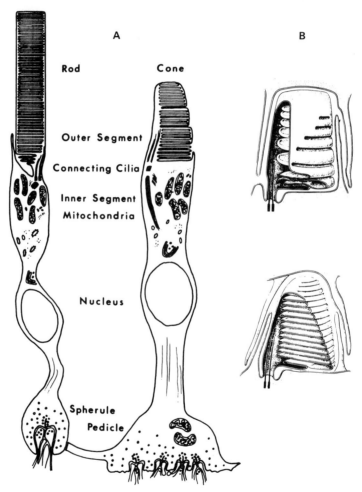

Fig. 10-12. Schematic diagram of rod and cone cells of the mammalian retina. The three-dimensional drawings in (B) show a cutaway view of a rod outer segment (top) and a cone outer segment (bottom). [(A) From Ripps and Weale, 1976 and (B) from Nilsson, 1964.]

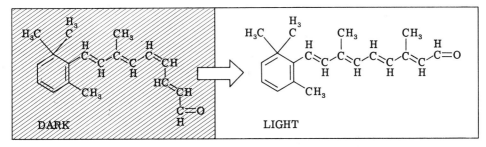

Fig. 10-13. Cis–trans isomerization of retinal.

twists its configuration as shown in Fig. 10-13). This in turn hyperpolarizes the receptor cell by a decrease in the sodium conductance (Wald, 1961). Normally, a rod is very leaky to sodium, and its response to light is a decrease in sodium permeability which results in a hyperpolarization of the membrane. It appears that the receptors are constantly releasing their transmitter in the dark, and this release is decreased or stopped by the hyperpolarization resulting from light stimulation. This seems to release other neurons from inhibition (Baylor *et al.*, 1971). It has been suggested that this odd situation minimizes the metabolic demands placed on the cells. Perhaps in the dark receptors have energy to spare only for making transmitters, while in the light it is all they can do to manufacture sufficient supplies of fresh pigment.

Illumination causes a polarization change, the size of which is graded with the intensity of the light flash. The receptors work like a light meter. They transmit information by means of graded potentials instead of action potentials. Since information is transferred only over a short distance, an action potential is not needed. Moreover, this keeps the signal graded at this point. A receptor cell is remarkably sensitive to light. The absorption of one or a very few photons by a rod will cause it to respond (Hecht *et al.*, 1942). The photon does not provide sufficient energy for this process, so somehow the energy is amplified. At present the nature of this key intervening process is largely unknown, but it may involve calcium and cyclic guanosine monophosphate (cGMP). Light causes a striking decrease in cGMP, and it has been proposed that cGMP may well be "the gatekeeper" of the rod outer segment permeability to sodium ions.

What property of the rods and cones is responsible for their differential sensitivity to light? The sensitivity of the receptor cells to light (rods to dim light and the cones to bright light and colors) is a direct result of the particular pigment they contain. Rhodopsin, the pigment of the rods, absorbs photons most efficiently at 507 nm, the blue region of the spectrum. The signal for the rods saturates (reaches its maximum) in fairly dim light so they are keenly sensitive. The different classes of cones, on the other hand, contain three different *visual pigments* with absorption maxima at 445 nm (blue), 535 nm (green) and 570 nm (red) (Fig. 10-14). Each cone contains only one of these pigments, so its response to light of a given wavelength depends precisely on the efficiency of its pigment to absorb light at that wavelength. The absorption curves of the three different pigments overlap, so that light of any wavelength will excite at least two classes of cones, but with an efficiency that depends on the height of each pigment's absorption curve at that wavelength.

All four photopigments are made of a protein (*opsin*) bonded to a chromophore molecule which is always a variant of vitamin A. The opsin differs in each of the four cell types, and this difference confers the specific light sensitivities to each photopigment, i.e., it determines whether a pigment responds to all light or it responds selectively to red, blue, or green.

Recall that color quality is a function of the wavelength of light and that by mixing red, green, and blue light (but not pigments) any color can be produced. Color vision, like the mixing of light, results from a synthesis of the signals from the different types of cones (Fig. 10-14). Green excites only certain cones, while red light excites others. Mixtures give us orange, blue-green, yellow, etc. The level of illumination at which the rods saturate is just barely sufficient to begin

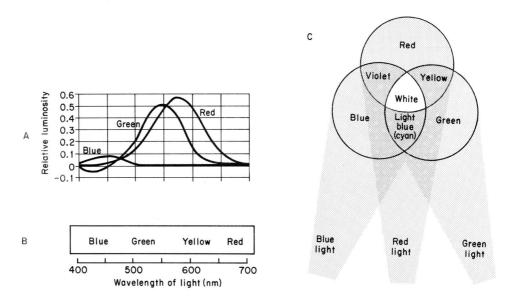

Fig. 10-14. Color response of the visual pigments of the cones. (A) The absorption curves for the color sensitive pigments. All colors seen are a mixture of these three pigments. By mixing three wavelengths of light (not pigments) widely spaced along the spectrum (B), any spectral hue can be produced by adjusting the relative intensities suitably. (C) The result of mixing color. White also can be made, but not black or nonspectral colors such as brown. In this way, the eye effectively mixes three colors to which it is basically sensitive. (After Gregory, 1972.)

exciting the cones, which respond rapidly to even very bright levels of illumination without saturating. Thus, the cones come into play when the light is strong. At night only the rods will work, and they do not respond to different colors. This explains why we cannot see colors at night and all things appear to be different shades of gray.

B.   Retinal Output Characteristics

Receptor cells influence the bipolar cells which in turn generate graded potentials and influence ganglion cell firing. What is the nature of the message the ganglion cells pass onto the brain? On the retina nearly 100 million receptor cells converge onto approximately 1 million ganglion cells so some type of data reduction must take place. Uniform illumination of the retina has very little effect on ganglion cell firing. Rather the ganglion cells prefer to respond to discrete stimulation such as small spots. The term used to define the area of the retina that when illuminated influences the activity of a single ganglion cell is the *receptive field* (Hartline, 1940).

A very simple experiment is done to analyze the receptive fields. A discrete light stimulus is shown on the eye, and the electrical activity from a single nerve fiber or ganglion cell is recorded (Fig. 10-15). How does the firing change when a

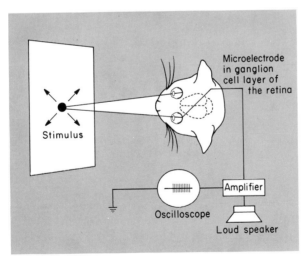

Fig. 10-15. Method used to determine receptive fields. An image (small spot, bar, edge, etc.) is projected on a screen and the electrical activity in the appropriate target cell under study is monitored for the best stimulus which evokes discharge. The signal is amplified, displayed on an oscilloscope and the amplified sound is monitored. As the image is moved about, investigators mark the point of best response on the screen creating a diagram that shows areas that produce increases in cell activity and others that cause decreases when stimulated (see Fig. 10-16).

small area of the retina is illuminated? Ganglion cells have a low spontaneous firing rate of about 5/second even in the dark, and their response to light is either to increase their firing rate or to decrease their firing rate. Small spots of light which illuminate certain parts of the retina have no effect whatsoever on the activity of certain ganglion cells. This light is outside their respective fields. However, once the light enters the receptive field of a cell, it has a marked effect.

Ganglion cell receptive fields have two key characteristics: (1) the receptive fields are circular with the ganglion cell in the geometrical center of its field and (2) the receptive fields are primarily of two types: the ON-center and the OFF-center.

Figure 10-16 shows the basic features of a ganglion cell's response to stimulation of its receptive field. Receptive fields of an _ON-center_ type have a central region where a light coming on makes the cell increase its firing rate. The response to central illumination is inhibited if the surrounding region is illuminated at the same time. An annulus (ring) of light illuminating only the surround

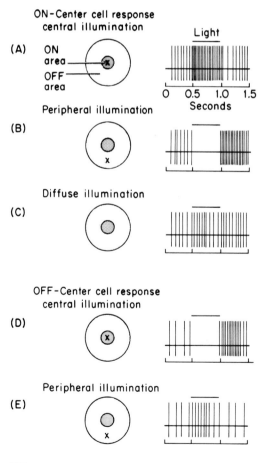

Fig. 10-16. Receptive fields of ganglion cells in the retina are grouped into two main classes: ON-center and OFF-center fields. Both are circular fields and a light shone anywhere in these fields increases cell discharge depending on the type of receptive field and where the light is directed. (A) ON-center cells give the best response to a light spot (X) directed to the center of the field. When this light comes on (indicated by the bar) cell discharge increases. (B) Light directed to the surround (X) suppresses cell firing when the light comes on. (C) Illumination of the entire field gives a relatively weak discharge because the center and surround oppose each other. (D) Light directed to the center of an OFF-center cell slows cell discharge. (E) Light directed to the surround increases cell discharge. (After Kuffler and Nicholls, 1976 and Kuffler, 1953.)

of the receptive field inhibits the spontaneous activity of the cell when it comes on and causes a burst of spikes when it goes off. This type of ganglion cell then has an ON-center and an opponent OFF-surround. Thus it signals with an increased rate of firing when the center is brighter than the average illumination of the surround.

The other main type of ganglion cell has exactly the opposite response to light, an _OFF-center_ response. It gives an OFF-response to illumination of the center of its receptive field, and an ON-response to illumination of the surround. This class of cell signals when the center is darker than the average of the surround.

We can now see why these two types of large ganglion cells do not effectively transmit information about the absolute level of light intensity. They respond best to information about the local grading of light intensity. ON-center and OFF-center cells also have different temporal adaptation curves, and they can signal how recently the center became brighter than the surround. Thus ganglion cells respond very markedly to spatial and temporal changes in light intensity.

It is a fact that the properties of the retina enable us to detect local differences in light intensities in the presence of background illumination which can vary over the tremendous range of 10^{11}. On the basis of cell discharge rate alone, the ganglion cells can signal over only a very limited dynamic range. The lowest useful rate in which they can signal is probably 1 spike/second while the highest (limited by the refractory period of the axons) is somewhat less than 1000 spikes/second. Thus the discharge frequently varies only over a range of 10^3, but we can detect differences over a range of 10^{11}. This is because the ganglion cells are very sensitive to the local gradient of light intensity. However, ganglion cells do discharge within the same receptive field in relation to light intensity. The greater the light intensity, the faster the firing rate. The relationship between intensity and firing rate is roughly logarithmic.

The OFF-surround of the ON-center cell is sharpened by the actions of the horizontal cells. In Figure 10-11 a _horizontal cell_ is shown between the receptor cells and the bipolar cells. Its processes course beneath the receptor cells and contact both the receptor and bipolar cells. Horizontal cells receive their input from the receptor cells and provide _lateral inhibition_ to adjacent bipolar cells and receptor cells; they inhibit adjacent receptor and bipolar cell activity (Naka and Witkovsky, 1972). In some species horizontal cells do not possess an axon and appear to be electrically coupled. These cells provide one of the best illustrations of local circuit interactions (see Chapter 6). Potentials in one horizontal cell spread electrotonically to other horizontal cells so that they can influence a large area of the retina. Since the horizontal cells sum signals from a large area, they respond best to diffuse fields of light. In this way the horizontal cells provide lateral inhibition and sharpen contrast (Kaneko, 1971).

In monkey and man, ganglion cells are sensitive not only to differences in light intensity between center and surround but also to differences in the wavelength of the light. Some cells may respond ON to red in the center and OFF to green in the surround, or vice versa. They also may respond to other OFF and ON combinations with blue or white. Such cells transmit information both about color and about spatial changes.

The rich system of retinal circuitry is not yet understood in complete detail, and the nature of certain interactions still must be worked out. Also many more complicated types of ganglion cell receptor fields need to be studied in more detail (Drujan and Svaetichin, 1972). Some are direction sensitive, others are sensitive to motion, and yet others are sensitive to the size of a stimulus.

In summary, at the retina a form is analyzed in terms of receptive fields, a series of closely spaced dots and contours. The image is captured on the retina and converted into a changing pattern of ganglion cell activity by the neuronal circuitry of the retina. Differences in ganglion cell response depend mostly on differences in illumination. A steady background illumination is largely discarded information. The retina is extremely refined in detecting contrasts, such as an edge moving and crossing the opposing regions of a receptive field. As an edge moves into the surround, impulse activity in the ganglion cell slows, and as it hits the ON-center impulse activity becomes most vigorous.

Position on the retinal surface is _place coded_ so that a ganglion cell fires in response to light in its receptive field. Thus an object (form) creates a mosaic of ganglion cell activity. Each cell sends the brain coded information about the nature of stimulation in its receptive field and the location of that receptive field in reference to others. The job of the brain then is to process this coded information, reassemble it, and translate it into something meaningful. The first processing station is the lateral geniculate nucleus.

C.   Lateral Geniculate Nucleus

After passing through the optic chiasma, the axons of the retinal ganglion cells travel in two bundles, one on each side of the brain. These bundles are known as the optic nerve (see Fig. 10-3). In primates the optic nerve runs up along the lateral surface of the thalamus to reach its main target, the lateral geniculate nucleus (called "geniculate" from the Latin for knee because in primates the pattern of cells bends, resembling a knee). Ganglion cell axons in most species project primarily to the opposite geniculate so that receptive fields are located in the geniculate on the opposite side. In the lateral geniculate nucleus of many primates, including man, there are six layers of cell bodies separated by thin bands of fibers. These layers contain cells organized as shown in Fig. 10-17. Each layer is predominately innervated by one or the other eye. Axons course radially through

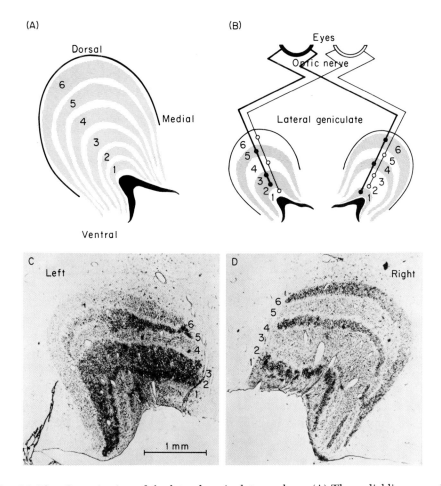

Fig. 10-17. Organization of the lateral geniculate nucleus. (A) The radial lines crossing the cell layers illustrate the column structure of the geniculate. In the lateral geniculate of the monkey there are six layers. (1–6). Particular areas of the retinal field project to particular columns in the lateral geniculate. Each layer is innervated by one eye. The lamination can be demonstrated by conventional silver degeneration methods or by autoradiography after injection of radioactive amino acids into one eye. The radioactive proteins are transported down the ganglion cell axons and label the terminal fields (B). (C) and (D) An autoradiogram showing the layers. (Data from Wiesel *et al.* 1974.)

the geniculate so that parts of lateral geniculate which respond to the same visual field are found on top of each other. Thus, the retinal fields are portrayed as neighboring columns which cut through cell layers (Guillery, 1970). The fovea and the area near the fovea, accounting for actually less than 5% of the total retinal surface, projects to half the lateral geniculate nucleus. This reflects the use of this area of the retina for high visual acuity and fine resolution (Hubel and Wiesel, 1961).

III. THE TRANSDUCTION PROCESS   421

What is the role of the lateral geniculate? The receptive fields of lateral geniculate cells are strikingly similar to those of the ganglion cells. The two main types of retinal ganglion cell receptive fields also have their counterparts in the lateral geniculate nucleus. There are both ON-center and OFF-center cells with their opponent surrounds just as at the retina.

It is surprising how little the receptive fields in the lateral geniculate nucleus differ from those of the cells in the retina. This suggests that perhaps the lateral geniculate nucleus functions merely as a passive relay station. Why then does the retina not send its axons directly to the cortex? The complete role of the lateral geniculate is not clearly understood at present, but one function seems to be to sharpen contrast. As we saw previously for retinal ganglion cells, diffuse light covering both the center and the surround of a receptive field is a much poorer stimulus than a spot which stimulates just the center of the receptive field. For lateral geniculate cells, diffuse light is an even poorer stimulus, often evoking no response at all (Hubel and Wiesel, 1961). Only those lateral geniculate cells that have their centers but not their surrounds lightened (for ON-center cells) or darkened (for OFF-center cells) appear to transmit information to the cortex; the cortex simply does not have to "listen to" regions of the visual field that are evenly illuminated (i.e., where nothing is happening).

The lateral geniculate also organizes visual information for further cortical reassembly. The other functions of the lateral geniculate are less clear. Some believe that it has a role in binocular interactions, mediated in part by a second input returning from visual cortex. It is also possible that input to the lateral geniculate from the brain stem serves to "reset" the visual system after each eye movement. Input to the geniculate from the brain stem may give the lateral geniculate a role in attention and eye movement. This, though, has not been definitely established, but it is important to note that at some point visual information must be intermixed with signals controlling attention and eye movement, and the lateral geniculate nucleus is a good candidate for such interactions.

D.   The Primary Visual Cortex

The cells in all layers of the lateral geniculate nucleus send their axons in a bundle of fibers, called the optic radiation, to the primary visual cortex (area 17) located in the back of the brain in the occipital lobe (see Fig. 10-3).

The cellular architecture of the visual cortex is quite complex. It is an intricate laminated structure consisting of a variety of cells forming six more or less discrete layers. Of all the regions of the cerebral cortex, the visual cortex has the most prominent layering. For this property it is often called striate cortex (Latin for striped) because when stained for fibers it appears striped with horizontal bands running through cell layers IV and V. Most of the lateral geniculate axons terminate in layer IV.

E. Cellular Feature Extractors

The general role of visual cortex is to reconstitute the visual image so features can be recognized. Neurons are sensitive to more and more general features of the stimulus. For example, cells respond to bars tipped at certain angles moving in particular directions. The first order of integration is primary visual cortex, (area 17), the next secondary visual cortex (area 18) and so on through higher centers. Eventually visual signals find their way to motor centers or other areas of brain concerned with nonmotor events. The secret to the function of the visual cortex is the integrative power provided by its circuitry.

As already mentioned briefly in Chapter 2, the visual cortex is neatly laid out so that the retina has point-to-point connections with it. Geniculate fibers terminate in the primary visual cortex in a precise topography creating a *retinotopic map* (Fig. 10-18). As previously discussed in Chapter 2, this retinal map beautifully displays one of the central organizing principles of the nervous system: the amount of a feature analyzing region devoted to a receptor surface is proportional to the importance of that surface. In the visual cortex the fovea (the area of the retina of sharpest focus) uses the largest area of cortex. Areas devoted to peripheral vision are much reduced. Each small area on the cortex then is entrusted with examining the world extracted by particular receptor cells on the retina. In turn each cortical area must have the neural machinery to analyze the features of stimuli on each small region of the retina. The organizing principle is the *cortical column*.

Unraveling the cellular organization of the visual cortex presents a formidable challenge. Much of our knowledge is due to the collaborative efforts of David Hubel and Torsten Wiesel at Harvard University. As is often the case, the initial discovery that started the research was a technical one. Hubel developed a new type of electrode that allowed long-lasting and stable recordings (Hubel, 1957). In the first application, he observed that a number of cells fired most effectively when a spot moved across the retina in a particular direction (Hubel, 1959). In a later paper that year, Hubel and Weisel (1959) mapped out the shape and polarity of the receptive fields and showed that they are organized in a side-by-side pattern so as to form barlike receptive fields in the cortex.

Hubel and Weisel called this first class of cortical cells *simple cells* because their responses to large, complicated moving stimuli are simple to predict from plots of their receptive fields made by using a tiny flashing spot as a stimulus. Figure 10-19 shows the receptive field plot of a typical simple cell studied with

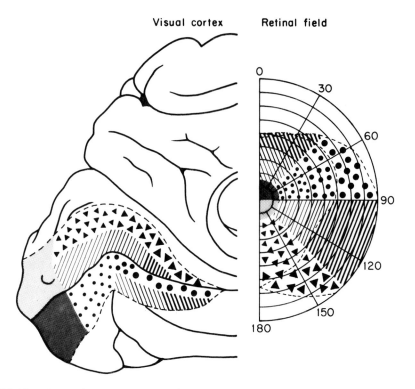

Fig. 10-18. Cortical representation of contralateral half of the field of vision. Areas of the right half of the visual field are marked corresponding to their areas of cortical representation. The central region of retina is represented posteriorly in brain and is relatively large; peripheral retina is represented anteriorly and is relatively small. (After Duke-Elder, 1952.)

stationary spots, and then shows its responses to a moving bar or edge stimulus. The receptive field of a simple cell can be subdivided into two parts; within one part it responds when a small spot of light comes on, and within the other it responds when the light goes off. The simple cell does *not* respond to diffuse light or to a large spot. In contrast to a lateral geniculate cell, a simple cell never responds very well to a small spot, unless it has a linear border whose orientation is the same as that of the line dividing the ON from the OFF area. A bar or edge stimulus is the best one to get a good response from the simple cell, but the edge must be parallel to the axis of the receptive field. This last property is called *orientation selectivity*, and it is the distinguishing characteristic of receptive fields in the visual cortex. It is now known that simple cells are those in layer IV which receive input directly from the lateral geniculate.

Microelectrode studies first revealed that cells of a particular orientation are

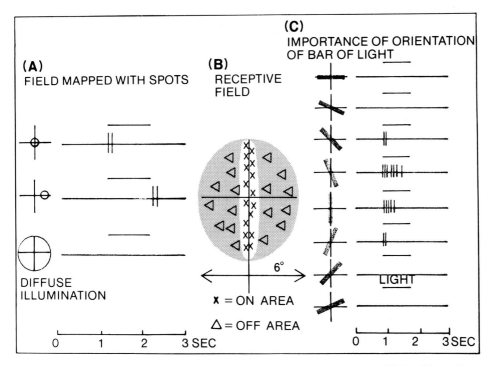

Fig. 10-19. Responses of a simple cell in cat visual cortex to spots of light (A) and bars (C). The period of illumination is indicated by a line above the recording. The receptive field (B) has a narrow central "on" area flanked by symmetrical antagonistic "off" areas. The sum of the spots predicts the best stimulus. The best stimulus for this cell is a vertically oriented light bar (1° to 8°) in the center of its receptive field [fourth record from top in (C)]. Other orientations are less effective or even ineffective. Diffuse light [third record from top in (A)] does not stimulate the cell. Illumination indicated by bar. Cortical receptive fields contrast to those of the retinal or lateral geniculate which are commonly either ON-center or OFF-center (see Fig. 10-10). (From Kuffler and Nicholls, 1976, as adapted from Hubel and Wiesel, 1959.)

grouped in columns. When a microelectrode penetration is made straight into the cortex, perpendicular to its surface, every cell in the entire column has the same preferred orientation for a stimulus (Fig. 10-20). When microelectrode penetrations are made nearly parallel to the surface of the cortex, the preferred orientation of stimulation of the cells changes gradually and progressively. As the electrode passes from cell column to cell column, the preferred orientation goes "around the clock" until a cell is encountered which has the same orientation preference as the first cell sampled (Fig. 10-21). Moreover, a group of cells dominated by the left eye is usually followed by a group driven better by the right eye. This suggests that neighboring columns of cells in the cortex represent similar preferred orientations and that there are also patches of cells dominated by either the left or right eye.

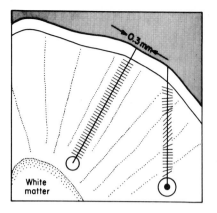

Fig. 10-20. Axis orientation of receptive fields of neurons encountered as an electrode traverses the cortex perpendicular to its surface. Cell after cell tends to have the same axis orientation, indicated by the angle of the bar to the electrode track. The electrode penetration to the right is somewhat more oblique, and the axis orientations of the cells encountered change more frequently. The electrode track is reconstructed by making a lesion at the end of the penetration (circle) and cutting serial sections through the brain. Such experiments have established that cortical cells with a similar axis of orientation are arranged in columns running at right angles to the cortical surface. (After Hubel and Wiesel, 1962.)

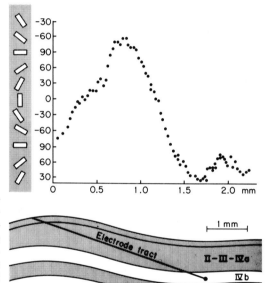

Fig. 10-21. Graph of orientation versus track distance for an oblique penetration through upper layers of the visual cortex of a normal monkey. Note the shifts and eventual reversals in direction of preferred orientation of the cells. (As adapted from Hubel and Wiesel, 1974.)

Only recently has it been possible to envision the orientation columns directly by an anatomical method. The arrangement of columns can be seen by using a novel technique—the measurement of glucose utilization by each small region of the brain. A large quantity of a radioactive deoxyglucose is given intravenously. Deoxyglucose, like glucose, is taken up and metabolized by cells (see Chapter 3) but it cannot be completely metabolized, so it accumulates in cells in proportion to their activity (Sokoloff *et al.*, 1977). If an animal sees vertical stripes over its whole visual field, the cells which are selective for vertical stripes will be more active and, therefore, take up more deoxyglucose in order to meet their energy needs. When an autoradiogram is made from sections of such an animal's visual cortex, the vertical orientation columns show up darker (indicating a higher rate of glucose utilization) than the rest of the cortex (Fig. 10-22).

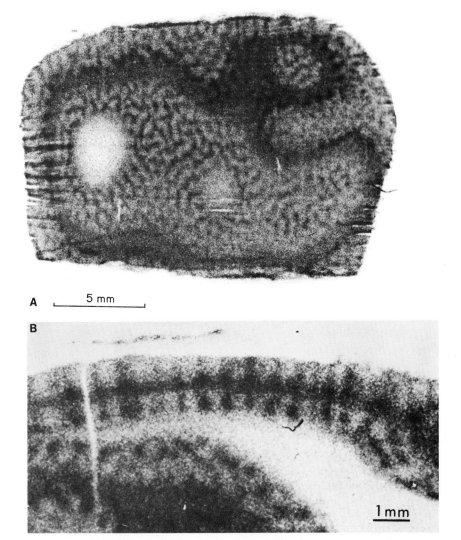

A ⊢—— 5 mm ——⊣

B

1 mm

Fig. 10-22.   Shape of orientation columns in the cerebral cortex as viewed by the [¹⁴C] deoxyglucose method. (A) Tangential section at low magnification through the primary visual cortex showing the orientation columns (dark areas). The pale areas are where the plane of section includes white matter (w). (B) Section perpendicular to the surface. Labeled areas are vertical and extend through the full cortical thickness except for layer IVc. The stimulus consisted of moving vertical, irregularly spaced white stripes presented to both eyes for 45 minutes. (From Hubel *et al.*, 1977b).

The property of ocular dominance is also organized in columns. As mentioned above, cells in neighboring areas with similar orientation preferences are driven by alternate eyes. Autoradiography has been used to visualize the pattern of *ocular dominance columns* in the cortex. If one eye is injected with radioactive amino acid, radioactive proteins are transported to lateral geniculate. There, a tiny amount of the radioactivity leaks out of the terminals, is taken up again by the nearby cells and transported to their own terminals in the cortex. When tissue sections are cut parallel to the surface of the cortex, it is found that the radioactive terminals in layer IV also form bands, like the stripes on a zebra (Fig. 10-23). The ocular dominance columns are like rows or parallel slabs. (It should be noted that the term column is probably somewhat inappropriate, since the actual geometrical shape is a slab; however, the term column is most generally used.)

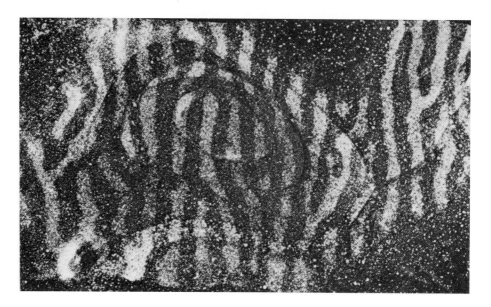

Fig. 10-23. Ocular dominance column. Autoradiogram following injection of the right eye with radioactive precursor illustrating ocular dominance columns. The radioactivity is transported via axoplasmic flow from the eye to the lateral geniculate where it is picked up again and transported to the geniculate terminals in the visual cortex. This section was tangential to layer IV. The columns are shown as a series of light strips representing the radioactivity transported from the injected eye and separated by dark strips where the travel of radioactive substances from the injected eye is absent. (From Hubel *et al.*, 1977a.)

Thus, at the most general level, the visual cortex is a topographical presentation of particular parts of the retina. In turn, the visual cortex is subdivided into ocular dominance columns and orientation columns. Cells representing each complete cycle of orientation cover 0.5 to 0.66 mm in the cortex, and each cycle,

10. SEEING

going from left ocular dominance cells to right ocular dominance cells and then back to left, covers 0.66 to 0.75 mm in a primate. The sector where these cross is called a *hypercolumn* (Fig. 10-24). It is an area a little smaller than 1 mm², which has all the cellular equipment used to analyze a region of the retinal field.

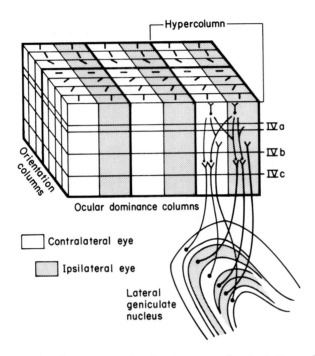

Fig. 10-24. Relationship between ocular dominance and orientation columns run at right angles to each other. In actual fact, this is apparently not quite the case. An example of a complex cell is shown in an upper layer, receiving its inputs from two simple cells that lie in two neighboring ocular dominance columns but share the same orientation column. (After Hubel and Wiesel, 1972.)

Most neurons in hypercolumns have great synthetic and reassembly properties. We have already described simple cells. Besides simple cells there are *complex* and *hypercomplex* cells, so called because the stimulation to which these cells respond becomes increasingly complex. Complex and hypercomplex cells are particularly sensitive to the length and thickness of a line as well as its orientation, and in some cases even the angle at which two lines meet. Receptive fields of complex and hypercomplex usually cannot be divided into separate regions corresponding to ON and OFF responses. Many *complex cells* do not respond at all to stationary spots of light, and those that do generally respond at both ON and OFF. It is not even possible to predict the response of a complex cell to bars and edges from the receptive field plots made with small spots of light. Even though the receptive fields of complex cells appear to be homogenous when studied using small spots of light, they are sensitive to orientation (Fig. 10-25). A complex cell responds well only when an edge or bar of light at a particular orientation enters or passes through its receptive field. Thus, like simple cells, complex cells care exquisitely about the orientation of an edge stimulus. But complex cells have larger receptive fields than simple cells, and, unlike simple cells, they are affected not so much by the precise position of a stimulus as by its orientation. A complex cell will respond to a stimulus that has the right orientation located anywhere within its receptive field (see Fig. 10-25J–L). Complex cells

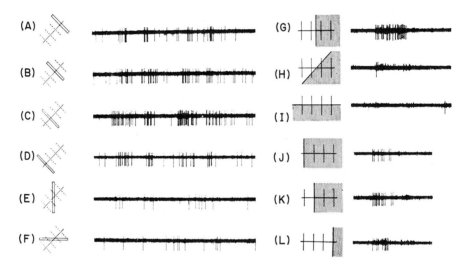

Fig. 10-25. Responses of complex cells. The best response of one cell is to a moving bar oriented diagonally (A)–(F). The optimum rate of movement is about 1°/second. If movement is stopped, discharge stops abruptly. The cell responds over a wide range of positions but is very sensitive to orientation. Diffuse light is ignored by this cell. Other cells will respond simply to an edge (a solid block object). These, too, care most about orientation (G)–(I) and less about position (J)–(L). (From Hubel and Wiesel, 1962.)

thus represent the next order of image analysis in the cortex. These cells appear to get their input from a number of simple cells having the same preferred orientation but different receptive field positions (Hubel and Wiesel, 1962, 1965a) (Fig. 10-26). Some evidence indicates complex cells also receive a direct projection from a special class of geniculate cell.

A further level of analysis is achieved by _hypercomplex cells_. These cells are much like complex cells, except that their responses are suppressed if a bar or edge stimulus projects out past the excitatory center of their receptive fields. Moreover, many of these cells respond best not to a bar stimulus of indefinite

10. SEEING

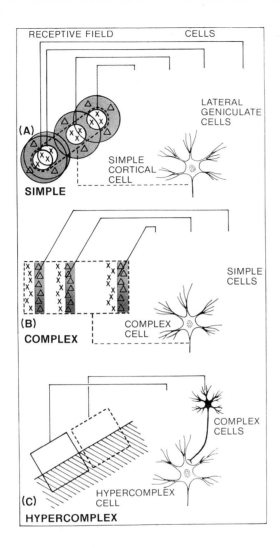

Fig. 10-26. Cellular hypothesis on the synthesis of receptive fields, by simple, complex and hypercomplex receptive fields. For each cell class, lower order neurons converge to form receptive fields of higher order neurons. (A) Fields of simple cells are created by the convergence of many geniculate neurons with concentric fields all arranged in a straight line on the retina corresponding to the axis of orientation of simple receptive fields. (B) The summation of simple cells responding best to a vertically oriented edge at slightly different positions is believed to account for the behavior of a complex cell, which responds well to a vertically oriented edge situated anywhere within its field. (C) In turn each of the two complex cells responds best to an obliquely oriented edge. But one cell is excitatory and the other is inhibitory to the hypercomplex cell so that an edge that covers both fields is ineffective, while a corner restricted to the left field excites. (From Kuffler and Nicholls, 1976, after Hubel and Wiesel, 1965.)

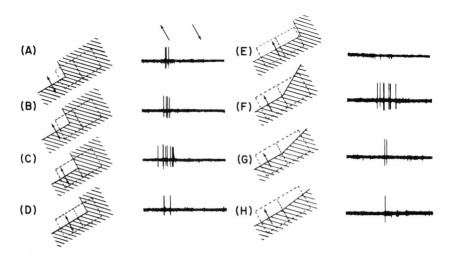

Fig. 10-27. Records from a hypercomplex cell in area 18 of a cat cortex. The best stimulus is a corner moving in the orientation shown in (C). Movements in an opposite direction are ineffective. Infringement upon the adjoining inhibitory portion (right side) of the field is antagonistic (D) and (E). Inhibition is optimum when the right half of the receptive field is stimulated with an edge of the same orientation as the optimum edge for the left (F)–(H). (From Hubel and Wiesel, 1965a).

length but to a corner (Fig. 10-27). It appears that hypercomplex cells receive excitatory inputs from a complex cell and inhibitory input from another complex cell within an adjacent receptive field (Fig. 10-26). Hypercomplex cells tend to reside in the upper layers of the cortex further away than simple or complex cells from the main area of lateral geniculate terminals.

Thus within the hypercolumn three feature extractor and analyzer cells are found—simple, complex and hypercomplex. Simple cells show some ocular dominance depending on the eye represented, whereas complex and hyper-complex cells are more binocular due to the interconnections of the cortical cells. Thus, signals from small sectors of retina are represented in the cortex and analyzed for orientation and shape of receptive fields. An adjacent hypercolumn then analyzes information in the same way for an adjacent part of the retinal field and so forth. Hypercolumns are one of the fundamental cortical units of perception: they analyze spatial–temporal relationships of stimuli.

In summary, the characteristics of the receptive field over successive levels of visual system processing have undergone a remarkable transformation. At the level of the receptor, light of any sort is the best stimulus and the diffuseness or orientation of the stimulus are completely irrelevant. By the time neural information reaches the ganglion cells, small spots are the best stimulus, and there are distinct ON and OFF centers within the receptive fields. Diffuse light is only a moderately effective stimulus in exciting ganglion cells, and the orientation of the stimulus is irrelevant. At the level of the lateral geniculate nucleus, again a small spot is an effective stimulus, but here diffuse light is extremely ineffective; otherwise, the properties of the receptive fields appear to be similar to those of ganglion cells. In the visual cortex we see a remarkable transformation and the beginnings of feature extraction. Diffuse light is irrelevant so that information about the background is completely extracted. And for the first time we see that orientation of the stimulus is a critical variable, and that the position of the stimulus can be unimportant as in the case of the complex cell responses. In general cells of the visual cortex respond to some extraordinarily complex forms. Finally, the interactions are binocular except for cells in layer IV.

IV. Building Blocks of Perception

In viewing an object we examine a whole range of properties: shape, size, movement and color. Such features are the cues of perception. The brain appears to use every possible cue in searching for meaning. It matches external cues against available information in memory and makes hypotheses on the basis of what is available.

Our brain makes the best decision. We can recall experiences when we first see someone. We may come to a conclusion which is rapidly revised as we acquire more cues as he or she approaches.

A. Rapid Scanning

When we view something, it is scanned quite aggressively in the search for meaning. In real life seeing is a scanning operation. We shift our gaze constantly. Besides slow drift conscious movements, there are rapid unconscious ones called *saccadic eye movements*. Saccadic eye movements are carried out at durations of about 60 msec and at amplitudes of 2 to 13 minutes of angle. Saccadic eye movements are essential for vision. If those movements are compensated for by artificial means, the stabilized images fade out. Though we are not aware of them, saccadic eye movements tend to trace out the prime contours of a picture. A person gazing at a picture of a girl's face, for example, for as little as 1 minute will trace out her facial features (Fig. 10-28). Eye movements directed by the motor system are an essential aspect of perception. It is necessary to think of retinal receptive fields as overlapping in distribution and as different in size.

In Section III, we discussed how orientation sensitive cells serve as feature detectors for elementary forms. It is not difficult to imagine, for example, how

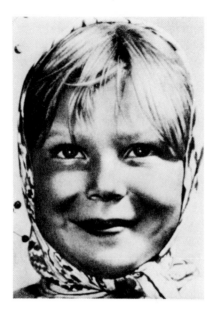 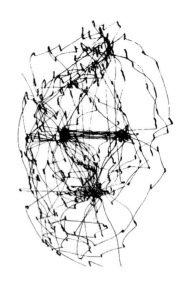

Fig. 10-28. Photograph of a girl's face and record of eye movements during free examination of the photograph for 1 minute. (From Yarbus, 1967. Reprinted with permission of Plenum Press.)

such cells might extract the essential features of the letter L. Such cells monitor the alignment of edges and shapes that fall within their receptive fields.

Objects are readily recognized independent of their size. A letter L is a letter L, a circle O a circle o, no matter what their size. It has been concluded that man and animals have the capacity to classify a shape as the same shape regardless of changes in size over a considerable range. Moreover, this capacity appears to be innate (Sutherland, 1968).

The presence of orientation selective channels would appear to demand that we recognize familar objects at the magnification at which they are learned. However, the brain is capable of a far less rigid interpretation of cues. How is it that we respond to size and are capable of generalizing for size?

B. Size Analysis

It now appears that the brain has another feature detecting system used for size analysis. The brain has size-sensitive cells and a system called *spatial frequency channels* for analyzing size (see Campbell, 1974; Granit, 1977). In order to study size, a grating with rectangular or sinusoidal alternating dark and bright parallels is used as the stimulus. The frequency of spacing is varied, while the

434

mean brightness of these gratings is kept constant. Various neurophysiological studies have been carried out in cats or monkeys at different levels of the visual system (Campbell et al., 1969a,b). At the retina there is little discriminative capacity. Geniculate cells respond to limited bands of frequency independent of the direction of movement of the grating. Like geniculate cells, cortical cells characteristically will discharge to a particular range in the spectrum of spatial frequencies. However, cortical cells respond to grating patterns only if they are moved at an optimal orientation. This is as expected based on orientational sensitivity of cortical cells described previously.

Spatial frequency channels can measure the dimensions of retinal images. Many investigators feel that spatial frequency channels appear to represent a fundamental, if not the most fundamental, feature detecting device where form and size are concerned (see Cambell, 1974; Granit, 1977). From sine wave patterns more complex forms can be constructed. All forms can be reduced to a composite of sine waves. Fourier analysis provides the fundamental mathematical means to decompose forms into their sine wave components. Accordingly, a square wave, for example, can be considered as the sum of a series of sine wave components whose frequencies are odd multiples of the fundamental frequency (see Fig. 10-29).

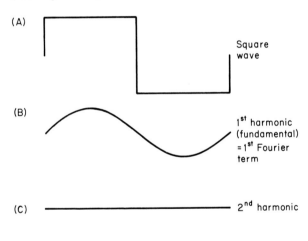

(A) Square wave

(B) 1st harmonic (fundamental) = 1st Fourier term

(C) 2nd harmonic

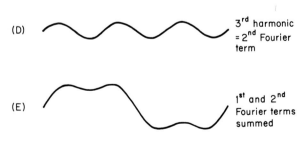

(D) 3rd harmonic = 2nd Fourier term

(E) 1st and 2nd Fourier terms summed

Fig. 10-29. A square wave(A) can be broken down into a series of sine wave components consisting of the fundamental harmonic (B) and higher order harmonics (C) and (D). When the fundamental and third harmonic are summated, the basic form of a wave results (E). Upon addition of higher order harmonics (not shown) the curves in the square wave disappear.

It has been proposed that spatial frequency channels allow the identification of objects independent of their absolute size (Campbell and Robson, 1968; Blakemore and Campbell, 1969). The information on an object might be stored solely in its harmonic content, i.e., the ratio of the fundamental to higher order harmonics. Such a mechanism, if used, could eliminate the need to store a memory of objects for each size, and it might account for the innate ability to recognize objects irrespective of their size. In this respect there is an interesting parallel to the auditory system. Musical intervals, the sound equivalent of image size, are identified by frequency ratios independently from their position in the auditory spectrum (see Chapter 9).

Do spatial frequency channels exist in man and are they sufficiently sensitive to provide the resolution consistent with perceptual data? Basic neurophysiological and psychophysical studies have been carried out and provide an exciting synthesis between basic physiology and psychophysics. One method used to study spatial frequency channels is that of selective adaptation (Blakemore and Campbell, 1969). Such data support the notion that there are many size-sensitive neurons in man.

You may try an adaptation experiment yourself (see Fig. 10-30).

First convince yourself that the two gratings on the right are identical in spatial frequency by looking from one to the other. Now place the illustration at a distance of about 2 m and look between the two gratings on the left for about a minute, allowing the gaze to wander back and forth along the horizontal bar. (This maneuver avoids the formation of a conventional after-image.) At the end of the period of adaptation, quickly transfer your gaze to the fixation point between the two gratings on the right. They should no longer seem identical in spatial frequency. The grating above the fixation point appears higher in spatial frequency because of adaptation of that retinal region to the low-frequency grating, and that below seems lower in frequency after adaptation to the high-frequency pattern (Blakemore and Sutton, 1969, pp. 245–246. Copyright 1969 by the American Association for the Advancement of Science.)

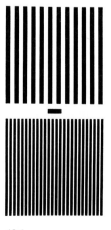 

Fig. 10-30. Follow the instructions in the text to observe the size adaptation aftereffect. (From Blakemore and Sutton, 1969. Copyright by the American Association for the Advancement of Science.)

Additional striking evidence that spatial frequency channels are operative in man comes from a simple experiment on binocular transfer. What does the observer see if the fundamental sine frequency of a square wave (see Fig. 10-29B) is presented to one eye and the third harmonic (Fig. 10-29C) is presented to the other? The observer actually sees a square wave (Maffei and Fiorentini, 1972). Such dynamic combinations also hold for color. Green light into one eye and red in the other gives the impression of yellow.

Measurement of evoked potentials allows the investigation of the properties of cortical neurons directly. Such a strategy removes the uncertainty associated with reporting. In a sense, the "psycho" is removed from psychophysics. As we saw in Chapter 8, an _evoked potential_ is the neural response to a discrete stimulus. It represents the local activity of a small population of neurons, most likely primarily their synaptic activity. In order to record evoked potentials to visual stimuli, a recording electrode is placed on the scalp overlying the occipital cortex. The indifferent electrode is generally taped to the forehead. Such evoked potentials are small and must be computer averaged many times in order to be reliable. Figure 10-31 shows an evoked potential recorded from the visual cortex of man in response to a sine grating.

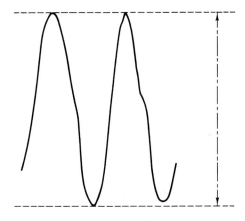

Fig. 10-31. Record of an averaged evoked potential recorded from the visual cortex of man. The stimulus was a grating moved across the visual field (4 cycles/degree at a contrast 1 log unit above the psychophysical threshold). The duration of the potential is 125 msec; amplitude of the potential is noted by the dashed line with arrows. The potential is the average of 1000 traces. (From Campbell and Maffei, 1970.)

Studies of evoked potentials confirm many of the expectations from psychological experiments. A linear relationship exists between the logarithm of contrast at a particular frequency and the amplitude of the evoked potential. This can be interpreted as if Fechner's law (see Chapter 9) is operating for visual contrast. Moreover, extrapolation of the line between the amplitude of evoked potential and log contrast predicts the psychological threshold (Campbell and Maffei, 1970). It can be shown that many separate channels exist for analyzing spatial frequency. If, for example, one pattern is presented to the visual field which is fixed while another is varied, the expectation is that for distinct frequencies two channels should be activated and result in distinct responses. As shown in Fig. 10-32, this is indeed the case. The optimal response to a particular frequency depends on the appropriate orientation of the grating. If one stimulus is an adapting one as another is presented, the responses will not summate unless one is rotated by about 15° (Campbell and Maffei, 1970). The orientation selectivity in these channels is high.

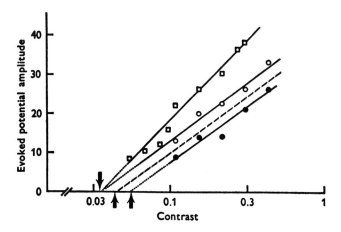

Fig. 10-32. Effect of stimulating with two different spatial frequencies. The open circles are obtained with the lower half of the screen filled with a spatial frequency of 4 cycles/degree; the closed circles were obtained with the upper half filled with 6 cycles/degree. The lines are parallel and the 6 cycles/degree is shifted to the right. Both frequencies presented together in their half-fields summate (open squares). This increase is not due to an overall increase in the area of stimulation, since, when the whole field is stimulated with a grating of intermediate frequency (5 cycles/degree), the response is intermediate (dashed line). (From Campbell and Maffei, 1970.)

Taken together these findings indicate the presence of size sensitive channels, endowed with orientation selectivity in man.

At present it appears as if spatial frequency channels are a fundamental device for the analysis of form. Just how the information is ultimately combined into the complete perception of complex forms is unknown at present.

C. Depth Perception

Another important aspect of perception is *depth perception*. How is the depth of an object determined? We use both eyes to judge the depth of objects. Objects form slightly different images on each of the eyes. Perceived depth is a function of the relative positions of the image of the object on the two retinas. If

438

these images are on corresponding parts of the retinas of the two eyes, then the object is in the *plane of fixation* (that is, in the same plane as the object at which the eyes are pointed). If the images are close together, then the object is farther away than the plane of fixation, and if the two images are far apart, then the object is nearer than the plane of fixation.

Cells in *secondary visual cortex* (area 18) appear particularly involved in depth perception. These cells respond not at all or very poorly to stimulation of one eye, and they respond very well only if the object is in the correct depth plane. If it is too near or too far from the animal (so that the images on the two retinas are too far apart or too close together) these cells do not respond. Thus, while the primary visual cortex extracts information about the configuration of edges from the two-dimensional retinal images, the secondary visual cortex puts the two eyes' separate images together into a three-dimensional picture of the visual scene. In accordance with its function, most of the area of this cortical region is devoted to representation of the more peripheral parts of the visual field (Allman and Kaas, 1976). It is presumed that fluctuations of ocular dominance within hypercolumns in area 18 are involved in providing the brain with cues for depth and solidarity. Exactly how this is achieved, however, is not understood at present.

D. Illusions

As we have emphasized, in order to accomplish what it does, the brain takes all cues and sorts out the significance of messages. Illusions illustrate the power of the brain to do this. The stimuli are the same, but we can see different meanings depending on our internal goals and/or external cues. What does Fig. 10-33 show? It shows the profile of an American Indian and a view from the back of an Eskimo. We can voluntarily switch back and forth by starting to build up cues (looking at the nose, or conversely looking at the left shoulder, for example).

Objects always exist in a frame of reference—our own internal reality and/or our multisensory external environment. In real life, many systems work in concert as part of a team effort. Orientation-sensitive cells, for example, are influenced by somatic and sensory inputs which help to differentiate a stable world from a moving one by providing a frame of reference. We move in reference to what we see. Our frame of reference is built over a lifetime and is constantly being revised. A new frame of reference can be built in some cases within days. For example, as we shall discuss in the next chapter, individuals can learn to move normally behind glasses which invert the world.

Finally, and certainly most difficult to even comprehend, there is a powerful subjective element to what we see. In part I of Fig. 10-34 it is clear that AG = GF.

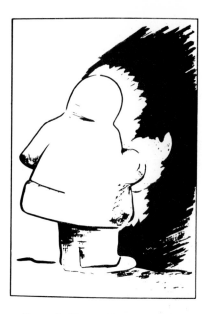

Fig. 10-33. The "Winson figure." (From Gregory and Gomrich, 1973. Reprinted by permission of Charles Scribners Sons. Copyright by Colin Blakemore, Jan B. Deregowski, E. H. Gombrich, R. L. Gregory, H. E. Hinton, Roland Penrose.)

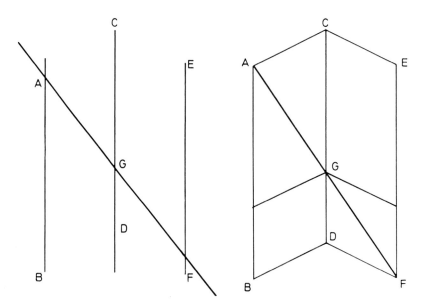

Fig. 10-34. An illusion from the work of the great Danish experimental psychologist Egar Rubin. See text for explanation. (After Rubin, 1950, reprinted from Popper and Eccles, 1977).

(The incline AF is cut in half by three parallel and equidistant lines). Now look at part II. You know that AG = GF as indicated by part I. Does AG look equal to GF? Most people admit it does not. In some way, subjective visual experience deviates from what we know and can objectively prove.

In summary, the brain uses what it can obtain and derives the best interpretation. It considers invariant size properties, form, color, contrast, depth and movement in the context of the scene and in relationship to past memories and finally to its own subject self. In Section V we shall explore the factors which determine how the visual system develops.

V. Development and Plasticity

The development of the visual system is a particularly exciting story since it allows us to examine the role of environment on the maturation of brain function. What is the relative importance of heredity versus environment in maturation of neuronal function? The question of the influence of heredity versus environment on growth and development is not a new one. It has concerned philosophers, physiologists and many others in one way or another for centuries. Aristotle, for example, entertained the idea that the creation of an organism depends on new factors from elsewhere. He wanted to know how beings come into being, and he looked at a chicken's eggs. Cracking eggs which had just been laid, he could see no chicken. At later stages he could see various parts and organs come into being and organize themselves into a chicken. From these observations, he drew the then reasonable conclusion that chickens were spontaneously generated from the nutrients in the egg, and extended his conclusions to the spontaneous generation of insects, etc., from piles of dung, etc. Of course, today such considerations are no more than history, but we are still searching to identify and understand the factors that can influence development. What are the consequences on CNS maturation of raising a child or animal in an environment with a poverty or imbalance of stimuli? The developing visual system has provided a particularly instructive system in which to examine the specific role of early experience on a sensory system.

In this section we shall examine the importance of environment on the maturation of the visual system particularly on the development of ocular dominance and orientation columns. In Chapter 15 we shall return to discuss development at a more mechanistic level. Perhaps the visual system develops independent from external influences, a kind of private assembly executed without interference from the outside world. Development might be protected from rather than dependent upon the world outside us. This certainly makes some sense. The world can be unreliably fickle, and in its wisdom the brain might not depend on it. The complete plans could come from the archives of the genes and their worldly information. Their knowledge of the past could be quite sufficient to guide the formation of key functions, such as ocular dominance columns, orientation columns and other similar key attributes of the visual system. On the other hand, experience may be necessary to reinforce certain attributes. Without such early experience, the system might mature abnormally and function inappropriately, out of tune with the world outside. The brain in its wisdom may tune itself to prominent patterns or objects early in life. In this way it maximizes the capacity to perceive and analyze important stimuli. Heredity may be important, but environment may be just as important. What do you think? The findings are relatively surprising.

Many studies have now examined the effects of the presence or absence of light and patterns on the development of vision. The initial clues that light and pattern deprivation might influence the maturation of the visual system came from clinical studies. People born with cataracts that are not removed until maturity show permanent perceptual defects. Such persons may require months to learn to differentiate a square from a circle and need to count corners to tell a square from a triangle. Studies on primates also point to the need for early visual experience. In the 1950's Riesen (1958) and co-workers carried out a series of insightful behavioral studies on chimpanzees which illustrated the role of early visual experience and inspired much subsequent research. Chimpanzees reared in the absence of light have great difficulty in recognizing simple objects. More recently, refined cellular analyses have now identified the quality and quantity of early visual experience which can disturb the development of ocular dominance and orientation columns, and, in many cases, the associated anatomical changes have been discovered.

A. The Role of Early Experience in the Development of Ocular Dominance Columns

In 1963 Hubel and Wiesel found that if an eyelid of one eye of a kitten is closed, even for a few days or weeks, during a particular period early in its life, that eye permanently loses its ability to drive almost all of the cells in the visual cortex. Only 13 out of 199 cells sampled responded to stimulation by the deprived eye. In monkeys, as well, visual deprivation in one eye produces devastating effects. Few, if any cells in the visual cortex respond to stimulation (Fig. 10-35). The effect of early monocular deprivation cannot be reversed even after 5 years of normal binocular experience. The eye deprived of visual experience early in life is truly nonfunctional. In contrast, closure late in life produces very little, if any, effect on ocular dominance columns.

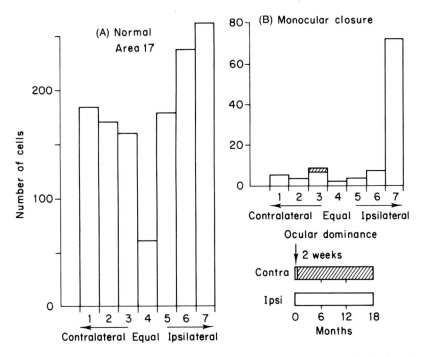

Fig. 10-35. Ocular dominance histograms in normal (A) and monocularly deprived (B) monkeys. The right eye was closed for 2 weeks to 18 months and recordings were made from the left hemisphere. Cells in group 1 are driven exclusively from the contralateral eye; those in group 7 exclusively from the ipsilateral eye; group cells are equally influenced whereas the remaining groups are intermediate. (From Hubel *et al.*, 1977a.)

The developmental period during which the visual system is particularly sensitive to the visual environment is called the *critical period*. During this period the visual system depends on appropriate binocular experiences in order to develop normally. The critical period in the kitten extends from about 3 weeks of age to possibly as many as 10 weeks of age (Hubel and Wiesel, 1963, 1970; Wiesel and Hubel, 1965a,b). Deprivation at 4 to 5 weeks of age has the maximal effect (Fig. 10-36).

One possible explanation for the change in ocular dominance is that the ocular dominance columns fail to develop properly. Autoradiography is an ideal way to evaluate this possibility. As previously described in this chapter, radioactive amino acid injected into the eye is incorporated into protein and transported to geniculate terminals, where the label is taken up by geniculate neurons and carried to their terminal fields in the visual cortex. Monkeys, raised with one eye closed early in life, were injected with radioactive amino acid as adults and audiograms prepared (Hubel *et al.*, 1977a). The autoradiograms clearly show that

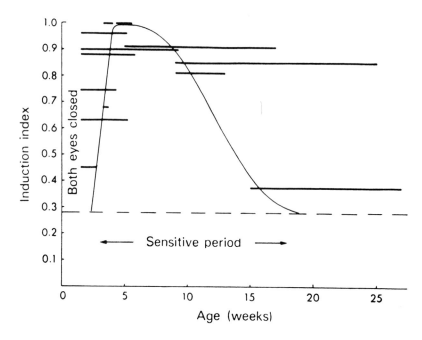

Fig. 10-36. Time course of the critical period for changes in ocular dominance in cortical cells of kittens. The kittens had one eye covered for varying lengths of time, shown by the length of each horizontal line. The scale that is labeled induction index is the ratio of cells dominated by the nondeprived eye compared to the total number of cells recorded. (From Blakemore, 1974.)

the ocular dominance columns of the undeprived eye are greatly expanded (Fig. 10-37).

In order to appreciate the mechanisms of this change, we need to describe briefly the state of visual system circuitry early in development. Is the visual system circuitry already developed and functional at birth? All major cells in the monkey's visual system undergo their final cell division at a time from one-third to a little more than halfway through gestation. Moreover, connections through the retina, between the retina and the lateral geniculate, and from the lateral geniculate to the visual cortex are also formed before birth. However, when a monkey is born, its ocular dominance columns have very fuzzy borders; the lateral geniculate terminals representing its two eyes are not yet segregated into separate bands in layer IV (Fig. 10-38A). This, of course, is a dramatic contrast compared to the brain of the adult. During the first 3 to 6 weeks after a monkey's birth, the ocular dominance columns segregate into their adult sharpness (Rakic, 1977).

So what happens when one eye is closed early in life? It appears that the cells in the layers corresponding to the deprived eye shrink, while those in the other

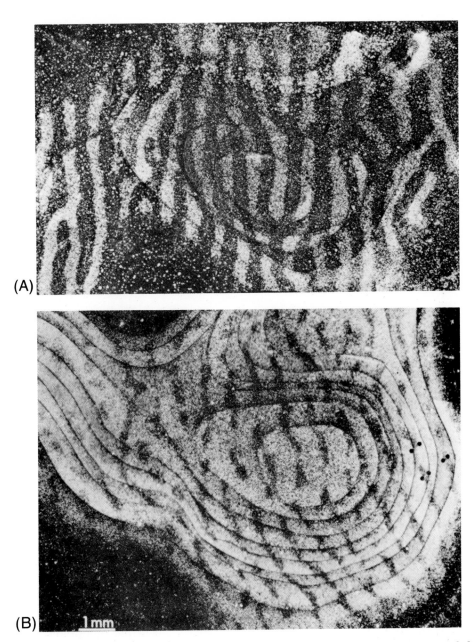

Fig. 10-37. Autoradiogram showing ocular dominance columns (light stripes) in left hemisphere of a normal monkey (A) and one whose right eye was closed from age 2 weeks to 18 months (B). The left eye (ipsilateral) is injected with radioactive amino acid when the animal is an adult and an autoradiogram prepared. The columns from the undeprived eye in the monkey whose eye had been closed appear wider than in the control animals. (From Hubel *et al.*, 1977a.)

layers expand slightly (Fig. 10-38B). The period when the monkey is most susceptible to the effects of deprivation corresponds to the 3–6 week period during which the ocular dominance columns assume their adult sharpness (Hubel *et al.*, 1977a). It seems that the process of segregation involves some type of competition between the terminals in layer IV representing the two eyes (Guillery and Stelzer, 1970). Significantly, a similar period of binocular deprivation seems to have little effect, suggesting that the effects of monocular deprivation are in some way related to competition between the two eyes in which visually triggered activity enhances a cell's ability to compete (Wiesel and Hubel, 1974). It is not known whether fibers from the geniculate of the undeprived eye expand into new territory, or whether they remove the deprived eye's terminals from cells which both eyes contact.

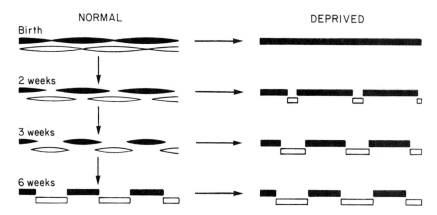

Fig. 10-38. Schematic illustration showing the development of ocular dominance columns. The columns are not segregated until some weeks after birth. The dark thick lines represent the terminations of geniculate afferents in layer IVc corresponding to input from one eye, while the open lines represent the termination of the other eye. Deprivation allows the undeprived eye to outcompete the deprived one and grow larger columns. The magnitude of its dominance depends on the developmental state of the columns at the time of disturbance (From Hubel *et al.*, 1977a.)

Lid closure, it should be emphasized, reduces but does not totally prevent light from stimulating the retina. Most remarkably, even blurring the image in one eye will interfere with normal visual development and produce an effect similar to eye closure (Wiesel and Hubel, 1963). Sewing the nictitating membrane, a thin tissue of the eye, over the eye creates functional blindness in cats. Thus the mere presence of light is insufficient to promote normal development. Form vision of some type is mandatory. Abnormalities in ocular dominance can also be produced by occluding one eye and then the other on alternate days (Hubel and Wiesel, 1965b)! This observation shows that normal function also depends on normal interactions between incoming fibers. Congruity of input from both eyes is essential. Thus there are strict requirements for sensory input.

It also appears that an animal must be able to match sensory input with motor behavior. Kittens had one eye sutured and the other rotated surgically in its orbit. The eye muscles were cut and the eye rotated and reattached (Singer, 1979). This causes a misalignment between visual input and other sensory and motor inputs. Animals experience the same amount of light, but the resultant visual signals are misaligned with other signals. In primary visual cortex, for example, the retinal map will not be matched with the appropriate motor signals. These animals fail to learn visually guided behaviors, and after a number of weeks they do not even use vision at all to guide their movements. Electrophysiological analysis of cortical cells showed that the shift in ocular dominance that usually occurs with monocular deprivation does not develop. A particular pattern of integrated sensory–motor activity is necessary for normal cortical maturation.

The fragility of the visual system seen in kittens and monkeys during early life probably exists in man as well. As mentioned earlier, a cataract that develops in a baby can lead to blindness without the possibility of recovery after surgery, whereas removal of cataracts in adults can restore vision even though the person has been blind for years (von Senden, 1960). In children, squint will also produce severe loss of vision or blindness. Squint (or _strabismus_) is a visual disorder characterized by an inability to direct both eyes to the same object due to a lack of coordination of the eye muscles. In squint, the eyes are misaligned so that they both receive approximately equal visual input, but the two eyes do not receive it at the same time. A moving object in the visual field is seen first by one eye and then by the other. Artificially produced squint in monkeys indicates that binocular representation in the visual cortex is largely deficient (Hubel and Wiesel, 1965b).

B. The Role of Early Experience in Development of the Orientation Columns

As described in Section IV, cells in the visual cortex are organized into orientation columns so that within each column all cells respond to only one stimulus orientation. Perhaps by examining the influence of environment on the development of these columns, the role of form (pattern) in early visual experience can be determined. There are two main questions. What is the status of the orientation columns prior to experience? How does experience affect the development of orientation selectivity?

Newborn monkeys (Wiesel and Hubel, 1974) and possibly kittens (Blakemore and Van Sluyters, 1975) appear to have at birth many neurons (but not necessarily all) with an already specified orientation preference. Moreover, monkeys reared in the dark without exposure to patterned vision still have orientation selective cells (Wiesel and Hubel, 1974). Thus cortical neurons have innate programs to develop orientation preferences.

What happens if kittens are raised with extremely restricted visual experience? Kittens were raised with opaque goggles so that they viewed stripes of a single orientation with each eye—horizontal with one eye and vertical with the other (Fig. 10-39). Thus their visual world is one of horizontal and vertical bars, a visual jail of sorts. What does this do to the physiology and anatomy of the cortex? In

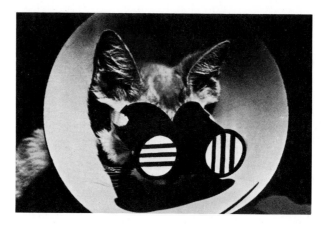

Fig. 10-39. In order to test the effect of restricted visual environment on development of the visual system, kittens are reared with opaque goggles with stripes going vertically over one eye and horizontally over the other eye. (Reproduced from *Science Year, The World Book Science Annual.* © 1971 Field Enterprises Educational Corp.)

normal adult cats all cells are selective to orientation as discussed, and 8% of these cells can be binocularly activated. In contrast, in goggle-reared kittens, about 60% of the cells are nonselective for stimulus orientation: they really do not care which way the bar is oriented. The remaining cells are monocularly driven and respond optimally only to the orientation to which the affected eye had been exposed. These neurons prefer the jail bars of their youth (Hirsch and Spinelli, 1971; Stryker and Sherk, 1975; Blakemore, 1977).

In a more natural situation, instead of goggles, kittens were reared where their early visual experience was a room of stripes going in one direction (Fig. 10-40). In one regime kittens begin to see stripes at the age of 20 days, and for an additional 2 months live in a world of horizontal black and white stripes (Blackmore and Cooper, 1970; Blasdel *et al.*, 1977). Upon casual observation these kittens appear normal when they emerge from their world of stripes and

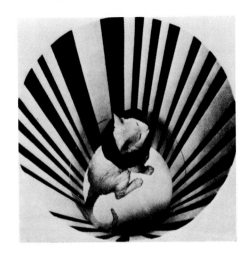

Fig. 10-40. Kittens reared in a world of vertical stripes develop so that they are particularly sensitive to vertical stripes but see horizontal stripes only very poorly. (From Blakemore and Cooper, 1970.)

adapt to a normal visual environment. However, detailed behavioral and physiological analysis shows that they are far from normal even when they are 1 to 3 years old. These cats can readily perform discriminations between a blank field and one containing stripes oriented like those in their early environment. But, they have some difficulty discriminating between a blank field and fine stripes with orientations orthogonal to the stripes of their early environment.

The deficit is clearly reflected in the operation of the brain circuitry in the visual cortex. A few of the neurons are nonselective, but most greatly prefer the orientation of the early environment (Fig. 10-41). It appears that neurons with orientation preferences orthogonal to the pattern in the early environment respond to a *broader* range of orientations. In addition, the normal development of binocularity is sensitive to the striped environment. In cats tested 3 years after having lived in an environment of stripes, only 30% of the cells could be activated to both eyes in contrast to normal cats where 80% are binocularly active (Blasdel *et al.*, 1977). All of these binocularly sensitive neurons preferred an orientation which is close to the orientation of the early environment.

At a neural level of analysis, it has been suggested that inhibitory interconnections in the cortex might be changing so as to increase the selectivity of neurons for certain orientations by inhibiting responses to non-optimally oriented stimuli (Blakemore *et al.*, 1970). Other evidence points also to a suppression of excitatory drive (see Singer, 1979).

Thus it appears that abnormal visual patterns early in life transform the primary visual cortex because they disrupt the maturation of certain cells with unrepresented innate preferences. That is, cells have an innate orientation but only the cells which receive appropriate visual stimulation early in life *maintain*

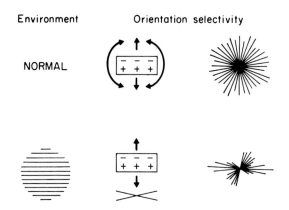

Environment   Orientation selectivity

NORMAL

Fig. 10-41. Influence of visual environment on the development of orientation selectivity. Kittens were raised either in a normal environment or in one consisting of horizontal stripes. Neurons in the visual cortex of the normal cats respond to all orientations, but those in cats raised in an environment of horizontal stripes show a strong bias for stimuli with the orientation present during rearing. The length of each line in the "star" diagrams corresponds to the proportion of the neurons sampled which are driven by a stimulus with that orientation. (After Blasdel *et al.*, 1977.)

their innate orientation. Cells not stimulated at their innate preferred orientation lose selectivity and become unresponsive or relatively nonselective. Genetic information then is sufficient to form the connections within the visual system, but this can be disrupted in immature animals during the critical period by abnormal environmental stimulation. It should be emphasized, however, that it cannot be shown at present that all neurons have innate preferences and some modification may occur in some cells. In fact, as mentioned above, it seems that neurons with orientations orthogonal to the pattern in the early environment may become more broadly tuned (Blakemore, 1977; Blasdel *et al.*, 1977), and in the course of normal development it has been reported that the orientation selectivity within a column sharpens (Imbert and Buisserct, 1975).

In order to develop normal behavior, normal sensory input is not all that is required. The development of visually guided movement depends on the appropriate visual stimuli in early life and on self-produced movement. Littermate kittens were raised so that they spent 3 hours a day in an apparatus which allows one kitten complete freedom to explore its environment. The other was suspended in a gondola that allows the kitten to see the same environment but not actively move in it (see Fig. 10-42). The inactive kitten cannot carry out movement along with visual experience. When not in the apparatus, the kittens are with their mother in darkness. After a few weeks of such limited visual experience, active kittens learn to use vision to guide effectively their movements. For exam-

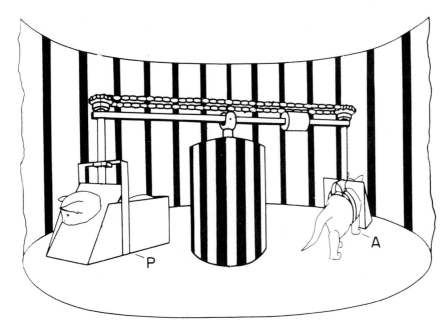

Fig. 10-42. Apparatus used to evaluate the effect of feedback from visual input on the development of normal motor patterns. One kitten is actively moving (A) while the other is passively carried about in a gondola (P) during the brief period of visual experience each day during development. (From Held and Hein, 1963.)

ple, a kitten placed on a shelf could either take a small step down on the side or fall off onto a visual cliff on the other side (the fall is actually prevented by an invisible glass barrier). Active kittens always chose the easy step down, whereas gondola-raised kittens randomly alternate between both sides. After a few days experience the gondola kittens learn to use their vision to guide their movements (Held and Hein, 1963).

The conclusion from these and other experiments is that an association of sensory experience and actual performance is necessary for the development of coordinated movement. Perceptual experience and behavior must go hand in hand.

C. Significance of the Critical Period

What is the role of the critical period for the development of the visual system? The critical period presents something of a paradox. Why should such a potential handicap be programmed into the development of an organism? Many believe that the early visual deprivation studies are but extreme cases of the normal processes that visual experience exerts on cortical development. One function may be to match the properties of feature detecting cells to the commonest features in the developing animal's world. In this way commonly encountered features of complex objects are programmed into the brain so as to maximize the capacity to perceive the more important components of the external world (Blakemore, 1974).

More importantly, however, it appears that the critical period may serve to finely tune the system so that all cells have well matched preferred orientations in the *two* eyes (Pettigrew *et al.*, 1973; Blakemore and Van Sluyters, 1975; Blakemore, 1977; Pettigrew, 1978). The development of the capacity to see depth, the stereoscopic visual system, probably requires visual experience. There are a number of reasons for this. First, very subtle discriminations are necessary to determine aspects of similarity and difference between the two visual images received on the two retinas. Second, the accuracy of detection of visual disparity is truly astounding, less than the diameter of one photoreceptor. It is likely that a system of this accuracy could not be coded genetically but rather develops through experience. Because there are slight abnormalities in every eye, and because eye size and eye position changes during development, it would be most adaptive if the capacity to rewire and develop this system would be the greatest during early development. And, indeed, the critical period corresponds to the period of greatest change in head size and eye conformation.

The phenomenon of the critical period during development is not strictly limited to the visual system. Social deprivation can as well have a devasting effect on social, intellectual and emotional development. Maternal and peer interactions are necessary prerequisites for the normal social and sexual development of young monkeys. The first year of life is a critical period. Isolation for more than 6 months has permanent and severe consequences on their social and sexual development (Harlow and Harlow, 1962). Perhaps here too the development of the requiste neuronal circuitry is influenced. No direct evidence is available, however.

VI. Summary

Visual stimuli are focused on the retina where rods and cones transform light into graded electrical signals. Photosensitive pigments (opsin plus a chromophore) capture light energy and cause a change in the electrical potential of the receptor cells. Receptor cells excite bipolar cells which in turn activate ganglion cells which send their axons to the lateral geniculate nucleus. Horizontal cells in the retina provide lateral inhibition to enhance contrast. The receptive fields of the retina are primarily circular, ON-center and OFF-center. Contrasts are better stimuli than diffuse light. The retinal ganglion cells terminate in a highly topographical pattern in the lateral geniculate nucleus. The receptive fields are similar to those of the retina. The geniculate enhances contrast, assembles stimuli for further cortical analysis and distributes and integrates signals for controlling eye movements. In the visual cortex, as in the geniculate, each part of the retina is processed by a specific area of cortex. In primary visual cortex, the fovea, the area of greatest visual acuity, covers the largest area of the cortex. Ocular dominance and orientation columns criss-cross in the cortex forming a unit of cortical organization called a hypercolumn. Each small area of retina is analyzed, and stimuli are reassembled for general features in a hypercolumn. Each hypercolumn contains simple, complex and hypercomplex cells. Simple cells in the column recognize lines and bars and their orientation, complex cells recognize edges more or less independent of the position and hypercomplex cells analyze corners and even more complex shapes.

A form on the retina which engages a number of receptive fields generates a mosaic of activity in ganglion cells. These send place and frequency coded information to the cortex via the geniculate, where the general features of the form are reassembled by the cellular feature detector in hypercolumns. Many hypercolumns analyze the form. Eventually the integrative power of the primary and secondary visual cortex and other cortical areas generate a neural map or representation which can be identified as the form in view. This last phase, that of perception itself, is not understood in specific terms at present. Spatial frequency channels appear to participate in the perception of object size.

Our survey of visual processing has progressed through seven synaptic relays. Many more neurons are involved, but progress to this point has taken us a long way. Our knowledge of the transactions has advanced so that we can understand the manner in which simple forms such as bars, squares and square waves are analyzed in neural terms. We can imagine at least how simple geometric forms can be recognized.

Most defects in vision are ones of the optical part of the eye. The lens and cornea fail to bring the image into sharp focus on the fovea. Nearsightedness, farsightedness, astigmatism and presbyopia are correctable by artificial lenses which bring the image back into focus on the fovea. Other eye conditions, such as cataracts (a clouding of the lens), are common and require corrective surgery. Glaucoma produces an increase in fluid pressure in the eye and may lead to retinal damage.

In the developing visual system, genetic factors appear to account for the retinotopic map, binocular interactions and to some degree orientation preference of cells. Binocular interactions are disrupted by monocular occlusion or squint during the critical period of development. Experiments on squint emphasize the role of synchronous timing rather than the quantity of light or its form on the proper development of binocular interactions. The anatomical changes produced by squint are unclear. Monocular occlusion produces an expansion of ocular dominance columns by fibers from the undeprived eye. Bilateral eye closure has a less severe effect on the development of binocular interactions. Abnormalities appear as a result of disturbances in congruity of input to the eyes. Competition between fibers is disturbed so that the normal segregation process of the columns is made unequal, and the undeprived eye prevails.

Many cells in the visual cortex of newborn animals display an innate preference to a linear stimulus having a specific orientation. Genetic information is sufficient for forming the correct connections, but this can be disrupted by abnormal visual stimulation during the critical period. Early visual experience appears to be essential for validating these orientation preferences. Deprivation of a certain orientation during early life has a destructive influence on those cells with innate preferences unrepresented in the environment. A normal (appropriately mixed) pattern of forms is essential for the maintenance and further growth of appropriate circuitry.

Clinical studies indicate that early ocular deficits such as cataracts can permanently alter the visual system. Animals reared in an environment of stripes respond behaviorally to patterns of their youth but are permanently blind to patterns with other orientations. In order to translate visual expression into movement effectively, movements must be practiced along with perceptual experiences. The critical period in the visual system may serve to imprint certain prominent forms, fine tune binocular interactions and learn various associations. Abnormal experience during this time can have a profound negative impact on visual system development.

Much more, however, is yet to be learned. Cells elsewhere in the brain may be unspecified early in life and acquire attributes, since obviously we learn many things that are not innate. It is clear that the same arguments will arise again at other levels of the nervous system. Plasticity must be understood and studied in the context of the functional role of each system. To what extent are other systems changed by "wrong" experiences stamping out potential innate capacities of the brain? Clearly, at present, we can say that extreme environmental changes can negatively affect a primary sensory system. However, the relative influences of heredity and environment may not be the same at all levels of the nervous system. Some intellectual attributes and morality, fear, etc., may in fact be imprinted into neuronal circuitry. In particular, unspecified cortical areas (see Chapter 18) characteristic of primates and humans may be exceptions to existing ideas. The next few years will provide some exciting insights toward understanding why we are what we are.

Key Terms

Accommodation: The automatic adjustments of the cornea which brings an object into sharp focus on the retina.

Astigmatism: Unequal optical power in two orthogonal axes.

Bipolar cells: A cell type of the retina interposed between the receptor cells and ganglion cells.

Complex cells: A class of cells in the visual cortex which respond when an edge or bar with a defined orientation passes through their receptive field. In contrast to simple cells, receptive fields are larger, and not as dependent on the precise position of the stimulus as on its orientation.

Cataracts: A clouding of the eye's lens.

Cones: A class of receptor cells of the retina which responds to color. In primates, cones are concentrated in the center of the retina (fovea).

Cornea: The clear, outer covering of the eyeball.

Cortical column: A grouping of cortical neurons sharing common properties (i.e., ocular dominance, orientation selectivity).

Critical period: The period during development when the visual system is particularly sensitive to the visual environment.

Evoked potential: Any transient change in the electrical activity of the brain that is elicited by a discrete stimulus.

Fovea: The center area of the retina where the image is focused and where visual acuity is greatest.

Ganglion cells: The output cells of the retina which give rise to the axons of the optic nerve.

Glaucoma: A disease accompanied by high intraocular pressure which results in damage to the retina if not corrected.

Horizontal cell: A retinal cell which serves to sharpen contrast through lateral inhibition.

Hypercolumn: A columnar sector of the visual cortex where the ocular dominance column for each eye and a complete cycle of orientations are represented.

Hypercomplex cells: A class of neurons in the visual cortex which responds to an edge or bar, preferably of a specific length and orientation. Their responses are suppressed if the edge or bar passes out of the excitatory center of the receptive fields. Hypercomplex cells carry out a higher order of image analysis than do simple or complex cells.

Iris: A ring of muscles on the lens which controls the amount of light entering the eye.

Lateral geniculate nucleus: A subdivision of the thalamus which receives its major input from the retina. It projects primarily to the visual cortex. It appears to sharpen contrast, organize visual information for further cortical assembly and participate in the control of eye movement.

Lateral inhibition: The process in the retina whereby horizontal cells inhibit the activity of bipolar and receptor cells outside the center of illumination. In general, lateral inhibition serves to sharpen contrast.

Lens: The transparent part of the eye which serves to adjust focus by changing shape. It becomes more curved for near objects and flatter for distant objects.

Myopia: Near-sightedness. Light rays from a distant object are focused in front of the retina.

Ocular dominance: Greater effectiveness of one eye over the other for firing simple, complex and hypercomplex cells.

OFF-center: A type of receptive field. Illumination of the center of the field inhibits a neuron while stimulation of the surround excites that neuron.

ON-center: A type of receptive field. Illumination of the center of the field excites neurons while stimulation of the surround inhibits the neurons.

Orientation selectivity: A property of receptive fields that requires that an edge or bar is oriented in an appropriate plane for a cell in the visual cortex to respond.

Presbyopia: Loss of the ability to focus or accommodate.

Pupil: A round region located in the center of the lens where light enters the eyeball.

Receptive field: An area on the retina which, when illuminated, influences the firing of a neuron.

Retina: The neural part of the eye composed of four major cell types (rods and cones, bipolar cells and ganglion cells) organized in discrete layers.

Retinotopic map: The orderly topographical projection of the retina to subsystems of the visual pathway.

Rhodopsin: The light-sensitive pigment which consists of a protein (opsin) and a chromophore of vitamin A aldehyde (retinal). It is located in the discs of rods.

Rods: Receptor cells of the retina which respond to light intensity but not color. Rods are concentrated at the periphery of the retina.

Saccadic eye movements: Very rapid unconscious movements of the eye.

Secondary visual cortex: The area of the cortex (area 18) which receives primary input from the primary visual cortex (area 17). It plays an important role in depth perception in addition to analysis of complex visual stimuli.

Simple cells: A class of cortical cell whose receptive field is a linear border of a specific orientation. Simple cells appear to reside in layer IV of the visual cortex.

Squint (strabismus):   A visual disorder characterized by an inability to direct both eyes to the same object due to a lack of eye muscle coordination.

Spatial frequency channels: A hypothetical system used for the analysis of image fundamentals independent of their size.

General References

Brown, K. T. (1974). Physiology of the retina. *In* "Medical Physiology" (V. B. Mountcastle, ed.), 13th ed., pp. 458–496. Mosby, St. Louis, Missouri.

Davson, H., ed. (1976). "The Eye," 2nd ed., Vol. 2A. Academic Press, New York.

Davson, H., ed. (1976). "The Eye," 2nd ed., Vol. 2B. Academic Press, New York.

Gregory, R. L. (1972). "Eye and Brain, The Psychology of Seeing." Weidenfeld & Nicolson, London.

Gregory, R. L., and Gombrich, E. H., eds. (1973). "Illusion in Nature and Art." Duckworth, London.

Grobstein, P., and Chow, K. L. (1976). Receptive field organization in the mammalian visual cortex: The role of individual experience in development. *In* "Studies on the Development of Behavior and the Nervous System: Vol. 3, Neural and Behavioral Specificity" (G. Gottlieb, ed.), pp. 155–193. Academic Press, New York.

Held, R., and Hein, A. (1963). Movement-produced stimulation in the development of visually guided behavior. *J. Comp. Physiol. Psychol.* **56**, 872–876.

Kandel, R. R. (1977). Neuronal plasticity and the modification of behavior. *In* "Handbook of Physiology," (E. R. Kandel, ed.) Sect. 1, Part 2, pp. 1137–1182. Am. Physiol. Soc., Bethesda, Maryland.

Pettigrew, J. D. (1972). The neurophysiology of binocular vision. *Sci. Am.* **227**, 84–95.

Poggio, G. F. (1974). Central neural mechanisms in vision. *In* "Medical Physiology" (V. B. Mountcastle, ed.), 13th ed., Vol. 1, pp. 497–535. Mosby, St. Louis, Missouri.

References

Allman, J. M., and Kaas, J. H. (1976). Representation of the visual field on the medial wall of occipital-parietal cortex in the owl monkey. *Science* **191**, 572–575.

Baylor, D. A., Fuortes, M. G. F., and O'Bryan, P. M. (1971). Receptive fields of cones in the retina of the turtle. *J. Physiol. (London)* **214**, 265–294.

Blakemore, C. (1974). Development of functional connexions in the manmalian visual system. *Br. Med. Bull.* **30**, 152–157.

Blakemore, C. (1977). Genetic instructions and developmental plasticity in the kitten's visual cortex. *Philos. Trans. R. Soc. London, Ser. B* **278**, 425–434.

Blakemore, C., and Campbell, F. W. (1969). On the existence in the human visual system of neurons selectively sensitive to the orientation and size of retinal images. *J. Physiol. (London)* **203**, 237–260.

Blakemore, C., and Cooper, G. F. (1970). Development of the brain depends on the visual environment. *Nature (London)* **228**, 477–478.

Blakemore, C., and Sutton, P. (1969). Size adaptation: A new aftereffect. *Science* **166**, 245–247.

Blakemore, C., and Van Sluyters, R. C. (1975). Innate and environmental factors in the development of the kitten's visual cortex. *J. Physiol. (London)* **248**, 663–716.

Blakemore, C., Carpenter, R. H. S., and Georgeson, M. A. (1970). Lateral inhibition between orientation detectors in the human visual system. *Nature (London)* **228**, 37–39.

Blasdel, G. G., Mitchell, D. E., Muir, D. W., and Pettigrew, J. D. (1977). A physiological and behavioural study in cats of the effect of early visual experience with contours of a single orientation. *J. Physiol. (London)* **265**, 615–636.

Boycott, B. B., and Dowling, J. E. (1969). Organization of primate retina: Light microscopy. *Philos. Trans. R. Soc. London, Ser. B* **255**, 109–184.

Campbell, F. W. (1974). The transmission of spatial information through the visual system. *In* "The Neurosciences: Third Study Program," (F. O. Schmitt and F. G. Worden, eds.), pp. 95–103. MIT Press, Cambridge, Massachusetts.

Campbell, F. W., and Maffei, L. (1970). Electrophysiological evidence for the existence of orientation and size detectors in the human visual system. *J. Physiol. (London)* **207**, 635–652.

Campbell, F. W., and Robson, J. G. (1968). Application of Fourier analysis to the visibility of gratings. *J. Physiol. (London)* **197**, 551–566.

Campbell, F. W., Cooper, G. F., and Enroth-Cugell, C. (1969a). The spatial selectivity of the visual cells of the cat. *J. Physiol. (London)* **203**, 223–235.

Campbell, F. W., Cooper, G. F., Robson, J. G., and Sachs, M. B. (1969b). The spatial selectivity of visual cells of the cat and the squirrel monkey. *J. Physiol. (London)* **204**, 120–121.

Drujan, B. D., and Svaetichin, G. (1972). Characterization of different classes of isolated retinal cells. *Vision Res.* **12**, 1777–1784.

Duke-Elder, S. (1952). "Textbook of Opthalmology," Vol. 1. Henry Kimpton, Publ., London.

Granit, R. (1959). Neural activity in the retina. *In* "Handbook of Physiology" (H. W. Magoun and V. E. Hall, eds.), Sect. 1, Vol. I, pp. 693–712. Am. Physiol. Soc., Washington, D. C.

Granit, R. (1977). "The Purposive Brain." MIT Press, Cambridge, Massachusetts.

Gregory, R. L. (1972). "Eye and Brain, The Psychology of Seeing." Weidenfeld & Nicolson, London.

Gregory, R. L., and Gombrich, E. H., (1973). "Illusion in Nature and Art." Duckworth, London.

Guillery, R. W. (1970). The laminar distribution of retinal fibers in the dorsal lateral geniculate nucleus of the cat: A new interpretation. *J. Comp. Neurol.* **138**, 339–368.

Guillery, R. W., and Stelzner, D. J. (1970). The differential effects of unilateral lid closure upon the monocular and binocular segments of the dorsal lateral geniculate nucleus in the cat. *J. Comp. Neurol.* **139**, 413–422.

Harlow, H. F., and Harlow, M. K. (1962). Social deprivation in monkeys. *Sci. Am.* **207**, 136–146.

Hartline, H. K. (1940). The receptive fields of optic nerve fibers. *Am. J. Physiol.* **130**, 690–699.

Hecht, S., Schlaer, S., and Pirenne, M. R. (1942). Energy, quanta and vision. *J. Gen. Physiol.* **25**, 819–840.

Held, R., and Hein, A. (1963). Movement-produced stimulation in the development of visually guided behavior. *J. Comp. Physiol. Psychol.* **56**, 872–876.

Hirsch, H. V. B., and Spinelli, D. N. (1971). Modification of the distribution of receptive field orientation in cats by selective visual exposure during development. *Exp. Brain Res.* **12**, 509–527.

Hubel, D. H. (1957). Tungsten microelectrode for recording from single units. *Science* **125**, 549–550.

Hubel, D. H. (1959). Single unit activity in striate cortex of unrestrained cats. *J. Physiol. (London)* **147**, 226–238.

Hubel, D. H., and Wiesel, T. N. (1959). Receptive fields of single neurones in the cat's striate cortex. *J. Physiol. (London)* **148**, 547–591.

Hubel, D. H., and Wiesel, T. N. (1961). Integrative action in the cat's lateral geniculate body. *J. Physiol. (London)* **155**, 385–398.

Hubel, D. H., and Wiesel, T. N. (1962). Receptive fields, binocular interaction, and functional architecture in the cat's visual cortex. *J. Physiol. (London)* **160**, 106–154.

Hubel, D. H., and Wiesel, T. N. (1963). Receptive fields of cells in striate cortex of very young, visually inexperienced kittens. *J. Neurophysiol.* **26**, 994–1002.

Hubel, D. H., and Wiesel, T. N. (1965a). Receptive fields and functional architecture in two non-striate visual areas (18 and 19) of the cat. *J. Neurophysiol.* **28**, 229–289.

Hubel, D. H., and Wiesel, T. N. (1965b). Binocular interaction in striate cortex of kittens reared with artificial squint. *J. Neurophysiol.* **28**, 1041–1059.

Hubel, D. H., and Wiesel, T. N. (1970). The period of susceptibility to the physiological effects of unilateral eye closure in kittens. *J. Physiol. (London)* **206**, 419–436.

Hubel, D. H., and Wiesel, T. N. (1972). Laminar and columnar distribution of geniculo-cortical fibers in the macaque monkey. *J. Comp. Neurol.* **146**, 421–450.

Hubel, D. H., and Wiesel, T. N. (1974). Sequence regularity and geometry of orientation columns in the monkey striate cortex. *J. Comp. Neurol.* **158**, 267–294.

Hubel, D. H., Wiesel, T. N., and LeVay, S. (1977a). Plasticity of ocular dominance columns in monkey striate cortex. *Philos. Trans. R. Soc. London, Ser. B* **278**, 377–409.

Hubel, D. H., Wiesel, T. N., and Stryker, M. P. (1977b). Orientation columns in macaque monkey visual cortex demonstrated by the 2-deoxyglucose autoradiographic technique. *Nature (London)* **269**, 328–330.

Imbert, M., and Buisseret, P. (1975). Receptive field characteristics and plastic properties of visual cortical cells in kittens reared with or without visual experience. *Exp. Brain Res.* **22**, 25–36.

Kaneko, A. (1971). Electrical connexions between horizontal cells in the dogfish retina. *J. Physiol. (London)* 213, 95–105.

Kuffler, S. W. (1953). Discharge patterns and functional organization of the mammalian retina. *J. Neurophysiol.* 16, 37–68.

Kuffler, S. W., and Nicholls, J. G. (1976). "From Neuron To Brain." Sinauer Assoc., Sunderland, Massachusetts.

Maffei, L., and Fiorentini, A. (1972). Processes of synthesis in visual perception. *Nature (London)* 240, 479–481.

Naka, K. I., and Witkovsky, P. (1972). Dogfish ganglion cell discharge resulting from extrinsic polarization of the horizontal cells. *J. Physiol. (London)* 223, 449–460.

Nilsson, S. E. G. (1964). Receptor cell outer segment development and ultrastructure of the disk membranes in the retina of the tadpole (Rana pipiens). *J. Ultrastruct. Res.* 11, 518–620.

Pettigrew, J. D. (1978). The paradox of the critical period for striate cortex. *In* "Neuronal Plasticity" (C. Cotman, ed.), pp. 311–330. Raven, New York.

Pettigrew, J. D., Olson, C., and Hirsch, H. V. B. (1973). Cortical effect of selective visual experience: Degeneration or reorganization. *Brain Res.* 51, 345–351.

Pirenne, M. H. (1967). "Vision and the Eye." Chapman & Hall, London.

Popper, E. R., and Eccles, J. C. (1977). "The Self and Its Brain." Springer-Verlag, Berlin and New York.

Rakic, P. (1977). Prenatal development of the visual system in the rhesus monkey. *Philos. Trans. R. Soc. London, Ser. B* 278, 245–260.

Riesen, A. H. (1958). Plasticity of behavior: Psychological series. *In* "Biological and Biochemical Bases of Behavior" (H. F. Harlow and C. N. Woolsey, ed.), pp. 425–450. Univ. of Wisconsin Press, Madison.

Ripps, H., and Weale, R. H. (1976). The visual photoreceptors. *In* "The Eye" (H. Davson, ed.), 2nd ed., Vol. 2A, pp. 5–41. Academic Press, New York.

Rubin, E. (1950). Visual figures apparently incompatible with geometry. *Acta Psychol.* 7, 365–387.

"Science Year: The World Book Science Annual" (1972). Field Enterprises Education Corp., Chicago, Illinois, p. 142.

Singer, W. (1979). Neuronal mechanisms in experience dependent modification of visual cortex function. *In* "Development and Chemical Specificity of Neurons" (C. Akert, M. Cúenod, and F. Bloom, eds.) (in press).

Sokoloff, L., Reivich, M., Kennedy, C., Des Rosiers, M. H., Patlak, C. S., Pettigrew, K. D., Sakurada, O., and Shinohara, M. (1977). The [^{14}C]deoxyglucose method for the measurement of local cerebral glucose utilization: Theory, procedure and normal values in the conscious and anesthetized albino rat. *J. Neurochem.* 28, 897–917.

Steinberg, R. H. (1973). Scanning electron microscopy of the bullfrog's retina and pigment epithelium. *Z. Zellforsch. Mikrosk. Anat.* 143, 451–463.

Stryker, M. P., and Sherk, H. (1975). Modification of cortical orientation selectivity in the cat by restricted visual experience: A re-examination. *Science* 190, 904–906.

Sutherland, N. S. (1968). Outlines of a theory of visual pattern recognition in animals and man. *Proc. R. Soc. London, Ser. B* 171, 297–317.

von Senden, M. (1960). "Space and Sight: The Perception of Space and Shape in Congenitally Blind Before and After Operation." Free Press, Glencoe, Illinois.

Wald, G. (1950). Eye and camera. *Sci. Am.* 183, 32–41.

Wald, G. (1961). Retinal chemistry and the physiology of vision. *In* "Visual Problems of Color" (National Physical Lab. Symposium) pp. 15–68. Chem. Publ. Co., New York.

Wiesel, T. N., and Hubel, D. H. (1963). Single-cell responses in striate of kittens deprived of vision in one eye. *J. Neurophysiol.* 26, 1003–1017.

Wiesel, T. N., and Hubel, D. H. (1965a). Comparison of the effects of unilateral and bilateral eye closure on cortical unit responses in kittens. *J. Neurophysiol.* 28, 1029–1040.

Wiesel, T. N., and Hubel, D. B. (1965b). Extent of recovery from the effects of visual deprivation in kittens. *J. Neurophysiol.* 28, 1060–1072.

Wiesel, T. N., and Hubel, D. H. (1974). Ordered arrangement of orientation columns in monkeys lacking visual experience. *J. Comp. Neurol.* **158,** 307–318.

Wiesel, T. N., Hubel, D. H., and Lam, D. M. K. (1974). Autoradiographic demonstration of ocular-dominance columns in the monkey striate cortex by means of transneuronal transport. *Brain Res.* 79, 273–279.

Yarbus, A. L. (1967). "Eye Movements and Vision." Plenum, New York.

11

Moving

I. Introduction

Our behavior consists of movement. We are constantly in motion. We walk, run and sit. We communicate through movement—speak, gesture, make facial expressions. These eloquent movements are sometimes instinctive, but often the consequence of our sensory experience. We see, hear, feel, smell and taste and we smile, speak, laugh, walk and reach. The control of movement is essential for our daily behavior. Without motor responses we would be but statues.

All our movements are direct consequences of neural control of patterns of muscular contraction. This chapter explores the basic organization and function of motor systems. The goal is to provide an understanding of the mechanisms of some quite complex processes which at first glance might seem simple. Take walking, for example. Initially it might seem that walking consists merely of a right–left oscillation of the legs directed by the brain. But it is much more than that. First of all it is not really necessary to initiate each and every movement by thinking about it. Most movements, it turns out, are run by centrally controlled programs for responding. It is almost as if there is an instructional tape in the nervous system which the brain turns on and which then plays out instructions to move the legs back and forth in order to walk. Walking, however, also requires control over balance, and it requires built-in sets of contingency plans to step over objects, change directions, etc. Each process requires highly sophisticated computing and control.

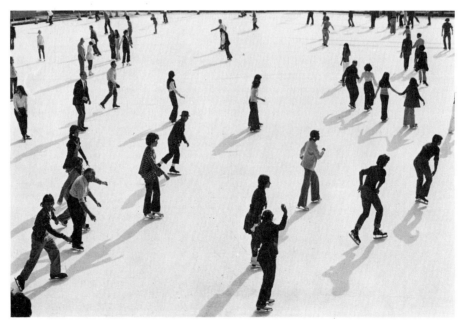

Courtesy of Michael Weisbrot and Family Photographers, Brooklyn, New York.

We shall start by describing some of the simple fundamental properties of motor systems. The first properties are the response characteristics of muscles driven by motor neurons. The motor system brings about contraction of muscles through neuromuscular transmission as discussed in Chapter 5, but the motor system also receives input or feedback from the muscles. Feedback is essential in some kinds of motor control, such as that involved in simply holding an arm outstretched. Without some type of feedback we could not keep an arm in the same position as different weights are placed in the hand, nor could we readjust with fatigue. Thus, Section II discusses receptor properties which provide feedback. We shall then progress to a discussion of more complex motor processes, such as walking, eye movements and how simple motor processes are modified by learning. It might prove helpful to scan the Summary prior to reading this chapter.

II.   The Output: Muscle Contractile Properties

We begin the discussion of control of movement with an analysis of the flexion and extension of the forearm. Figure 11-1 illustrates the organization of the muscles. A contracting muscle exerts a force on the bone through its connecting tendons. When the pulling force of the biceps is great enough, the forearm flexes.

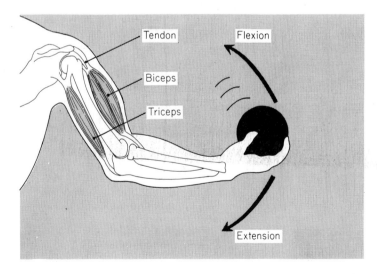

Fig. 11-1.   A simple movement, the flexion or extension of the forearm. When the biceps contracts the forearm flexes. Contraction of the triceps extends the forearm. When one muscle is active, the antagonist is relaxed.

Conversely when the contractile power of the triceps is sufficient, the forearm extends. _Flexion_ is a bending or movement toward the body, and _extension_ is a straightening or movement away from the body. Pairs of muscles, such as the biceps and triceps, which produce oppositely directed movements of a limb are known as _antagonists_.

Each motor neuron connects to several muscle fibers. The motor neuron and those muscle fibers it innervates is known as a _motor unit_. A motor unit is the quantal element of organized motor activity (Fig. 11-2).

The total _tension_ in a muscle depends upon two factors: (1) the number of muscle fibers in the muscle that are contracting at any given time which depends on the number of active motor neurons and (2) the contractile properties of the individual motor units. The contractile properties of motor units may be described in relation to twitch time, twitch tension, and fatigability. In order to evaluate these properties, the axon of a single motor neuron is stimulated while the tension from the resulting contraction of the motor unit's muscle fibers is recorded. The contractile properties of a motor unit are related both to the biochemical characteristics of the muscle fibers making up the motor unit and the

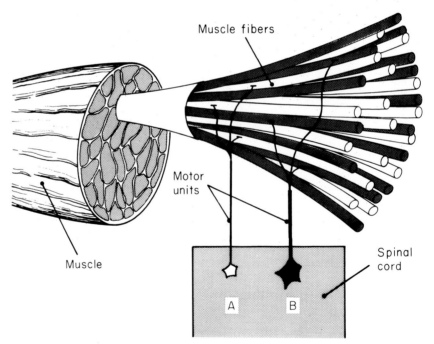

Fig. 11-2. Muscle fibers associated with two motor neurons forming two motor units within a muscle. There are two distinct types of motor units: slow twitch motor units which are innervated by small motor neurons and which connect to slow twitch muscle (A) and fast twitch motor units which are innervated by large motor neurons and which connect to fast twitch muscle (B).

properties of the spinal motor neuron whose axon innervates these muscle fibers. Table 11-1 summarizes the factors determining the properties of motor units.

Table 11-1 Factors determining the properties of motor units

1. Motor neuron characteristics
   a. Synaptic inputs
   b. Membrane properties
   c. Axonal diameter
2. Muscle fiber characteristics
   a. Size and membrane properties
   b. Biochemical characteristics of contractile proteins

More than one type of motor unit makes up a given muscle. At one extreme are the "*slow twitch*" motor units; they are small, have relatively long duration twitches and are resistant to fatigue. They tend to be innervated by small motor neurons that usually generate relatively small peak twitch tensions. At the other extreme in the distribution of motor units are "*fast twitch*" units; they are larger, generate large peak tensions but fatigue rapidly. These fast twitch, fast fatigue units tend to be innervated by larger motor neurons with axons of greater diameter and high conduction velocity. Within a given muscle the hundreds of fibers of one motor unit are intermixed with fibers of other motor units (Fig. 11-2).

It is possible to identify individual motor units histochemically by the disappearance of glycogen stores after intense stimulation. Activated motor units do not stain for glycogen, since their store of glucose is depleted with repeated contractions (Kugelberg, 1973). The fast twitch, fast fatigue motor units stain more intensely for myofibrilar ATPase (an energy utilizing enzyme in their constituent fibrils) than do the slow twitch motor units (Fig. 11-3). The difference in ATPase activity illustrates only one of the key biochemical properties of muscles associated with differences in twitch times of the two extreme types of motor units.

The importance of these motor unit properties for movement is seen in the sequence in which different motor units of a muscle come into play. This sequence, called *recruitment order*, refers to the successive calling up (or "recruiting") of individual motor units as the tension generated by the muscle rises. In flexing the biceps of the arm, slow twitch units, which are fatigue resistant and which generate relatively small tensions, are the first to be called into action. Last to be recruited are the fast fatigue, fast twitch units which generate large peak tensions. These units are brought into play only under conditions which require extreme tensions as, for example, the presence of a heavy ball in one's hand. The fast twitch units are called up last and put to rest first; they are the power units

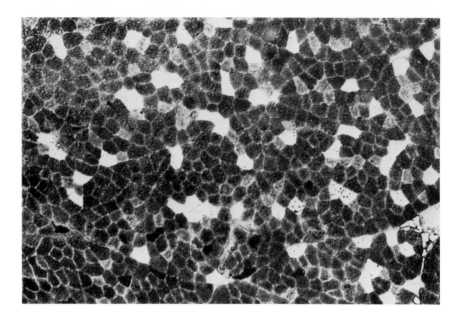

Fig. 11-3. Cross section of a muscle stained for ATPase. The fast twitch units have high ATPase activity so they stain darkly. × 150. (From Kugelberg, 1973.)

called in when the slow twitch units need reinforcement. The fast twitch units are innervated by bigger motor neurons, and their muscle fibers are bigger. They are the "bulge" in the weight-lifters' muscles. The largest motor unit in some muscles (e.g., the medial gastrocnemius or calf muscle) can develop approximately 240 times as much tension as the smallest unit.

Sometimes we need to move quickly with a great deal of force, while at other times we must slowly grade the force of response. Under conditions in which the overall tension of a muscle must rise abruptly, little recruitment order is seen. Virtually all motor units are activated simultaneously. However, when an order of recruitment takes place, it is always the smaller fatigue-resistant units which become active first and the fast twitch high-tension units last. Small tensions are produced and precisely controlled by selective mobilization of various numbers of small motor neurons. When the total output must be increased, larger motor neurons are activated, as previously described. But such neurons never become active without prior or simultaneous participation of the small units. This order of recruitment is called the "*size principle*" (Henneman, 1968).

In summary, much of the fine control of movement comes from the properties of motor units. The mechanical force generated is set by their tension generating properties, their recruitment order and the tension generating capabilities of the individual muscle fibers that make them up. These properties

11. MOVING

combined with the efficient rigging of the individual muscles on the skeleton and the lever arm skeletal characteristics are the foundations of movement. Next we shall turn to the nature of receptor properties of the muscles.

III. The Input: Muscle Receptor Properties

Much of the input which drives the motor neurons arises from feedback from the muscles. Embedded within skeletal muscles are *receptors* which monitor muscle length and tension. Information from these receptors passes into the central nervous system to mediate local reflexes which provide a negative feedback control over muscle length and tension. The knee jerk (or patellar tendon) reflex commonly used by physicians as a test of spinal reflexes is an example of a local reflex. Information from muscle receptors, however, is also relayed to higher centers, such as the cerebellum, where it is integrated with other types of input. The maintenance of muscle stretch through these local reflexes is extraordinarily important. Without muscle tension in our legs, for example, we would fall in a heap upon the floor. We must always fight the pull of gravity.

Muscle receptors are of two types. One type (the *Golgi tendon organ*) senses tension; the other type (the *muscle spindle*) senses muscle length. The organization of these receptors in a muscle is shown in Figs. 11-4 and 11-5. Muscle has embedded within it slender modified muscle fibers within a fusiform bag of connective tissue called a muscle spindle. Each of these little fibers, which contribute nothing to the tension developed by the muscle, has a spiral-like ending called a *primary ending* wrapped around its center (Fig. 11-4). When stretched, the primary ending sends a volley of impulses to the spinal cord. Primary endings from muscle spindles are excitatory for the motor neurons sending axons back to the muscles in which the receptors are located. Thus, an increase in the length of a muscle stretches the spindles located in the muscle. This gives rise to increased activity of spindle receptors, which in turn monosynaptically activate motor neurons innervating the stretched muscle. Activation of these motor neurons causes contraction of the muscle, and thus opposes the increase in length which initiated the sequence.

The Golgi tendon organ is a very different type of muscle receptor. It is located on the muscle tendon (Fig. 11-5), and it is exquisitely sensitive to tension (or force) rather than length. Its central connections lead to disynaptic inhibition through spinal interneurons of the motor neurons supplying the muscle where the tension receptor lies. Increased muscle tension increases Golgi activity, which is then fed back to motor neurons to reduce muscle tension. The Golgi activity activates an inhibitory interneuron, which in turn decreases the firing of the motor neuron and relieves muscle tension. Thus, both length and tension recep-

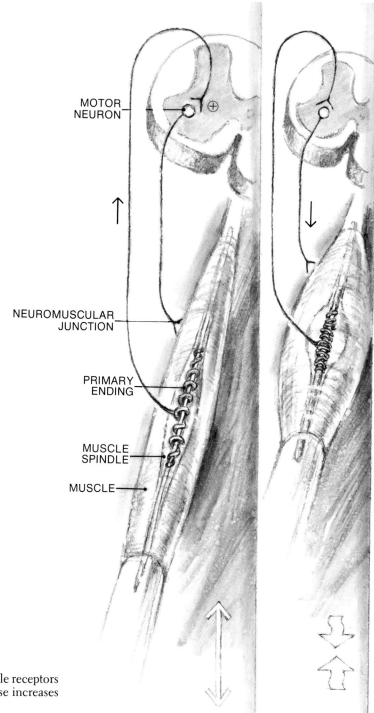

MOTOR
NEURON

NEUROMUSCULAR
JUNCTION

PRIMARY
ENDING

MUSCLE
SPINDLE

MUSCLE

Fig. 11-4. Spindle receptors which act to oppose increases in muscle length.

468

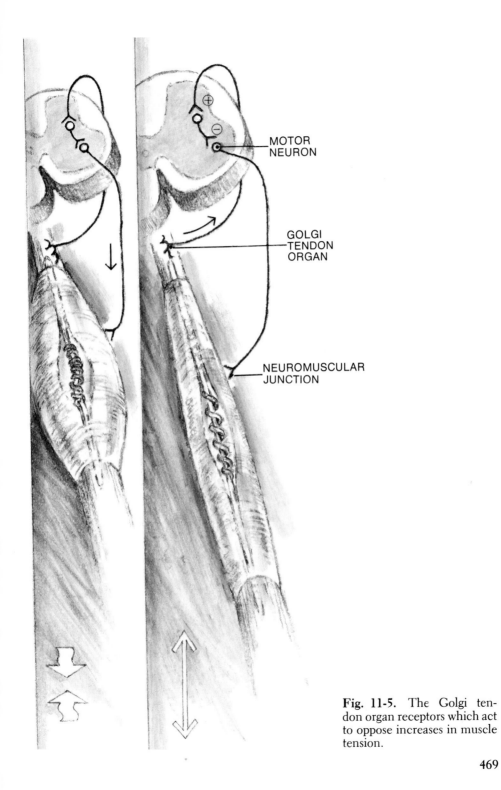

MOTOR
NEURON

GOLGI
TENDON
ORGAN

NEUROMUSCULAR
JUNCTION

Fig. 11-5. The Golgi tendon organ receptors which act to oppose increases in muscle tension.

469

tors may be viewed as components in a negative feedback control system—a servo system—which tends to maintain postural *stability* by resisting changes of muscle length and muscle tension.

To clarify the operation of this servomechanism, let us consider a person trying to hold his arm out straight (Fig. 11-6). In this situation a decrease of tension in the muscles opposing the forces of gravity will be followed by an increase in muscle length. The result will be decreased activity in tension receptors and increased activity in length receptors. Although these represent opposite changes in impulse frequencies, their ultimate effects on muscle activity reinforce each other. The decreased activity of the tension receptors (which are disynaptically inhibitory) relieves the motor neuron pool from inhibition, while the increased discharge in muscle receptors directly excites the same motor neuron pool. Both of these effects (reduced inhibition and increased excitation) will lead to increased discharge frequency of motor neurons and thereby cause increased contraction of the muscle. The muscle will thus act to correct the transient decrease in tension which gave rise to the process in the first place. In this way, we overcome a transient decrease in tension and maintain the outstretched arm in a stable position.

Conversely, increased tension during maintained tonic contraction will produce the opposite pattern of change in muscle receptors: an increase in tension resulting in a decrease in muscle length will lead to increased discharge of tension receptors and decreased discharge of muscle length receptors. The central consequences of this pattern of change will be decreased excitation of the motor neuron pool by length receptors and increased inhibition of the motor neuron pool by way of the inhibitory interneuron mediating the disynaptic inhibitory effects of the tension receptors. These two effects (decreased excitation and increased inhibition) will diminish the discharge frequency of the motor neuron pool, and the result will be decreased muscle activity. Again, the arm stays in a stable position.

Causes for variations in muscle tension may lie within the muscle itself or within the motor pool. Within a muscle, tension may fall with fatigue. From the motor neuron pool, fluctuations of output arise as a result of variations in regulating drive to motor neurons from many other parts of the nervous system. These variations occur even when the subject seeks to remain motionless. The servo action of the muscle receptors continuously "clamps" and "damps" the muscle against instabilities of all these kinds.

These servo actions controlling muscle activity thus seem well designed to maintain postural stability rather than to allow motion. So how is movement achieved? To see how the muscle and its receptors are used during motion, we have to consider the systems which control, and are in turn controlled by, events in the muscle and its receptors.

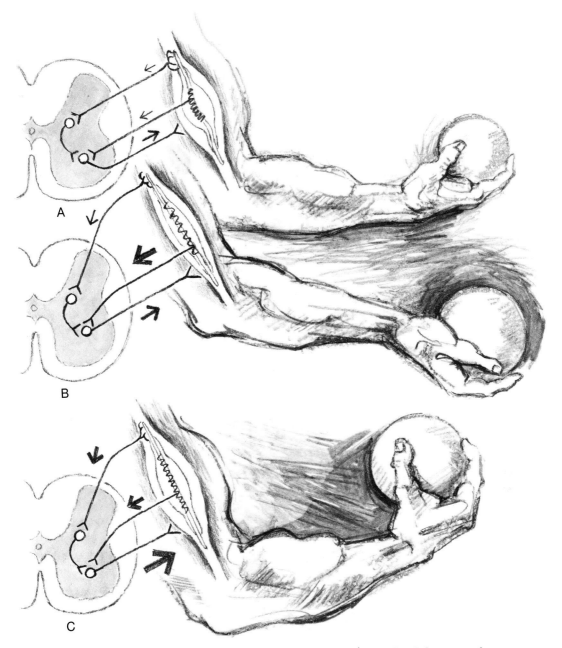

Fig. 11-6. Control of forearm stability through local reflexes by feedback from muscle receptors. When the arm drops (B) stretch receptors send more impulses (thick arrow) to the spinal cord and drive the motor neuron. Tension receptors send fewer impulses and reduce the inhibition on the motor neuron. Both actions work to increase muscle tension (C).

IV. Concepts in Motor Control

Our understanding of mechanisms involved in control of movement began almost a century ago. The concepts evolved from the work of Sherrington and his students (e.g., Eccles and Granit) on the spinal cord. We shall see that motor systems are called upon to direct a continuum of movement. The patterns of movement are rich and varied as in walking and writing, and the classes of movement are far-ranging. There are three classes of movements. Some are brief, swift and darting; others are continuous and slow. Finally, just maintaining stability—holding still and maintaining skeletal position—is a motor task. The neural systems behind the scenes commanding movements commonly involve central programs and feedback and feedforward design concepts. We shall discuss how these organizing principles serve movement. The general principles revealed by studies of spinal cord motor neurons apply, as well, to operations throughout the nervous system. This section considers some of these basic concepts and general principles.

A. Motion and Stability

Motor systems have a dual purpose: they maintain stability and they generate motion. These two contrasting purposes of motor systems, stability and motion, are illustrated by the operation of the *oculomotor system*, the system that controls eye movement. The function of this system is to bring the fovea of the retina (the region where vision is sharpest) into alignment with a visual target of interest and to maintain this alignment. In even such a seemingly simple movement such as the control of the eye there are distinctive movements: rapid search or saccadic eye movements, smooth pursuit tracking, and movements governed by the semicircular canals (the vestibulo-ocular reflex).

1. SACCADIC EYE MOVEMENTS. We are constantly shifting our eyes from position to position from one object to another, often without a head movement. There are alternate periods of fixation and shift, fixation and shift, etc. These shifts of fixation, of which we are usually unaware, are saccadic eye movements. They represent a scanning of the field of view—a search for targets. The magnitude of *saccadic eye movements* varies widely. Fixation is not always perfect and is sometimes marked by small corrective shifts and drifts of eye position. As shifts reach a certain critical magnitude, the misalignment off the *fovea* (called retinal slip) leads to a correction which brings about a tiny corrective saccadic eye movement. The angular velocity of this movement may reach 500°/second. This is the fastest movement the body performs.

2. SMOOTH PURSUIT TRACKING. This voluntary eye movement is used in tracking an object (a fly or an airplane, for example) as it moves in the visual field. The signal for tracking arises from the retina. _Smooth pursuit movement_ involves detection of retinal slip. Movement of the eyes is also required to track a visual object which changes in its depth of field. As an object comes closer the eyes turn inward and as it recedes the eyes turn outward.

3. VESTIBULO-OCULAR REFLEX. The _vestibulo-ocular reflex_ (VOR) is a response that serves to maintain a stable retinal image in response to head movement. The VOR, as the name implies, is a simple reflex. In discussing saccadic eye movements, we referred to situations in which there may be no associated head movement. However, in viewing an object, the target on the fovea must be maintained under conditions in which the subject is voluntarily moving the head. Stability of the retinal image during head movements is achieved in the following way. As the head is moved, input from the vestibular organs corresponding to head velocity generates an equal but oppositely directed eye movement. For example, for a given change in head position of 10° there is an equal 10° movement of the retina in the opposite direction (Fig. 11-7). The net effect of equal and opposite head and eye movements will be to stabilize the retinal image on the fovea—to keep the eyes on target.

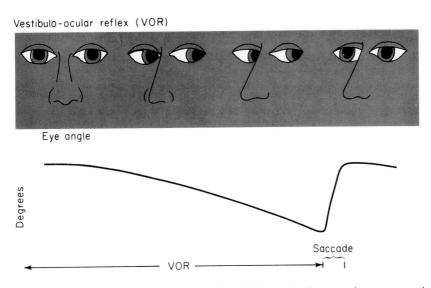

Fig. 11-7. Vestibulo-ocular reflex (VOR). The VOR maintains gaze in compensation for small rotations in head position. As the head turns slowly in a horizontal plane the eyes move slowly in the opposite direction (first three sequences). With large head rotations the eyes shift upon a new center position. This ballistic shift is called saccadic eye movement (fourth sequence). The VOR does not depend on visual input, since it occurs in the dark; it is a vestibular reflex, since it is absent when there is no vestibular input.

IV. CONCEPTS IN MOTOR CONTROL   473

The oculomotor system is truly a remarkable system. It moves the eye slowly or rapidly, and it generates motion to maintain a fixed gaze when the head moves. It elegantly demonstrates the concepts of motion and stability. We shall return again to the VOR in subsequent sections on plasticity of reflexive movement.

B. Ballistic and Continuously Controlled Movements

In a very general way, there are two types of movement: (1) ballistic or rapid movements and (2) continuously controlled movements. The concepts of ballistic and continuously controlled movement have for the most part evolved in relation to movements of the legs and arms, but they are at least parallel to the concepts of saccadic and smooth pursuit eye movements. A *ballistic movement* is like the flight of a cannon ball: its trajectory is determined by a brief initial application of energy, without the possibility of subsequent controlled modification of the flight. Thus, a ballistic movement is predetermined by the initial forces applied—the die is cast so to speak.

Continuously controlled movements, on the other hand, are subject to continuous modification throughout their course, either by fluctuations in the drive to the motor neuron pool from higher systems or by feedback from peripheral receptors. Although these two idealized concepts have proved useful, we should keep in mind that in the real world of movement they are not mutually exclusive. Even ballistic movements are subject to continuous control by reflex action. Saccadic eye movements, for example, are ballistic movements par excellence, and yet when movement of the head occurs concurrently, vestibular feedback will continuously control their magnitude by way of the VOR. Figure 11-8 illustrates that a saccadic eye movement can be modified by concurrent inputs from the vestibular system.

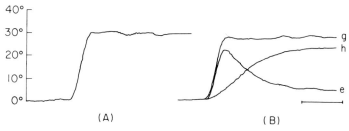

Fig. 11-8. Comparison of saccadic eye movements and gaze. (A) Saccadic eye movements to a suddenly appearing target with head fixed. (B) Coordinated saccadic eye movements (e) and head movement (h) to the same target with head free. The gaze movement (g) represents the sum of e and h. Note the remarkable similarity of saccadic eye movements in (A) and gaze trajectory in (B) as well as reduced saccadic amplitude in (B). Time calibration 100 msec. (From Morasso *et al.*, 1973.)

C. Centrally Programmed and Peripherally Driven Movements

Thus, so far we have seen that movements lie on a continuum. At one extreme are movements whose functions are to maintain stability; at the other extreme are movements whose functions are to produce change. Many of the neural mechanisms underlying stability continue to operate during periods of change and thereby allow the change to be smooth and accurate. We have also seen that movements are, in essence, of two types—ballistic (brief, swift, darting, predetermined) or continuously controlled (continuous and slow with the possibility of continuous modification). Next, we shall examine the concept of centrally programmed movements.

Consider chewing for a moment. Chewing is a type of movement pattern which illustrates the concept of centrally programmed movement. Imagine having to think about every movement in chewing. It would, indeed, be unfortunate if we had to devote our mental activities to each and every minute routine movement. Central programs provide mechanisms so that we can carry out certain action patterns on "automatic pilot." Central programs, once triggered, play out a complex movement pattern much as a musical tape plays a particular song when it is started.

In 1899, Woodworth noted that ballistic limb movements could not be modified by changed visual inputs and was led to the concept that such movements were driven by a central program which, once generated, was uninfluenced by feedback. This concept of a centrally programmed movement was contrasted with the concept of a peripherally driven movement. In its extreme form, the peripherally driven movement was viewed as a slavish response of the motor neuron pool to a peripheral input. However, as early as 1917, Lashley attacked the concept of the peripherally driven movement by noting that human subjects carried out movements even though they lacked sensory feedback because of damage to afferent neural systems. More recently, experiments in invertebrate preparations have reinforced the view that central neural structures can produce motor output in the absence of peripheral input.

Real movements are both centrally programmed and peripherally controlled. Controlled interaction is more often the case than either pure centrally programmed movement or pure peripheral control.

One class of movements in which sensory input and central programs interact is the class of movements which involve "triggering" of a central program by a peripheral stimulus. A number of such triggered movements have been studied in invertebrate preparations. Such research has led to the important concept of *command interneurons*, as discussed by Delong (1971).

Larimer and Kennedy (1969a,b), for example, have identified a specific interneuron in the crayfish abdominal cord that produces a complex cyclic series of movements in the tail appendages even when stimulated at constant frequencies; the rhythm of the movements is unrelated to the rhythm of the stimulation. The output to the individual muscles is patterned in a rhythmical manner, with dozens of motor neurons discharging, each at a particular phase of the cycle. The output follows the same "motor score" from one animal to another, and is undisturbed by total deafferentation. Again, central connections automatically determine the output.

Examples of triggered central patterning in mammals are less numerous than in arthropods. However, swallowing in mammals provides an excellent example. Doty and his colleagues have shown that the act of swallowing involves the coordination of nearly 20 different muscles whose motor neurons are distributed from mesencephalic to posterior medullary levels (Doty, 1968; Doty and Bosma, 1956; Doty et al., 1967). The patterning of muscular contractions is independent of the stimulus used to evoke the response, i.e., touching the pharynx, rapid injection of water into the mouth or electrical stimulation of the superior laryngeal nerve. Attempts to alter the pattern by disturbing feedback loops, i.e., by excision of the participating muscles, fixation of the hyoid mass, or traction on the tongue, fail to bring about any significant change in the patterning. The neurons responsible for the coordination have been shown to be situated bilaterally just dorsal and rostral to the rostral pole of the inferior olive. These neurons form a "swallowing center," which is viewed as a "functional neuronal grouping interconnected in such a manner as to produce automatically, when it is effectively excited, the inhibitory and excitatory sequences in appropriate motor neurons" (Doty, 1968).

The triggering or initiation of most behavioral acts of any complexity requires a "decision" by the CNS that certain criteria have been met. The "decision" in the case of triggered movements is of an "either-or" nature. One possibility, as exemplified by the Mauthner cell or the giant fiber system of arthropods, is that a single neuron may act as a decision-maker. Convergence of appropriate input on a single cell may initiate a single impulse that releases a complex behavioral response. A second possibility for decision-making within the CNS is a network of mutually interacting neurons, with a threshold for the network that is different from that for any one cell. The excitability of the network as a whole must reach a definite level before it becomes active (Bullock and Horridge, 1965) (Delong, 1971, pp. 18–19).

While the concept of the command neuron evolved from work on invertebrates, it is now applied widely to other systems. One may even think of the output neurons of the cerebral motor cortex in primates as analogues of the command neurons of invertebrates. Such neurons, as described in Chapter 2, send axons through the corticospinal tract and other routes to many different levels and stations in the nervous system, just as the axons of command neurons in invertebrates fan out to activate and coordinate the many elements involved in a complex pattern of motor activity. We know that these neurons in the motor cortex can act as command elements in the absence of any peripheral input, but these same cells, which can be discharged by internal events (thoughts?) in the absence of peripheral signals, also receive strong inputs from the receptors located in the body part which they control. This feedback of sensory input onto command elements has been demonstrated in a number of recent studies in invertebrates. Thus, the concept of a command neuron operating independently of feedback from the movements that it controls has now been replaced by a concept of command elements which control patterns of neuronal activity and which receive feedback from the systems they control.

D.   Feedback and Feedforward Control

The next basic concept is feedback and feedforward control. Feedback and feedforward control, as emphasized in Chapter 2, are common features of the nervous system. They are widely used principles in the spinal cord, vestibular system, cerebellum and throughout the rest of the brain. In *feedback* the output acts back on the system (Fig. 11-9A). The simplest type of feedback control is one in which a disturbance of the controlled output generates nerve impulses whose central connections are such as to overcome the disturbance and thereby to nullify the nerve activity induced by the disturbance. Feedback influences are illustrated, for example, by the *vestibulospinal reflex*, which maintains stability of head position in space. The vestibulospinal reflex is activated whenever a subject moves while seeking at the same time to maintain the head in a stable orientation. In this situation, impulses arising in the inner ear (vestibular apparatus) as a result of movements of the head pass to neurons in the vestibular nuclei. These, in turn, connect with motor neurons of the neck muscles, whose reflex activation controls the muscles which oppose head movements. Such opposition tends to reduce the output of the vestibular system which generated the correction and, thus, promotes head stability. The overall effect is to eliminate the vestibular signal which generated the reflex. Feedback thus promotes stability by arresting the disturbance.

In contrast to this closed-loop negative feedback system, there are other systems which operate *"open loop"* and in which feedback, in the sense referred to in the previous paragraph, does not exist. A controller is introduced in the circuit which modifies the output as illustrated in Fig. 11-9B. One such open-loop system is the VOR. Here the reflex output (movement of the eyes) has no effect at all on the vestibular activity which generates the reflex. Thus, the VOR is an open-loop control system (i.e., it has no feedback); whereas the vestibulospinal reflex is a closed-loop control system.

In summary, feedback systems operate when the output acts back on the system in a way to modify the output. In accord with the concepts of systems analysis feedback systems, as the name implies, are *closed-loop systems*. Feedforward systems are those in which controllers within the system can modify the output. Feedforward systems are open-loop systems.

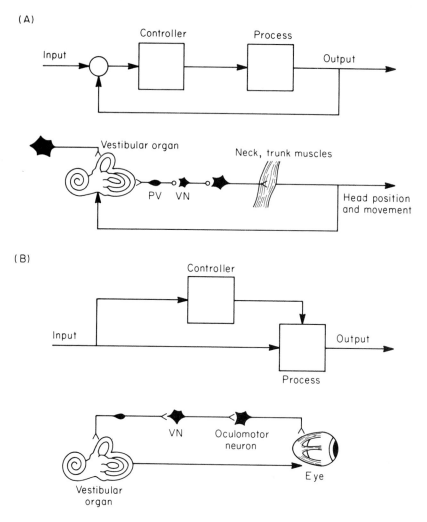

Fig. 11-9. Feedback and feedforward control systems. (A) Block diagram for a feedback system. The vestibulospinal reflex makes use of this principle. PV, primary neuron; VN, vestibular nuclei cell. (B) Block diagram for a feedforward system. The vestibulo-ocular reflex arc illustrates this concept.

At birth the VOR is relatively ineffective in stabilizing the retinal image, but it is gradually and accurately calibrated as maturation takes place. The improvement in effectiveness depends on the visual experience of the developing animal. But, how can the reflex be calibrated? The answer is that it uses a memory system. The calibration cannot be achieved by simple negative feedback, since the VOR is an open loop. A different type of regulation must operate, which is referred to as

478

"feedforward" control. The term *feedforward control* implies that with each occurrence of the VOR a central "memory" records the consequences of the particular pattern of activity associated with the reflex. The success or failure of each reflex will be measured in terms of the extent to which the VOR has prevented "slip" of the fovea image, i.e., the extent to which head movement is exactly counterbalanced by an equal and opposite eye movement. If the reflex has overcorrected eye position in relation to movements of the head, then the memory system provides a feedforward signal which reduces the effectiveness of the synaptic contacts between the vestibular afferent fibers and links in the VOR. Alternatively, if the reflex has undercorrected, then the feedforward control system receives information from the memory system concerning retinal slip in the opposite direction and provides a control signal which increases effectiveness of vestibular inputs.

In summary, we have emphasized the four basic concepts of motor control. First, we learned that motor systems have a dual purpose. They generate motion and they maintain stability. We used the oculomotor system to illustrate this dual purpose. The VOR maintains stability while saccadic eye movements and smooth pursuit tracking movements generate change. Second, we have identified that movements can be considered ballistic or continuously controlled; these are the extremes in a continuum of motility. In the real world of motion, the output of the motor neuron is under a number of different controls simultaneously. Third, we have discovered that movement may be centrally programmed, "driven" by command neurons and, yet at the same time, peripherally controlled. Some movements, moreover, have central programs which have been built-in with experience. Fourth, we have identified two of the fundamental features of circuit design in the CNS: feedback and feedforward control. Feedback control gives the system stability by damping a reaction to a disturbance after the response. Feedforward control introduces a controller into the circuit so that a response can be modified.

With this foundation we are well prepared to discuss the ways the brain, spinal cord and peripheral motor circuitry command muscles and deliver motion. We shall begin, as did early physiologists, at the level of the spinal cord.

V. Spinal Cord Control and Organization

The motor system can be conveniently divided into spinal and supraspinal centers. Supraspinal centers include the basal ganglia, cerebellum and motor cortex.

The traditional experimental approach to studying the motor system has been to separate spinal from supraspinal centers by spinal transection, creating the so-called "spinal animals." It was in spinal preparations, in fact, that Sherrington made many of his important observations on the integrative action of the nervous system. His studies, together with more recent experiments have uncovered the principles of neural organization which apply to all levels of the nervous system.

Sherrington (1947) spoke of transsection of the spinal cord as creating two animals: one a spinal reflex creature, the other an animal which sees, smells, hears and has emotions but cannot move. It would be easy to conclude that the creature below the spinal transsection is inert. In fact, however, this is not the case. The spinal dog, for example, displays scratching, certain forms of reflexive locomotion, and sucking, carried out without obvious abnormality.

In elucidating the capacity of the spinal cord to generate and control movement, two forms of motor activity exhibited by the spinal animal have been particularly useful: scratching and locomotion.

A.   Scratch Reflex Organization in the Spinal Animal

Sherrington (1947) found that within a few months following transsection of the cervical spinal cord, a scratch reflex could be elicited by mechanical stimuli (e.g., tickling the skin, pulling lightly on the hair) applied within a large saddle-shaped region over the upper part of the body. The scratching movements consisted of rhythmic alternate flexion and extension at the hip, knee and ankle. One of the first questions investigated was the neural mediation of this intraspinal reflex. By making lesions at various levels within the spinal cord, Sherrington discovered that severance of a lateral region of white matter within the spinal cord permanently abolished the reflex. The intrinsic fibers mediating the reflex pass through this region directly connecting the gray matter of the spinal segments from the shoulder with the spinal segments for the leg.

The scratch reflex in the chronic *spinal animal* is triggered by a cutaneous stimulus, and, while intact afferents from a particular spot on the skin are essential to initiate the reflex, subsequent input from the rhythmically moving hindlimb is not necessary for the scratching. Sherrington demonstrated that the deafferented hindlimb could participate almost normally in the scratch reflex. This finding was one of the first to demonstrate what we now refer to as *centrally programmed movement*.

The clearest demonstration that scratching is under executive control of a central program comes from studies on the scratch reflex in spinal animals

(Arshavsky *et al.*, 1975a,b). In such experiments the scratch reflex is elicited by electrical stimulation within the spinal cord, and the detailed agenda of muscle activity underlying the scratch reflex is examined (Fig. 11-11). Even in the absence of afferent inflow, the spinal mechanism is capable of generating the main features of the scratching movements—the frequency of oscillating movements and phases of activity of individual muscles. Since the frequency of oscillation and phase relations do not change after deafferentation, these characteristics are determined by the central program of scratching and not by tonic afferent inflow or peripheral feedback. In this respect, scratching is similar to other highly patterned movements, such as chewing and swallowing.

Does the rhythmical process originating in the isolated spinal cord have any importance to the nervous system acting as a whole? It would seem that the brain should know what business the spinal cord is about, lest the brain call for walking while the spinal cord is orchestrating scratching. Some pretty confused limb movements could result! In order to sudy such interactions, the animal may be curarized (given curare which blocks neuromuscular transmission) so that all movement is prevented. In such a preparation the neural activity which would ordinarily accompany the scratch reflex occurs relatively normally, but there is no movement. The term *"fictive scratching"* has been employed in reference to the central events of scratching without the actual movement (Fig. 11-10).

By studying "fictive scratching" it has been possible to determine the consequences for the nervous system as a whole of a rhythmical process originating within the spinal cord and occurring without any afferent feedback. Studies of the activity of neurons of the *ventral spinocerebellar tract* (VSCT) during "fictive scratching" show that such upwardly communicating neurons are rhythmically modulated in phase with the scratching movement. Since there is no afferent input during the "fictive scratching," it follows that the rhythmical discharge of these neurons must have been set up through intraspinal connections. Furthermore, since the rhythmical activity in VSCT neurons is sent to the cerebellum, it follows that this tract carries information about events within the spinal cord itself. This observation (that VSCT activity is driven by internal spinal mechanisms) provides a clear example of what has come to be called *"corollary discharge."*

Rhythmical activity in VSCT generates cerebellar rhythms which in turn will have consequences for the brain as a whole. An example of this spread of rhythmical activity from a spinal generator to other parts of the nervous system has been seen in the rhythmical activity of vestibulospinal neurons sending axons to the lumbosacral spinal cord. In the intact animal, activity of the vestibulospinal neurons might be expected to play a role in the postural stability necessary to maintain upright posture during scratching. If we were to observe such discharge

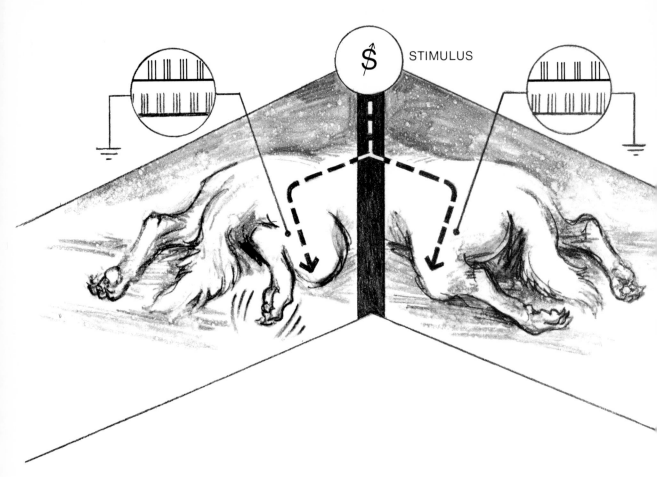

STIMULUS

FICTIVE SCRATCHING

Fig. 11-10. Direct electrical stimulation of certain places in the spinal cord elicits a rhythmic pattern of efferent activity to the muscles and causes scratching (*left*). The record shows the alternate activation of the flexor and extensor muscles which generates the muscle movement underlying scratching. This efferent activity is generated by central programming since the pattern is independent of peripheral feedback. The same pattern is present in the absence of movement (*right*). Scratching in the absence of movement is called "fictive scratching."

of vestibulospinal neurons in the intact animal, we might assume that the discharge was due to inputs from the vestibular system. Now we can see, however, how the periodic modulation of activity in vestibulospinal neurons can be achieved by rhythmical activity coming up from the spinal cord, even without afferent input from the vestibular system.

How does the rhythmical activity originating in the spinal cord reach the vestibulospinal neurons? It has been shown that it reaches the vestibulospinal neurons by way of the cerebellum. During scratching, a pattern generator within the spinal cord sends correlated signals to the cerebellum via the VSCT and, from that information, the cerebellum transmits modulatory signals to the neurons of the vestibular nuclei. The entire sequence, we should remember, is mediated by internal connections and occurs in the absence of afferent signals from the periphery.

The observed changes in discharge of VSCT neurons and vestibulospinal neurons in "fictive scratching" provide two examples of instances in which central programs modify the discharge of elements which are *also* modulated by peripheral sensory inputs. This "*dual modulation*" turns out to be a cardinal feature of centrally programmed movement; central programs modify the activity not only of motor neurons but also of the sensory elements which will receive feedback as a result of the movements resulting from motor neuronal discharge. A centrally programmed movement thus involves *coordinated* control of excitability in both afferent and efferent systems.

B.   Locomotion in the Spinal Animal

How does our nervous system direct walking? Walking is a typical repetitive sequence of limb movements. It is, however, highly complex. Just as we had to learn to walk in stages, so we need to analyze the mechanisms of walking in stages. We shall initially need to use a relatively simple preparation, the spinal animal, to analyze the features of walking.

Rhythmical progression, stepping, and other repetitive limb movements can be elicited in spinal animals whose weight is supported and whose feet are placed on a treadmill. Just as experiments employing curarization and deafferentation have shown that scratching can be centrally programmed, so too such experimental manipulations have demonstrated intrinsic spinal generators for locomotion. Of course, locomotion in a spinal animal is far from normal, but its existence and the principles by which it is controlled provide an understanding of the elementary mechanisms of motor organization that underlie walking. Before considering these principles, however, it will be useful to consider locomotion as it exists in the spinal animal in the proper relation to locomotion in the intact animal. During ambulation a person or animal has to deal with at least three different tasks (Grillner, 1975) (Fig. 11-11).

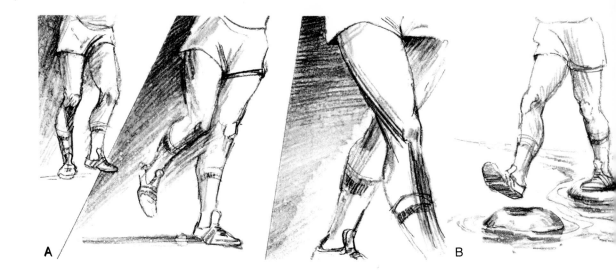

WALKING

Fig. 11-11. (A) The actual locomotor movements of the different limbs must proceed according to a rather stereotyped plan, back and forth, for example.

(B) These movements must adapt to external conditions in order to accomplish purposeful locomotion so as to achieve various goals. Furthermore, we must continuously anticipate where to put down our foot and make adjustments. We must place the limb properly on a stone and not in a hole.

(C) Equilibrium must be maintained during the movements. The projection of the center of gravity must fall in an optimally stable point between the moving points of support and be maintained within rather narrow limits. In order to accomplish this, a whole set of different compensating mechanisms operates to enable us to counteract various types of unexpected perturbations.

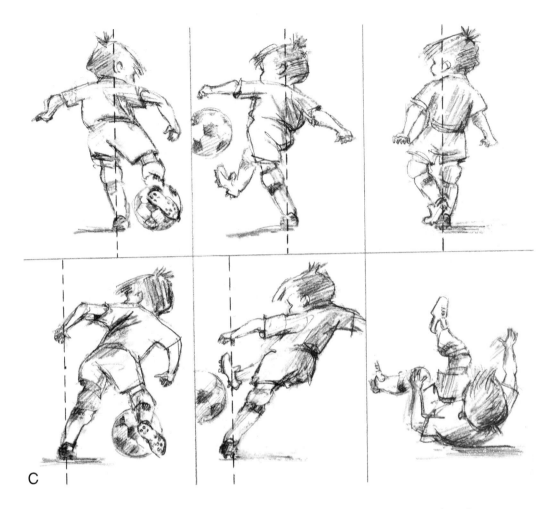

C

1. CENTRALLY PROGRAMMED RECIPROCAL INHIBITION   Walking is analyzed in its simplest form as a back and forth movement of the legs achieved through reciprocal muscle movements (Fig. 11-12). Excitation of the extensors and inhibition of flexors in the left leg move the left leg forward, at the same time excitation of flexors and inhibition of extensors move the right leg back. In the next step, the pattern is reversed, and this cycle repeated many times moves the legs back and forth. There are many details to this movement. *Reciprocal inhibition* and excitation of flexors and extensors in one leg, for example, is achieved by a process called *centrally programmed inhibition*.

A group of large sensory fibers, the so-called IA afferents, arising from muscle spindles have monosynaptic excitatory connections with the very motor neurons that send axons out to the extensor muscles in which these spindles lie. In addition, the IA afferents send branches to interneurons which inhibit the motor

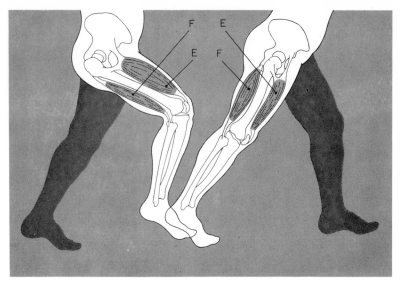

Fig. 11-12. Reciprocal limb movement involved in walking. E, extensors; F, flexors.

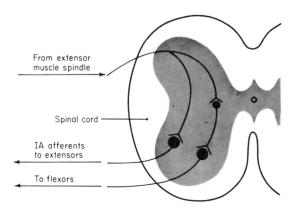

From extensor
muscle spindle

Spinal cord

IA afferents
to extensors

To flexors

Fig. 11-13. Circuitry used in reciprocal inhibition. Receptor input from the extensor muscle spindle excites the extensor but inhibits the flexor muscles.

neurons that supply flexor antagonist muscles (Fig. 11-13). Thus, spindle IA discharges excite the muscle in which the spindle lies and inhibit the antagonist. Both of these effects underlie the negative feedback, stability-reinforcing properties of a servo loop of which the IA afferent fiber forms the afferent side.

Studies of locomotion in spinal animals have clarified the way in which the inhibitory interneuron activated by the IA fiber is simultaneously modulated by central programs. Studies of such modulation were carried out during "fictive locomotion," a situation in which the central program for locomotion occurred but in which actual movement was blocked [either by curare or by severing the ventral (motor) roots of spinal neurons]. In such preparations, IA interneurons in the spinal cord were identified by their response to muscle stretch. Then their activity was studied during centrally programmed locomotion. Remember, variations of IA input will not occur, since the motor roots had been cut. Any changes in electrical discharge of IA interneurons in phase with locomotion in such a preparation would have to be based on central driving. The observations showed that, during locomotion, signals coming to IA interneurons from central networks can modulate their activity in the same way as the IA input from the periphery. Thus, just as IA and centrally programmed inputs to motor neurons are combined during locomotion, so too these inputs are combined to inhibitory interneurons at the same time. The central program for locomotion in the spinal animal sets up coordinated patterns of excitation and inhibition in motor neurons and particular interneurons.

2. RESPONSES TO AFFERENT INPUT IN SPINAL PREPARATIONS. The foregoing discussion on locomotion and scratching in deafferented limbs might suggest that the spinal cord makes rather poor use of sensory input! But the capacities of intrinsic spinal cord machinery to generate rhythmic patterns in the absence of afferent information does not mean that such input is of relatively little importance. On the contrary, when afferent input is present, it can control the operation of the spinal cord circuits. A number of investigations in spinal animals have shown that reactions to sensory input are highly organized. One of these involves the demonstration of *"phase-dependent reflex reversal"* during walking in chronic spinal cats.

A demonstration of such interaction between intrinsic spinal machinery and afferent input is seen in studies on chronic spinal cats which are supported and placed on a treadmill. Tactile stimuli are then applied to the hindlimbs at different phases of the step cycle (Fig. 11-14). When the limb is being flexed in the swing phase, a tactile stimulus applied to the upper surface of the foot enhances flexion, causing the limb to be elevated so as to pass over the obstacle which delivered the

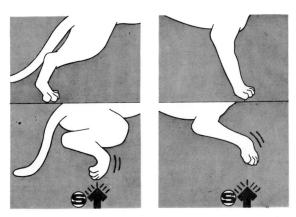

Fig. 11-14. Phase-dependent reflex reversal during walking in chronic spinal cats. The reflex (flexion, left or extension, right) depends on the phase of the step cycle in which the stimulus is applied.

V. SPINAL CORD CONTROL AND ORGANIZATION   487 tactile stimulus. In contrast, the same tactile stimulus applied during the extension phase results in a large response in the extensor muscles and none in the flexors. Thus, an identical tactile stimulus applied to the dorsum of the foot can give rise either to marked flexion or a marked extension, depending entirely on the *phase* of the step cycle in which the stimulus occurs (Forssberg *et al.*, 1975). The mechanism is not well understood, but it appears as if a central generator phasically switches between reflex pathways, while activating appropriate muscle groups sequentially throughout the step cycle.

More generally, these observations on reflex reversal point to the way in which centrally programmed movement depends upon afferent triggers to generate one sort of response modification at one phase of the program and a different type of modification at another phase. While it is sometimes thought that centrally programmed movement should be independent of sensory input at the time of program readout, the results just described suggest that such programs may include contingency plans to cover a variety of different sensory inputs, which then generate subroutines of the program. Such built-in planning would clearly seem to be the case for the response of the hindlimb to an obstacle; the central program includes the contingency of meeting such obstacles and stepping over them.

C. Significance of Experiments on the Isolated Spinal Cord

The experiments just described, then, show that intrinsic mechanisms within the spinal cord can give rise to rhythmical scratching and locomotion. Of course, the "locomoting" spinal animal must be supported and must be on a treadmill. The spinal animal has lost the mechanisms necessary for maintenance of upright posture and, for this reason alone, locomotion is impossible. Thus, studies on locomotion in the spinal animal reveal the existence of neuronal mechanisms but not systems which can subserve independent, useful function.

If we now think of locomotion in the intact animal, we immediately realize that it involves the utilization of a variety of cues which must arise from supraspinal components of the CNS. Let us consider the act of running on a surface in which each individual step must be determined by visual inputs (for example, running among large rocks). In this situation, each successive step must vary in direction and magnitude according to the target of the next footfall. Every aspect of the running cycle now must be amenable to information coming from neural systems which utilize these inputs.

Therefore, results of work on the isolated spinal cord must be taken in proper perspective. Such work uncovers neuronal circuitry which not only provides for reciprocal coordinated activity but which can also utilize afferent input appropriate to the phase of motor output. And higher centers must be able to operate via this circuitry. As we have emphasized in Chapter 2 and throughout much of this text, the fundamental principles used at lower levels of the nervous system appear to be repeated again at higher levels. The nervous system is a multilayered hierarchical organization in which the same general principles are utilized at each layer and, in which, in the intact animal, all layers function simultaneously and in harmony.

VI. Supraspinal Control: Basal Ganglia, Cerebellum and Motor Cortex

As we learned when we examined the motor system in Chapter 2, movement in the intact subject involves an interaction between the spinal cord and three interconnected components of the brain's motor control system: (1) the cerebral motor cortex, (2) the cerebellum, and (3) the basal ganglia. Figure 11-15, the figure we saw already in Chapter 2, recalls again some of the interconnections between these structures.

A central problem in studying motor control is that of understanding the interrelationships between these major components. Much of the progress in this field is due to the development of techniques which allow the recording of single cell discharges in the awake behaving monkey (see Evarts, 1973).

A.   Timing of Brain Activity in Relation to Movement

When do cells in the motor cortex discharge in association with a simple volitional movement? To answer this question Evarts (1966) trained monkeys to depress a telegraph key and watch for a light which came on at unpredictable times. The monkeys were rewarded by a drop of fruit juice for releasing the telegraph key promptly after onset of the light. By simultaneously recording the brain cell discharges and muscle responses, it was possible to determine the temporal relationship between them (Fig. 11-16). Cells in the motor cortex discharged approximately 60 msec prior to muscular contraction.

When do cells in the cerebellum discharge in relation to movement? When the activity of cerebellar Purkinje neurons of monkeys was recorded during rapidly alternating arm movements, such activity was modified (Thach, 1970) (Fig. 11-17). Thus, the _cerebellum_ is active during movement, but is it involved prior to volitional movement? It is. Records of the discharge patterns of cerebellar cells related to prompt movements triggered by the appearance of a light demonstrate that cerebellar neurons change their firing patterns well in advance of

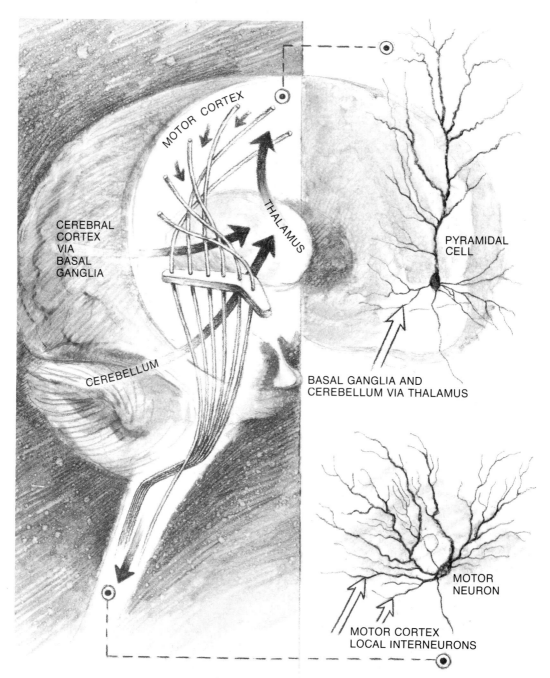

Fig. 11-15. Cortical pyramidal cells (inset) collect reports from basal ganglia and cerebellum (which come via thalamus) on their apical dendrites while adjusting their firing rates by feedback circuits through local interneurons. From the motor cortex fibers of varying length run directly to their targets, the motor neurons (inset) or small subordinate cells.

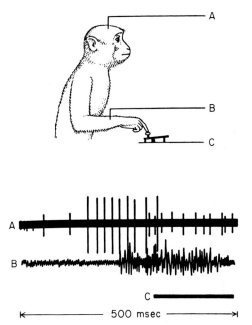

Fig. 11-16. Temporal relation between the discharge of a nerve cell in the motor cortex and a simple hand movement is shown above. A monkey was trained to depress a telegraph key and then to release it within 350 msec after a light came on. The upper trace (A) shows the activity of a single nerve cell in the arm region of the motor cortex, which was recorded by a microelectrode. The trace starts at the onset of the light signal. In a series of trials the nerve cell became active first, usually within 150 msec of the signal. There followed a contraction of arm muscles (B), which was detected by an electromyograph. Trace (C) shows when the telegraph key opened. (From Evarts, 1973.)

volitional movements (Fig. 11-17C). In addition, however, cerebellar neurons discharge in relation to feedback from the moving part as well as prior to the movement.

The axons of the Purkinje cells of the cerebellar cortex pass to deep nuclei within the cerebellum, and axons from these cell clusters then pass to a nucleus in the front half of the thalamus which, in turn, "reports" to motor cortex (see

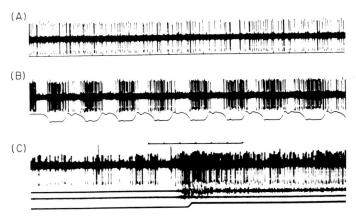

Fig. 11-17. Discharge patterns of a Purkinje cell (A) in the absence of movement and (B) during rapidly alternating movement of the ipsilateral wrist (C) to a wrist movement triggered by a light (top bar). A pause in firing and rapid firing preceded the movement. (From Thach, 1970.)

Chapter 2). This thalamic waystation is the _ventral lateral nucleus_ (VL), which represents a major point of convergence between the cerebellum and the basal ganglia. It turns out that in both VL and the basal ganglia neurons are active _prior_ to movement.

Thus, all three major components of the brain's motor system (motor cortex, cerebellum, and the basal ganglia) discharge prior to movement. This is important because we know that the basal ganglia and cerebellum receive information from the somatosensory, visual, auditory and associative regions of the cerebral cortex. Traditionally, the cerebral cortex was thought of as the highest level of motor integration, but now it appears that both the cerebellum and basal ganglia are important in the early stages of motor programming.

How do these observations on activity of single neurons in the monkey compare to the transactions of single nerve cells in humans? Recordings in man have been obtained by placing microelectrodes into the brain of patients undergoing stereotaxic surgery for the relief of motor disorders (Hongell _et al._, 1973). Activity of thalamic VL neurons is strikingly related to volitional movements carried out by the patient, whereas passive movements have relatively little effect on neuron discharge. Similar observations have been made in monkeys (Strick, 1974). We can conclude that these observations in monkeys and human patients are consistent with the view that the activity of thalamic VL neurons is of importance in relaying and integrating cerebellar and basal ganglia motor programs to motor cortex, but such activity is relatively uninvolved in bringing sensory impulses from the periphery to that cortical region, even though other thalamic nuclei are critically important in conveying sensations to other regions.

B. The Control Mechanisms of Cerebellar Motor Systems

In Section VI,A we emphasized the coordinated activity of a trio—the motor cortex, cerebellum, and the basal ganglia. Now we must look at the special functional roles of the cerebellum and basal ganglia. Each has its own special function. Their outputs are of importance in determining motor cortex discharge, but in what particular way does the cerebellum contribute to motor control, and how does this contribution contrast to the contribution of the basal ganglia?

Understanding of the role of the cerebellum in motor control has been greatly advanced by the work of the Japanese physiologist, Ito, who discovered that the entire output of the cerebellar cortex (by way of the Purkinje cell axons) is inhibitory: the cerebellar cortex functions exclusively like a brake—by inhibiting and disinhibiting rather than by exciting and not exciting. In this respect, the output of the cerebellar cortex is different from the output of the motor cortex, whose axons descending to the spinal cord are excitatory.

THE VESTIBULO-OCULAR REFLEX ARC AND THE VESTIBULOCEREBELLUM. Much of the work of Ito and of other investigators currently studying the role of the cerebellum in motor control has utilized the vestibulo-ocular reflex (VOR). Recall that the VOR serves to maintain a stable retinal image during head movements. Vestibular signals generated by head movements lead to motor neuron discharges which activate eye muscles and maintain gaze fixed as the head rotates. As summarized by Ito (1974), the major pathway for the VOR is a well-defined three-neuron arc: primary vestibular neurons, secondary vestibular neurons, and oculomotor neurons (Fig. 11-18A). Studies of the relationship between this arc and the cerebellum showed that one part of the cerebellum is linked with it. This part is the flocculus, a small lobule intimately connected with the vestibular nuclei beneath it. This so-called "*vestibulocerebellum*" receives collaterals from the same primary incoming vestibular fibers that lead to the secondary neurons in the vestibular nuclei. On the output side, Purkinje cell axons in the flocculus descend to the vestibular nuclei, directly or indirectly, to inhibit activity of the neurons there. Thus, as shown in Fig. 11-18A, the flocculus

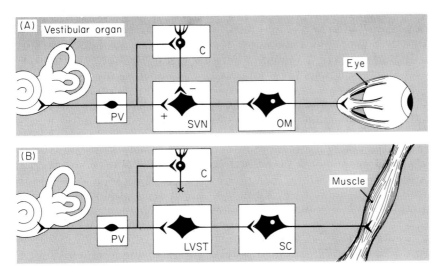

Fig. 11-18. (A) The central pathway for the VOR is a three neuron circuit. The primary vestibular neurons (PV) connect to secondary vestibular neurons (SVN) which in turn drive the oculomotor neurons (OM) and control eye movement. The cerebellum (C) is a sidearm of the central pathways and acts as a feedforward control center. It places a negative bias on the passage of information on its way to the eye muscles. The VOR is an example of an open loop system. (B) The control pathway for the vestibulospinal reflex is also a three-neuron arc going from the primary vestibular neuron (PV) to the lateral vestibulospinal tract (LVST) to the spinal cord (SC) where spinal motor neurons drive various muscles. Although the vestibulospinal part of the cerebellum receives afferent vestibular input, it does not influence either the LVST or SC. It is a closed-loop system.

forms a side path in the VOR arc. Ito proposed that the flocculus functions in the feedforward control of the arc by processing the primary vestibular information.

An understanding of the way in which the cerebellum improves the VOR by feedforward control may be gained by contrasting the VOR with the vestibulospinal reflex, a reflex that (unlike the VOR) is a closed-loop system. The vestibulospinal arc involves a three-neuron chain composed of primary vestibular afferents, secondary neurons in the vestibular nuclei and spinal motor neurons (Fig. 11-18B). The axons of the secondary vestibular nuclei neurons mediating the vestibulospinal reflex reach the spinal cord via two separate fiber bundles, the lateral and medial vestibulospinal tracts. In neither of these tracts is there Purkinje cell inhibition from the vestibulocerebellum. Thus, in spite of the fact that VOR and vestibulospinal reflex have similar trineuronal construction, the vestibulospinal reflex arc is free of inhibitory influences from the vestibulocerebellum, whereas the VOR arc is subject to inhibition mediated by the flocculus.

Reflexes based on closed-loop feedback control, such as the vestibulospinal, do not seem to require assistance by the cerebellar cortex, whereas open-loop systems utilizing feedforward control do require cerebellar participation. In essence, then, the cerebellum is a neuronal system performing a feedforward control function that provides complex input–output relationships not possible with more elementary closed-loop feedback systems.

C. The Basal Ganglia

Theories on the role or roles of the basal ganglia are not as highly developed as are those concerning the cerebellum. This difference stems in part from their great diversity of structure. One of the striking features of the cerebellar cortex is a uniform architecture: the numerous functionally different zones of the cerebellum have different external connections but a virtually invariant cortical architecture. In view of its highly defined and formalized structure and well-understood pathways of input and output, neurophysiological hypotheses as to the role of the cerebellum have been formulated with considerable precision. In contrast, the basal ganglia are still somewhat enigmatic in function.

The basal ganglia play a major role in movement as judged by the consequences of basal ganglia disease. In Chapter 6 we saw that an abnormality in basal ganglia dopamine metabolism, particularly in the dopaminergic pathway from the substantia nigra to the striatum (see also Chapter 2), is one of the primary causes of _Parkinson's disease_, a disease characterized by tremor, rigidity and poverty of movement with particular difficulties in generating continuous, regular movements spontaneously. Why? The answer lies in the mysterious functions of the basal ganglia. Studies on Parkinsonian patients have revealed much about the functions of the basal ganglia, although much is still unknown.

Imagine for a moment that you were asked to track a sine wave with your finger. You would probably start by moving your finger with visual information as your guide, and your movements would lag behind the target because of delays from visual input to corresponding motor output. However, gradually, as you got the idea, you would develop a strategy or an internal model of the pattern of movement. The sine wave is regular, and it is easy to predict the appropriate moves. Accordingly, with practice, you could predictively track the waves with less and less lag. Parkinsonian patients, on the other hand, would find this predictive tracking task very difficult. They make many errors at all frequencies of the sine wave, and at the highest frequencies are unable to track any better than if they were making no movements at all. There is little, if any, improvement with practice (Lee and Tatton, 1975).

A part of the problem is that Parkinsonian patients have a greater than normal reaction time, but this is not the only cause of their poor performance. Even after correction for this, Parkinsonian patients do more poorly.

Sensory input is extremely important to Parkinsonian patients for the control of movement. If a patient is asked to hold out an arm and touch an object he can do so easily, but if he closes his eyes his arm will fall, much to the surprise and dismay of the patient. It appears as if these patients cannot develop a satisfactory strategy for movement. They lack a dynamic internal model of their own movements from which to control them predictively. The patients tend to be tied more to sensory information. They respond to, rather than act in anticipation of, such information. They have great difficulty producing continous movements when movements are executed with infrequent corrective monitoring (Flowers, 1978a,b).

A normal individual's movements are a mixture of voluntary and programmed movements. Normal subjects perform visually aimed movements, for example, with the entire movement executed ballistically as a large open-loop period with little, if any, feedback. Characteristically, such movements do not require continuous correction from sensory input. Such movements are thought to be directed by central programs as suggested in the example for tracking a sine wave. Peripheral feedback, on the other hand, comes into play for movements that require constant monitoring and correction. The closed-loop mode operating with feedback serves to clamp and damp such movements as appropriate. Most movements in normal individuals are executed by a dynamic interplay between open- and closed-loop modes. It is necessary to shift in and out of both modes as appropriate.

It seems that damage to the basal ganglia results in an inappropriate readout of central programs. An oscillation in motor output is created due to incorrect integration, the details of which are largely unknown. The ability to create and draw upon central programs appropriately is essential for normal movement. Inappropriate readout of central programs causes problems, and the dependence on peripheral feedback compounds the difficulties. The constant need of correction from the periphery promotes jerky movements since the system over- and undercompensates and it can do this only slowly. The open-loop mode used in movement control is not executed effectively in Parkinsonian patients.

One observation in line with this model is that Parkinsonian patients at times invent devices to provide sensory cues just to continue functioning. A patient who finds that his gait becomes frozen may be able to start walking again by placing a stick a few inches before him to help initiate the first step. It appears as if the basal ganglia fail to operate appropriately prior to and during open-loop voluntary movements. This produces responses of longer duration, since they cannot be executed ballistically from central programming. It also results in a strong dependence on peripheral feedback. As a result continuous and progressive movements tend to be slower, more jerky and more difficult.

Thus, in summary, it appears as if damage to the basal ganglia results in a situation in which people are deficient in some "internal model" of their own actions by which to generate movements spontaneously and to control them predictively (Flowers, 1978a,b).

VII. Plasticity, Learning and Volition

The most challenging questions in neuroscience concern mechanisms underlying neuronal plasticity, learning and volition. What features distinguish volitional movements from reflexes? How are learned movements acquired, and how do they differ from innate motor patterns? What is the link between changes in function and changes in structure underlying motor plasticity?

A.   Plasticity of the Vestibulo-ocular Reflex

Ito's work pointed to a role for the cerebellum in the VOR, and many current studies on CNS plasticity use the VOR as a model. A major impetus to such work came from exciting discoveries showing VOR plasticity in human subjects as a result of long-term reversal of vision during free head movement (Gonshor and Jones, 1976a,b). The subjects wore head-mounted "dove prisms" or mirrors constantly, and for days all their visual experience, whether moving or at rest, involved seeing left as right and right as left. Normally, as we know, the VOR drives the eye muscles so that the eyes rotate in a direction *opposite* to the head movement; this action stabilizes the retinal image on the fovea and keeps this point of keenest vision on target. In a prism experiment this relationship is disrupted. Prisms can reverse the direction in which the world appears to move so that, if the head moves to the left, the world appears to move to the left! In order to compensate for the unfortunate change introduced by the prisms, it would be necessary to eliminate or reverse the VOR, which is now a maladaptive response.

To better consider the action of the VOR we need to define two terms: *gain* and *phase*. As described earlier, the VOR keeps the image centered on the fovea as the head moves. Movement of the head is compensated by equal and opposite movement of the eyes. *Gain* is a measure of eye velocity to head velocity; a gain of 1 means that the image is kept centered. However, such measure does not specify the relationship with respect to time: the velocities need to be in phase. The *phase* relationship describes the ability of the VOR to maintain head-to-eye position constant. It is a dynamic measure.

With reversing prisms, optimal adaptation would be a 180° phase shift with gain equal to the normal value for 100% of the 180° of phase-shifted head movements. Further, the associated VOR-produced eye movements should now be in the *same* direction, rather than in the opposite direction. Under the viewing conditions imposed by dove prisms, head and eye movements in the same direction would stabilize the retinal image.

Four volunteer subjects were studied. All subjects showed substantial reduction of the VOR gain during the first 2 days of vision reversal. After removal of the prisms, VOR gain then recovered along a time course which approximated that of the original adaptive attenuation. In one subject in a 27-day experiment, there was a large phase change observed. It progressed to a 130° phase lag relative to normal by the beginning of the third week, so that this aspect of the VOR was essentially eliminated. Accompanying this was a restoration of gain from 25 to 50% of normal. The phase shift observed in the long-term experiment was maintained until return to normal vision on day 28. Thus, over a period of a few weeks, a change in the VOR occurs so that as the head moves the eyes do not move nearly so completely in the opposite direction.

The VOR changes were adaptive, in the sense that they tended to keep the eyes on target during head movement. Furthermore, they were plastic—there was extensive (and retained) remodeling of the reflex toward this goal. These findings aroused great surprise and excitement; the VOR had been viewed as a "hard wired" elementary reflex. When it was shown that such a reflex could be *reversed* as a result of reversed visual experience, a door was opened to explore the mechanisms of motor plasticity. It was hypothesized that such changes in gain and phase might derive from a neural network involving vestibulo-ocular projections by way of brain stem and cerebellar pathways. The reversed visual tracking of the subjects was suspected to produce plastic modulation of efficacy in the cerebellar limb of these pathways. [This pathway is the "cerebellar side-loop" discussed earlier (see Fig. 11-18).]

In order to investigate the brain mechanism underlying VOR plasticity it is necessary to use a number of animal models. One such model is the study of monkeys wearing telescopic spectacles (Miles and Fuller, 1974). These spectacles present a different challenge to the VOR systems. They magnify or diminish the monkey's view of the world and, hence, alter the magnitude of the compensatory eye movements required to maintain a stable retinal image. Telescopic lenses require a change in gain *without* a change in phase. Normally a 10° head movement produces a 10° retinal movement which is described as a gain of 1. However, if the image is magnified, say two times, a 10° movement of the head can create a 20° movement or slippage on the retina! In order to compensate for this, the VOR has to increase its gain twofold (Fig. 11-19). Over the course of a

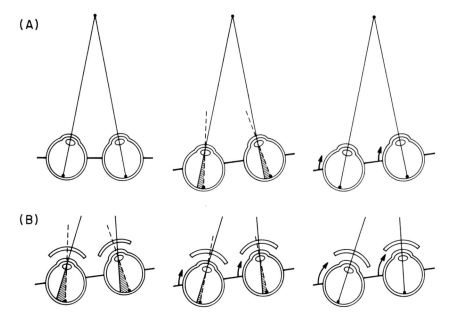

Fig. 11-19. Effect of telescopic lenses on the vestibulo-ocular reflex (A) normal VOR. For sideways head movement (middle panel) the VOR drives the eyes an equal amount in the opposite direction (far right panel). (B) VOR with telescopic lenses. With the lenses, a sideways movement and compensating eye movement is insufficient to realign the image on the fovea. The VOR must increase and move the eyes further.

few days, animals wearing magnifying lenses did, in fact, show an increase in gain. Adaptation required 2 to 3 days. Following removal of the spectacles, recovery to original gain took a similar period of time. Hence, the change was reversible.

Where do the adaptive changes take place? What is modified and how? One possibility is that the cerebellum provides an inhibitory loop—a variable gain element able to adjust performance levels within the system. The hypothesis that changes in the cerebellum underlie VOR plasticity implies that such plasticity would fail to occur in animals without a cerebellum. Indeed, the VOR remains fixed in animals with lesions of the vestibulocerebellum (Robinson, 1976). Thus, it seems that the adaptive plasticity of this reflex depends upon the cerebellum. In fact, lesions of a brain stem nucleus in the medulla, which has powerful excitatory input to the cerebellum (the inferior olive), will prevent VOR adaptation. Studies on the electrical response of single units have confirmed the key role of cerebellar circuitry in VOR plasticity and provided important insights into the events monitored there, and the nature of the changes. The results of these studies suggest that the cerebellum has a special role in the on-line stabilization of retinal images for both moving and stationary targets (Miles, 1977).

The emerging picture is not yet complete, but cerebellar events may be viewed as follows (Miles, 1977). The VOR is a three-neuron arc whereby the eyes use vestibular information to maintain visual fixation despite movements of the head. In this arc the cerebellum acts as a feedforward system: it places a negative bias on the vestibular nuclei. The side-loop vestibular input to the cerebellar Purkinje cell is a velocity signal for head movements. The greater this input, the faster such movements should be. As for the long-term consequences of wearing telescopic spectacles, there should be long-term adaptive changes in the strength of the head velocity component of Purkinje cell firing.

The cerebellum appears not to be a fixed system. Rather, optimum performance requires a "fine tuning" circuit. The fine tuning may depend on a pathway in which the Purkinje cell inhibits these same vestibular nuclear cells. Fine tuning of this inhibitory effect could be achieved if fibers from the brain stem (the climbing fibers) originating in the inferior olive were controlled by information indicating inappropriate eye movement during head movement (e.g., by visual feedback). The Purkinje cell might then learn to "tune" the basic circuit to appropriate performance by changing the vestibular input–oculomotor output relations within the vestibular nuclei. The inferior olive might be seen as a comparator, detecting the discrepancies between what was intended (ocular fixation despite head turning) and what was achieved. If this is so, then an "error signal" based on the comparison of command and response might generate climbing fiber inputs to the cerebellar cortex that could "teach" the Purkinje cells to "tune" the command–response relationship, gradually perfecting the VOR as required by changes in the optical media through which the world was viewed.

These data strengthen the view that the cerebellum is an important, if not the principal, structure in learning motor skills. It has also been pointed out that "the cerebellum may be able to detect and repair defects of movement resulting from accumulation of lesions, large and small, that naturally occur in the nervous system over the years" (Robinson, 1976).

B. Motor Learning

The gradually appearing and disappearing changes of VOR gain occurring with altered visual inputs provide a powerful model for investigating processes underlying synaptic modification. In some ways these gain changes are akin to the hypertrophy and atrophy associated with muscle use and disuse. They are probably not the same as motor learning, as the term is commonly understood. We usually think of motor learning as involving volition, whereas changes of VOR and muscle are involuntary processes involving "will power" only insofar as the subject must be willing to be active. A subject (man or monkey) wearing dove prisms or telescopic spectacles may prefer to remain immobile, and it therefore takes will power for him to move about. Without such movement, VOR adaptation will *not* occur. Likewise, a subject wearing lead boots will find it easier to sit still than to walk, and lead boots will not cause muscle hypertrophy in an immobile subject! However, given sufficient activity, the mental attitude of the subject will not determine the amount of muscle hypertrophy or of VOR gain change, for that matter. In these respects then VOR plasticity differs from what we understand by the term "motor learning."

To point out some additional differences between VOR plasticity and motor learning, let us take an example of motor learning which bears a superficial similarity to VOR plasticity but which is really very different. Consider learning to steer a bus. As most of us know, the steering column of a large vehicle such as a bus or a truck must be turned through a greater angle for a given change in tire orientation than is the case for a smaller vehicle such as an automobile. A driver confronted with a given angular deviation of the road ahead must, therefore, effect a greater angular deviation of the steering wheel when driving a bus than when driving a car. The sort of learning which takes place when a person who can already steer a car learns to steer a bus is one form of motor learning. The learning requires no new concepts, but does involve setting up new proportionalities between a visually perceived angular deviation of the road and arm movements which will produce a proportional movement of the steering wheel. There is a superficial similarity between VOR adaptation to magnifying telescopic spectacles and learning to steer a bus; both spectacles and bus will require a greater motor output for a given magnitude of sensory input. However, the differences are more important than the similarities. Perhaps the most fundamental difference is that in the case of the VOR the afferent input from the semicircular canals has a strong genetically patterned linkage to oculomotor neurons, with only the vestibular nuclei intervening, whereas the visual inputs which guide steering have no such direct linkages to the arm motor neurons which are used in steering. A second important difference between VOR adaptation and motor learning is seen in the processes which occur when the subject returns from the recently learned task to the previously familiar motor performance (i.e., from telescopic spectacles to normal vision or from car to bus). For the adapted VOR, the return to normal gain may take almost as long as the original adaptation process! For acquired motor skills this is not the case: the bus driver has no trouble steering his automobile home from work each day.

In considering these differences between adaptive VOR gain changes and motor learning, it is useful to think in terms of the "central motor program"—a concept mentioned earlier in this chapter in connection with locomotion and scratching in the spinal animal. An essential feature of the centrally programmed movement is that information controlling the movement arises from *within* the nervous system rather than from peripheral receptors. Of course, sensory inputs can initiate or trigger program readout (as in the scratch reflex) and can modify programmed movements during their occurrence (as in phase-dependent reflex reversal in locomotion), but the template controlling the programmed movement lies within the CNS. For the VOR, the information controlling the eye movements arises continuously from vestibular receptors, and VOR adaptation requires a change in the synaptic efficacy of these vestibular inputs. In contrast, learning to steer a bus, boat, airplane or bicycle requires establishing new sets of motor programs. Following motor learning, subjects can "switch programs" in a second or less! This virtually instantaneous switching sharply contrasts to the slow adaptations of VOR gain. Perhaps we can say that changes of VOR gain seem to require changes of "hardware" rather than of "software."

C. Centrally Programmed Movement

What are the neural circuits involved in "switching programs"? How can a subject respond to a sensory input with a given motor output and then an instant later respond to the same sensory input with an opposite motor output? It is now clear that a considerable amount of *preprogramming* of movement is involved in switching motor programs. This can be illustrated by considering the effect of intention on motor responses to arm displacements in human subjects. An abrupt pull on the elbow, for example, which stretches the biceps muscle, elicits a 25-msec latency (delay) biceps tendon jerk which is then followed by a 50-msec latency second biceps response if the subject is instructed to resist. However, when the subject has been instructed *not* to resist, the tendon jerk is still present, but the second response is absent (Hammond, 1961). It now seems clear that following the instruction (during the second or so before the triggering arm displacement), the subject *"preprogrammed"* the appropriate movement and that the arm displacement is able to elicit the desired motor program very soon after the tendon jerk. Preprogramming is very beneficial for motor responses. For example, as a result of knowing that an event is impending, a person's response is much quicker than when he or she simply has to respond without any preinstruction. Moreover, preprogramming is not only beneficial in responding faster but also in responding more accurately.

Studies on monkeys have provided the key insights into the neural mechanisms of motor preprogramming. The situation used is similar to that employed in human subjects. Monkeys are trained to react to an arm displacement according to a prior instruction (Fig. 11-20). The monkey grasps a rod and holds it in a control zone midway between a pull and push position. Correct position is signaled by a white light. After the position is held briefly, a red or green light comes on. The red light instructs the monkey to pull the handle toward itself when a perturbation (torque) is applied to the handle. (The handle is connected to a motor which drives it in either direction.) Thus, the instruction (light) tells the monkey *how* to move, whereas the trigger (torque) tells him *when* to move. A key goal in the design of this experiment was dissociation of the reflex from the intended components of motor activity. It was in this respect that this study in monkeys differed from previous experiments in monkey (Evarts, 1973) or in man (Hagbarth, 1967; Hammond, 1956). To achieve this dissociation, either of the two possible instructions, pull and push, was followed by either of the two possible directions of perturbation, pull or push. For example, when a monkey was given an instruction to push in response to a subsequent perturbation of its arm, the perturbing trigger could move the arm in either of two possible directions: either toward the monkey (pull) or away (push). When the instruction "push" was followed by the perturbation "pull" (thus stretching the triceps and opposing the intended push movement), the reflex response in the stretched triceps muscle was of the same sign (+) as the intended response, and there was association of the reflex and intended components of the muscle response. But when the instruction "push" was followed by the perturbation "push," which shortened triceps and assisted the intended push movement, the reflex response in the shortened triceps muscle was opposite (−) to the intended response: now the reflex response of triceps (to becoming shorter while its antagonist was being stretched) was to become less active, and the triceps discharge which occurred when the monkey carried out the intended push movement was in spite of, rather than because of, muscle inputs.

This dissociation of reflex from intended response components by the combination of two sorts of instructions with two sorts of triggering perturbations was seen in motor cortex *pyramidal cells* as well as in muscle, as illustrated in Fig.

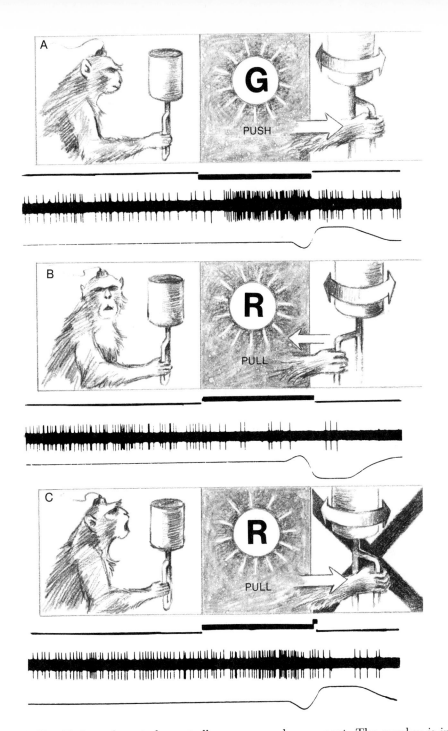

Fig. 11-20. Task used to study centrally programmed movement. The monkey is instructed to push the lever forward when the green light comes on (A) and pull the lever back when the red light comes on (B). Records of activity in the motor cortex shows that the movements are preprogrammed. Prior to the actual movement (lower thin line) the discharge frequency of pyramidal tract neurons changes. (C) shows that when the monkey makes an error the pyramidal cell activity gave inappropriate instructions. (Data from Evarts and Tanji, 1976.)

11-21. This figure shows the change of perturbation-evolved activity in a pyramidal cell as a result of a change of the prior instruction. This neuron was reciprocally related to push–pull movements, becoming active with push and silent with pull. The pull perturbation (which moved the handle toward the monkey, opposing the intended push movement in association with which the neuron discharged) excited the pyramidal cell at short latency. Although this excitation was evoked by the perturbation regardless of the prior instruction, the magnitude and the duration of the excitation were greater when the perturbation followed the push instruction than when it followed the pull instruction. The effect here is analogous to the enhanced triceps tendon jerk when triceps stretch follows instruction push. Comparison of the perturbation-evoked responses of this pyramidal cell for the two different instructions (Fig. 11-21) reveals that the two responses had the same initial onset latency but very different magnitudes and durations. When the prior instruction was pull, the excitation was very brief, terminating after about 10 msec.

Indications as to how strongly the instructions for neuronal discharge correlated with subsequent motor performance could be seen when the monkey made a mistake (Fig. 11-19B). Such errors underscore the idea that a neuron's correct response to the instruction is a necessary precondition for the animal's correct motor response. For one trial with pull instruction, the cortical cell fails to become less active, but instead becomes more active. On this occasion the cell responds to the pull instruction as if it had been a push instruction, and the following perturbation elicits the wrong movement. Thus, the response of the cell to the instruction reliably predicted the subsequent motor response. The mistake originated from the brain's instructions.

Cortical output neurons which respond correctly upon presentation of the instruction show further (and usually more intense) changes when the perturbing trigger is delivered. Some type of facilitation strengthens the anticipatory response when it is correct.

D. Contrasts between Reflex and Intended Activity in Motor Cortex

The discharge of corticospinal neurons in the arm area associated with a contralateral arm movement (triggered by input to that arm) has two components: (1) a relatively short latency reflex component which depends on the nature of the input and (2) a longer latency component which depends on the movement the subject intends to perform. The first component of discharge appears comparable to discharges which a number of previous investigators have described for motor cortex neurons in response to stimulation of cutaneous, muscle, or joint receptors

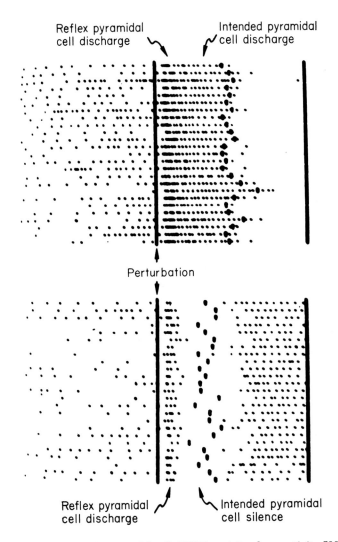

Fig. 11-21. Raster display of pyramidal cell (PTN) activity show activity 500 msec before and 500 msec after a perturbation which occurred at the center line of the display. A raster plot shows the discharge patterns of neurons over many trials. Each line represents the behavior of a cell over time and each point on that line a discharge. The single heavy dot in each row following the perturbation shows when the handle reached the intended push or pull zone. The pyramidal cell discharged with intended push movement and fell silent with intended pull movement. In the raster at the top, the heavy dot marking completion of the push movement is followed by pyramidal cell silence as the monkey pulls back into the "hold zone" to initiate a new trial. In the lower raster the heavy dot occurs during pyramidal cell silence as the monkey pulls, and then becomes active as the monkey pushes back to the hold zone to start a new trial. (From Evarts and Tanji, 1976.)

(Albe-Fessard and Liebeskind, 1966; Albe-Fessard *et al.*, 1965; Brooks *et al.*, 1961; Oscarsson, 1966; Porter, 1973; Rosén and Asanuma, 1972; Towe *et al.*, 1964; Wiesendanger, 1969). The second component is related to the nature of the intended output and would seem to depend on a central program rather than on the nature of the triggering input. When an excitatory perturbation triggers a movement involving quiescence of the cortical output neurons, only the first (or reflex) component of discharge occurs. Conversely, when a movement involving discharge of the neuron is triggered by a perturbation which previously suppresses the cell's activity, only the second (or intended) component occurs.

E. The Intended Component of Cortical Output Neuron Discharge

The initial short latency reflex component of corticospinal neuron discharge depends in large measure on the nature of the kinesthetic input. It appears to reach motor cortex from the postcentral gyrus, where the sensory homunculus lies. A second component depends primarily on the intended movement. This discharge can occur at latencies as short as 50 msec, even when the initial effect of the perturbing stimulus is to *reduce* the activity of the neurons. Excitation of output neurons during this intended phase of discharge must involve very different pathways from those involved in the first phase. The second phase of discharge depends on learning and seems to be the sign of a central program, while the first phase appears to be automatic and is thus more akin to a reflex. The animal has learned to set up the control program and, upon its wish, it can retrieve and use it to facilitate its response.

It now appears that neurons in the VL nucleus of the thalamus have properties consistent with playing a role in mediating this second phase of discharge: these neurons are related to the intended movement and, unlike cells in more posterior regions of the thalamus, are relatively independent of the specific features of the sensory input (Strick, 1976). Further studies of VL are needed to provide more information as to its possible role (and perhaps that of the cerebellum, which also connects with it) in programming the changes of input–output relations which occur as a result of changes of the "set" or "intention" of subjects performing learned movements.

VIII. Summary

All our bodily movements are controlled by motor neuron innervation of muscle fibers. Small motor neurons generally activate small motor units which exhibit long-lasting muscle twitches, have small peak tensions and show resistance to fatigue. Larger motor neurons innervate larger "fast twitch" units, which develop large peak tension and fatigue rapidly. As a muscle is contracted, the slow twitch units are activated prior to the recruitment of the more powerful fast twitch units.

Motor systems are designed to maintain stability and to generate movement. To illustrate these contrasting roles of motor systems, we have studied the oculomotor system. The oculomotor system, which controls eye movements, initiates three types of movement: rapid ones (saccades), smooth pursuit tracking, and the vestibulo-ocular reflex. Saccadic movements are swift darting eye movements. Smooth pursuit tracking allows tracking of an object moving in the visual field. The VOR maintains a stable retinal image in response to head movements by moving the eyes in the opposite direction.

There are two types of movement, ballistic and continuously controlled movements. Ballistic movements are predetermined by initiating influences—the die is cast. Continuously controlled movements, on the other hand, are modulated by continuous input or feedback from receptors. While movements may be controlled by central programs or peripheral input, most are subject to both types of influences.

Receptors in a muscle monitor muscle length and tension. Stretching of a muscle activates muscle spindles, which monosynaptically activate motor neurons and thus cause contractions. Tension is sensed by the Golgi organ in the muscle tendon. When activated, this receptor inhibits the motor neuron and thus reduces tension. These two receptors thus initiate negative feedback control to resist changes in muscle length and tension.

Motor systems in the spinal cord or brain are feedback and feedforward systems. Feedback maintains stability by correcting, through excitation or inhibition, disturbances in input. Feedforward exerts control by recording in some way the consequences of the movement and, then, through memory, producing changes in the response.

The motor system can be divided into spinal and supraspinal centers. The latter includes the basal ganglia, cerebellum and motor cortex. Simple responses such as the scratch reflex can be produced in spinal animals. Feedback from the moving hindlimb is not essential for occurrence of the scratching—the scratch reflex is centrally programmed. Electrical stimulation of the spinal cord that elicits scratching innervates rhythmic activity ("fictive scratching") in the ventral spinocerebellar tract even if the animals are paralyzed with curare. This tract activity brings about cerebellar modulation that affects other brain regions, including the vestibulospinal neurons which normally play a role in maintaining posture during scratching. Such modulation of output centers, including pools of motor neurons by central programs, as well as by continued resulting peripheral input, is an example of the principle of dual modulation. Principles of motor organization elucidated by studies of spinal animals seem to apply to all levels of the nervous system.

VIII. SUMMARY   507

Studies of spinal animals have also helped to provide understanding of the neural control of locomotion. The reciprocal pattern of excitation of extensors and inhibition of flexors in one leg and the converse in the other leg during walking is centrally controlled. Feedback from the legs is *not* required for locomotion. However, responses in spinal animals are influenced by peripheral stimulation. In spinal cats supported and placed on a treadmill, stimulation of a foot can enhance either flexion or extension, depending upon the phase of the step cycle in which such stimulation occurs. Centrally programmed movement appears to consist of subroutines, or "contingency plans," to deal with variations in afferent input such as running between rocks.

In normal animals, movement involves an interaction between the spinal cord and a trio of brain structures—the cerebral motor cortex, cerebellum and basal ganglia. Studies of cells in all three brain regions indicate that the cells fire *prior* to movement. All three regions appear to be involved in motor programming. The cerebellum may be part of a feedforward control system, as well as greatly concerned with rapid movements. The basal ganglia appear to be involved in generating movements spontaneously and controlling them predictively. Parkinsonism, a disease accompanied by tremor, rigidity and difficulty in initiating movements, is related to disturbances in them.

Studies on human volunteers and monkeys indicate that the vestibulo-ocular reflex can be modified by experience. Ordinarily the VOR produces eye rotation in a direction opposite to head movement to stabilize the retinal image. Prisms can reverse the direction in which the world appears to move. Under these conditions the subjects learn to change the direction of eye movement during head movement. Studies with monkeys indicate that the plasticity of the VOR can be disrupted by cerebellar lesions. Unlike other motor skills, the appropriate VOR has to be relearned when the prisms are removed. In other forms of motor learning, we appear to develop programs which can be switched quickly when the environmental circumstances change. Studies of the activity of motor cortex cells in monkeys indicate that the type of movement which would occur in a learned task could be predicted from the neuronal activity. The "instructions" given appeared to activate programs for responding. The thalamus and cerebellum seem to be importantly involved in the programs controlling intentional learned movement, and such involvement reminds us again of the never-ending team work of brain components.

Key Terms

Antagonist muscles: Pairs of muscles that produce oppositely directed movements (i.e., flexion and extension).

Ballistic movements: Rapid movements that lack the possibility of control once started by a brief application of energy. Such movements are predetermined by the force applied.

Centrally programmed movements: Movements that are centrally preprogrammed and do not depend on peripheral feedback.

Cerebellum: A specialized brain area involved in motor control. It performs feedforward control. It appears to provide an inhibitory loop with a variable gain which can adjust performance levels within the system, as in the normal and adapted vestibulo-ocular reflex.

Closed-loop system: A circuit with feedback.

Command interneurons: Neurons which, when stimulated, trigger a defined complex movement pattern.

Continuously controlled movement: Movements which are continuously controlled by feedback. Such movements contrast to ballistic movements, which are predetermined by the forces applied. Most movements are a combination of continuously controlled and ballistic ones.

Corollary discharge: Information about events, passed to areas of the central nervous system that are not directly involved in the event itself. Corollary discharge serves to inform critical systems of the CNS of ongoing events. Sometimes called internal feedback or efferent monitoring.

Dual modulation: The concept that centrally programmed movement involves the coordinated control of excitability in both afferent and efferent systems, i.e., motor neurons and sensory elements.

Extension: Straightening or movement of a limb away from the body.

"Fast twitch" motor units: Motor units made up of motor neurons and muscle fibers that are larger than "slow twitch" motor units; "fast twitch" motor units develop more tension than "slow twitch" units.

Feedback control system: A type of control where a portion of the output is returned to the system thus modifying the output, e.g., as in the vestibulospinal reflex. A feedback system is a closed-loop system; feedback may be negative or positive.

Feedforward control system: A circuit which introduces a controller so that output is modified through adjustments in the controller, e.g., as in the vestibulo-ocular reflex.

Fictive scratching: CNS events of scratching without the actual execution of the movement itself.

Flexion: Bending or movement of a limb toward the body.

Fovea: The region of the retina where the image is focused and vision is sharpest.

Golgi tendon organ: A type of sensory receptor located on muscle tendons which monitor tension. Their stimulation activates motor neurons.

Motor unit: A single motor neuron and the muscle fibers with which it synapses. Motor units may be "slow twitch" or "fast twitch."

Muscle spindle: A slender modified muscle fiber, embedded in a muscle, which has a primary ending wrapped around its center.

Muscle spindle receptors: A type of sensory receptor located on muscle spindles which monitors muscle fiber length. Stimulation of this receptor increases motor neuron activity, promotes muscle contraction and thus opposes increases in muscle length.

Muscle tension: The tautness of a muscle. Muscle tension depends on the number of muscle fibers and the contractile properties of the individual motor units.

Oculomotor: The motor system that controls eye movement.

Open-loop control system: A circuit with no feedback.

Parkinson's disease: A chronic progressive disease characterized by muscular rigidity, tremor and poverty of movement. It appears to be due, in part, to the degeneration of dopaminergic neurons in the substantia nigra region.

Phase-dependent reflex reversal: A term which describes the finding that, during walking, a given stimulus to the bottom of the foot can cause different responses depending on the phase of the step cycle in which the stimulus occurs.

Preprogramming of movement: Neural activity in the brain precedes that of the actual movement when it is known that a movement is impending. Preprogramming allows faster and more accurate responses.

Primary ending: A sensory process located on a muscle spindle which, when stretched, sends impulses to the spinal cord.

Purkinje cells: The large output neurons of the cerebellum; they are inhibitory.

Pyramidal cells: A type of large neuron in the brain, named for its pyramid shape. Pyramidal cells in the motor cortex are the output cells which innervate spinal motor neurons as well as other neurons.

Reciprocal inhibition: A process whereby excitation of one muscle (an extensor muscle, for example) is accompanied by inhibition of its antagonist (a flexor) muscle. This inhibition is mediated by a spindle inhibitory interneuron.

Recruitment order: The successive calling up of individual motor units. "Slow twitch" units are recruited prior to or simultaneously with "fast twitch" motor units. This recruitment of small, before large, neurons is called the size principle.

Saccadic eye movements: Involuntary darting movements of the eye, which occur to shift the point of fixation and scan the field.

Size principle: *See* Recruitment order.

"Slow twitch" motor units: Motor units which consist of motor neurons and muscle fibers smaller than "fast twitch" motor units. The slow twitch units are fatigue resistant and generate small tensions; they are recruited prior to or simultaneously with fast twitch units.

Smooth pursuit tracking: A term used to describe the voluntary movements of the eyes used to track an object.

Spinal animal: An animal in which the spinal cord is surgically separated from supraspinal centers. Such preparations are used to study spinal functions independent of supraspinal ones.

Ventral lateral nucleus: A nucleus of the thalamus which represents a major point of convergence between the cerebellum and basal ganglia.

Ventral spinocerebellar tract (VSCT): A bundle of nerve fibers in the spinal cord which project to the cerebellum.

Vestibulocerebellum: A subdivision of the cerebellum (also called the flocculus) which connects with the vestibular nuclei and is dedicated to processing vestibular signals.

Vestibulo-ocular reflex (VOR): A reflex that serves to maintain a stable retinal image. As the head moves it causes an equal and opposite compensatory movement of the eyes so that the image remains stabilized on the fovea.

Vestibulospinal reflex (VSR): A reflex which serves to promote head stability. A head movement causes a signal from the vestibular system to activate neck muscles and restore head position. This reflex is an example of a closed-loop control system.

General References

Evarts, E. V. (1973). Brain mechanisms in movement. *Sci. Am.* **229**, 96–103.
Ito, M. (1974). The control mechanisms of cerebellar motor systems. *In* "The Neurosciences: Third Study Program" (F. O. Schmitt and F. G. Worden, eds.), pp. 293–303. MIT Press, Cambridge, Massachusetts.
Sherrington, C. S. (1947). "The Integrative Action of the Nervous System." Yale Univ. Press, New Haven, Connecticut.

References

Albe-Fessard, D., and Liebeskind, J. (1966). Origine des messages somato-sensitifs activant les cellules du cortex moteur chez le singe. *Exp. Brain Res.* **1**, 127–146.
Albe-Fessard, D., Liebeskind, J., and Lamarre, Y. (1965). Projection au niveau du cortex somato-moteur du singe d'afférences provenant des récepteurs musculaires. *C. R. Hebd. Seances Acad. Sci.* **261**, 3891–3894.
Andrews, C. J., Burke, D., and Lance, J. W. (1973). The comparison of tremors in normal, Parkinsonian and athetotic man. *J. Neurol. Sci.* **19**, 53.

Arshavsky, Yu. I., Gelfand, I. M., Orlovsky, G. N., and Pavlova, G. A. (1975a). Activity of neurones of the ventral spinocerebellar tract during "fictive scratching." *Biophysics* **20**, 762–764.

Arshavsky, Yu. I., Gelfand, I. M., Orlovsky, G. N., and Pavlova, G. A. (1975b). Origin of modulation in vestibulospinal neurons during scratching. *Biophysics* **20**, 965–967.

Brooks, V. B., Rudomin, P., and Slayman, C. L. (1961). Peripheral receptive fields of neurons in the cat's cerebral cortex. *J. Neurophysiol.* **24**, 302–325.

Bullock, T. H., and Horridge, G. A. (1965). "Structure and Function in the Nervous Systems of Invertebrates," Vol. I. Freeman, San Francisco, California.

DeLong, M. R. (1971). Central patterning of movement. *Neurosci. Res. Program, Bull.* **9**, 10–30.

Doty, R. W. (1968). Neural organization of deglutition. *In* "Handbook of Physiology" (C. F. Code and W. Heidel, eds.), Sect. 6, Vol. IV, pp. 1861–1902. Williams & Wilkins, Baltimore, Maryland.

Doty, R. W., and Bosma, J. F. (1956). An electromyographic analysis of reflex deglutition. *J. Neurophysiol.* **19**, 44–60.

Doty, R. W., Richmond, W. H., and Storey, A. T. (1967). Effect of medullary lesions on coordination of deglutition. *Exp. Neurol.* **17**, 91–106.

Evarts, E. V. (1966). Pyramidal tract activity associated with a conditioned hand movement in the monkey. *J. Neurophysiol.* **29**, 1011–1027.

Evarts, E. V. (1973). Brain mechanisms in movement. *Sci. Am.* **229**, 96–103.

Evarts, E. V., and Tanji, J. (1976). Reflex and intended responses in motor cortex pyramidal tract neurons of monkey. *J. Neurophysiol.* **39**, 1069–1080.

Flowers, K. (1978a). Some frequency response characteristics of Parkinsonism on pursuit tracking. *Brain* **101**, 19–34.

Flowers, K. (1978b). Lack of prediction in the motor behaviour of Parkinsonism. *Brain* **101**, 35–52.

Forssberg, H., Grillner, S., and Rossignol, S. (1975). Phase dependent reflex reversal during walking in chronic spinal cats. *Brain Res.* **85**, 103–107.

Gonshor, A., and Jones, G. M. (1976a). Short-term adaptive changes in the human vestibulo-ocular reflex arc. *J. Physiol. (London)* **256**, 361–379.

Gonshor, A., and Jones, G. M. (1976b). Extreme vestibulo-ocular adaptation induced by prolonged optical reversal of vision. *J. Physiol. (London)* **256**, 381–414.

Grillner, S. (1975). Locomotion in vertebrates: Central mechanisms and reflex interaction. *Physiol. Rev.* **55**, 247–304.

Hagbarth, K.-E. (1967). EMG studies of stretch reflexes in man. *Recent Adv. Clin. Neurophysiol., Electroencephalog. Clin. Neurophysiol. Suppl.* **25**, 74–79.

Hammond, P. H. (1956). The influence of prior instruction to the subject on an apparently involuntary neuromuscular response. *J. Physiol. (London)* **132**, 17P–18P.

Hammond, P. H. (1961). An experimental study of servo action in human muscular control. *Proc. Int. Conf. Med. Electron., 3rd, 1960* pp. 190–199.

Henneman, E. (1968). Peripheral mechanisms involved in the control of muscle. *In* "Medical Physiology" (V. B. Mountcastle, ed.), Vol. 2, pp. 1697–1716. Mosby, St. Louis, Missouri.

Hongell, A., Wallin, G., and Hagbarth, K.-E. (1973). Unit activity connected with movement initiation and arousal situations recorded from the ventrolateral nucleus of the human thalamus. *Acta Neurol. Scand.* **49**, 681–698.

Ito, M. (1974). The control mechanisms of cerebellar motor systems. *In* "The Neurosciences: Third Study Program" (F. O. Schmitt and F. G. Worden, eds.), pp. 293–303. MIT Press, Cambridge, Massachusetts.

Kugelberg, E. (1973). Properties of the rat hind-limb motor units. *In* "New Developments in Electromyography and Clinical Neurophysiology" (J. E. Desmedt, ed.), Vol. 1, pp. 2–13. Karger, Basel.

Larimer, J. L., and Kennedy, D. (1969a). Innervation patterns of fast and slow muscle in the uropods of crayfish. *J. Exp. Biol.* **51**, 119–133.

Larimer, J. L., and Kennedy, D. (1969b). The central nervous control of complex movements in the uropods of crayfish. *J. Exp. Biol.* **51**, 135–150.

Lashley, K. S. (1917). The accuracy of movement in the absence of excitation from the moving organ. *Am. J. Physiol.* **43**, 169–194.

Lee, R. G., and Tatton, W. G. (1975). Motor responses to sudden limb displacements in primates with specific CNS lesions and in human patients with motor system disorders. *J. Can. Sci. Neurol.* pp. 285–293.

Miles F. A. (1977). The primate flocculus and eye-head coordination. *In* "Eye Movements" Arvo Symp. (B. Brooks and F. Bajarandas, eds.), pp. 75–92. Plenum, New York.

Miles, F. A., and Fuller, J. H. (1974). Adaptive plasticity in the vestibuloocular responses of the rhesus monkey. *Brain Res.* **80**, 512–516.

Morasso, P., Bizzi, E., and Dichgans, J. (1973). Adjustment of saccade characteristics during head movements. *Exp. Brain Res.* **16**, 492–500.

Oscarsson, O. (1966). The projection of group I muscle afferents to the cat cerebral cortex. *In* "Muscular Afferents and Motor Control" (R. Granit, ed.), pp. 307–316. Wiley, New York.

Porter, R. (1973). Functions of the mammalian cerebral cortex in movement. *Prog. Neurobiol.* *(Oxford)* **1**, 1–51.

Robinson, D. A. (1976). Adaptive gain control of vestibuloocular reflex by the cerebellum. *J. Neurophysiol.* **39**, 954–969.

Rosén, I., and Asanuma, H. (1972). Peripheral afferent inputs to the forelimb area of the monkey motor cortex: Input–output relations. *Exp. Brain Res.* **14**, 257–273.

Sherrington, C. S. (1906). On the proprio-ceptive system, especially in its reflex aspect. *Brain* **29**, 467–482.

Sherrington, C. S. (1947). "The Integrative Action of the Nervous System." Yale Univ. Press, New Haven, Connecticut.

Strick, P. L. (1974). Activity of neurons in the ventrolateral nucleus of the thalamus in relation to learned movement in the monkey. *Abstr., 4th Annu. Meet. Soc. Neurosci.* p. 442.

Strick, P. L. (1976). Cerebellar neuron response to imposed limb displacement: Dependence of short latency dentate acitivity on intended movement. *Neurosci. Abstr. (Soc. Neurosci.)* **2**, 533.

Tanji, J., and Evarts, E. V. (1976). Anticipatory activity of motor cortex neurons in relation to direction of an intended movement. *J. Neurophysiol.* **39**, 1062–1068.

Thach, W. T., Jr. (1970). The behavior of Purkinje and cerebellar nuclear cells during two types of voluntary arm movement in the monkey. *In* "The Cerebellum in Health and Disease" (W. S. Fields and W. D. Willis, Jr., eds.), pp. 217–230. Green, St. Louis, Missouri.

Towe, A. L., Patton, H. D., and Kennedy, T. T. (1964). Response properties of neurons in the pericruciate cortex of the cat following electrical stimulation of the appendages. *Exp. Neurol.* **10**, 325–344.

Wiesendanger, M. (1969). The pyramidal tract. Recent investigations on its morphology and function. *Ergeb. Physiol., Biol. Chem. Exp. Pharmakol.* **61**, 73–136.

Woodworth, R. S. (1899). *Psychol. Rev., Monogr. Suppl.* **3**, No. 13.

12

Internal States of the Body: Autonomic, Neuroendocrine and Pain Functions

I. Introduction

The nervous system has three major effector systems. The motor system which we have just studied in Chapter 11 is one. It drives the skeletal muscles and moves us. The other two are the autonomic nervous system and the neuroendocrine system. They are the housekeepers and energizers of our body. They keep body state constant and most importantly adapt it to new situations. The autonomic nervous system innervates the *viscera*—the digestive system, reproductive system, urogenital system, the heart, the blood vessels, etc., and helps coordinate visceral activities. It is the system that aids in maintaining fluid balance, ionic composition of the blood and temperature as well as other processes. The neuroendocrine system influences body state via hormones. Hormones are released into the bloodstream, find their way to various tissues and affect them in highly specific ways. The control of sexual behavior and reproduction is but one of the many functions of the neuroendocrine system. In general, the neuroendocrine system is the means by which the brain and endocrine glands integrate body function and behavior. The viscera must be controlled, but they must also give feedback to the brain in time of distress. Pain serves this role. It also tells us when our bodies have met injurious or unpleasant stimuli.

In this chapter we shall explore the functions of the autonomic nervous system and the neuroendocrine system. We shall also discuss the perception of pain. Lest any misconceptions arise, it is appropriate to emphasize that this chapter does not cover all aspects of internal body state. Entire physiology texts are devoted to the subject. The focus of this chapter is to illustrate how the nervous system acts to control body state and how, in turn, body state is conveyed to the nervous system. Besides the normal maintenance functions, we will illustrate how the regulation of internal body state brings the body in line with behavior.

II. Autonomic Nervous System

The complex task of integrating the work of the vital organs, the heart, lungs, blood vessels, digestive system and urogenital system with all their associated glands, is delegated to the *autonomic nervous system* (ANS). It regulates aspects of gastrointestinal activity, modulates cardiovascular functions, regulates body temperature and controls pupillary dilation to cite a few of its many assignments (Table 12-1). It looks after many "housekeeping" functions of the body, and it brings all this in line with outward body activities. At one time it was thought that the autonomic nervous system went its own way, hence the curious term autonomic nervous system. It does, in fact, largely mind its own affairs, but it is still a part of the harmonious unity of the nervous system.

PARASYMPATHETIC
NERVOUS SYSTEM

Fig. 12-2. (*right*). The parasympathetic division of the autonomic nervous system. The parasympathetic nervous system consists of a subset of autonomic motor neurons in the spinal cord and brain stem which connect to parasympathetic ganglia located close to the peripheral targets. It serves primarily to conserve, maintain and restore bodily resources. As Walter Cannon, the pioneering physiologist and theorist on autonomic functions said in 1929, "a glance at these various functions of the cranial division (of the parasympathetic system) reveals at once that they serve for bodily conservation; by narrowing the pupil they shield the retina from excessive light; by slowing the heart rate they give the cardiac muscle longer periods for rest and invigoration; and by providing for the flow of saliva and gastric juice, and by supplying the necessary muscular tone for the contraction of the alimentary canal, they prove fundamentally essential to the processes of proper digestion and absorption, by which energy-yielding material is taken into the body and stored. To the cranial division belongs the great service of building up reserves and fortifying the body against times of need and stress." The parasympathetic division also rids the body of urinary and intestinal wastes.

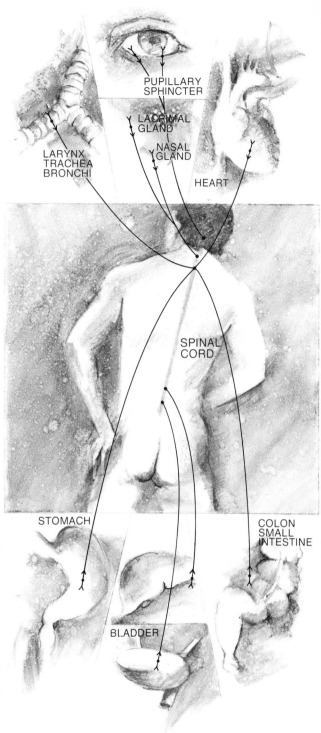

Fig. 12-1. (*left*). The sympathetic division of the autonomic nervous system is concerned with mobilizing the resources of the body in stressful situations, such as emergencies or periods of emotional crisis. It consists of a column of small motor neurons in the spinal cord connecting to a chain of sympathetic ganglia. The efferents from these ganglia innervate many tissues. Activation may deepen respirations, increase the rate and force of cardiac contractions, constrict blood vessels in the skin, increase blood supply in skeletal musculature, dilate the pupils, and decrease gastrointestinal secretion and mobility. All these activities prepare the body for the possibility of intense motor activities involved in attack, defense or escape.

In general, for both divisions the central control structures for the ANS lie within the *hypothalamus*. Afferent fibers from a variety of sources converge there carrying information about the general state of various internal organs, and about the adaptive requirements imposed by the external environment. From this information neural control signals are generated by the hypothalamus and sent out along the appropriate autonomic efferent fibers. Many of these autonomic projections from the hypothalamus proceed to cell groups in the spinal cord, while others project to nuclei in the brain stem. The many fibers of the ANS do not run directly to smooth or cardiac muscle but pass instead to another group of little motor neurons en route to their myriad targets. These subordinate motor cells lie in *ganglia* either close to the neural trunk or far away in the wall of the target organ.

The two divisions of the ANS function in a reciprocal manner, and their activities are integrated to produce coordinated responses that maintain an appropriate internal environment to meet the demands of whatever situation may be encountered at the moment. It appears that parasympathetic activity is initiated by changes in the internal organs themselves, while a considerable amount of sympathetic activity is initiated by changes detected in the external environment. The sight of a grizzly bear while hiking will activate the sympathetic system, for example.

There are a number of morphological differences between the two divisions of the ANS. One important difference is the location of the *preganglionic* cell bodies. The preganglionic cell bodies of the sympathetic division are all found in the spinal cord in a cell column located above the ventral horn (Fig. 12-3). Most preganglionic cell bodies of the parasympathetic system are found within nuclei located in the brain stem, although some are found in the spinal cord.

The ganglia of the sympathetic and parasympathetic divisions also differ in their gross morphology. Sympathetic ganglia tend to be located away from their target receptors, and one class of sympathetic ganglia are located parallel to the spinal cord (Fig. 12-1). The *postganglionic* axons of the sympathetic system are thus quite long. In addition, each postganglionic cell of the sympathetic division usually receives inputs from a number of preganglionic axons arising from several different levels of the spinal cord. Such a diffuse pattern of connections suggests that activity in the sympathetic division will probably not be confined just to a single target organ, but will have widespread effects. In fact, the sympathetic division often produces high levels of arousal, and this is quite consistent with the notion of the sympathetic division as a system that prepares an organism for "fight or flight." Clearly, high stress situations are best met by simultaneous and coordinated responses from many different visceral muscles and glands.

On the other hand, the parasympathetic ganglia are generally located close to the peripheral parasympathetic effectors, and hence these cells have relatively short postganglionic axons, usually ranging from 1 mm to no more than several

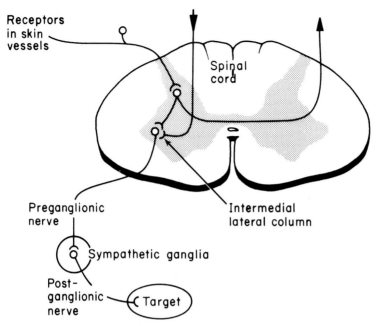

Fig. 12-3. Simplified circuitry for sympathetic nervous system reflexes. Unlike skeletal muscles, which are activated by neurons that project directly from the CNS, autonomic effectors do not receive direct central projections. Rather, the axons from autonomic cell bodies in the CNS go to various autonomic ganglia where they synapse on cells that project to the peripheral autonomic targets. The cells that extend from the CNS to the autonomic ganglia are called preganglionic neurons, those that project from the ganglia to the autonomic effectors are called postganglionic neurons.

centimeters in length, which spread into the body of the organ. In contrast to the pattern of sympathetic anatomy, neural connections within the parasympathetic division are much more specific. The preganglionic axons of the parasympathetic division project from more isolated cell groups of the spinal cord and connect with fewer postganglionic cells. As a result, parasympathetic activity is often relatively more discrete than sympathetic activity. Indeed, there would seem to be little reason for the simultaneous activation of such diverse parasympathetic functions as pupillary constriction, cardiac deceleration, and stimulation of gastrointestinal secretions and activity. However, often there is an association between various parasympathetic responses. For example, salivary, gastric, and pancreatic secretions often occur at or about the same time. This is certainly an example of parasympathetic coordination. In both divisions, the post-ganglionic fibers are quite small (0.3 to 1.3 μm in diameter), are unmyelinated, and conduct impulses relatively slowly (0.7 to 2.3 m/second).

In both divisions autonomic actions are generally slow and diffuse as they need to be. This is in striking contrast to the skeletal motor system where the action is fast and specific. This distinction between skeletal muscle and autonomic systems is a result of the organization and properties of the cells.

Unlike skeletal muscle innervation, there is little specificity in the way in which preganglionic axons of either division terminate on their postganglionic neurons. These axons branch repeatedly before they form axosomatic and axodendritic synapses on a number of different postganglionic cells. In addition, a single postganglionic axon usually influences a number of gland or muscle cells, and each of these cells may, in turn, be influenced by many postganglionic axons. Brief stimulation of autonomic efferents usually produces a prolonged response by the innervated organ, and responses of several seconds duration are typical. In contrast, similar brief stimulation of somatic nerves produces skeletal muscle responses lasting for only a few milliseconds. Smooth muscle fibers of the viscera are much smaller than skeletal muscle fibers, and the fibers are so crowded together that their membranes almost fuse together. Thus, when one part of visceral smooth muscle tissue is stimulated, the action potential generated there is electrically conducted to neighboring fibers and excites them also. This allows current to flow from one smooth muscle cell to another and causes the action potential to be distributed over the entire surface of the muscle mass. In the intestine, for example, once an action potential begins, it spreads along the intestinal wall consecutively stimulating adjacent areas. This, in effect, creates a ring of constriction that travels down the intestine pushing the internal contents along.

There are a variety of sensory afferents closely associated with the ANS. They are involved in sensing such diverse kinds of information as visceral pain, the amount of stretch in the walls of hollow organs (such as the bladder and blood vessels), the acidity of the contents of the digestive tract, and the amount of dissolved oxygen in the blood. These afferents enter the central nervous system through the spinal cord and through the vagus nerve. Much of the information carried by these afferents is unavailable to conscious experience, and when such information is available, it is nearly always in the form of diffuse and poorly localized sensations such as nausea or hunger. Even fairly severe visceral pain may not be subjectively localized at the diseased or injured organ, but as we shall describe in the end of this chapter it is often "referred" to (or feels as if it is located at) areas of the skin which send somatic afferents to the same segment of the spinal cord as the affected visceral organ.

B. Neurotransmitters

The neurochemistry of synaptic transmission is perhaps better understood in the ANS than in any other portion of the nervous system. In the ANS, synaptic transmission is mediated primarily by two substances—acetylcholine and norepinephrine. In both the sympathetic and parasympathetic divisions of the ANS, the transmitter at preganglionic synapses is acetylcholine—the same transmitter found at somatic neuromuscular junctions. Acetycholine is also the only known transmitter in the postganglionic parasympathetic neurons. In postganglionic neurons of the sympathetic division, norepinephrine is the most important, but not the only, transmitter substance. Some sympathetic postganglionic fibers release acetycholine as, for example, projections to the sweat glands and some of the projections to perivascular musculature. In addition, there is some evidence that histamine may function as a sympathetic transmitter, and other evidence suggests that several other substances may be involved as well.

Adrenaline or epinephrine—the call to action chemical of the adrenal gland—is of central importance to sympathetic function. Epinephrine excites or inhibits various peripheral organs. It is produced by the adrenal medulla, a peripheral gland which is innervated by sympathetic *preganglionic* fibers (Fig. 12-1). When the adrenal medulla is stimulated by sympathetic activity, it secretes epinephrine into the blood (along with smaller quantities of norepinephrine) and quickly reaches and influences many sympathetic target organs, which are exquisitely sensitive to epinephrine. A denervated mammalian heart, for example, can be accelerated by as little as 1.4 *parts per billion* epinephrine in the blood. One of the most important effects of circulating epinephrine is to increase blood flow to skeletal muscles, brain, and liver—all of obvious importance in "fight or flight" situations.

In the ANS, a single neurotransmitter substance sometimes has opposite effects on different target organs, or exhibits strong action at one site and acts weakly at another. For example, epinephrine causes relaxation of bronchial muscles, but causes constriction of pulmonary perivascular muscles. Why? The answer is deceptively simple and in fact we have discussed the principle before (Chapter 4). The effect of a neurohumoral substance on an organ depends not only on the substance itself but also on the nature of the receptors. In the ANS, there are three distinct types of adrenergic (norepinephrine and epinephrine) receptors and two types of cholinergic receptors. The net response of the organ or organ systems to sympathetic activity is thus not merely a simple function of the amount of one neurohumoral substance, but is a function of both the relative balance of two substances and their absolute levels. This additional complexity gives the sympathetic system more flexibility and a broader range of control of bodily functions than it would have otherwise.

C.   ANS Control Functions

In many respects the ANS can be thought of as a very elegant control system. Consider, for example, the way it functions to regulate body temperature. The maintenance of vital organs at an appropriate temperature, of course, is critically important to us, since we will suffer injury and eventually death if body temperature fluctuates excessively.

The autonomic thermoregulatory system monitors body temperature with two sets of temperature sensors. One set is located in the anterior portion of the hypothalamus and senses arterial blood temperature. This temperature is very closely related to the temperature of the vital organs, or the core zone temperature. The other set of receptors is widely distributed in the skin where they sense skin or peripheral zone temperature. Both sets or receptors send projections to the posterior portion of the hypothalamus where their outputs are compared to the optimum or *set point* temperature. In a normal, healthy organism the temperature set point is essentially constant and can be considered an inherent characteristic of the nervous system.

If the core zone temperature sensor indicates that core temperature is rising above the optimum range, the posterior hypothalamic comparator activates two heat emitting processes—both mediated by the sympathetic division of the ANS. First, sweat glands are stimulated causing heat to be removed by evaporative cooling. Second, blood vessels near the body surface dilate, thus increasing the surface blood flow and increasing the amount of heat lost through the skin. Recall that we noted earlier that these two autonomic effector systems are innervated by cholinergic synapses, while the rest of the sympathetic division is primarily adrenergic. Because of this we can consider these heat emitting effectors to constitute a relatively distinct subdivision of the sympathetic system.

The second set of temperature receptors, the peripheral zone receptors, respond primarily to cold. If the peripheral temperature falls below the optimal range, the posterior hypothalamic comparator activates sympathetically mediated heat production and heat conservation processes. These heat conservation and production processes include peripheral vasoconstriction, increased skeletal muscle tone, shivering, and increased metabolic breakdown of fats and carbohydrates. The first three functions are accomplished primarily by direct sympathetic innervation, while the last is controlled primarily by hormonal secretions from the adrenal medulla and the adrenal cortex.

In achieving thermoregulation the ANS brings into action two important design features: it consists of two independent and antagonistic processes. It uses not only a feedback circuit (core temperature sensors—heat emission), but a feedforward circuit as well (peripheral temperature sensors—heat conservation). This means that the body can respond to a cold environment, as sensed by the peripheral receptors in the skin, even before there is any appreciable core temperature change. This combination results in a control system that is more responsive, and much more accurate, than a simple single process feedback system might be.

We will illustrate one other vital function of the ANS, the regulation of *arterial blood pressure*. Overly high blood pressure will damage the circulatory system; excessively low blood pressure will deprive the body and brain of its necessary blood supply. Arterial blood pressure is regulated by the resistance to blood flow offered by the vessels and the cardiac output. The resistance to blood flow in the circulatory system is determined primarily by the diameter of the arterioles, which in turn is determined by the degree of contraction of the smooth muscles in arteriole walls. This perivascular musculature is innervated only by sympathetic neurons (except in the genital region). These fibers are continuously active so that they normally maintain the arterioles in a state of partial contraction. By decreased or increased autonomic activity the muscles can either be relaxed so the vessels dilate or contracted so they constrict.

Sensory input for blood pressure regulation comes from baroreceptors and chemoreceptors. *Baroreceptors* monitor arterial blood pressure by sensing the amount of stretch of the arterial vessel walls. An increase in arterial pressure produces an increase in the discharge rate of these cells, while a decrease in pressure produces a decrease in their discharge rate. The principal baroreceptors are located in the vascular walls of the aortic arch and carotid sinus. The chemoreceptors are also located in walls of the aorta and carotid arteries near the baroreceptors. The *chemoreceptors* are sensitive to the amount of dissolved oxygen in the blood. A decrease in blood oxygen level produces an increase in the discharge rate of these cells. Both of these receptor sets send projections into a region of the medulla known as the cardiovascular center. This region is also the major site of origin of cardiovascular efferent fibers.

Cardiovascular efferent fibers activate the spinal autonomic motor cells which pass the message to the ganglia and to the appropriate targets. The two autonomic divisions exert opposite effects on heart rate. Parasympathetic activity mediated by acetylcholine produces a decrease in cardiac activity, while sympathetic activity mediated by norepinephrine produces an increase. (It should be noted, lest any confusion arise, that the heart will beat just fine without autonomic input. However, it cannot be regulated).

The control loop is now complete. Receptor information converges on the *medullary cardiovascular center* where it is compared with the *set point*, and if there is sufficient mismatch between actual and optimal conditions, the appropriate efferents are activated to reduce the discrepancy. The response patterns of the various components of this system are illustrated in Fig. 12-4.

How might high blood pressure be treated? Most drugs act to decrease the activity of the noradrenergic sympathetic input to the heart. Thus receptor blockers or reserpine (which reduces the catecholamine stores available for release) are effective drugs.

We are still left with the problem of how the set point conditions are deter-

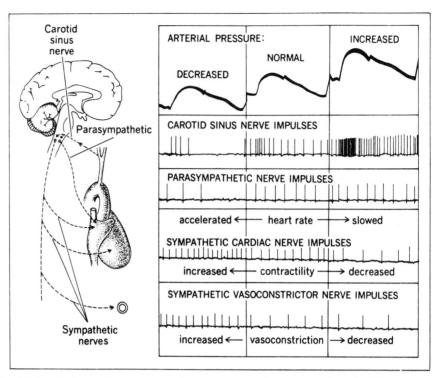

Fig. 12-4. Autonomic nervous system responses to changes in arterial pressure. An increase in arterial pressure causes an increase in the rate of firing of carotid sinus baroreceptors. This causes a reflex stimulation of the parasympathetic nerves to the heart and an inhibition of the sympathetic nerves to the heart, arterioles and veins. The net result is a decreased cardiac output and peripheral resistance which causes arterial pressure to drop. A decrease in blood pressure results in an opposite event. (From Vander *et al.*, 1970, *Human Physiology*, p. 288. Reprinted with permission of McGraw-Hill Book Company.)

mined. Unlike the set point in temperature regulation, the blood pressure set point must change since cardiovascular demands are not constant. It is common knowledge that blood pressure is often significantly elevated in stressful situations. Some people turn very red! However, changes in blood pressure and blood flow do not occur in response to physical stimuli alone. Merely anticipating or imagining a stressful situation can also cause such changes. The answer to this problem appears to be that set point determination is primarily a function of the hypothalamus, which is, in turn, interconnected with the medullary cardiovascular center. For example, electrical stimulation of the posterior lateral hypothalamus produces immediate blood pressure elevation, while immediate depression occurs upon stimulation of anterior portions of the hypothalamus. The hypothalamus, as we noted earlier, receives information from a wide variety of sensory receptor systems as well as inputs from the cerebral cortex, the reticular activating system, and the limbic system. Precisely how all of this information is integrated to generate appropriate set points for cardiac output (and for many other regulatory systems) is still largely unknown.

The mechanisms that control the amount of cardiac output are very sophisticated and specific as they need to be. Cardiac output must constantly change to meet the metabolic demands of various tissues. For example, during exercise, cardiac output increases and blood flow to muscles rises to meet their oxygen demands, while blood flow to other areas, such as the skin, gastrointestinal system, and even the inactive muscles, decreases. However, while exercise promotes more cardiac output and blood flow to contracting muscles, changes in posture impose different demands. When we move from a prone to an upright posture, cardiovascular adjustments must assure adequate circulation to the brain and prevent blood from pooling in the lower body in response to the pull of gravity. This change does not generally require increased cardiac output as does exercise; rather, it involves increasing blood flow to the brain and restricting vascular flow to the body. Temperature regulation, described earlier in this section, provides yet another illustration of a basic cardiovascular reflex pattern. In this case the primary adjustment is in the amount of flow through the blood vessels of the skin—increased flow for heat loss and decreased flow for heat conservation.

These are but a few examples of many basic cardiovascular reflex adjustments in which the brain participates (Cohen and MacDonald, 1974; Cohen and Obrist, 1975). They represent the changes in cardiac output and its distribution that are required to meet the differing metabolic demands of such situations as exercise, postural adjustment, temperature change, agonistic behavior, sexual activity, feeding, etc. In each of these situations, a highly specific and appropriate pattern of adjustment is made. This indicates considerable specificity in central autonomic control.

There are probably only a limited number of such basic reflex patterns, and each is activated by a specific set of stimuli. These stimulus–response connections are programmed into the organism and need not be learned (Cohen and Obrist, 1975). However, it is possible through various well-established training procedures to produce _learned cardiovascular responses_. That is, by employing various learning systems, one can couple cardiovascular responses to stimuli that do not normally elicit a cardiovascular change. For example, if one trains an animal to run on a treadmill (exercise) in response to a tone, then that tone will gradually gain the capacity to elicit those cardiovascular adjustments generally seen during exercise. Similarly, if one associates a stimulus such as light or tone with a painful or stressful stimulus, then the light or tone will acquire the capacity to produce those cardiovascular changes that generally occur in painful or stressful situations

(Cohen, 1974). These changes can include rather dramatic increases in arterial blood pressure, and this finding has been used as a basis for developing various behavioral models of hypertension in animals.

Thus, it is possible for stimuli that do not naturally affect cardiovascular activity to acquire some control over various basic cardiovascular reflex patterns. Through such learning, the nervous system is capable of expanding the set of stimuli that activate autonomic reflex patterns. In this sense, central autonomic control can be viewed as plastic in the same way as control of skeletomotor activity is plastic. An important finding is that an organism can learn to make the appropriate cardiovascular adjustments in anticipation of, or in preparation for, metabolic demands. So, for example, a trained runner will increase his cardiac output and muscle blood flow at the starting line, prior to the actual metabolic demand produced by running a race. Also, cues associated with threatening situations will elicit substantial increases in arterial blood pressure before the actual need for this response occurs. While this is generally adaptive, it must also be recognized that such learned or anticipatory adjustments can occur without the actual metabolic demand ever materializing, as in the case of fear or anger with no ensuing action. Although still an hypothesis, it may be that such a mismatch between adjustment and demand may lead to various cardiovascular pathologies such as hypertension (Cohen and Obrist, 1975).

In the end then we see that visceral activities are regulated in a harmonious manner. They are brought in line with the oneness of the body by the autonomic nervous system. At many levels in the spinal cord, brain stem and hypothalamus, visceral and somatic functions are brought together in comprehensive strategies. The performances of many organs during times of stress provide eloquent examples of total body function. Moreover, visceral sensations and communications may intrude deeply upon our thoughts and feelings. Although the autonomic nervous system is constructed to allow for overall responses we can see that it can be very specific. Its plasticity shows that it does not merely respond reflexively to changes in visceral conditions, but that it has adaptive versatility.

III.   The Neuroendocrine System: Chemical Integration

The autonomic nervous system, however, is not the only intrinsic influence on the body. The other major one is the neuroendocrine system, the system entrusted with regulating hormone levels in the body.

If you accidentally touch a hot surface you will quickly withdraw your hand from the heat. This "reflex withdrawal" involves a noxious sensory stimulus, central integration and the activation of the appropriate flexor muscles. The response is mediated by the sensory and motor systems described in Chapter 11. The total response pattern of the organism is not over, however, when the flexor muscles have contracted. The painful stimulus is also followed by a complex pattern of hormonal secretions. For example, the painful stimulus causes the anterior pituitary gland to secrete *adrenocorticotropic hormone* (ACTH) which is carried by the vascular system to the *adrenal cortex* which then secretes a class of hormones called glucocorticoids. The principal glucocorticoid which is secreted in man, cortisol, is then carried by the blood to the burned tissue where it has an antiinflammatory effect. Thus, the painful stimulus has two major kinds of effects, a rapid neuromuscular effect and a slower *neuroendocrine* effect. This is just one example of the constellation of roles played by the endocrine system.

In general, hormones are involved in such processes as basic cellular metabolism, the development and differentiation of several organ systems including the brain, and in several behaviors such as maternal, sexual and aggressive behavior. As we saw in Chapter 8, hormones are even involved in the modulation of learning and memory processes. Whereas the ability to reproduce is totally dependent on the endocrine system, other functions do not absolutely require it. However, without the endocrine system our effectiveness in adapting to the environment would be extremely impaired. Our bodies would require the attention given a hothouse plant. The neuroendocrine system works right along with the nervous system to integrate body function and adapt it to new challenges through the controlled release of many hormones which act in specific ways on many targets. New discoveries are still being made about the nature of neuroendocrine integration, but the basic concept of hormonal control is quite ancient. Aristotle had compared the effects of castration in birds and men some 300 years before Christ.

What is a hormone? A *hormone* is a chemical substance which is synthesized and secreted by specialized cells and which is carried by the vascular system to target tissues, where it may have its primary effect or where it may cause the secretion of another hormone. In the example, ACTH is secreted by the pituitary gland and has its effect on the *adrenal gland* (see Fig. 12-5), which in turn secretes cortisol, the hormone which then affects the tissue that was burned. The important distinction between hormones and neurotransmitters is that hormones are carried by the blood to their target tissues, whereas neurotransmitters have their effect directly on the target cell at the synapse. There are many hormones: each has a special assignment and produces essential changes in body functions. Table 12-2 gives a comprehensive view of hormone actions.

Chemically there are three types of hormones: (1) the polypeptides or proteins, such as ACTH; (2) the derivatives of the amino acids, such as thyroxine, which is produced by the metabolism of the amino acid tyrosine; and (3) the

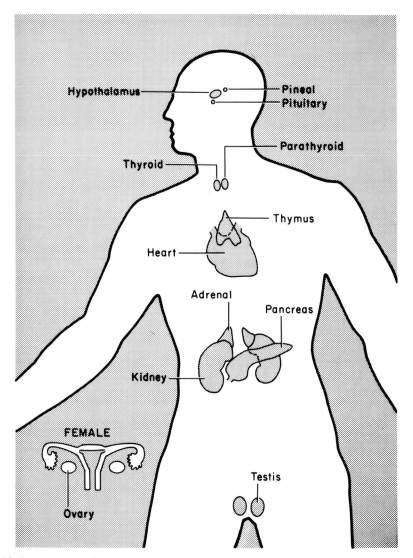

Fig. 12-5. Location of endocrine glands and certain tissues. (Redrawn from Frieden and Lipner, 1971. Copyright 1971. Reprinted by permission of Prentice-Hall, Englewood Cliffs, New Jersey.)

steroid hormones, such as the male hormone testosterone, which are derivatives of cholesterol. The structures of some of these hormones are illustrated in Fig. 12-6.

Figure 12-7 illustrates the primary sources of hormones. The brain is the master gland—it is command central—having its own hormones which directly control the secretion of other hormones from various glands. This idea, de-

Table 12-2 The vertebrate hormones: classes, targets, and effects[a]

Hormone	Target	Effects
I. Peptides, Protein hormones		
1. Pituitary gland (Hypophysis)		
A. Adenohypophysis		
a. Pars distalis growth hormone (GH, somatotropin)	All tissues	Growth of tissues (easily seen in long bones, metabolism of protein, mobilization of fat)
		Lipolysis
Adrenocorticotropin (ACTH, corticotropin)	Adrenal cortex	Synthesis and release of gluco-corticoids
Thyroid-stimulating hormone (TSH, thyrotropin)	Adipose tissue	Lipolysis
	Thyroid gland	Synthesis and secretion of thyroxine and triiodothyronine
Male		
Follicle-stimulating hormone (FSH)	Seminiferous tubules	Production of sperm
Interstitial-cell-stimulating hormones (ICSH, luteinizing hormone, LH)	Testes	Synthesis and secretion of androgens
Female		
FSH	Ovary (follicles)	Follicle maturation
LH	Ovary (interstitial cells)	Final maturation of follicle, estrogen secretion, ovulation, Corpus luteum formation, Progesterone secretion
Prolactin	Mammary glands (alveolar cell)	Milk production in prepared gland
	Crop gland of pigeons	Crop gland "milk" production
b. Pars intermedia		
Melanocyte-stimulating hormones (α- and β-MSH, Intermedin)	Melanophores	Pigment dispersal in melanophores (darkening of skin)
B. Neurohypophysis (Posterior lobe)		
Oxytocin (Let-down factor, milk-ejection factor)	Uterus	Contraction of smooth muscle, milk ejection
	Mammary glands	

(Continued)

Table 12-2 (*Continued*)

Hormone	Target	Effects
Vasopressin (antidiuretic hormone, ADH)	Kidney Arteries	Reabsorption of water Contraction of smooth muscle
2. Pancreas		
Insulin	All cells	Carbohydrate, fat and protein metabolism, hypoglycemia
Glucagon	Liver	Hyperglycemia
3. Ovary		
Relaxin	Pelvic ligaments	Separation of pelvic bones
4. Thyroid		
Thyrocalcitonin (calcitonin)	Bones, kidney	Excretion of calcium and phosphorus, inhibited calcium release from bones, decreased blood calcium levels
5. Parathyroid		
Parathyroid hormone	Bones, kidney	Elevated blood calcium and phosphorus levels, mobilization of calcium from bone, inhibited calcium excretion from kidney
6. Kidney[b]		
Erythropoietin	Bone marrow	Increased erythrocyte production
Renin	Adrenal cortex	Aldosterone synthesis, secretion
7. Stomach and Duodenum		
Gastrin	Stomach	Acid secretion
Enterogastrone	Stomach	Inhibited gastric mobility
Cholecystokinin	Gallbladder	Contraction of the gallbladder
Secretin	Pancreas	Secretion of water and salts
Pancreozymin	Pancreas	Secretion of digestive enzymes
II. Amino Acid Derivatives		
1. Thyroid		
Thyroxin Triiodothyronine	Most cells	Increased metabolic rate, growth, and development

Table 12-2 *(Continued)*

Hormone	Target	Effects
2. Adrenal medulla Norepinephrine Epinephrine	Most cells	Increased cardiac activity, elevated blood pressure, glycolysis, hyperglycemia
3. Pineal gland Melatonin	Melanophores	Dispersion of melanin
4. Argentaffin cells, platelets, nerves Serotonin (5-hydroxytryptamine)	Arterioles, central nervous system	Vasoconstriction
III. Steroids and Lipids **1. Testes** Androgen (testosterone)	Most cells	Development and maintenance of masculine characteristics and behavior
2. Ovary Estrogen (17β-estradiol)	Most cells	Development and maintenance of feminine characteristics and behavior
3. Corpus luteum Progesterone	Uterus, mammary glands	Maintenance of uterine endometrium and stimulation of mammary duct formation
4. Adrenal cortex Hydrocortisone Cortisone	Most cells	Balanced carbohydrate, protein, and fat metabolism; anti-inflammatory action
Aldosterone	Kidney	Reabsorption of Na^+ from urine
5. Prostate, Seminal Vesicles, Brain, Nerves Prostaglandins	Uterus, rabbit duodenum	Contraction of smooth muscle

[a] From Frieden and Lipner (1971). Copyright 1971. Reprinted by permission of Prentice-Hall, Englewood Cliffs, New Jersey.

[b] The renal hormones appear to be enzymes that activate plasma substrates which act on the target organ.

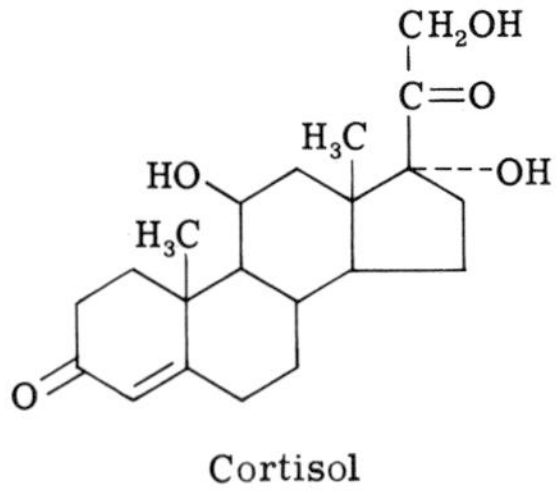

Cortisol
[glucocorticoid]

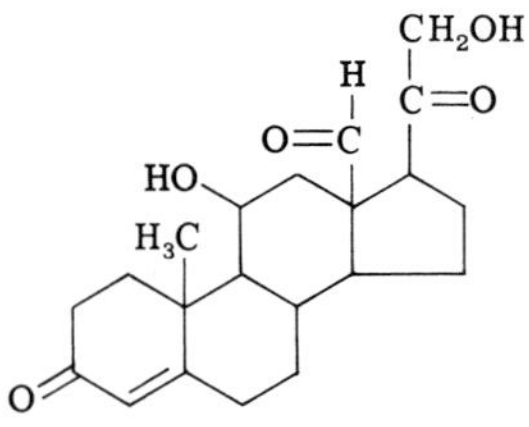

Aldosterone
[mineralocorticoid]

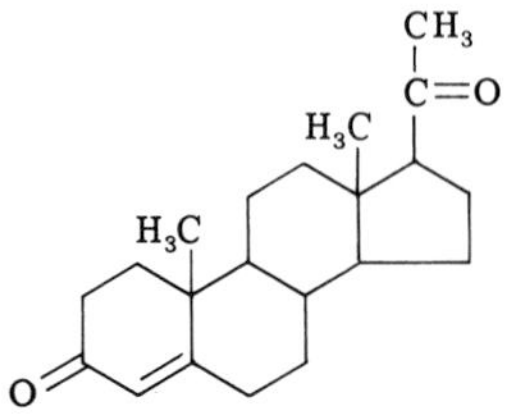

Progesterone
[progestin]

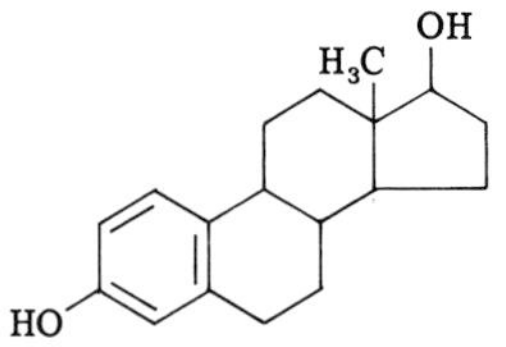

β-Estradiol
[estrogen]

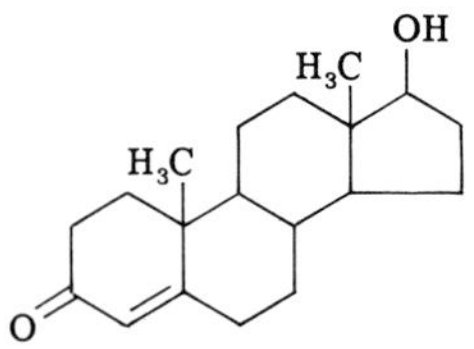

Testosterone
[androgen]

Ser -Tyr-Ser -Met-Glu -His -Phe-Arg-Tyr-Gly -Lys-Pro-Val -Gly -Lys-
 1   2   3   4   5   6   7   8   9   10   11 12   13   14   15

Lys-Arg-Arg-Pro-Val -Lys-Val -Tyr-Pro-Ala -Gly -Glu -Asp-Asp-Glu -
16   17   18   19   20   21   22   23   24   25   26   27   28   29   30

                    NH₂
                    |
Ala -Ser -Glu -Ala -Phe-Pro-Leu-Glu -Phe
31   32   33   34   35   36   37   38   39

Adrenocorticotropic hormone
(sheep)

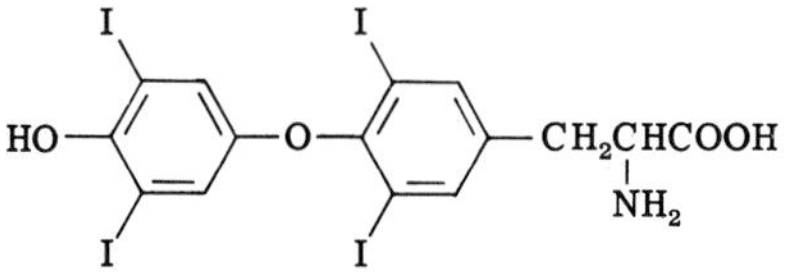

Thyroxine
(3,5,3′, 5′-tetraiodothyronine)

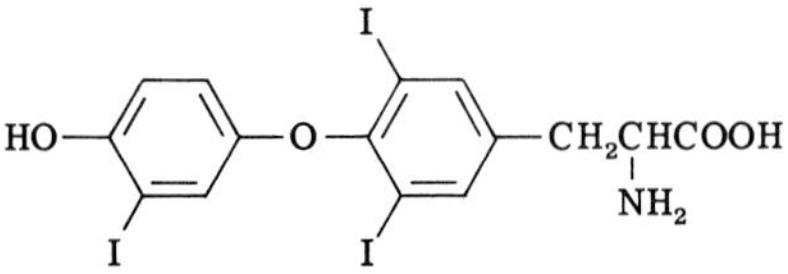

3,5,3′-Triiodothyronine

Fig. 12-6. Chemical formulas of hormones. (From Frieden and Lipner, 1971.)

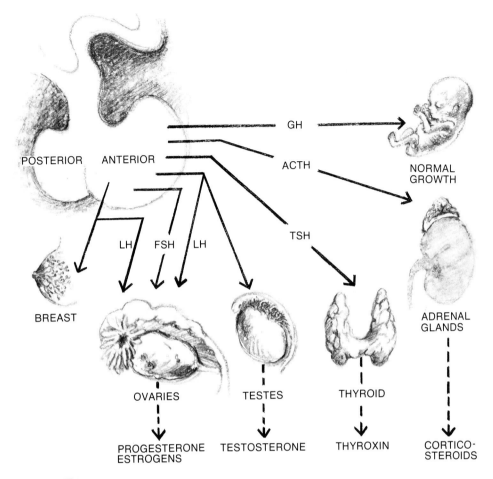

PITUITARY GLAND

Fig. 12-7. The pituitary gland, located in the brain underlying the hypothalamus, secretes a variety of hormones, LH, FSH, TSH, ACTH and GH which act on various parts of the body to regulate body functions.

veloped only during the past decade, has led to exciting new developments in our understanding of how hormones influence physiology and behavior.

Specific hormones have a major role in regulating behavior. In most vertebrates, for example, the _gonadal hormones_ play a critical and often unsuspected role in reproductive behavior; _gonadectomy_ results in the decline and disappearance of mating responses in nonhuman animals. These behaviors can be reinstituted either by the systemic administration of the gonadal hormones or by the application of small amounts of hormone directly to limited regions of the brain.

Gonadal hormones are also important in regulating the maternal behavior shown by mammals. Nest-building, retrieving and huddling behaviors exhibited by maternal animals are regulated by gonadal hormones. In all mammals the stimuli provided by the young are important in regulating the hormones controlling milk production and release. Gonadal hormones also regulate aggressive behaviors. In most mammalian species, the male is more aggressive than the female. Castration of the male usually leads to a decrease in fighting behavior, and this can be reinstituted with _testosterone_, the primary hormone secreted by the testes. Female mammals may also be aggressive but usually only in limited circumstances, for example, during pregnancy and when caring for newborn young. While it is not yet entirely clear which hormone or group of hormones modulates "maternal" aggression, it is clear that ovarian and/or placental hormones are involved.

Communication behaviors are also regulated by gonadal hormones. These may involve the development of hormone controlled visual signals such as the red wattles of the rooster, the fat pads about the shoulders of male squirrel monkeys during the breeding season (making them look like miniature football players), or the brilliantly colored sex skin which appears at the time of ovulation in several species of primates including baboons, macaques and chimpanzees. Gonadal hormones also control olfactory stimuli, odors called _pheromones_, which are produced by secretory glands and which appear in as many as 40 different positions of the body including the chin, belly, anus and forearms in different species. Pheromones appear to give information about sexual receptivity, dominance status, territorial boundaries and the like and are clearly important in regulating social interactions between members of the species. Indeed, the perfume industry is based on the notion that odors are important social stimuli (see also Chapter 9).

Central to the entire endocrine system is the _pituitary gland_ located at the base of the brain in a bony cavity called the _sella turcica_. Hormones [ACTH, TSH (thyroid-stimulating hormone), LH (luteinizing hormone) and _FSH (follicle-stimulating hormone)_] from the _anterior pituitary_ (or the _adenohypophysis_) control the secretion of hormones by the adrenal cortex, thyroid gland and gonads, while two other adenohypophyseal hormones (prolactin and growth hormone) have various direct effects on somatic tissues such as the mammary gland and the bones. The hormones oxytocin and vasopressin of the _posterior pituitary_ (or the _neurohypophysis_) have a variety of direct effects upon tissues such as the uterus and kidney. The anterior and posterior pituitary lie together, but embryologically, like nonidentical twins, they have very different origins. The anterior pituitary develops from epithelial cells arising from the roof of the mouth, while the posterior pituitary develops as an outgrowth of the brain.

In the 1940's it was discovered that the nerve endings which make up the posterior pituitary contain granules which hold _oxytocin_ and _vasopressin_. The

536

cell bodies of these neurons originate in two areas of the hypothalamus, the supraoptic nucleus and the paraventricular nucleus. Release of milk during nursing exemplifies how this system functions (See Fig. 12-8). The tactile stimulus of a sucking baby activates receptors which activate the appropriate supraoptic and paraventricular neurons in the hypothalamus. When these cells are stimulated, they release oxytocin from their nerve endings in the posterior pituitary, much in the way that a neurotransmitter is released. The oxytocin is carried by

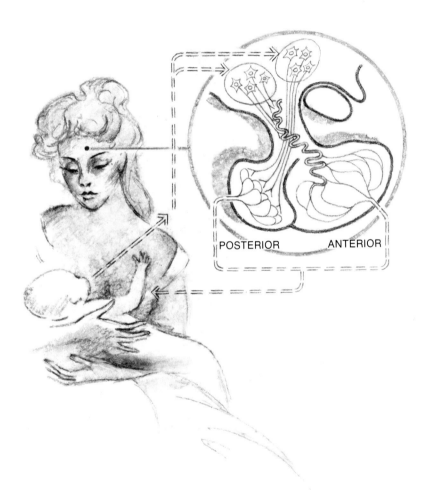

POSTERIOR   ANTERIOR

NEUROENDOCRINOLOGY

Fig. 12-8. The basic events in neuroendocrine mediated release of milk. Sucking stimulates receptors which activate neurons in the hypothalamus causing them in turn to stimulate oxytocin release from the posterior pituitary into the bloodstream. Prolactin secretion from the anterior pituitary stimulates the development of the breast and milk.

the vascular system to the mammary gland where it causes milk let-down. Result—happy baby! In a similar way, internal osmotic stimuli produced by dehydration cause the secretion of vasopressin which increases blood pressure and causes the kidney to retain water.

In the anterior pituitary we run into a problem. It is clear that stimuli, such as the burn used in the earlier example, cause the secretion of the hormones of the anterior pituitary. The problem is that there are no neural connections between the brain and the adenohypophysis. How then does the brain control the secretion of the hormones of the anterior pituitary? Geoffrey Harris in England reasoned that the only possible connection between the brain and anterior pituitary must be chemical rather than electrical and must be mediated by a vascular link. Harris then showed that the rich vascular interface between the hypothalamus and the anterior pituitary (see Fig. 12-9) carried blood from the region of the hypothalamus to the anterior pituitary. (Many years earlier it had been proposed that the blood flowed in the opposite direction).

The implication of this theory was that the brain secretes chemicals into the vascular system and that these are carried into the anterior pituitary where they cause the release of the hormones which are synthesized in the anterior pituitary (see Table 12-2). The first indication that this theory might be correct came when it was shown that extracts from the hypothalamus, but not from the cortex, caused the secretion of ACTH from the pituitary (Guillemin and Burgus, 1972). In the 20 odd years since this discovery, developments have been rapid. It has been established that the brain does indeed synthesize and secrete chemicals which are carried by the blood to the anterior pituitary where they cause the secretion of the

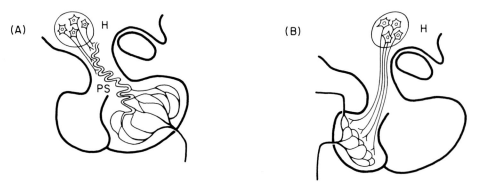

Fig. 12-9. Organization of hypothalamus and anterior and posterior pituitary. (A) The anterior pituitary is linked to the hypothalamus (H) by a rich vascular bed [the hypothalamohypophyseal portal system (PS)]. Hypothalamic neurons secrete releasing hormones into the bloodstream which stimulate the release of anterior pituitary hormones. (B) Posterior pituitary hormones are released by the direct action of hypothalamic neurons.

12. INTERNAL STATES OF THE BODY

tropic hormones. In 1970 the first of these *"releasing hormones,"* *thyroid-releasing hormone* (TRH), was identified and synthesized. This brain hormone causes the anterior pituitary to secrete *thyroid-stimulating hormone* (TSH) (see Fig. 12-7). TRH is a simple molecule made up of three amino acids in the following sequence: glutamine, histidine, and proline (Fig. 12-10). Since the discovery of the chemical structure of TRH, the structure of the hormone which releases luteinizing hormone has been discovered, as has the structure of somatostatin, the brain hormone which *inhibits* the secretion of growth hormone.

As illustrated in fig. 12-7, secretion from the anterior pituitary controls hormonal secretions from many glands. Figure 12-6 and Table 12-2 describe hormones released and their many functions. Here we will discuss only a couple of examples.

The adrenal glands, for example, secrete such an array of steroid hormones (a number of different corticoids, plus androgens, estrogens and progestins) that it has been difficult to determine all of the behavioral effects of this complex gland. The *adrenal corticoids*, however, appear to be quite involved in stress-related behaviors, such as those that accompany crowding, e. g., fighting, and competition for food and mates. The adrenal *androgens* and *progestins* also appear to interact in intricate ways with the gonadal hormones in the control of reproductive states. The adrenal hormones also modulate learning and memory storage processes. Adrenalectomized animals show greatly reduced performance on some learning tasks and these deficits can be remedied by replacement corticoids. Adrenal steroids may also help to influence learning processes through their feedback control of ACTH secretion.

The thyroid gland manufactures and secretes two hormones, thyroxine (T4) and triiodothyronine (T3). The *thyroid gland* is located on the ventral surface of the trachea just below the Adam's apple (see Fig. 12-5). The thyroid hormones are involved in regulating metabolism of all cells (particularly to increase energy production and oxygen consumption) and in the development of the brain (see Chapter 15).

A.   Control of the Pituitary

It is now clear that hormones secreted by the brain actively cause or inhibit the release of anterior pituitary hormones, but it has also been learned that other factors influence the secretion of anterior pituitary hormones. For example, if for some reason the thyroid gland stops functioning (it might be removed surgically because of a tumor) there is a rapid increase in the secretion of TSH from the pituitary. If one then gives thyroxine to the individual, TSH secretion declines. Similar events happen if the adrenal cortex is removed (ACTH secretion in-

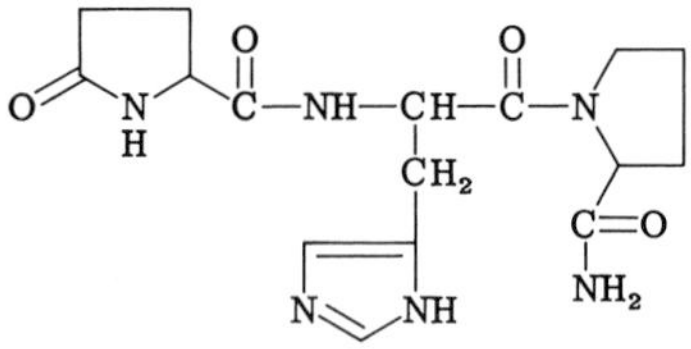

Thyroid-releasing hormone

Fig. 12-10. Structure of thyroid-releasing hormone (TRH). This was the first hypothalamic releasing hormone to be isolated and synthesized in a test tube.

creases), or if the gonads are removed (FSH and LH secretion increase). This phenomenon is known as the *"negative feedback" effect* of glandular hormones. Sensory stimuli stimulate (or inhibit) the secretion of anterior pituitary hormones, these hormones stimulate the adrenal cortex, thyroid gland and gonads to secrete their hormones, and these latter hormones, in addition to having effects on their target tissues, "feedback" to influence the subsequent secretion of anterior pituitary hormones. This feedback sequence is illustrated in Fig. 12-11 in terms of our earlier description of hormonal changes induced by a burn. Cortisol not only has an effect upon the burned skin, it also "feedsback" to control the subsequent secretion of ACTH by the anterior pituitary.

The action of birth control pills provides another example of how the feedback system works. These pills, by producing relatively high and constant levels of estrogen, inhibit the secretion of FSH and LH. Ovarian follicles therefore do not mature (FSH) and ovulation is prevented (LH). Because these pills are used not only in this country, but in developing countries with emerging population problems, there are important social, moral, ethical, economic and political implications involved in research about how hormones control the brain and the secretion of anterior pituitary hormones.

There is still controversy about *where* the adrenal, thyroid and gonadal hormones act to inhibit the secretion of pituitary hormones. Figure 12-11 suggests

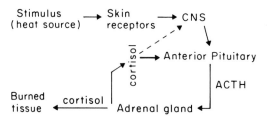

Fig. 12-11. Flow chart illustrating feedback sequence in the hormonal response to a burn. Feedback is a general principle used in neuroendocrine control processes.

12. INTERNAL STATES OF THE BODY

that the hormones could feedback to the CNS and/or the anterior pituitary. While it is generally accepted that thyroxine can inhibit the secretion of TSH by a direct action on the anterior pituitary, it is likely that thyroxine and the adrenal and gonadal hormones inhibit the secretion of pituitary hormones by their action on the brain.

The adrenal, gonadal and thyroid hormones thus help to regulate the rate of their own secretion via their negative feedback actions. Neither growth hormone nor prolactin from the pituitary, however, cause the secretion of peripheral hormones. Prolactin, for example, stimulates the production of milk by the mammary gland, but the milk has no way of exerting a negative feedback action. Rather, control is provided, in these cases by a dual secretion at different times of releasing and inhibiting hormones by the brain. The brain secretes prolactin releasing hormone and prolactin inhibiting hormone, growth hormone releasing hormone and growth hormone inhibiting hormone (somatostatin). These brain hormones stimulate or inhibit the release of prolactin or growth hormone by the anterior pituitary. Thus, organisms have developed two different ways of regulating the anterior pituitary, one which utilizes negative feedback control by peripheral hormones, and one which utilizes both releasing and inhibiting hormones (Schally et al., 1973).

One might next ask how the secretion of the releasing hormones is controlled. It appears that the secretion of these hypothalamic hormones is regulated by neurons whose synaptic transmission is accomplished by the same biogenic amines which regulate other behaviors. For example, norepinephrine seems to be the major transmitter involved in the release of LRH, TRH and somatostatin. Serotonin may inhibit the secretion of prolactin inhibiting hormone (PIH) and TRH, and there appears to be an inhibitory noradrenergic mechanism involved in the release of corticotropic releasing hormone. In addition, prolactin inhibiting hormone is stimulated by the secretion of dopamine with a resultant decrease in prolactin secretion. This role of dopamine in the control of prolactin secretion is perhaps the best understood of the endocrine effects of the biogenic amines. Dopamine releases PIH and inhibits prolactin secretion; serotonin, on the other hand, stimulates the release of prolactin; and L-dopa, a precursor of dopamine, also inhibits prolactin secretion (Ganong, 1974).

Because of these monoamine control mechanisms, it is possible to modulate the release of anterior pituitary hormones by a number of drugs which affect biogenic amine metabolism. This is especially true for the psychopharmacological agents (such as chlorpromazine, which through its effect on dopamine can cause increases in the release of prolactin) and for the anti-Parkinson's disease drug, L-dopa (a precursor of dopamine) which causes a release of growth hormone and a concomitant decrease in prolactin.

B. Interaction between Anterior and Posterior Pituitary

A good example of the interaction between anterior and posterior pituitary hormones as a part of an organized behavior is found in the physiology of lactation (Fig. 12-8). The anterior pituitary hormone, _prolactin_, is increased during pregnancy and parturition. This hormone stimulates the development of the breast and milk production. A baby sucking the breast of its mother maintains high concentrations of the mother's prolactin through reflex pathways in the spinal cord. This sucking activity has been found to cause the release of _TRH_ which is also a potent stimulator of _prolactin_ secretion. There is also an increase in _growth hormone release inhibiting hormone (somatostatin)_ which blocks the TRH-stimulated production of _TSH_ without blocking the effect on prolactin. Thus, a nursing mother does not become hyperthyroid. The same sucking stimulus is monitored by the paraventricular and supraoptic nuclei of the hypothalamus and causes release of _oxytocin_ by the posterior pituitary, and the resultant "let-down" of milk to the infant. Finally, sucking causes an _inhibition_ of _gonadotropin_ release and subsequent infertility during nursing. Thus, both the anterior and posterior pituitary glands, modulated by neural input from the periphery, maintain the production and delivery of milk during breast feeding.

C. Episodic Secretion and Biological Rhythms

A recent advance in the understanding of control mechanisms of the anterior pituitary and hypothalamic releasing hormones has been the discovery that all these hormones are released in _pulses_, resulting in patterns over extended time periods of _episodic secretion_. This secretion has important rhythmic characteristics as well. There have now been found to be both _ultradian_ (less than 24 hours) and _circadian_ (about 24 hours) rhythms in the secretion of all anterior pituitary hormones. The CNS-controlled temporal sequence of these episodes determines the periodicity of the biological rhythm. For example, the central nervous system program for episodic release of ACTH determines the 24-hour periodicity of the cortisol cycle, with lowest values appearing in the plasma early in the nocturnal period, and the highest values in the morning hours. Growth hormone and prolactin, on the other hand, are released predominantly as a function of sleep, with some as yet unknown mechanism linking their nocturnal release to states of consciousness. The biological significance of these relationships is as yet unknown. A very interesting relationship between sleep and hormone output is seen in the sleep-related release of luteinizing hormone during puberty but not during childhood or adulthood. Most of the other pituitary, target gland, and hypothalamic hormones will undoubtedly also be found to be episodic in their appearance in the circulation.

D. Hormonal Action on the Brain

The central nervous system not only controls the output of hormones, but it is itself a target tissue for these hormones. The peripheral hormones, and even the peptide hormones of the anterior pituitary, have actions on the brain which serve to regulate both behavior and subsequent hormone secretion. This is particularly true for the steroid hormones, such as cortisol from the adrenal cortex and the androgens, estrogens and progestins from the gonads, which readily pass the blood–brain barrier and are selectively accumulated by specific cell groups in the brain. For example, the hippocampus accumulates radioactive corticosterone (Fig. 12-12), whereas the hypothalamus and cerebral cortex accumulate very little. On the other hand, estradiol (the primary estrogen secreted by the ovaries) is incorporated into an extensive cell system running from the septum posteriorly through the hypothalamus. Relatively little of it is retained by the hippocampus (McEwen, 1976). Progesterone is accumulated predominantly by mesencephalic structures, although some is retained in the hypothalamus (Whalen and Luttge, 1971). These studies show that different brain structures selectively extract particular steroid hormones from the blood and retain them for several hours.

How do cells recognize particular hormones, and what do they do with hormones once they enter the cell? When steroid hormones enter their target cells they are rapidly bound to special proteins in the cytoplasm, called "*receptors.*" The hormone–receptor complex then undergoes a conformational change which allows the complex to be transferred to the cell nucleus. Within the nucleus the hormone–receptor complex binds to the chromatin material which is made up of the genetic material DNA plus histones and nonhistone proteins. It is currently thought that the DNA and nonhistone proteins are primarily involved in the binding process. The hormone activates the genes and stimulates the production of *messenger RNA* (mRNA). The mRNA then migrates to the cytoplasmic compartment where protein synthesis is initiated. The production of new proteins is considered a critical event in the action of the hormone (Chan and O'Malley, 1976).

This sequence of events (see Fig. 12-13) was established in studies of the effects of gonadal hormones on peripheral target tissues such as the uterus and prostate. The model is thought to hold true for the effects of hormones on all other tissues including brain. With respect to the brain, at least the initial steps in the sequence have been established. Estradiol, for example, enters hypothalamic

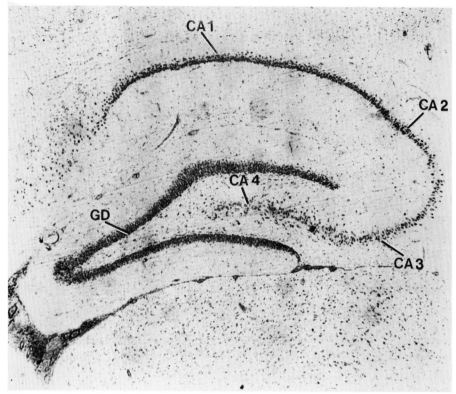

Fig. 12-12. Accumulation of radioactive corticosterone by hippocampal neurons. Radioactive corticosterone is administered to the animal, and a short while later the animal is sacrificed, hippocampal tissue is sectioned and coated with a photographic-type emulsion sensitive to radioactivity. The presence of the dark dots indicates the sites of radioactivity. Hippocampal neuronal nuclei are heavily labeled in the various regions (GD, CA1, CA2, etc.). Only certain neurons in brain bind radioactive steroids. (Courtesy of J.L. Gerlach and B.S. McEwen.)

neurons. These neurons have binding proteins in their cytoplasm called receptors. The estradiol–receptor complex is transferred to the nucleus where it binds to the chromatin material. Estradiol also enters nonhypothalamic neural cells, such as those of the cortex. However, adult cortical cells do not possess the protein receptors so the hormone diffuses out of these cells as rapidly as it diffuses into them. As a result, in cortical cells, the hormone is neither translocated to the nucleus nor bound to nuclear chromatin.

Thus it appears that some brain cells, like other target tissue cells for hormones, recognize their appropriate hormone on the basis of the nature of the cytoplasmic protein receptor. It is this receptor which initiates the molecular action of hormones. It is not understood, however, how the production of new

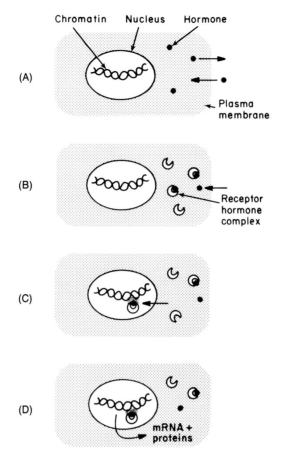

Fig. 12-13. Action of steroid hormones is dependent on receptor molecules which are only present in hormone sensitive cells. Free hormone in the blood freely enters cells. In nontarget cells (A) the hormone diffuses in and out of the cell so its concentration is very low. In target cells (B) the hormone binds to a receptor protein which concentrates the hormone and carries it to the nucleus (C). The hormone–receptor complex binds to nuclear chromatin and stimulates the synthesis of messenger RNA (mRNA) corresponding to the gene of the effector site. mRNA enters the cytoplasm (D) where it codes for the production of specific proteins.

proteins is involved in regulating the electrical or metabolic activity of the neuron's cells.

The available evidence shows us that the brain controls the secretion of hormones and that these hormones can return to the brain where they are selectively accumulated by particular neurons. These morphological and biochemical studies do not prove that the cell groups so identified do indeed participate in the regulation of hormone secretion and behavior. To obtain appropriate answers to these questions, investigators have applied small amounts of hormones directly to brain tissue. In the case that has been most thoroughly studied to date, namely, the effect of estrogen, it has been found that the cells which are involved in the control of FSH and LH secretion (see Fig. 12-6) are located primarily in the posterior hypothalamus. Implants in the cortex have no effect. The cells which control mating behavior are located primarily in the anterior hypothalamic–preoptic region. Estrogen implanted in the region of the ventromedial nucleus of the posterior hypothalamus can also stimulate mating behavior, but implants in other regions are quite ineffective. Thus, the cells which regulate the pituitary and those which mediate behavior are anatomically distinct. The cells which respond to testosterone and which control male mating responses are found primarily in the preoptic region.

We can begin now to see how hormones perform their integrative function. Hormones act at various tissues in multiple loops and elicit or modulate metabolic and behavioral responses (Fig. 12-14). On the left side of Fig. 12-14 can be seen the typical, nonhormonal control of behavior. A stimulus, for example, the burn discussed at the beginning of this chapter stimulates pain receptors. The central nervous system is activated and the individual withdraws his hand. Withdrawing the hand changes the stimulus–receptor interaction. When the receptors are activated, they also excite different cells in the CNS, namely, those which cause the release of corticotropin releasing hormone. This agent travels to the anterior pituitary causing the release of ACTH. The ACTH travels via the vascular system to the adrenal cortex which then secretes cortisol, and the cortisol travels to the burned area where it has its antiinflammatory effects, thereby changing the burned area such that pain is reduced. At the same time, the cortisol from the adrenal cortex is carried to the brain, where it inhibits the further secretion of ACTH. Thus, the total system starts in some steady state, is activated by a sensory stimulus, and finally returns to a steady state when the neural and hormonal messages have completed their task.

Reproductive events are also illustrated by Fig. 12-14. For example, the

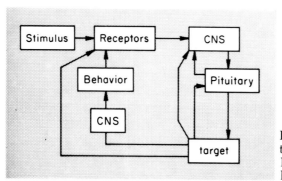

Fig. 12-14. Generalized model for the control of neuroendocrine systems. Note the feedback effects of dual behavior of hormones on the CNS.

female rat shows a 4-day *estrous cycle* in which the hormones of the ovary, estradiol and progesterone, are secreted in sequence and in which mating behavior follows the estrogen–progesterone stimulation. Stimuli from the external world, such as regular changes in light and darkness, initiate the secretion of the pituitary gonadotropins. These in turn stimulate the ovary to secrete *estrogen*. Approximately 6 hours after the peak of estrogen secretion, there is a surge of progesterone secretion. Maximal sexual receptivity occurs some 8 hours later. At the same time that the ovarian hormones are stimulating the neural systems which underlie the behavioral response, they also feedback to the brain and/or pituitary to inhibit the release of gonadotropins and terminate the estrous cycle (Fig. 12-15).

In conclusion, the model presented in Fig. 12-14 thus illustrates how hormones are controlled by the brain and how the hormones help to regulate neural activity. This interaction between neural activity and hormone secretion is continual and even shows cycles of activity. Many types of external and internal stimuli and many types of hormones are involved in this process of neuroendocrine integration.

E. Uses and Abuses of Endocrinology

Earlier it was noted that if the thyroid gland is removed, an increase in the secretion of TSH follows. Behavioral changes also follow. Hypothyroid individu-

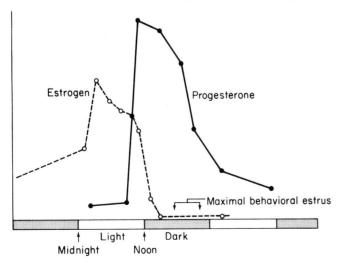

Fig. 12-15. Temporal patterns of estrogen and progesterone secretion preceding behavioral estrus in female rats displaying 4-day estrous cycles. Measurement units were nanogram/milliliter plasma for estrogen and μg/hour/ovary for progesterone. (From Powers, 1970.)

als are lethargic, show reduced reactivity to environmental stimuli and demonstrate generally reduced mental activity. These symptoms can be ameliorated by the proper dosage of thyroid hormones.

In cases of adrenal cortical insufficiency, as occurs in Addison's disease, striking behavioral changes occur. Such individuals show thresholds for the detection of taste stimuli which are 100 times lower, i.e., more acute, than those of normal individuals. Similarly, olfaction may be as much as 100,000 times more acute than in normals. Addison's patients are also more sensitive to sound stimuli, when the sounds are pure tones, but these same individuals show a reduced ability to discriminate words. Treatment of these patients with synthetic corticoids returns these sensory thresholds to the normal range.

In men with reduced testicular function, sexual drive or libido, as indicated by sexual dreams and fantasies as well as by sexual activity, often declines. Treatment with testosterone restores these functions, although in cases of severe testicular dysfunction, spermatogenesis and, therefore, reproductive capacity may continue to be impaired.

These examples illustrate how an understanding of the neuroendocrine system, including its biochemistry, physiology and psychology, can be utilized to identify and correct the effects of glandular *malfunctions*. The use of synthetic steroids for contraceptive purposes provides an example where such an understanding of hormone action has been used effectively in the control of *normal endocrine function*. In some cases, however, "therapeutic" manipulation of the neuroendocrine system has far outdistanced a scientific understanding of the neuroendocrine integrative system. For example, several clinics have attempted to cure sexual deviation, homosexual pedophilia in particular, by placing electrolytic lesions into the ventromedial nucleus of the hypothalamus under the belief that this region of the brain comprises the "sex center." Such a belief is not warranted based on our current understanding of neuroendocrine systems.

Others are trying to achieve the same end by administering antiandrogens to men who have sociosexual problems. These antiandrogens are thought to reduce or eliminate sexual libido by interfering with the actions of the male hormone, testosterone. Although positive results have been reported, this treatment seems doomed to failure, since even castration fails to suppress completely sexual desire and activity in men, although such surgery does reduce sexual activity to some degree in many cases. Moreover, so little is yet known about the precise biochemical effects of the antihormones that therapeutic usage of these agents is premature.

Synthetic hormones are also widely used today in women who are entering menopause. *Menopause* involves a cessation of ovarian function with a consequent loss of estrogen and progesterone secretion and is often accompanied by psychophysiological symptoms such as hot flashes, uncontrolled sweating, dizzi-

12. INTERNAL STATES OF THE BODY

ness and so forth. Estrogen eliminates these symptoms to a large degree, and it has become quite common to prescribe estrogen treatment at the time of menopause. The problem is that we still do not understand the effects of long-term estrogen treatment (and this concern applies to long-term usage of birth control pills as well). However, we do now know that estrogens can have effects which are not evident until many years later. For example, women have been administered estrogens during pregnancy, for presumed therapeutic reasons. The daughters of many of these women are now found to develop a highly malignant form of vaginal cancer at the time of or shortly after puberty. This type of cancer was almost unknown until the advent of estrogen treatment during pregnancy. Moreover, evidence is being collected which indicates that prenatal estrogen stimulation has later behavioral effects as well.

These few examples illustrate how hormone treatment can be used to ameliorate physiological and behavioral problems associated with defects in the neuroendocrine system. They also indicate that treatments become instituted on occasion which are beyond our understanding of this system and which can lead to foolish or detrimental treatment programs.

F.   Summary

The endocrine system provides a form of integration of physiological systems underlying cellular metabolism, organ function and behavior. The brain is the "master gland." It regulates the secretion and inhibition of secretion of the protein hormones of both the anterior and posterior pituitary. The pituitary hormones regulate the secretion of the steroid and amino acid hormones of the peripheral glands. The peripheral hormones influence the function of a wide variety of tissues, including the brain. They serve self-regulating functions through their negative feedback control of pituitary secretion, and they activate and inhibit a number of behavioral and physiological systems. The neuroendocrine system is a major regulator of homeostasis, but it also plays a significant role in the development and differentiation of organisms as we shall discuss in Chapter 15.

In many situations, such as our reactions to stress, the ANS and neuroendocrine systems work in a coordinated way. A sprinter in the starting blocks reacts to the stress of competition by consciously tensing his muscles. Unconsciously, the hypothalamus begins its task to control glands and organs to prepare the body for stress. Directed by the hypothalamus, the sympathetic nervous system widens the pupils, nostrils and throat; adjusts the blood supply; and relaxes the stomach, intestine and bladder. The hypothalamus also signals the pituitary gland to send hormones to the thyroid and adrenal glands, which release their own hormones. Thyroid hormones step up energy production; adrenal hormones increase fuel supplies by regulating the liver, pancreas, spleen and large blood vessels. After the stress is over, the parasympathetic division helps quell the stress reactions.

So far in this chapter we have described how body states are adjusted to myriad situations through the action of the ANS and the neuroendocrine systems. We have also emphasized how the changes in body state strongly influence many behaviors. Sometimes, however, some acts damage the body, and sometimes disorders of the organs occur which are outside the control of the body's normal homeostatic mechanisms. Pain processes provide a continuing and ever so powerful report on our well being.

IV. Pain

Pain is our body's message that something biologically harmful is happening to it. Pain reports a wound, a burn, a bruise and its location on the body surface to us. Pain warns us when our internal organs are malfunctioning and, as we all know too well, pain tells us when we are sick. Pain is the nervous system signaling that its partner, the body, is in trouble. Our job in turn is to initiate an appropriate behavior to relieve the pain—escape, go see a doctor, find out what is wrong. Pain enables both people and animals to protect their bodies from mortal harm. Pain is also an excellent teacher. It protects us by teaching us to avoid further contact with painful stimuli. Many experiments in physiological psychology use painful stimuli as a conditioning agent. Everybody learns quickly what hurts and how to avoid it.

Those unfortunate enough to be born without an ability to feel pain illustrate all too dramatically the need for pain mechanisms.

> The best documented of all cases of congenital insensitivity to pain is Miss C., a young Canadian girl who was a student at McGill University in Montreal. Her father, a physician in Western Canada, was fully aware of her problem and alerted his colleagues in Montreal to examine her. The young lady was highly intelligent and seemed normal in every way except that she had never felt pain. As a child, she had bitten off the tip of her tongue while chewing food, and had suffered third-degree burns after kneeling on a hot radiator to look out of the window. When examined by a psychologist (McMurray, 1950) in the laboratory, she reported that she did not feel pain when noxious stimuli were presented. She felt no pain when parts of her body were subjected to strong electric shock, to hot water at temperatures that usually produce reports of burning pain, or to a prolonged ice-bath. Equally astonishing was the fact that she showed no changes in blood pressure, heart rate, or respiration when these stimuli were presented. Furthermore, she could not remember ever sneezing or coughing, the gag reflex could be elicited only with great difficulty, and corneal reflexes (to protect the eyes) were absent. A variety of other stimuli, such as inserting a stick up through the nostrils, pinching tendons, or injections of histamine

under the skin—which are normally considered as forms of torture—also failed to produce pain.

Miss C. had severe medical problems. She exhibited pathological changes in her knees, hip and spine, and underwent several orthopaedic operations. Her surgeon attributed these changes to the lack of protection to joints usually given by pain sensation. She apparently failed to shift her weight when standing, to turn over in her sleep, or to avoid certain postures, which normally prevent inflammation of joints (from Melzack, 1973, p. 15).

The intensity of pain is generally related to the extent of damage. However, pain has important subjective elements. It differs between individuals and obeys strict cultural determinants. It is now agreed that in many cases the psychology of pain is as important as the type of actual damage (Melzack, 1973).

The perception of pain varies with the *culture*. A most striking example is the hook hanging ritual practiced in parts of India (Kosambi, 1967). A man who is chosen to represent the power of the gods goes around to the villages at particular times of the year blessing the crops and children. He is pierced in the back muscles and travels from place to place partially suspended from the hooks. At the end of the ceremony he swings freely by the hooks in his back. He feels no pain and appears to be in a state of exaltation. Afterward he heals quickly.

Pain also depends on *past experience*. Scottish terriers, for example, raised in isolation and deprived of the normal bodily abuses experienced in growing up, will endure pin pricks with no evidence of pain or emotion. Although their reflexes are normal and they jerk away from the pin, they make no attempt to avoid repeated pricks. Their perception of actual damage is abnormal. Their socially reared littermates usually do not allow themselves to be pricked more than once. Some aspects of pain must be learned (Melzack and Scott, 1957).

Pain also depends on *anxiety, attention and suggestion*. Football players can endure extreme pain in competition. Soldiers under attack can fail to notice severe wounds until after the battle. Pain is not a simple sense produced by a specific stimulus. The qualities of pain are abstracted from mental states.

A.   Types of Pain

Pain due to noxious stimuli on our body surface is sharp and easy to locate precisely. Visceral pain, on the other hand, is generally more widespread and not as readily localized. Pain, however, can be deceptive, and can be felt at places other than its origin.

1.   REFERRED PAIN.   Visceral disorders frequently cause pain that is felt in the skin as well as the viscera. This is commonly called *referred pain*. Angina

pectoris is the classic example of referred pain. It is a horrible burning pain felt in the underside of the upper arm. It is actually the result of heart trouble, but it is experienced in the arm. Visceral afferents from the heart are anatomically mixed with those of the skin. Through experience we learn to sort out the signals and recognize the different sensations, but in times of trouble the brain does not correctly interpret the pain and registers it as originating from the arm. Referred pain is important in the diagnosis of visceral disorders. Appendicitis in its early stages may be felt just below the sternum; a kidney stone passing down the ureter may be referred to the back of the groin. Physicians are trained to recognize referred pain and interpret it correctly.

2. PROJECTED PAIN. *Projected pain* is a type of pain that is projected beyond the area where the stimulus is applied. For example, hitting the funny bone (striking the ulnar nerve at the elbow) causes a pain that radiates down the forearm. A stimulus applied to a peripheral nerve causes impulses that are indistinguishable from those that originate at the receptors.

A most striking example of projected pain is *phantom limb pain*. It is an unfortunate and miserable, but curious phenomenon. Most people who have lost a limb report feeling a phantom limb almost immediately afterward. About 30% of them feel pain in the missing limb, and in 5–10% of amputees the pain may be persistent and excruciating.

Phantom limb pain is more likely to develop in patients who have suffered pain for a while prior to amputation. It may closely resemble the quality and location of pain present before amputation. Soldiers who have lost a limb suddenly usually do not experience it. In phantom limb pain, trigger zones on the stump may spread to surrounding areas of the body or to the opposite side of the body. The most likely explanation of phantom limb pain is that traumatic and abnormal inputs produce a change in information processing in the CNS (Melzack, 1973).

Pain experiences are so diverse it is exceedingly difficult to develop a formal definition. In fact, there is really not a generally accepted one. Pain is a complex personal, but at the same time universal, experience. As C. S. Lewis once wrote

> When I think of pain—of anxiety that gnaws like fire and loneliness that spreads out like a desert, and the heartbreaking routine of monotonous misery, or again of dull aches that blacken our whole landscape or sudden nauseating pains that knock a man's heart out at one blow, of pains that seem already intolerable and then are suddenly increased, or infuriating scorpion-stinging pains that startle into maniacal movement a man who seemed half dead with his previous tortures—it "quite o'ercrows my spirit." If I knew any way of escape I would crawl through sewers to find it. But what is the good of telling you about my feelings? You know them already: they are the same as yours. I am not arguing that pain is not painful. Pain hurts. That is what the word means (Lewis, 1962, p. 105).

12. INTERNAL STATES OF THE BODY

If an injury or noxious stimulus does not cause a negative effect or aversive drive, the experience cannot be called painful. The problem in defining pain is describing that feeling in objective terms to others. A true understanding of the sensation of pain will depend on understanding its mechanisms.

B.   Treatment of Pain

The controlled relief of pain is, of course, one of the universal goals of medicine. People go to the doctor when they hurt. For minor relief of pain, aspirin or similar medications are most frequently prescribed. *Aspirin* is a vasodilator and antiinflammatory agent. The site of aspirin's *analgesic* action against inflammation is the peripheral nervous system (Lim *et al.*, 1964). It interacts specifically with the process of pain reception at the site of injury. Aspirin is a potent inhibitor of the synthesis of certain *prostaglandins*, a class of molecules related to unsaturated fatty acids (Fig. 12-16). When prostaglandins are slowly infused under the skin at concentrations similar to those found in areas of inflammation, a sensitization of the area to mechanical and chemical stimuli is produced. By inhibiting prostaglandin synthesis, aspirin prevents the sensitization of pain receptors, a necessary event in the transduction of pain signals from inflamed tissue (Ferreira, 1972). One of the side effects of aspirin is that it reduces the ability of blood to clot.

Anesthetics are of major clinical importance and provide temporary relief of pain. Local anesthetics such as novocaine "deaden" nerves by increasing their firing thresholds. Barbiturates act on central synaptic transmission.

In 1680 an English physician wrote: "Among the remedies which it has pleased Almighty God to give man to relieve his suffering none is so universal and so efficacious as opium" (quoted in Snyder, 1977). Opium and other narcotics effectively relieve severe pain, but they are also toxic and addictive (see Chapter 17).

Surgery is sometimes used for treatment of severe pain. A cordotomy is performed in which the anterolateral quadrant of the spinal cord is removed. This destroys most pain fibers ascending to the brain. Initially, the patient experiences

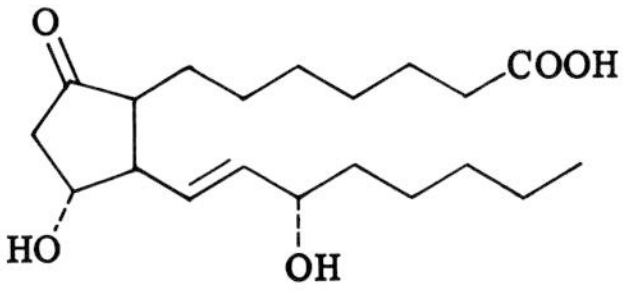

Prostaglandin (PGE₁)

Fig. 12-16.   Prostaglandin (PGE₁). Prostaglandins sensitize pain receptors. They are present in small quantities in many tissues. In general they serve as modulators of hormone activity.

less pain, but after 8–9 months pain returns, worse than ever. Axon sprouting may recreate pain circuitry, although the time course appears too slow to be due solely to such processes.

The most fascinating of all ways to relieve pain is the practice of *acupuncture*. When, after centuries of use in China, acupuncture came to the attention of Western scientists it instantly created skeptics. According to Chinese philosophy disease and pain occur because of a poor balance between two principles of nature, Yin and Yang. Acupuncture, the practice of inserting long, thin needles into various parts of the body, is believed to improve this balance. It is traditionally used to treat numerous conditions varying from arthritis to asthma.

Since the 1960's perhaps as many as 90% of the patients in China have undergone surgery with the acupuncture procedure (Brown, 1972). Many Western scientists have witnessed operations, and the procedure has been successfully performed in the United States. Acupuncture is not analogous to hypnotic analgesia for two main reasons: (1) Hypnosis is effective in creating analgesia in only about 20% of people; acupuncture apparently nearly always works. (2) Patients under hypnotic analgesia rarely speak or act spontaneously, while acupuncture patients chat and even show an interest in the operation (Melzack, 1973). It is now clear that the acupuncture procedure produces genuine anesthesia by some means or other. For acupuncture procedures, the body is divided into meridians associated with the major internal organs (Fig. 12-17). There are specific sites for insertion of needles for different operations. After insertion of the needles (two or more), electric current is passed through the needles for a period of almost 20 minutes. The analgesic effect develops slowly and requires continuous current. For example, an operation on the stomach was carried out with four acupuncture needles inserted into the lobe of each ear.

The patient was a slender fifty-year-old man with a non-healing ulcer of the lesser curvature of the stomach. The procedure was to be a gastrectomy (removal of the stomach). This patient had not had medication at bedtime the previous night. He was given sixty mg of meperidine hydrochloride (an analgesic drug) in 500 cc of 5 per cent dextrose during surgery. Acupuncture anaesthesia was introduced by placing four stainless steel needles in the pinna of each ear at carefully identified points. . . . The needles were connected to a phasic direct current battery source, delivering six volts at 150 cycles per minute. The patient remained awake, alert, and chatted throughout the procedure. A subtotal gastric resection was done by skilful surgeons, scrubbed, gowned, and disciplined thoroughly in modern or Western surgical practice. This patient required no additional anaesthesia but did note some sensation associated with visceral traction (Dimond, 1971, p. 1560. Copyright by the American Medical Association).

The basis of the acupuncture effect is not well understood at present. Injection of a local anesthetic into the acupuncture points prevents analgesia. Acupuncture may be the result of a peripheral effect on central biasing mecha-

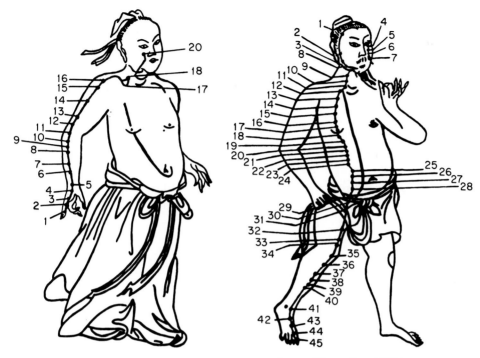

Fig. 12-17. Typical acupuncture charts. (From Lu, 1973.)

nisms. That is, acupuncture can be considered in a sense the reverse of the mechanism we saw in referred pain. Specific stimulation acts on central analgesic processes which refer the analgesia to specific organs. After the needles are removed, the analgesia lasts a few hours. Still, acupuncture is a most mysterious subject.

C.   Mechanisms of Pain Perception

Receptors for pain are everywhere. They are in the skin, joints, muscles, all tissues except bone and brain and nonliving parts of the teeth, hair and nails. It is generally believed that pain receptors are the bare nerve endings of primary sensory afferents. No one has ever identified a pain receptor in the electron microscope, however, since there is no way at present to identify those sensitive to pain versus other stimuli. The structure and active mechanism of pain receptors is still open to debate. Some feel that mechanical stimuli activate pain receptors. Others argue that chemicals from destroyed tissue activate pain receptors. Perhaps it is a little of both.

We do know, however, that all pain receptors report to the spinal cord. *Primary sensory pain fibers* terminate in an area of the dorsal horn of the spinal cord called the <u>substantia gelatinosa</u> (Fig. 12-18). Fibers from neurons in the substantia gelatinosa course through the contralateral anteroventral quadrant of the spinal cord and ascend to the brain along with the spinothalamic tract. The reticular pathway, another ascending spinal pathway, also reports pain. However, it is slower and more diffuse. No pain information is carried by lemniscal pathways, the other main ascending system in the cord. This pathway, you may recall, conveys only somatosensory information (Chapter 2). In fact, it can actually turn off pain to a degree.

What happens in the brain? The story is not all in but the developments are truly exciting. The discovery of endorphins and enkephalins (see Chapter 6) has revolutionized pain research. These small peptides are the brain's own built in analgesics with opiate-like actions (Snyder, 1977).

Let us look at an experiment. If these peptides have analgesic actions, it should be possible to inject them into the brain and increase pain thresholds. Analgesic activity in rats can be measured by the *tail flick test*. A rat's tail is placed on a hot plate and the degree of analgesia measured by the time it takes the rat to

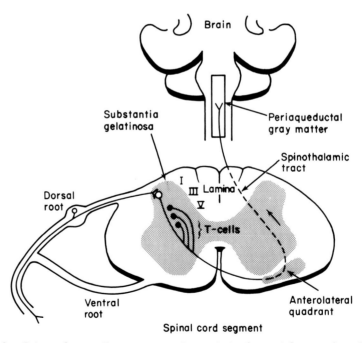

Fig. 12-18. Pain pathways. Receptors monitor pain in the periphery and send messages to neurons in the substantia gelatinosa in the spinal cord. These neurons send ascending projections via the spinothalamic tract to the brain stem.

12. INTERNAL STATES OF THE BODY

remove it. The more analgesia the peptide produces, the greater the latency. A cut-off time (usually about 12 seconds) is necessary to avoid permanent damage to the tail. Figure 12-19 shows the analgesic action of human β-endorphin injected into the brain of rats measured by the tail flick test. There is a dose-dependent increase in the tail flick latency. Analgesia is reversed by the morphine antagonist, naloxone. This is compelling evidence that the brain has its own analgesics that act like morphine. Recent clinical tests indicate endorphins are effective analgesics in humans too.

The sites of *in vivo* analgesic activity of *β-endorphins* have been determined by microinjection of the peptide at various brain regions. Those most sensitive to β-endorphin are located in the periaqueductal gray area, medial preoptic area, anterior hypothalamus and nucleus accumbens. This correlates very well with those regions sensitive to morphine.

About the same time as endorphins were making scientific headlines, another key story was in the making. A number of workers, mainly Liebeskind and co-workers at the University of California, Los Angeles, were scanning the brain looking for stimulation sites which affected pain (Liebeskind *et al.*, 1974). Pulses of electric current were delivered through electrodes to specific brain areas. Most remarkably, stimulation at some sites caused a powerful analgesia. Many of the most sensitive electrode locations were in the same locations in which endor-

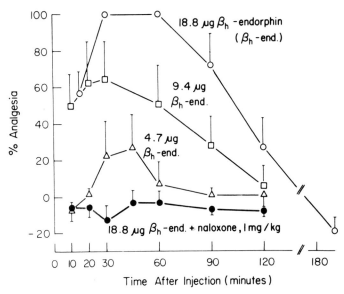

Fig. 12-19. Inhibitory effect on tail flick response following the intraventricular injection of human β-endorphin and its blockade by naloxone. Various doses of β_h-endorphin were injected at 0 time. In the naloxone experiment the drug was injected 10 minutes before the injection of β_h-endorphin. (From Tseng *et al.*, 1977.)

phins and enkephalins were most effective (the *periaqueductal gray*, for example). Is it possible that electrical stimulation released the brain's endorphins and enkephalins? In order to test this intriguing possibility naloxone was administered. It blocked or reversed electrically produced analgesia, clearly demonstrating an involvement of endorphins and enkephalins.

Circuits must exist which suppress the perception of pain. It appears that connections from the periaqueductal gray matter go to *raphé nuclei* in the medulla (Rhodes and Liebeskind, 1977). Perhaps you will recall that raphé nuclei are rich in serotonergic neurons (see Chapter 6). These neurons send slow conducting unmyelinated fibers to the substantia gelatinosa in the spinal cord. There they inhibit lamina I neurons and suppress the entry of pain signals into the cord (Fig. 12-20). It appears as if these raphé neurons mediate analgesia produced by opiates or electrical stimulation of the brain stem (Basbaum *et al.*, 1976; Fields and Basbaum, 1978).

Basic research is providing important clues on how pain can be treated. In patients with intractable pain, narcotics are often ineffective and neurosurgical lesions produce serious side effects. One of the recent developments is the treatment of chronic intractable pain in humans through electrical stimulation of the brain. The results are astonishing. Most patients with electrodes implanted in

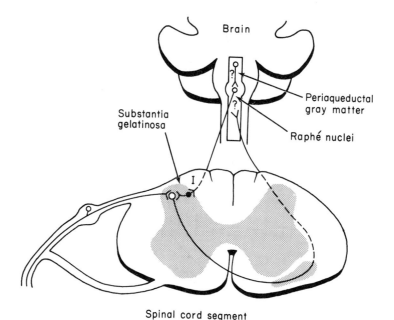

Fig. 12-20. An endogenous analgesia circuit. Descending fibers from the brain stem block pain reports where they enter the spinal cord. Descending fibers appear to act on enkephalin interneurons, which in turn act to block synaptic transmission at primary afferents.

12. INTERNAL STATES OF THE BODY

the periventricular or periaqueductal gray matter experience long lasting relief from pain through intermittent stimulation. Intravenous naloxone totally reverses the pain relief produced by electrical stimulation. Excessive repetitive stimulation produces tolerance to both stimulation produced pain relief and the analgesic action of narcotics. Fortunately, however, abstinence from stimulation for a few days leads to a return of the beneficial effects (Hosobuchi *et al.*, 1977). In some cases stimulation becomes more and more effective in relieving pain over time. In one patient, for example, a stimulation electrode was implanted in the thalamus. At the first session, after a rather prolonged stimulation period, pain gradually disappeared, only to return again very shortly when the stimulus was turned off. After repeated use, however, the amount of stimulation required decreased and the benefits lasted longer until finally the patient needed only minimal stimulation (Hosobuchi *et al.*, 1973, 1975). Somehow the patient had learned to alter his brain to almost permanently remove the pain. How? This is only one of the continuing mysteries in the field of pain research.

D. Summary

Pain is a hurting feeling telling us the body is in danger from noxious stimuli or internal disorders. It is a distress call. The feeling of pain is generally related to the actual amount of damage, but it also depends on cultural attitudes, past experience, the meaning attached to the situation, one's attention and anxieties. Pain's qualities are abstracted from our total mental state. Accordingly there is an important learning aspect to pain. Pain can be experienced in many ways. It can be experienced simply as a hurt in the viscera or skin area directly affected, but in referred pain sensations due to visceral malfunction are transferred to the skin. In phantom limb pain the person feels the ghostly sensation of a lost arm or leg.

Pain receptors synapse in the substantia gelatinosa of the spinal cord. Pain messages travel to the brain via ascending tracts (spino-thalamic and reticular) and terminate primarily in the periaqueductal gray matter and midbrain areas. Direct electrical stimulation in these areas will produce analgesia which is blocked by naloxone. The endorphins and enkephalins are the built-in mediators of CNS analgesia. Raphé neurons, which project to the cord, converge with afferent pain fibers in the substantia gelatinosa to inhibit arriving reports.

Pain is most commonly relieved by aspirin, which desensitizes pain receptors in the periphery, or narcotics which act centrally on endorphin or enkephalin receptors. The benefits of direct surgical intervention are temporary.

Pain must be controlled over a narrow range and kept there if we are to function effectively. Absence of perceptual processes for pain at birth is disastrous; chronic pain is debilitating. Pain processes modeled to our culture, our past, and our other feelings are essential. Together with autonomic and endocrine functions, pain processes look after the body in which we live.

Autonomic, neuroendocrine and pain processes are entrusted with care of body state and with preparing it to meet the challenges and necessities of the world it faces. They are not mere custodial robots, however. They respond to and intrude upon our behavior. They are in close communication with the commanding and planning brain and work as part of a concerted program to deliver more oneness, more flexibility and more reliability to the total being.

In Chapter 13 we will analyze the way in which the nervous system serves to deliver day in and day out fluid, energy and material needs for itself and the body.

Key Terms

Acupuncture: The practice of inserting long, thin needles into specific areas of the body in order to treat pain and certain diseases.

Adenohypophysis: The anterior pituitary.

Adrenal cortex: The outer part of the adrenal gland. Its secretory products are corticoids (e.g., cortisol), androgens, estrogens and progestins.

Adrenocorticotropic hormone (ACTH): A protein hormone secreted from the pituitary gland that causes the release of cortisol from the adrenal cortex.

Adrenal gland: An endocrine gland comprising two components, an inner medulla and an outer cortex, located near the kidney. It secretes epinephrine (adrenalin) and smaller quantities of norepinephrine upon sympathetic activation. In addition, ACTH stimulates the release of an array of steroid hormones (adrenal corticoids). Products of the adrenal gland are involved in stress-related behaviors.

Adrenal medulla: The inner part of the adrenal gland. The medulla secretes epinephrine and smaller amounts of norepinephrine.

Analgesia: Relief from pain.

Androgen: A male sex hormone (e.g., testosterone).

Anterior pituitary gland: A specialized part of the pituitary gland which synthesizes and releases various hormones (LH, FSH, TSH, ACTH, GH, prolactin). The release of these hormones is controlled by releasing factors from the hypothalamus. In addition release is controlled by negative feedback.

Baroreceptors: Receptors which monitor arterial blood pressure by sensing the amount of stretch in the arterial vessel walls.

Chemoreceptors: Receptors located in the walls of the aorta and carotid arteries which are sensitive to the amount of dissolved oxygen in the blood.

Episodic secretion: Release of hormones in discrete pulses rather than continuously.

Estrogen: A generic term for hormones which produce estrus; specifically, the female steroid hormone (a derivative of cholesterol). It is secreted by the ovaries, adrenal gland and placenta. It promotes the development of female sexual characteristics and behaviors.

Follicle-stimulating hormone (FSH): A hormone secreted by the anterior pituitary. It promotes the maturation of egg cells in the ovary; together with luteinizing hormone (LH), it stimulates synthesis of estrogens by the ovary in the female and androgens and the production of sperm in the male.

Gonadal hormones: Hormones secreted by the gonads (primarily estrogen and testosterone).

Gonadectomy: The process of removing the gonads (ovaries or testes).

Gonadotropin: Any hormone which has a direct effect on the gonads.

Growth hormone: A hormone secreted by the anterior pituitary which promotes growth.

Hormone: A chemical substance synthesized by specialized cells and secreted into the circulatory system which carries it to the target cells elsewhere in the body where it may have its primary effect or where it may cause the secretion of another hormone.

Hypothalamus: A group of nuclei near the base of the brain which regulates the secretions of the pituitary gland and which is involved in a variety of behaviors (feeding, drinking, reproduction, sleeping, etc.).

Learned cardiovascular responses: A change in cardiovascular responses produced by coupling them to stimuli that do not normally elicit a cardiovascular change.

Messenger RNA: The RNA species which codes for protein synthesis.

Negative feedback: In neuroendocrinology, the inhibition of secretion of a hormone (e.g., FSH) by another hormone (e.g., estrogen).

Neurohypophysis: Posterior pituitary gland. A neural extension from the base of the brain with cell bodies in the hypothalamus.

Oxytocin: A hormone secreted by the posterior pituitary which causes contractions of the uterus and release of milk from the mammary gland.

Parasympathetic nervous system: A division of the autonomic nervous system. Preganglion cell bodies are located in the brain stem and spinal cord; the ganglia are located close to their peripheral targets. The parasympathetic nervous system responds primarily to changes in the internal organs.

Periaqueductal gray: An area in the brain stem running along the midline which appears critically involved in pain mechanisms. (See Chapter 6.)

Pituitary gland: A gland located at the base of the brain comprising two parts: the anterior pituitary secretes hormones which have direct effects on tissues (e.g., growth hormone or prolactin) or regulate other glands (e.g., adrenal cortex), and the posterior pituitary secretes oxytocin and vasopressin which have effects on various tissues.

Projected pain: A type of pain that is projected beyond the area where the stimulus is applied (e.g., phantom limb pain).

Prolactin: A hormone of the anterior pituitary which controls the development of the breast and production of milk.

Prostaglandins: A class of molecules related to unsaturated fatty acids. They appear to sensitize pain receptors. Aspirin inhibits prostaglandin synthesis.

Receptor protein: In endocrinology, specific protein(s) contained in the cytoplasm of target cells which bind hormones. The hormone-receptor complex is then translocated to the nucleus where it activates the genes and stimulates the production of specific messenger RNAs.

Referred pain: Pain that is felt at places other than at its origin. Visceral disorders may cause pain that is felt in the skin as well as the affected organ (e.g., angina pectoris).

Set point: A desired level of activity established by a feedback system as in thermostatic regulation of body temperature.

Somatostatin: A hormone which inhibits the release of growth hormone by the anterior pituitary.

Substantia gelatinosa: An area of the dorsal horn of the spinal cord where primary sensory pain fibers emanate.

Sympathetic nervous system: A division of the autonomic nervous system. Preganglionic cell bodies of the sympathetic division are located in the spinal cord; the ganglia are organized in a chain. The sympathetic nervous system responds primarily to changes in the external environment and functions in a manner reciprocal to the parasympathetic chain. Its activities prepare the body for the possibility of intense motor activities involved in attack, defense or escape.

Testosterone: A male steroid hormone (derivative of cholesterol). It is the primary hormone secreted by the testes and responsible for the development of male sex characteristics.

Thyroid gland: A gland which secretes thyroxine (T_4), a hormone involved in the regulation of cell metabolism and brain development.

Thyroid-releasing hormone (TRH): A hypothalamic hormone which causes the anterior pituitary to secrete thyroid stimulating hormone (TSH).

Thyroid-stimulating hormone: The hormone released from the anterior pituitary which causes the thyroid gland to release the thyroid hormones.

Thyroxine: A hormone secreted by the thyroid gland.

Vasopressin: A hormone secreted by the pituitary gland which increases blood pressure and decreases the flow of urine.

General References

Brown, P. E. (1972). Use of acupuncture in major surgery. *Lancet* **1,** 1328–1330.

McEwen, B. S. (1976). Interactions between hormones and nerve tissue. *Sci. Am.* **235,** 48–58.

Melzack, R. (1973). "The Puzzle of Pain." Basic Books, New York.

Snyder, S. H. (1977). Opiate receptors and internal opiates. *Sci. Am.* **236,** 44–56.

References

Basbaum, A. I., Clanton, C. H., and Fields, H. L. (1976). Opiate and stimulus-produced analgesia: Functional anatomy of a medullospinal pathway. *Proc. Natl. Acad. Sci. U.S.A.* **73,** 4685–4688.

Brown, P. E. (1972). Use of acupuncture in major surgery. *Lancet* **1,** 1328–1330.

Cannon, W. B. (1929). "Bodily Changes in Pain, Hunger, Fear, and Rage," 2nd ed. Appleton, New York.

Carpenter, M. B. (1976). "Human Neuroanatomy," 7th ed., p. 206. Williams & Wilkins, Baltimore, Maryland.

Chan, L., and O'Malley, B. W. (1976). Mechanism of action of the sex steroid hormones. *N. Engl. J. Med.* **294,** 1322–1328.

Cohen, D. H. (1974). The neural pathways and informational flow mediating a conditioned autonomic response. *In* "Limbic and Autonomic Nervous Systems Research" (L. V. DiCara, ed.), pp. 223–275. Plenum, New York.

Cohen, D. H., and MacDonald, R. L. (1974). A selective review of central neural pathways involved in cardiovascular control. *In* "Cardiovascular Psychophysiology" (P. A. Obrist *et al.*, eds.), pp. 33–59. Aldine, Chicago, Illinois.

Cohen, D. H., and Obrist, P. A. (1975). Interactions between behavior and the cardiovascular system: A brief review. *Cir. Res.* **37,** 693–706.

Dimond, E. G. (1971). Acupuncture anaesthesia. Western medicine and Chinese traditional medicine. *J. Am. Med. Assoc.* **218,** 1558–1563.

Ferreira, S. H. (1972). Prostaglandins, aspirin-like drugs and analgesia. *Nature (London), New Biol.* **240,** 200–203.

Fields, H. L., and Basbaum, A. I. (1978). Brain stem modulation of spinal pain transmission neurons. *Annu. Rev. Physiol.* **40,** 217–248.

Frieden, E., and Lipner, H. (1971). "Biochemical Endocrinology of the Vertebrates." Prentice-Hall, Englewood Cliffs, New Jersey.

Ganong, W. F. (1974). Brain mechanisms regulating the secretion of the pituitary gland. *In* "The neurosciences: Third Study Program" (F. O. Schmitt and F. G. Worden, eds.), pp. 549–563. MIT Press, Cambridge, Massachusetts.

Guillemin, R., and Burgus, R. (1972). The hormones of the hypothalamus. *Sci. Am.* **227,** 24–33.

Hosobuchi, Y., Adams, J. E., and Rutkin, B. (1973). Chronic stimulation for the control of facial anesthesia dolorosa. *Arch. Neurol. (Chicago)* **29,** 158–161.

Hosobuchi, Y., Adams, J. E., and Rutkin, B. (1975). Chronic thalamic and internal capsule stimulation for the control of central pain. *Surg. Neurol.* **4,** 91–92.

Hosobuchi, Y., Adams, J. E., and Linchitz, R. (1977). Pain relief by electrical stimulation of the central gray matter in humans and its reversal by naloxone. *Science* **197,** 183–186.

Kosambi, D. D. (1967). Living prehistory in India. *Sci. Am.* **216,** 105–114.

Lewis, C. S. (1962). "The Problem of Pain." Macmillan, New York.

Liebeskind, J. C., Mayer, D. J., and Akil, H. (1974). Central mechanisms of pain inhibition: Studies of analgesia from focal brain stimulation. *Adv. Neurol.* **4,** 261–268.

Lim, R. K. S., Gusman, F., Rodgers, D. W., Goto, K., Braun, C., Dickerson, G. D., and Engle, R. J. (1964). Site of action of narcotic and non-narcotic analgesics determined by blocking bradykinin-evoked visceral pain. *Arch. Int. Pharmacodyn. Ther.* **152,** 25–58.

Lu, H. (1973). "Chinese Version of Modern Acupuncture." Academy of Oriental Heritage, Vancouver, B. C.

McEwen, B. S. (1976). Interactions between hormones and nerve tissue. *Sci. Am.* **235,** 48–58.

Melzack, R. (1973). "The Puzzle of Pain." Basic Books, New York.

Melzack, R., and Scott, T. H. (1957). The effects of early experience on the response to pain. *J. Comp. Physiol. Psychol.* **50,** 155–161.

Powers, J. B. (1970). Hormonal control of sexual receptivity during the estrous cycle of the rat. *Physiol. Behav.* **5,** 831–835.

Rhodes, D. C., and Liebeskind, J. C. (1977). The central mode of action of narcotic analgesic drugs. *In* "Psychopharmacology in the Practice of Medicine" (M. E. Jarvick, ed.), pp. 143–152. Appleton, New York.

Schally, A. V., Arimura, A., and Kastin, A. J. (1973). Hypothalamic regulatory hormones. *Sci.* **179,** 341–350.

Snyder, S. H. (1977). Opiate receptors and internal opiates. *Sci. Am.* **236,** 44–56.

Tseng, L., Loh, H. H., and Li, C. H. (1977). Human β endorphin: Development of tolerance and behavioral activity in rats. *Biochem. Biophys. Res. Commun.* **74,** 390–396.

Vander, A. J., Sherman, J. H., and Luciano, D. S. (1970). "Human Physiology." McGraw-Hill, New York.

Whalen, R. E., and Luttge, W. G. (1971). Differential localization of progesterone uptake in brain, role of sex, estrogen pretreatment and adrenalectomy. *Brain Res.* **33,** 147–155.

13

Thirst and Hunger

I. Introduction

The cells of our bodies are maintained in a relatively constant state by a complex set of physiological processes. Blood vessels carry oxygen, water, nutrients, and hormones to the cells where specialized metabolic activity is carried out. As we saw in Chapter 12, body temperature, blood pressure, and other states are very precisely regulated. None of these homeostatic processes is under our direct "voluntary control," but in order for these processes to work we must behave. In a fundamental sense we behave in order to maintain constant internal states. We must drink water, eat a variety of foods, avoid some foods, and protect ourselves from excessive heat and cold. Such behavior is generally referred to as motivated or goal-directed behavior. Motivated behavior may be contrasted with reflexive behavior. A reflex is triggered by some stimulus. Motivated behavior is initiated by stimuli, involves goal-directed behavior, and is maintained until terminated by other stimuli. Motivated behavior thus involves feedback. The important feature of motivated behavior is goal-directedness or selectivity.

This chapter is concerned with the neural basis of two types of motivated behavior, drinking and feeding. Thirst and hunger can become so intense that they dominate our behavior. We all know what it is like to be thirsty on a hot day after vigorous exercise and to be hungry when we have not eaten for many hours. When we need water we become thirsty, and we seek and drink liquids. When we need food, we become hungry, and we seek and eat food. While these facts are obvious, their causes are not. What processes cause us to seek and drink water and eat food? What processes cause us to stop drinking and eating? When we consider thirst or hunger we usually think about peripheral sensation, such as a dry mouth or hunger pangs. While there is no doubt that we have such sensations, eating and drinking are not explained by reference to them. Research on hunger or thirst has attempted to determine the physiological conditions and neuronal processes that initiate, maintain, and terminate drinking and feeding. We see in experimental studies on feeding and drinking a vivid illustration of integrative physiological mechanisms expressed in simple defined behaviors essential to the maintenance of life.

II. Drinking

The intensity of the thirst drive is second only to that for air. All living tissues depend on water for maintenance of metabolic processes. In land animals water is continuously being lost during respiration, waste removal, and temperature regulation. Thus, water must be taken in. The intake of water must be directly proportional to the amount lost so that the cells of the body neither dehydrate or overhydrate.

Thirst, expressed as motivated drinking behavior, is one of a variety of mechanisms that work together to maintain body fluid balances. Thirst interacts with the renal functions of the kidney and other mechanisms that maintain electrolyte balances in the blood to sustain a constant amount of water in the body. The contribution of the kidneys to this system is to eliminate excess fluids and metabolic waste products while conserving those fluids and metabolites that are in demand. The kidneys, however, cannot add new water to the bodily fluid reserves. Behavior, particularly drinking, is required to restore body fluid deficits. In Fig. 13-1 we can see the cooperative action of kidney function and behavior. In Fig. 13-1A, the kidney is shown to compensate for both the behavioral excess of ingesting too much liquid, and the behavioral deficit of not taking in enough. Figure 13-1B illustrates the behavioral precision of water intake in rats with diabetes insipidus. These rats lack the ability to synthesize antidiuretic hormone, and, as a result, cannot conserve water efficiently. In the following sections we will describe some of the conditions that cause an animal to start drinking, the mechanisms that detect body fluid losses, and finally, those events that terminate drinking.

A.   The Distribution of Water in the Body

Mammals are 67% water by weight. Body water is distributed by both osmotic and hydrostatic gradients into two unequal phases. One phase, the *cellular phase*,

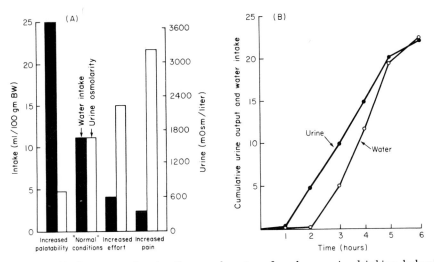

Fig. 13-1. (A) Compensation by the renal system for changes in drinking behavior. When the liquid is highly palatable, drinking increases above normal rates, and the osmolarity of the urine decreases. On the other hand, when drinking decreases because of increased effort required to obtain water, or because of punishment, then drinking decreases and the kidneys compensate by retaining water. The result is an increase in urine osmolarity. (B) Rats with diabetes insipidus have a genetic defect that prevents them from synthesizing antidiuretic hormone. As a result, they cannot retain water in the body and excrete large quantities of urine. Here it can be seen that the rat behaviorally compensates for this water loss by increasing its intake to match the amount that was lost. (From Blass, 1973.)

contains all the water located within cells, and it is about twice the volume of the extracellular phase. However, it is through the *extracellular phase*, which includes water in the blood, that fluid exchanges occur with the external environment. Fluids are lost through the extracellular phase, and ingested fluids enter it first before they move into the cellular phase. The extracellular phase, therefore, is the more labile of the two. It is the first to lose water during periods between drinking and its relative loss is greater.

B. Thirst and Drinking

One form of drinking, *primary drinking*, is observed following an actual loss of body fluids. Primary drinking occurs following hemorrhage, sweating or some redistribution of fluids, such as edema, that makes water unavailable to the general circulation. The sensation of thirst precedes primary drinking. Drinking may also occur when animals are in a state of positive fluid balance, that is, when they have sufficient or even an excess of fluids. In this case an animal may drink because the fluid is very palatable, because of habit, or because the liquid may serve as a lubricant to help swallow dry food. These forms of drinking are all called *secondary drinking*. In secondary drinking the animal does not have a water deficit but, in fact, has a positive fluid balance when drinking begins. We will not discuss secondary drinking here mainly because its causes are many and poorly understood. For a review of the factors that influence secondary drinking, see Kissileff (1973).

If water balance is to be maintained, there must be mechanisms to measure and regulate fluid content of the body. Research on thirst mechanisms has centered on three topics: (1) Identification of the stimuli and the receptor systems which measure fluid content and promote thirst. (2) The manner in which these receptor systems act on brain centers. (3) The mechanisms which terminate the drinking response.

STIMULI WHICH PROMOTE THIRST.   Body fluids are either inside of cells (the cellular compartment) or outside of cells (the extracellular compartment). The extracellular compartment is vast and complex, consisting of the blood (vascular compartment) and the interstitial tissues and lymph fluids (nonvascular compartment). When body fluids are decreased, usually due to lack of water intake, the salinity of the fluids increases and changes in cellular osmotic pressure* occurs. Certain cells in the brain are sensitive to changes in osmotic pressure which results in cellular dehydration. As the osmotic changes are detected, thirst

---

* The relative tendency of dissolved substrates to diffuse or move to regions of lower concentration.

and drinking behavior are elicited. In addition, there are receptors in the blood vessels and kidneys that respond to changes in blood volume and blood pressure. These changes promote the production of angiotensin, which circulates in the blood and acts on brain thirst centers to stimulate drinking. When water is ingested, the fluid balance in the cellular and extracellular compartments returns to normal, and the blood volume and blood pressure no longer activate receptors that initiate drinking. An imbalance in water is clearly extraordinarily detrimental to the organism. Thus, it is no wonder that specialized mechanisms which involve strong motivated behaviors are present to maintain this balance.

C. Thirst Promoted as a Result of Cellular Dehydration

1. NATURE OF THE STIMULI. As early as 1918 Leschke showed that the intravenous injections of a hypertonic salt solution (one more concentrated than body fluids) causes immediate thirst in man. This result, which has been confirmed many times, was unexpected, since it showed that thirst does not depend upon the commonly felt sensation of dryness of the mouth. Gilman (1937) investigated the properties of the fluid stimulus in greater detail and found that the stimulus is quite specific. Intravenous injection of _hypertonic_ saline in dogs causes twice as much drinking as, for example, an osmotically equivalent amount of urea which is twice as concentrated. Hypertonic saline, sodium sulfate, sodium bicarbonate, sucrose, or sorbital all stimulate drinking, whereas hypertonic urea, glucose, or isomannide do not. Gilman concluded that _cellular dehydration_, and not an increase in osmotic pressure, is the stimulus to thirst. In general, it appears that hypertonic solutions composed of solutes which do not penetrate cells stimulate thirst because they cause cells to dehydrate: water leaves the cells in order to reestablish the _osmotic pressure_ equilibrium across the cell membrane. On the other hand, hypertonic solutions such as glucose that are composed of permanent solutes do not stimulate thirst because the solutions can equilibrate across the membrane. This type of mechanism imparts a desirable selectivity to thirst and may indicate the significance of the _cell dehydration mechanism_. It is essential to balance water loss due to salt accumulation. Thirst should not be stimulated automatically whenever a solute increases its concentration in the body fluids, as is the case when blood glucose is elevated in response to energy demands.

When body fluids are reduced and drinking occurs, the net intake of water is fairly precisely that amount needed to dilute the body fluids to their normal tonicity. The time course of this return varies according to species and also with the degree of contribution of both renal and behavioral factors. When water is totally unavailable, the task of osmoregulation falls entirely on the kidney. When an animal is made anuric by either nephrectomy (kidney removal) or tying off the ureters, the task of regulation falls entirely on the behavior of drinking. It is important to note that the cellular thirst mechanism does not habituate. Nephrectomized rats drink as much water after a 24-hour period of water deprivation as they do when water is made available shortly after cellular dehydration (Fitzsimons, 1963). It would be maladaptive indeed if under natural circumstances thirst habituated before a source of water could be reached. In addition to causing thirst and drinking, cellular dehydration strongly inhibits feeding. Inhibition of feeding has the obvious beneficial effect of preventing the animal from aggravating the cellular deficit by adding additional dry material (including solutes) to an already dehydrated system.

2. MECHANISMS OF DETECTION. Early theories of cellular thirst maintained that because all cells of the body lose water when osmotic pressure rises, then the sensation of cellular thirst is also of a general origin. This view is no longer accepted. Recent research has provided us with strong evidence for the existence of detectors of cellular dehydration in the brain. Although cellular water is lost more or less uniformly throughout the body under conditions of water deprivation, it is the water lost from these specialized receptors located in the basal forebrain that causes drinking.

Andersson (1971) demonstrated that injections of hypertonic saline into the third ventricle of the goat produces vigorous drinking. Moreover, intraventricular injections of hypertonic sucrose do not cause drinking. The drinking response to NaCl is very reliable and substantial. On the basis of these studies and others, Andersson concluded that cells sensitive to intracellular sodium concentration are the receptors mediating cellular dehydration (thirst) and that they may be found in the walls of the third ventricle. While there is clear evidence that intracranial injections of hypertonic solutions can cause drinking, questions about the exact location of these receptors and their mechanism of action are the focus of lively debate. One problem with Andersson's view is that NaCl is a nonspecific excitatory agent. Whether drinking is initiated by specific Na^+ receptors, or whether NaCl nonspecifically excites cells that mediate drinking has not as yet been determined.

Other investigators (Blass and Epstein, 1971; Peck and Novin, 1971) suggested that cellular thirst is detected by _osmoreceptors_ (cells sensitive to changes in osmotic balance) located in the lateral preoptic area. Evidence for this position follows the criteria proposed by Gilman (1937) for the identification of systemic thirst mechanisms. These criteria are that intracranial injections of those solutions that are normally excluded from cells should cause drinking, while injection of solutions that cross cell membranes to enter cells should not. Recent findings (shown in Fig. 13-2) indicated that microliter injections of hypertonic saline and hypertonic sucrose into the lateral preoptic area of the hypothalamus

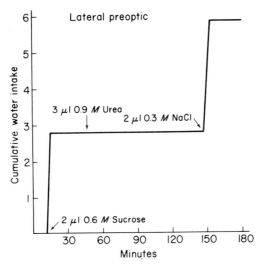

Fig. 13-2. The effectiveness of injections of microliter quantities of various substances into the lateral preoptic area of the rat in eliciting drinking. Injections of either sucrose or salt solutions (both substances that cannot cross the cell membranes and enter the cell) cause the rapid onset of drinking. However, an injection of urea solution (which can enter the cells) at even higher concentrations than the sucrose or salt, does not elicit a bout of drinking. (From Blass and Epstein, 1971.)

causes drinking in rats while injection of hyperosmotic urea, which can enter the cells, is totally ineffective at provoking drinking even though the urea solution was more concentrated than the sucrose or saline solutions. Clearly the elicitation of drinking is selective. These findings also fulfill a second major criterion for the identification of a thirst mechanism. Drinking can be induced by intracranial injections of hypertonic substances that are in the normal physiological range. However, there are also some problems with the _osmorecepter hypothesis_. First, there seem to be relatively few effective injection sites in the lateral preoptic region. Second, the drinking response obtained by this method, although quite reliable, is usually small.

In conclusion, the currently available evidence favors the notion that osmoreceptors in the brain can detect imbalances in osmotic pressure in brain fluids, the extracellular thirst mechanism. However, the controversy is far from resolved. It should be stressed that current views are consistent with the available data on drinking following systemic cellular dehydration. It is possible that there may be two sets of detectors that cooperate to induce drinking: osmoreceptors and another as yet unidentified one which is influenced by the salinity imbalance. We shall see in fact that changes in blood can stimulate release of angiotensin which is a powerful stimulus for inducing drinking.

II. DRINKING

571

3. THIRST RESULTING FROM EXTRACELLULAR DEHYDRATION.   Because maintenance of blood volume is absolutely vital for the health of any animal, it is not surprising that there are elaborate mechanisms that ensure a fairly constant circulating volume and pressure of blood. The circulatory system is generously endowed with receptors that constantly monitor blood pressure. Activation of these receptors releases a host of vascular and hormonal changes involving pituitary, adrenal, and kidney responses. Reduction of extracellular volume, particularly intravascular volume, called _hypovolemia_, causes thirst and drinking.

Because many of the adjustments of the body to extracellular water depletion have been understood for years, it is rather surprising that a clear-cut demonstration of _extracellular thirst mechanisms_ was provided only recently (Fitzsimons, 1961). It was known that patients suffering fluid loss caused by burns or excessive bleeding often complain of severe thirst. However, it proved to be very difficult to perform a convincing experimental demonstration of an extracellular thirst mechanism. Historically, two forces worked against its discovery. First, there was the belief that cellular mechanisms alone could account for all drinking behavior. Second, those intrepid few researchers who attempted to demonstrate an extracellular control mechanism met with frustration. Animals go into shock when too much blood is removed. Modest blood depletions are quickly corrected by the animal's intrinsic hemodynamic mechanism. In the early 1960's Fitzsimons overcame these problems by injecting rats with large molecular weight colloids (MW 20,000) which remained in the interstitial space and slowly absorbed water from the blood. When animals are treated in this way they drink an amount of fluid proportional to the severity of the extracellular deficit (Fig. 13-3). When these findings were confirmed and extended (Stricker, 1966), the existence of an extracellular thirst mechanism was on a firm experimental footing. This thirst mechanism is a by far more complex and less well understood control than the cellular thirst mechanism. Its major receptors have not yet been identified.

Unlike the drinking that follows cellular water loss, water intake resulting from a reduction in extracellular volume terminates well before the deficit has been restored (Stricker, 1969). This incomplete rehydration may be understood by considering the fate of the ingested water. Only about 10% of the ingested water remains in the vasculature, where the deficit is. About 67% of the water moves out of the vasculature and enters the cells, overhydrating them. Thus, if water intake were to continue unabated until extracellular volume was completely restored, severe water intoxication would result. It appears that drinking in response to extracellular thirst stimuli is inhibited by cellular overhydration. It is interesting to note that rats allowed to drink a saline solution will drink only an amount of saline that will correct an extracellular deficit. The reason for this is that isotonic saline remains in the extracellular phase and does not overhydrate

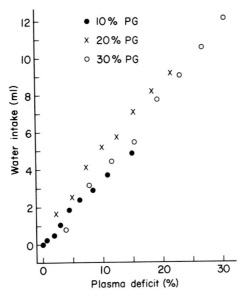

Fig. 13-3. Polyethylene glycol when implanted into the interstitial space of a rat will absorb water from the blood producing a decrease in blood volume. In this figure, the three different concentrations of polyethylene glycol (PG) tested produced varying degrees of blood plasma volume deficits. In each case, water intake increased with the decrease in blood volume. (From Stricker, 1968, by permission of publisher.)

the cells. This suggests that when unopposed by cellular overhydration, extracellular mechanisms are very sensitive.

D.   The Role of Angiotensin II

One mediator of extracellular thirst mechanisms has been identified with some degree of certainty. Following a variety of manipulations influencing extracellular fluids (such as decreasing blood volume, blood pressure, or sympathetic activation), _renin_, a proteolytic enzyme, is released from the juxtaglomerular cells (JG) of the kidneys. Renin alters a blood plasma protein (angiotensinogen) to form the decapeptide _angiotensin I_. This peptide is then rapidly hydrolyzed to the octapeptide angiotensin II, the most potent drinking stimulus known. _Angiotensin II_ then enters the cerebrospinal fluid where it stimulates receptive structures. For example, an intracranial injection of picogram (10^{-12} gm) quantities of angiotensin II into the subfornical organ, an ependymal structure located near the roof of the third ventricle, elicits marked drinking (Simpson and Routtenberg, 1973). Although the subfornical organ is clearly very responsive to angiotensin II, there may be a number of angiotensin II-sensitive structures, all bathed by cerebrospinal fluid, which are involved in the control of drinking (Buggy *et al.*, 1975).

Release of renin in the kidney is triggered by the kidney itself, which possesses receptors and by sympathetic activity which is stimulated by venous pressure receptors. Figure 13-4 illustrates the control of drinking involving peripherally released angiotensin.

Recent research has indicated that under normal physiological conditions the peripheral renin–angiotensin system may be of only minor importance (Stricker *et al.*, 1976). Although injections of renin administered to nephrectomized rats can produce drinking, the quantity of renin in the injections is well above the physiological range. Additionally, when blood pressure is experimentally lowered in normal rats renin is released, angiotensin II is produced, and the rats drink. However, the levels of renin activity are not high enough to provide the basis for the increases in water intake (Stricker *et al.*, 1976). While it is clear that renin–angiotensin will evoke drinking, it is not yet clear that peripherally released angiotensin is the only stimulus. Recently, it has been discovered that the brain contains another renin–angiotensin system that may be "independent" of the peripheral system and that this system may also influence drinking.

E.   Mechanisms of Normal Drinking

Up to this point we have considered drinking in response to the reduction of water in each of the major fluid compartments alone. However, purely cellular or extracellular depletion occurs only rarely in nature. Under normal circumstances when water is not available, fluids are lost by both phases. These losses are then detected by the mechanisms we have described, and behavior related to the search for water and finally drinking ensues. However, many animals, including humans, do not completely restore their fluid losses in a single drinking session (Adolph *et al.*, 1954). This fact does not seem surprising in the light of what is now

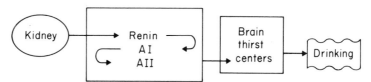

Fig. 13-4.   The role of renin in the initiation of drinking. When a fall in blood pressure or blood volume is detected, renin is released into the bloodstream from the kidney. In the bloodstream, renin splits a plasma protein into angiotensin I. (AI). When this decapeptide passes through the lungs, a converting enzyme located there splits it further into the octapeptide angiotensin II. (AII). The angiotensin II is then carried to the brain where it enters the cerebrospinal fluid and stimulates structures located near the ventricles to induce drinking.

known about extracellular controls of drinking. The events that underlie drinking termination do not simply reflect cellular overhydration per se. Rather, cellular overhydration interacts with peripheral controls, such as those originating in the mouth and throat, to halt drinking in water-deprived animals (Blass and Hall, 1976).

The major feature of the Blass and Hall approach was to study the drinking behavior of rats in situations where the ingested water could not be absorbed. Thus, to evaluate the control exerted by oral factors, they created a fistulous opening in the stomach so that the ingested water was immediately lost through a small tube. To study gastric control, ingested water was trapped in the stomach (Hall, 1973). In addition, these manipulations permitted rats to be preloaded with measured amounts of water or isotonic saline, at various times before a drinking test. Thus following a given level of water deprivation, oral and gastric controls over drinking could be studied singly and in conjunction with various degrees of cellular or extracellular rehydration. The findings of such studies indicate that orogastric mechanisms alone exert rather little control over normal water intakes. Yet they become extremely sensitive following absorbed water preloads which for the most part improved cellular, but not extracellular, balance. Conversely, isotonic saline preloads restore extracellular balance but have little effect on drinking.

The model offered by Blass and Hall (1976) emphasizes drinking termination, but it highlights the major points dealing with the control of water balance. According to their model, cellular and extracellular fluid balances are integrated over time and give rise to specific commands. These individual commands feed into a single command to drink. When drinking begins, the ingested water quickly finds its way into the cellular phase (Novin, 1962), and the alteration in cellular fluid balance reduces the strength of the command to drink in four important ways. First, by helping remove the cellular deficit and, ultimately, by causing a degree of cellular overhydration, absorbed water directly reduces the command to drink. Second, improved cellular balance sensitizes the mechanisms of mouth metering which reflect the volume and quality of the fluid being ingested. Third, a signal reflecting gastric fill is sensitized reducing the command to drink. Fourth, in order for cellular overhydration to be most effective, it must occur close in time to the act of drinking. Figure 13-5 summarizes some of these regulatory processes.

We know a great deal about why we become thirsty and feel driven to drink. However, there are still many interesting questions which are in need of study. Aside from the identification of some structures thought to be receptors, the details of the neural system controlling thirst remains virtually unknown. How do those specific cells stimulated finally act on other brain centers to drive the animal to drink? Research techniques, particularly those related to mapping specific pathways and those which allow the recording of electrical activity in the brains of

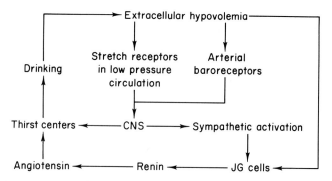

Fig. 13-5. A schematic model outlining some of the events that lead to drinking following extracellular fluid loss. A fall in blood volume is detected by stretch receptors, arterial baroreceptors, and by the juxtaglomerular cells (JG cells) of the kidney. Activation of the stretch receptors and baroreceptors stimulates the CNS which, in turn, activates the thirst centers in the hypothalamus and the sympathetic division of the ANS. This, in turn, adds additional stimulation to the JG cells which release renin into the bloodstream. Renin is converted to angiotensin II which also stimulates thirst centers to induce drinking. Drinking behavior then reduces the extracellular volume deficit. (From Thompson, 1975.)

behaving animals, offer exciting new hope that these mechanisms will soon be understood.

III. Feeding

A. Homeostatic Behavior

Feeding is basic to all living animals and, for all but the most primitive, feeding involves characteristic behaviors. Some animals that live in water may use circulating currents to bring them fuel for their metabolism, but most animals must work for their food.

Reptiles, insects, birds, and mammals all struggle with the problem of finding water, salt, warmth, and food in ecological niches that are as varied as the Death Valley desert and the glaciers of Mt. McKinley. Even where the climate is the same, such as Harlem, New York and Pleasantville, New York, the problems of obtaining food require enormously different and adaptable behavioral repertoires.

Homeostatic behavior is a useful term to describe actions that an animal exerts in order to achieve internal stability. Vincent Dethier, a behavioral biologist who studies homeostatic behavior, has described its essential features as seen in the feeding behavior of the common fly.

Insects are among the most successful animals on earth. In terms of numbers, at least, they dominate the world. They live almost everywhere; they have existed in forms so well adapted that some species have not changed appreciably from times of fossil records to the present. How have they done it? What is the homeostatic behavior that so successfully finds food for such tiny beasts, generation after generation? In this section we will first discuss some of the essential factors that control feeding in a simple system, a fly, and then discuss more complex controls on feeding, such as taste and the consequences of eating as seen in mammals.

B. Feeding Mechanisms in the Fly

Dethier (1967a,b) and his colleagues have studied factors controlling the initiation and termination of feeding behavior in the fly (Fig. 13-6). In brief, feeding in a fly consists of first flying at random and then, when a food odor is detected, flying upwind. Upon landing in the odor's vicinity, the fly walks about until it tastes the food with its feet where its taste organs are located (Fig. 13-7). Neural recordings made by inserting an electrode through a hole drilled in the side of a taste hair of a fly (clearly a technical tour de force!) demonstrated the existence of a neuron sensitive to sugar and another neuron sensitive to salt (Fig. 13-8). These neurons fire in proportion to the concentration of the stimulus

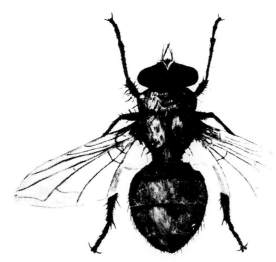

Fig. 13-6. Blowflies belong to the family Caliphoridae, of the order Diptera. Blowfly is a name given to several kinds of flies. Many have bodies that are metallic blue or green, and they range in size from that of a housefly to three or four times larger. Like the housefly they are found practically everywhere. They are scavengers and pests. (From D. Borror, 1971.)

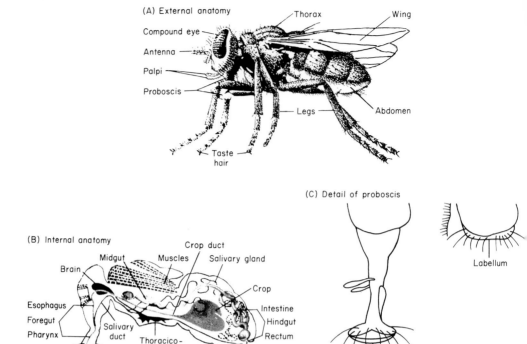

(A) External anatomy

Thorax

Wing

Compound eye

Antenna

Palpi

Proboscis

Legs

Abdomen

Taste hair

(C) Detail of proboscis

Labellum

(B) Internal anatomy

Crop duct

Midgut · Muscles · Salivary gland

Brain

Crop

Esophagus

Intestine

Foregut

Hindgut

Pharynx · Salivary duct

Rectum

Thoracico-abdominal ganglion

Labellum

Labellum

Taste hair

Fig. 13-7. Anatomy of a blowfly. (A) External anatomy. (B) Internal anatomy. (C) Details of proboscis. When an odor is detected by a fly, he flys upwind and lands. Upon landing he walks around until he tastes the food with the taste hairs located on his feet. These hairs are sensitive to sugar, salt and water. If the stimulation is appropriate, the fly then extends its proboscis. The taste hairs on the labellum of the proboscis also contain receptors for sugar, salt, and water. If the appropriate signal is received from the taste hair, then the fly sucks up the food. The food travels from the labellum into the foregut, which is comprised of the pharynx and esophagus. It then goes into the crop via the crop duct. Located in the wall of the crop are stretch receptors. When the crop is distended a signal is sent to the brain relaying the message that the fly is full. When the fly is full, feeding stops. (Modified from *The World Book Encyclopedia*, Vol. 7, Copyright 1978 World Book-Childcraft International, Inc.)

solution and trigger extension of the proboscis which also has sensory receptors. Each taste hair on the labellum, or "lip" of the proboscis contains two sugar receptive cells, two salt cells, and one water cell. If the taste signal is appropriate, the fly then sucks up food until the sensory receptors become adapted to the stimulus and cease firing. This defines the end of a meal. A new feeding sequence will start as soon as a fresh stimulus is encountered.

This process continues until internal physiological factors stop feeding, that is until the animal is satiated. The signal to stop eating is generated by stomach

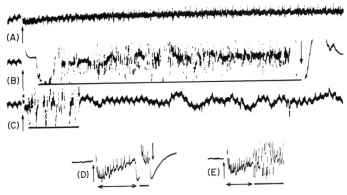

Fig. 13-8. Recordings from the labellar hair of blowfly proboscis demonstrating the differential sensitivity of sugar and salt receptors. (A) Water pretest showing no muscle activity of the proboscis after introduction of water stimulus (↑). (B) After sugar stimulation (↑) the large spikes (—) show muscle activity of the moving proboscis, resulting in proboscis extension (↓). (C) Water posttest. After sugar the fly will now respond to water stimulation (↑) with muscle activity of the moving proboscis (—) and extension (↓). This altered response is due to a change in the central excitatory state of the fly's nervous system. (D) 0.2 M NaCl stimulation (↑). After the sensory spikes from the salt (↔) there is proboscis muscle activity (—) resulting in extension (↓). (E) 0.5 M NaCl stimulation (↑) with the proboscis in the extended position. The fly will not drink this concentrated solution. After the salt spikes (↔) the muscle activity (—) is proboscis retraction. (Modified from Dethier, 1976. Copyright 1968 by the American Association for the Advancement of Science.)

distension. Flies have a food storage crop, or stomach, with stretch receptors in the crop wall. When the fly is full, literally full, feeding stops (Fig. 13-9). If the nerve carrying this inhibitory information from the crop to the brain is cut *hyperphagia* (overeating) results. Hyperphagic flies sometimes eat until they burst. Hyperphagia in a fly can also be produced by cutting the ventral nerve cord, which is analogous to cutting the spinal cord of a vertebrate. This causes the fly to eat one huge meal. Apparently, sensory adaption that normally brings a meal to an end is lost. This type of hyperphagia is different from the hyperphagia following loss of the internal signal from the crop. In that case the fly eats and stops eating normally, but then starts eating again very soon. In other words, there is more than one possible reason for overeating—a fact which is too often forgotten in the treatment of human overeaters. These studies demonstrate the importance of both external and internal sensory signals in the control of feeding. There are other, however, important principles of homeostatic behavior in the fly.

The smell and taste of food generate locomotor activity. Activity is one sign of what is often called *arousal*. Dethier termed this process of the nervous system a central excitatory state which is operationally defined in terms of behavior. A fly

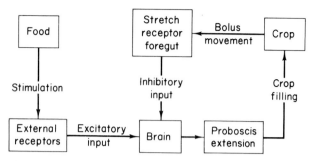

Fig. 13-9 Regulation of homeostatic feeding behavior in the blowfly. When a fly's external receptors are stimulated by food nerve impulses are sent to the brain. If the concentration of the original solution is found unfavorable, a no eat signal is sent to the proboscis and there is no extension. If the concentration and quality of the solution is favorable a message is sent to the proboscis causing proboscis extension. The food is then sucked up and sent down the esophagus by a pumping action to the crop. There is movement of digested food, as a bolus, from the crop to the foregut. When the stretch receptor, located in the wall of the crop, receives stimulation that it is fully distended it sends a nerve impulse to the brain to stop feeding. When the brain receives this signal it triggers proboscis retraction and feeding stops. (Modified from A. Gelperin, 1966. Reprinted with permission from *J. Insect Physiol.* **12.** Copyright 1966 by Pergamon Press, Ltd.)

that tastes water but does not drink it at that time may drink the same water immediately after a taste of sucrose. Thus the sucrose raised the central excitatory state. The central excitatory state is opposed by a central inhibitory state. The inhibitory process can be shown by inserting a taste of strong salt between the first water test and the sucrose. When this is done the fly refuses to drink water. The inhibitory aftereffect of the salt taste cancels the excitatory effect of the sucrose.

So far we have discussed factors that start feeding and stop it, with associated long lasting effects on excitability, but there is more to ingestive behavior than starting and stopping. Sometimes the food becomes aversive. There is some evidence that proboscis withdrawal may be a sign of an active escape response that is more than just satiety, that is, more than just cessation of eating. Moderate concentrations of salt may cause extension of the proboscis or "acceptance," while slightly higher concentrations of the same salt will cause withdrawal or "rejection." A difference of only three sensory nerve impulses initiated during the first 100 msec can make the difference between acceptance and rejection (Dethier, 1968).

The same switch-over from acceptance to rejection can occur for a given concentration depending on whether the fly is tested when deprived or satiated. The switch-over concentration is not fixed, but instead can vary with the homeostatic state of the animal. This variability or shift in the switch-over from acceptance to rejection is a function of the central nervous system. The firing rate of the sensory receptors does not change before and after the switch-over. Therefore, some central mechanism must compare the sensory signal from the external world with internal sensory signals from stretch receptors in the stomach and then adjust motor output accordingly.

It does not require a complex nervous system such as ours to engage in homeostatic behavior. The fly has only a simple trigger system (three sensors: water, sugar, salt) and such an incredibly simple brake system (stretch receptors) that one can only marvel at the effectiveness of it in a complex environment. After all, flies live with us and share our food when they can get it.

The fly's greatest complexity in feeding behavior, and a hint of what is to come when we discuss vertebrates, lies in the CNS "shifty switch-over"—that sliding threshold for palatability. A machine with a fixed set point for go, no-go decisions would be relatively simple. For example, a thermostat controlling the furnace on the basis of a fixed unadjustable set point is relatively simple and may be adequate, but a machine with a sliding set point (how often do you change your room thermostat?) is better. Not all food is equally filling, equally caloric, equally nutritious, equally hydrated, nor equally rapidly digested. Therefore, it seems appropriate that an organism be able to adjust its response to its sensors accordingly. Given that arousal will lead to food tasting, and food tasting will trigger eating, then we may judge that a sliding set point for eat, no-eat decisions is useful for survival. If it were not useful, flies would probably not have it.

C. Feeding Processes in Mammals

The account of feeding in the fly sets the stage for our study of feeding in mammals. The basic mechanisms and basic issues have been outlined. Most of what we know about feeding in mammals comes from studies of the rat, and all that follows refers to research with rats unless otherwise specified.

1. TASTE FACTORS. External sensory factors are extremely important in initiating and maintaining feeding. These include taste, smell, temperature and texture of the food. Animals express clear preference based on these qualities. Some of these preferences are innate, such as a preference for sweetness in some species, and are termed *specific hungers*. Others are learned and easily modifiable. For example, a rat that eats a meal of food with a novel flavor is more likely to develop a preference for that flavor if hungry at the time. Satiety induced by preloading the animal with glucoses tends to block the development of a taste preference.

Garcia discovered that rats can develop strong taste aversions. Rats faced with a novel food usually sample only a little taste of it. If the animal is made sick by X irradiation, nausea-producing drugs, or even a wide variety of drugs including amphetamine and alcohol, the rat will refuse to eat any more of a recently tasted novel food (Garcia *et al.*, 1974). This phenomena has been called "*bait shyness*." Similarly, it can be shown that a sick rat which tastes a new food and then improves in health will later display a learned preference for taste. This is called a *medicine preference effect* (Fig. 13-10). The development of learned preferences explains some of the astounding food self-selection behavior first described in rats by Richter. Thiamine-deficient rats in a cafeteria choice situation will develop a learned preference for thiamine-containing foods. This is a medicine preference effect, not an innate specific hunger for thiamine (Rozin, 1967). However, specific hungers do exist. Salt hunger is the clearest example. Salt-deprived animals spontaneously prefer salty food. There are also built-in mechanisms which shift taste preference at different stages of development. Notably, sex hormones modulate taste preference. All of these taste aversions and preferences have been shown to involve the CNS. They are not just a function of changes at the peripheral receptor level. For example, a salt-deprived rat *prefers* higher concentrations of salt, but is no better than a nondeprived rat at *detecting*

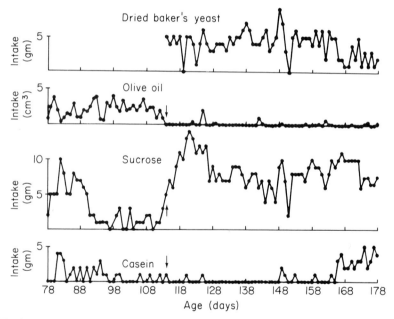

Fig. 13-10. An animal given a deficient diet will choose from the available food sources one which makes him feel better. This is called the medicine preference effect. If thiamine-deficient rats are given a choice only between fat (olive oil) carbohydrate (sucrose), or protein (casein), they will select fat since this is best for their health. When food containing thiamine (baker's yeast) is added to the choice, the rats consume the baker's yeast, resume a normal carbohydrate intake and decrease their consumption of fat. This shows a medicine preference effect not a specific hunger for thiamine (From Richter *et al.*, 1938.)

salt. The hypothalamus is one area that has been strongly implicated. Lesions in the medial region of the hypothalamus affect salt preference. Lesions in the lateral hypothalamus have been reported to block learning of taste aversions (Roth *et al.*, 1973; Schwartz and Teitelbaum, 1974).

The role of the CNS in learned taste aversions is bound to be one of the challenges for future research. This research is forming an interface between feeding studies and experiments exploring brain mechanisms in learning and memory. It is a phenomenon researchers can work with easily because the effects are so pronounced and intriguing. Some of the questions that have already come up are: Does the brain have built-in linkages that associate gastric illness with tastes better than with sounds? Is it possible to destroy the brain's capacity to make new taste preference associations without destroying the memory of old ones? Can simple animals display this kind of learning, and if so, can we hope to find the synapses that mediate it? There are investigators who have answered yes to each of these questions, and others who have expressed doubts. The study of learned taste aversion is one of the current frontiers in the study of feeding and brain research.

When a meal begins rats eat rapidly, and for a time they may even gradually accelerate their rate of eating, but then gradually slow down and stop. The effect of taste alone can be seen in animals fixed with an *esophageal fistula* that prevents food from entering the stomach (Fig. 13-11). Under this condition animals eat or drink tremendous quantities of palatable food—triple normal amounts in a 1 hour test. However, they still display a preference. The sweeter the food the more they eat, up to a point, then the preference curve turns downward. Rats consume less of a supersweet solution, even when it never reaches their stomachs (Epstein, 1967; Mook, 1963). Even in the case where everything eaten passes into the stomach, animals show a *"preference–aversion function"*; that is, an inverted U-shaped curve relating intake to concentration. This preference–aversion function allows researchers to compare different concentrations of the same taste. Given that palatable tastes can cause additional eating, it is reasonable to ask if a palatable taste, all by itself, can lead to obesity. This has been shown clearly in rats using highly palatable additives such as sugar or vegetable oil to the rat chow. Obesity was also produced by feeding rats American grocery store foods: sweetened cereal, salami, cookies, etc. This was called *"dietary obesity"* (Sclafani, 1976). We leave it to you to judge whether this occurs in humans. Actual controlled experiments are lacking, but the answer seems to be fairly obvious.

Even normal plain food can trigger excessive feeding if the animal lacks certain regulatory signals. As we will show further on, brain damaged rats that have trouble monitoring internal energy signals rely unduly on taste. This may save their lives if they are starving, but, on the other hand, it may contribute to gross obesity if they have trouble tearing themselves away from food.

Oral factors including taste and smell play a very large role in feeding in

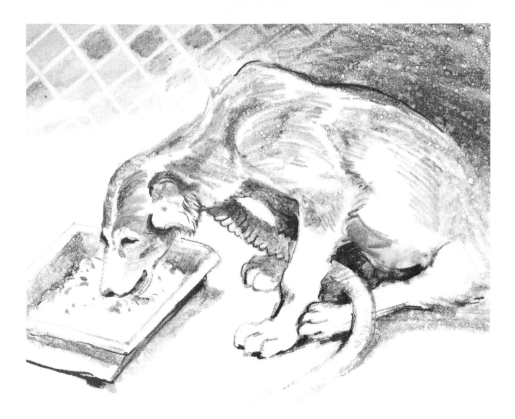

Fig. 13-11. An esophageal fistula. A tube is inserted in the throat of an animal preventing all food from reaching the stomach for digestion. The animal may eat up to three times the normal amount of food, but will still display a taste preference. The sweeter the food the more it will eat up to a point, and then it will decrease its eating. Animals given a supersweet solution eat less of it, even when it never reaches their stomachs.

mammals. However, animals can also regulate food intake without oral stimulation. In studies demonstrating this, rats were prepared with a plastic tube which led from a liquid food pump to an overhead swivel joint, down to the rat's head, in through the nasal passage to the back of the mouth, and down the esophagus to the stomach. The rats could activate the pump by pressing a level (Fig. 13-12). The animals learned to feed themselves intragastrically, and even compensated by pressing about twice as often when the liquid food was diluted in half with water (Teitelbaum, 1971; Epstein, 1971). Another example of regulation without taste is provided by a study in which monkeys were tube-fed a preload of food 15 minutes before regular mealtime. The monkeys compensated for the preload by eating less in that next meal even though they had not tasted the preload. Compensation was found to be within a few calories regardless of the caloric density of the preload (McHugh *et al.*, 1975).

584   **13. THIRST AND HUNGER**

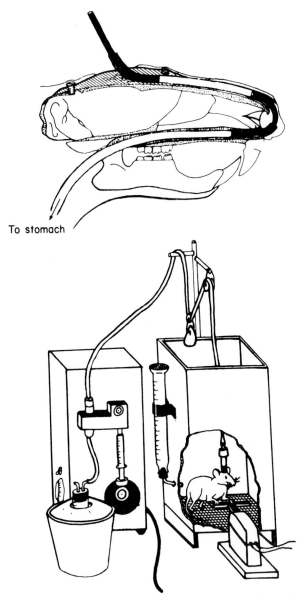

To stomach

Fig. 13-12. Intragastric feeding. Shown in the top panel is the course of the nasopharyngeal gastric tube in a midsagittal plane through the rat's head. A hole is drilled in the skull and tubing is inserted through the nasal passages and pharynx into the stomach. Shown on the bottom is the apparatus for intragastric self-injection. A plastic tube leads from a liquid food pump to an overhead swivel joint, down to the rat's head, and in through the esophagus to the stomach. The rat can activate the pump by pressing a lever located in front of him. The rat learns to feed itself and even compensates by pressing twice as often when the food is diluted in half with water. (From Epstein and Teitelbaum, 1962.)

An interesting series of related experiments with human volunteers shows that they do not do so well under the kinds of experimental conditions one can establish for people. Subjects did not respond to caloric dilution within one meal when taking food intragastrically. If they received food by mouth simultaneously with food intragastrically, they overate (Jordan, 1969). The degree of overeating depended on the nature of the administration. An intravenous carbohydrate–amino acid solution somewhat shortened oral meals, but the addition of a fat emulsion to the injection completely blocked eating.

For a long time there has been no doubt that postingestional factors serve as satiety cues. However, there is as yet no convincing evidence that any one factor is primarily responsible for controlling the cessation of eating. In flies it was mechanical distension. What is it in mammals?

2.   POSTINGESTIONAL FACTORS.   Physiologists have tried to study feeding in the same way that they have so successfully studied other homeostatic control systems, such as the control of respiration. Perhaps taking in food is analagous to taking in air and so appetite control centers can be compared to inspiratory control centers and satiety centers to expiratory control centers. Just as inspiration is inhibited by stretching of the lungs when filled with air, stomach distension also inhibits ingestion. Just as fine adjustments in breathing are regulated on the basis of a by-product of inhalation, CO_2, fine adjustments in feeding may be regulated on the basis of a by-product. Although it is at first surprising that our life support systems may rely on monitoring by-products, not just fuel inputs, it is sensible if one considers that end products are better evidence of moment to moment functioning than are fuel supplies. Mammals are so much bigger than a fly that fuel distribution is an enormously more complex logistic task. Moment to moment supply of glucose to the brain, for example, is certainly not adequately signaled by gastric distension.

All basic regulatory systems, breathing, temperature control, drinking, and feeding, involve both automatic reflex adjustments and voluntary behavioral components. For example, you shiver or sweat automatically, but you also turn on a heater or put on a coat through behavioral acts. Likewise, feeding involves both reflex actions and complex behavior. This discussion is limited arbitrarily to the neural control of complex behavior. Our problem is to find the physiological signals which potentiate feeding behavior and those which inhibit it. The following seven metabolic by-products have been repeatedly suggested as major signals: glucose utilization, insulin levels, fat availability, body weight, body temperature, overall energy flux, and most recently the hormone cholecystokin.

Glucose utilization measured as an arterial–venous *difference* in glucose levels correlates rather well with hunger, much better than does overall glucose level. This difference is highest when the tissue is absorbing large amounts of glucose from the blood. *Insulin* is necessary for efficient transport of glucose across cell membranes and therefore necessary for its utilization. An animal that lacks either a supply of glucose, for example a starved animal, or an animal that lacks insulin, for example an untreated diabetic, should also lack this satiety signal and tend to eat. Untreated diabetics tend to overeat, even though they have high blood sugar. Hyperglycemia will not trigger glucoreceptor cells for satiety unless insulin is also available.

The primary location of satiety *glucoreceptors* is thought to be in the *medial region of the hypothalamus*. The firing rate of cells in that region is increased by iontophoretic application of glucose, especially glucose plus insulin (Oomura, 1976) (Fig. 13-13). Systemic administration of insulin also increases firing. Conversely, *lateral hypothalamic* cells tend to decrease firing under those conditions that produce increased firing in medial hypothalamic cells. Researchers find many exceptions to this pattern, but the trend is strong enough to support the *glucose utilization theory* and also the concept of dual reciprocally related systems.

Insulin may be involved in long term control of feeding (Woods and Porte, 1976). This possibly is implied by a very strong correlation between body weight and insulin level. Insulin and other hormonal factors in the blood are too variable to account for weight regulation, but their levels are stable in the cerebrospinal fluid. Therefore, it is conceivable that brain receptors may monitor hormonal factors in the ventricular fluid. Such effects have been shown only for the control

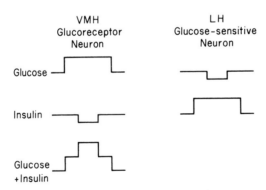

Fig. 13-13. Schematic representation of the effects of glucose, insulin and their combined effects on the neuronal discharge frequency in the ventromedial hypothalamus (VMH) and the lateral hypothalamus (LH) of the rat. The VMH is the primary location of glucoreceptors. Insulin is necessary for transport of glucose across cell membranes and therefore is needed for its utilization. Application of glucose, especially glucose plus insulin, increases the frequency of discharge in the VMH. Conversely, the LH neuronal discharge decreases under the same conditions that increase firing in the VMH. (Modified from Oomura, 1976, *in* "Hunger: Basic Mechanisms and Clinical Implications." Copyright 1976 by Raven Press, New York.)

of thirst, but it is a good possibility that brain receptors involved in feeding are sensitive to hormonal factors.

Another theory, the *lipostatic hypothesis*, proposes that satiety receptors measure fat availability (LeMagnen, 1976). It is well known that force-fed rats will display undereating (*anorexia*) until their weight returns to normal. Of course they cannot weigh themselves, but they can sense some correlate of the excess fat. It may or may not be fat itself. Conversely, it is conceivable that fatty acid is released into the blood when the animal is in energy deficit and consequently signals the rat to eat. In support of this view, Oomura (1976) found cells in the lateral hypothalamus that fire in response to iontophoretic application of free fatty acids.

Part of the problem in identifying metabolic satiety signals is that carbohydrates, fats, and proteins are all interconvertible through intermediary metabolic pathways. This suggests the control signal may not be any one of them, but rather some overall measure of total fuel utilization. The *thermostatic theory* maintains that energy homeostasis is temperature regulated. There is no doubt food intake can be reduced by sufficient environmental temperature on a summer day, sufficient body temperature as in a fever, or sufficient hypothalamic temperature produced by an implanted thermoprobe. The metabolism of food could also produce an increase in temperature. However, thermoreceptors in the brain with activity that corresponds precisely to feeding patterns have not yet been found. It is possible that the crucial receptors do not fire in proportion to temperature but rather to their own rate of metabolism regardless of the energy source, be it carbohydrates, fat or protein. In this case energy flux would be the signal (Booth *et al.*, 1976). In any of these theories the receptors need not be just in the hypothalamus or, for that matter, even in the brain. For example, Russek (1970) proposed that glucoreceptors in the liver send their information to the brain via the vagus nerve.

Most recently, a hormone manufactured in the wall of the upper intestine has been implicated. This hormone, *cholecystokinin* (CCK, a peptide hormone) is known to cause gallbladder contraction to aid in digestion of food recently arrived in the gut. Cholecystokinin may be transported to the brain by the blood and act as a satiety signal informing the brain of food in the gut. Cholecystokinin injected intraperitoneally produces satiety even if the vagus nerve is cut (Smith and Gibbs, 1976). It also causes satiety when injected directly into the medial hypothalamus. Moreover, radioactive CCK turns up preferentially accumulated in the hypothalamus as if there were specific CCK binding sites there. Recently, it was found that CCK is present in certain fibers in the brain (Dockray *et al.*, 1978) and may act in a neurotransmitter capacity.

It should be clear now that the body has neural receptors that monitor fuel availability and fuel consumption at all or most stages of the utilization process, from nose to tongue to stomach to intestine to liver to blood to cerebrospinal fluid. Integrated factors, such as heat production and perhaps total energy flux, may also be monitored. All this suggests that the brain must receive many different receptor signals and funnel them onto integrative cells. Presumably such cells would be close together so they could mutually interact. If so, this area would be a "satiety center." Where is it?

3.   OVEREATING FOLLOWING BRAIN DAMAGE.   Most evidence points to the medial hypothalamus as a satiety center. This theory was proposed by Anand and Brobeck (1951) who suggested that it inhibited a lateral hypothalamic "feeding center." This _dual center theory_ has been immensely useful in designing experiments, but it has met with increasing resistance on several grounds. True, medial hypothalamic lesions disinhibit feeding. True, lateral hypothalamic lesions or lesions of both areas cause loss of feeding, but are the effects _specific_, behaviorally, anatomically, or neurochemically? Many researchers think not. Let us look at where the pendulum of opinion started, where it swung, and then try to guess whether it will swing back or just turn into a bygone issue.

Lesions of the ventromedial hypothalamus can cause overeating which leads to obesity. Lesioned rats may even double their weight. This phenomenon is called hypothalamic hyperphagia. However, that is a misnomer because the lesions do not necessarily cause overeating. It depends on the rat's starting weight. If the animal was forced to gain weight before the lesion was made, it will not overeat afterward. Rats lesioned at a normal weight rapidly gain weight and then stabilize at a new and obese plateau. If subsequently force-fed or starved, they will undereat or overeat to bring their weight back to this plateau. In other words, lesioned rats regulate their weight like a normal animal, but at a higher level. It is as if more weight is necessary to provide enough of the long-term satiety signal to activate what is left of the damaged medial hypothalamus or some other structure (Hoebel and Teitelbaum, 1966).

Many factors may be involved in this phenomenon. In addition to altering sensitivity to internal satiety signals, metabolic functioning, and endocrine balance, the lesions also alter sensitivity to external stimuli. Rats often become hyperresponsive to tastes. This was originally called "finickiness" and, like a gourmand, they overeat palatable food and undereat unpalatable foods. On a diet of free tasty food, they become especially fat. Given food with bitter quinine added, they spurn it even more than a normal rat would. Recently, this phenomenon has come to be called "_sensory enhancement_," and is demonstrated clearly in rats with a medial hypothalamic lesion on just one side of the brain. These rats do not become fat, but they do prefer to eat tasty food presented to the contralateral side of their face. Apparently contralateral sensory fields are enhanced by the lesion.

Schacter, a social psychologist, suggests that obese rats with sensory enhancement may provide a model to help us understand obese people (Schacter and Rodin, 1974). His group found that Columbia University students who were 15% or more overweight were hyperresponsive to food-related stimuli. They overate crackers during a flavor-ranking task, and tended to eat when the experimenter's clock said lunchtime regardless of the real time. We can be reasonably sure that body weight correlates with sensory reactivity, but we cannot be sure of a causal relationship, nor do we have any independent definition of a person's natural weight level. Weight is generally held constant, barring any sudden brain damage, but weight level depends on genetic factors, the composition and diet palatability. Insurance companies refer to an "ideal weight range" defined in terms of longevity, not neuroscience considerations. People live the longest if they die weighing what they weighed in their 20's. By this definition, in the industrialized nations a large portion of people over 30 years old are already overweight.

In rats the tendency toward obesity can be produced in many ways. In addition to electrolytic (direct current) lesions and electrothermal (radio frequency current) lesions, obesity has also been produced by knife cuts along the lateral and dorsal borders of the medial hypothalamus, local cooling or local procaine anesthetization of the medial hypothalamus, and in mice, by destruction of the medial hypothalamus with intraperitoneally administered gold thioglucose. The gold thioglucose is preferentially concentrated in this brain region if insulin is available to transport it into hypothalamic cells. The gold, which is very toxic, then kills the glucose-concentrating cells in the medial hypothalamus, and the mouse becomes obese. This is a *functionally* produced lesion.

The biggest problem with this series of experiments is that the effect of medial hypothalamic damage is often not specific to feeding, and researchers have reported hyperactivity, hypoactivity, emotionality, rage, and general hyperreactivity. Cats, in particular, show aggressiveness, and one woman with a hypothalamic tumor had outbursts of violence that could only be stopped by excessive feeding. Small, localized lesions in rats tend to produce fewer side effects. Some lesions cause hyperphagia without finickiness, but this technique clearly cannot produce as selective a lesion as one would like.

D. Hypothalamic Injection of Neurochemicals

Recent work has attempted to identify those neurochemical factors that mediate feeding and satiety. Grossman (1969) discovered that norepinephrine injected into the hypothalamus through an implanted cannula caused feeding. This effect has been localized in the midline areas of the hypothalamus. Lebowitz

(1972) has localized the satiety effect in the lateral hypothalamus. Neurotransmitters with β-adrenergic potency, such as epinephrine, or β-adrenergic drugs, such as isoproterenol, inhibit feeding in this region (see Chapter 5 for discussion on β receptors). Amphetamine injected into the lateral hypothalamus also inhibits feeding. Perhaps these β-adrenergic-type synapses inhibit part of the lateral hypothalamic feeding system we described earlier. There is some evidence that there may be two types of satiety systems, but the details are still unresolved (see Margules, 1970).

One way to test the effects of norepinephrine or epinephrine on feeding behavior is to deplete the amount of them in the brain. As described in Chapter 6, fluorescent histochemical mapping of monoamine pathways showed that noradrenergic neurons extend from their several cell body nuclei in the brain stem to the forebrain in two main bundles (Ungerstedt, 1971). Both bundles of nerve fibers travel in the lateral regions of the hypothalamus; one of them, the ventral bundle, has many terminations in various parts of the hypothalamus as well as the rest of the limbic system. The dorsal bundle projects to higher reaches of the brain, the hippocampus and cortex.

Local injection of the drug *6-hydroxydopamine* into the ventral and dorsal bundles selectively poisons adrenergic and noradrenergic neurons. This treatment causes a marked loss of noradrenergic and adrenergic fluorescence in the hypothalamus and elsewhere. Total forebrain norepinephrine drops to less than 10% of normal. The 6-hydroxydopamine injected into the dorsal bundle eliminates fluorescence in the cortical regions, but not the hypothalamus.

The behavioral result when the ventral bundle was depleted was hyperphagia leading to mild obesity. This new means of producing obesity is interesting because it was additive with the obesity of classical medial hypothalamic lesions. This finding suggests that the hyperphagia resulting from depletion of the ventral bundles is of a different origin. Moreover, the depleted rats have not yet proved to be finicky, and they only overate at night (Alhskog *et al.*, 1975). These findings with 6-hydroxydopamine have yet to be confirmed, and some authors question whether the hyperphagia is due to norepinephrine depletion or to nonspecific damage at the injection site. Another difference led to a new finding. It was well known that medial hypothalamic lesions do not block the appetite-killing properties of amphetamine. However, adrenergic depletion does do this. 6-Hydroxydopamine treatment also potentiated the action of fenfluramine, which is a different appetite suppressant. Fenfluramine is serotonergic. Perhaps serotonin also plays some role in satiety. If so, serotonin depletion should cause yet another form of hyperphagia. Serotonin depletion with various drugs [*p*-chlorophenylalanine (PCPA) or 5,7-dihydroxytryptamine (5,7-DHT)] injected into the ventricles produces hyperphagia. As with medial hypothalamic lesions, the female rats displayed marked obesity; they overate both day and night. Thus, it appears that serotonin depletion or some other unknown depletion caused by PCPA causes yet another form of hyperphagia. The various effects of the agents discussed above are summarized in Table 13-1.

In summary, electrolytic lesions proved to be too gross for a fine analysis of satiety functions. Knife cuts are helping to discern the route of satiety pathways in and out of the region (Sclafani *et al.*, 1975; Gold, 1973). Neurochemical injections have the advantage that they are selective, but they suffer from the criticism that the treated regions may not ever receive these chemicals under normal circumstances. Neurochemical depletions at least eliminate endogenous stores. Perhaps some obese animals lack a proper balance of these neurochemical systems. Unfortunately, whole forebrain depletion of some neurochemical may be almost as gross as the old lesion procedure. At least a lesion totally eliminates terminals and their postsynaptic receptors in a given area. Of course, lesions also damage countless fibers of passage. A depletion almost totally eliminates terminals of the given system, but it does so all over the brain, and the receptor cells are left to become supersensitive and eventually reinnervated. Perhaps in the future we will be able to combine the best of both; localized, selective total depletion of specific fields with marked changes in satiety as a result.

Future research is also sure to focus on the recently discovered role of the vagus nerves and its input from the liver and other gut organs. Vagotomy somehow blocks hyperphagia and obesity after ventromedial hypothalamus (VMH) lesions (Powley and Opsahl, 1976).

E. Starvation Following Brain Damage

It has been known for many years that lesions of the lateral hypothalamus result in a marked suppression of feeding behavior. Once the phenomenon of starvation after lateral hypothalmic (LH) lesions had been described, investigation

Table 13-1 Summary of the effects of various agents on feeding behavior

Agent	Injection site	Effect
Norepinephrine	Hypothalamus	Causes feeding
β-Adrenergic agonists (e.g. epinephrine, isoproterenol)	Hypothalamus, particularly lateral areas	Causes satiety
6-Hydroxydopamine	Ventral midbrain	Hyperphagia leading to mild obesity
p-Chlorophenylalanine	Ventricles	Hyperphagia leading to marked obesity

began in detail with the description of the *"LH syndrome,"* a series of stages that a rat goes through in the process of recovering the ability to eat and drink in response to homeostatic requirements (Teitelbaum, 1971; Epstein, 1971). Stage 1 consists of no eating (*aphagia*) and no drinking (*adipsia*). Often the rat must be force fed or it will die. Stage 2 is undereating (anorexia) and adipsia. The rat eats wet palatable food without regulation. In stage 3 the rat eats dry food if hydrated or given sweet liquids to drink. Stage 4 was originally called the "recovery stage" because the animal could regulate its body weight on dry food and plain water; however, recently, it was found that the rats were still not drinking normally under the stress of experimentally induced thirst, nor eating normally under the stress of a potentially lethal drop in blood sugar level following insulin injection.

In several ways the advancement of our knowledge of the LH syndrome has paralleled the medial hypothalamic story. The phenomenon was discovered, then carefully described in behavioral terms, a weight regulation shift was demonstrated, a role for ascending monoamines was reported, incoming sensory nerves were shown to play important roles, and overall changes in reactivity to stimuli were emphasized.

The weight regulation shift in this case is downward instead of upward (Boyle and Keesey, 1975). A rat that is starved before a small LH lesion is made may eat immediately after the lesion and lose no more weight. Thus, in a rat lesioned at normal weight, aphagia functions to lower weight to a new balance point. That is to say, a rat with LH lesions acts as if normal weight were overweight. Apparently bilateral LH lesions upset the balance between feeding and satiety systems such that the animal loses weight until the systems are back in balance, assuming this can be accomplished without starving to death (Fig. 13-14). What neural systems are damaged by LH lesions? We know only a very incomplete answer. One of them is the ascending projections of the trigeminal complex which bring in information from the oral region. Damage to the trigeminal nerve before it enters the brain produces many of the same symptoms as an LH lesion (Zeigler, 1975). Another system involved is identified by its neurotransmitter, dopamine. The dopamine path from the substantia nigra in the midbrain passes through the LH on its way to the striatum. Ungerstedt (1971) found that depletion of dopamine by 6-hydroxydopamine injected into the pathway or into the ventricles caused the LH syndrome.

This is the same dopaminergic system involved in Parkinson's disease in humans. People with this disease can sometimes be cured with L-dopa treatment to replete the lacking neurotransmitter. In fact, there is a similarity between dopamine-deficient people and dopamine-depleted rats (Striker and Zigmond, 1976). Both have great difficulty initiating movement under normal circumstances, but both can fly into action in a severe emergency. In a fire, the human patient will leap from a wheelchair and manage to run outside before collapsing

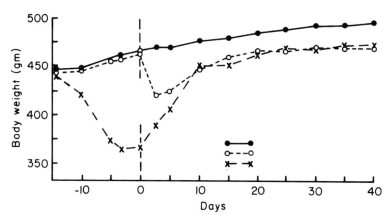

Fig. 13-14. Body weight in rats with LH lesions as a function of lesion parameters and weight at the time of lesioning. Control animals feed *ad libitum* and not lesioned (●) maintain a relatively constant weight. One group of rats (○) was allowed to eat *ad libitum* and was then given a lesion. This group showed a time of aphagia after the lesion which resulted in a reduction in their weight and when they started eating again they had adjusted to a new set point. Another group (×) was starved until the time of lesion and therefore had a marked decrease in weight prior to the lesion. Animals in this group were force-fed immediately after the lesion and ate until they reached the same weight as the *ad libitum* group. Both groups never reached the weight of normal unlesioned rats. Rats with LH lesions act as if normal weight is overweight. (Modified from Keesey *et al.*, 1976, *in* "Hunger: Basic Mechanisms and Clinical Implications." Copyright 1976 by Raven Press, New York.)

again. A dopamine-depleted rat that does not ordinarily walk well and cannot swim in a tank of water, will swim, leap and run from a tank of hot water. Therefore, according to this theory, a major part of the LH syndrome is an inability to react appropriately to normal mild homeostatic stress. It may take a stronger stimulus or a more prolonged stimulus to get a dopamine-depleted animal organized for action.

As a result of such studies, it is generally agreed that the LH is not a unique brain site for producing the starvation phenomenon. It is seldom called a feeding "center" anymore. And yet the LH is still the best locus to obtain adrenergic feeding inhibition with cannulated drugs. Therefore, there must be some synapses there that inhibit part of an LH feeding system. The LH is more than a region of passing nerve fibers and may yet prove to be an area of integration.

F.   Electrical Stimulation-Induced Feeding

Feeding can be initiated by electrical stimulation of the LH through implanted electrodes. Ravenous feeding has been elicited in numerous species of laboratory animals. This behavior was initially called stimulus-bound feeding, but it was changed to stimulation-bound feeding and is now referred to as stimulation-elicited or -induced feeding. *Stimulation-induced feeding* was first seen in cats by the Nobel Prize winner W. R. Hess (1957) and his colleague M. Brugger in the 1940's. Animals will start to eat within moments after the current is turned on and stop when the current goes off (Fig. 13-15). Hess believed that specific behavioral functions are located in circumscribed regions of the limbic system, but with overlapping and intermingling of fiber systems. In the opposum, stimulation can clearly induce fractions of a complete behavioral pattern (Roberts, 1969). Recently, Valenstein (1973) and his colleagues pointed out that an electrode which induced feeding could also induce drinking or some other behaviors just as well. The size and exact location of the electrode, the prior experience of the animal, the calmness of the animal, and the testing environment all seem to make a big difference in the behavior that emerges.

The most amazing thing is that any sensible, recognizable behavior emerges at all. The brain must somehow channel the artificial excitation into a normal behavior pattern, while at the same time inhibiting competing behaviors. Of course, that is similar to real life, but to obtain it with a gross stimulation electrode was revolutionary.

The feeding behavior induced by hypothalamic stimulation is under normal external physiological and pharmacological controls. It is potentiated by sweet tastes and diminished by bitter tastes. Food in the stomach or an anorexic drug inhibits induced feeding more than induced drinking; whereas water in the stomach inhibits induced drinking (Hoebel, 1974). Stimulation-induced feeding and drinking are both blocked by dopamine blockers, such as spiroperiodol, indicating that they probably depend, at least in part, on activation of the nigrostriatal dopamine pathway. Thus there are nonspecific activation components that involve many behaviors, but when the behavior observed is feeding it is under appropriate homeostatic control.

As one could predict, stimulation of the medial hypothalamus inhibits feeding. Stimulation of this region is quite noxious to a rat and might disrupt any behavior, but true inhibition was demonstrated in goats when they ate at the rebound, or offgo, of medial stimulation. Stimulation resulted in inhibited feedings followed by a rebound disinhibition when the current was turned off (Wyrwicka and Dobrezecka, 1960; Wyrwicka, 1976). As always we are not quite sure how much the specificity of this effect depended on situational factors. Medial hypothalamic stimulation might have inhibited and then disinhibited other behaviors too if they had been tested. In rats, dorsolateral hippocampal stimulation produces rebound feeding, but not drinking, demonstrating a degree of specificity.

This matter of inducing behaviors of questionable specificity is very curious. In humans an injection of adrenaline causes a feeling of arousal and will lead to

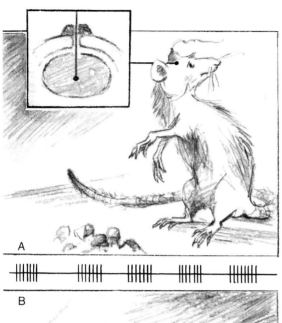

A

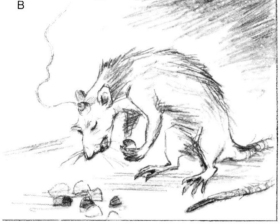

B

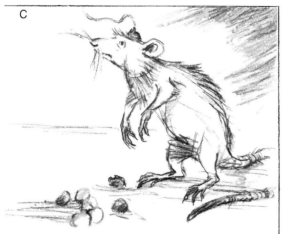

C

STIMULATION-INDUCED FEEDING

Fig. 13-15. Ravenous feeding is induced when the lateral hypothalamus is stimulated. An electrode is placed in the lateral hypothalamus (inset) and anchored to the skull so the animal can be stimulated in the awake state by a train of pulses (A). The rat starts eating when the current is turned on (B) and stops eating when it is turned off (C).

SELF-STIMULATION

Fig. 13-16 (facing page). The rewards of self-stimulation are related to the natural rewards of eating. Neural processes are rewarding when the energy balance is low, as in a thin, hungry rat, so animals repeatedly self-stimulate (A). However, when the energy balance is high, self-stimulation at the same electrode placement decreases and can even become aversive. An overweight well-fed rat, for example, will lever press just to terminate hypothalamic stimulation. This behavior, called stimulation escape behavior, is shown in (B). The stimulus is on constantly and the rat will lever press to obtain time out from the stimulus. Self-stimulation experiments dramatically illustrate that the brain controls the animal's willingness to eat by shifting between reward and aversion. The animal gets rewarded for eating when it needs energy and is punished when there is an energy surplus.

reports that the injection increased happiness in subjects that are in the presence of a euphoric companion and reports of disgruntlement if they share the room with a grouch (Schacter and Singer, 1962). Rats aroused by mild, steady tail pinch will eat in the presence of food, copulate in the presence of a mate, carry objects, chew, or whatever (Rowland and Antelman, 1976). Whatever they do, it is done under appropriate control. For example, appetite suppressant drugs inhibit the feeding that is induced by tail pinch. As another example of nonspecific, or environmentally determined behavior, rats given a bite-size food pellet once every minute will engage in "adjunctive" behavior right afterward. They will drink more water than they need, chew on shavings, or generally do whatever consummatory behavior is available.

Nonspecific arousal or the nonspecific priming of reinforcement processes clearly plays an important role in motivated behavior. The dopamine nigrostriatal system is clearly one link in this system. Not only do dopamine-depleted rats require stronger stimuli to motivate them, it is also known that dopamine blockers prevent lateral hypothalamic stimulation-induced feeding and drinking. The dopamine (DA) system seems roughly analogous to the setting of the idling mechanism in a car. The lower it is set, the harder one must step on the accelerator to set the car in motion. Set too high, the car moves out in response to the slightest input or wanders aimlessly. If we assume for the sake of argument that a lateral hypothalamic electrode taps into a DA system that activates motivated behavior, the next question is, "does it also tap into a system that can steer behavior?"

There are two basic ways to steer consummatory behavior. One is to home in on a food stimulus as a fly does. The other is to reinforce arbitrary acts, like a bar press, that are far removed from the actual sensory signal, but which are instrumental in obtaining it. This is the difference between literally "following one's nose" to reach food and learning an instrumental task by imitating a teacher or by response shaping. Unlike fly behavior, rat behavior is easily shaped. A rat can

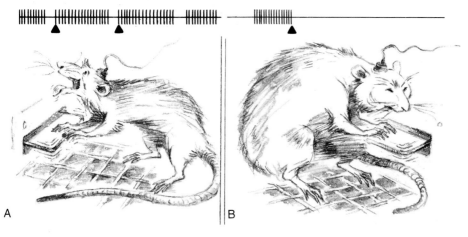

A   B

learn an arbitrary response such as pressing a bar for food in just a few minutes if the teacher is clever. Of course, the rat must be food deprived and then rewarded for approaching and pressing the bar. With extensive training the animal can learn to respond 100 times just to get one pellet. We can presume that somewhere in that rat's CNS there exists a "reward process" which becomes associated with bar pressing. If one could electrically stimulate that reward process it should be possible to train an animal to do anything.

SELF-STIMULATION.   Olds (1962) reported that electrodes implanted in certain regions of the brain can reward virtually any behavior, from pressing a bar to crossing an electrified grid. Thus the animals work to stimulate themselves. _Self-stimulation_ has been demonstrated in fish, rats, cats, dogs, monkeys, and humans. Although carefully controlled studies are lacking in humans, people variously report pleasure, relaxation, or sexual inclination. Most areas of the limbic system support self-stimulation. A rat will self-stimulate the lateral hypothalamus by pressing for a 0.5 second train of stimulation 3000 times an hour for hour after hour (Fig. 13-16). If the response requirements are made simple enough, a rat with its entire brain surgically removed above the thalamus will still self-stimulate.

What is the nature of this potent reward? Olds found that rats self-stimulated faster at some electrode locations when they were food-deprived and at other electrodes when given androgen injections. These relations have been studied extensively in the hypothalamus. Lateral hypothalamic self-stimulation not only increases during food deprivation, it also increases if the rat tastes sugar. On the other hand, it decreases after stomach distension, force feeding, forced weight gain, or small appetite suppressant doses of insulin (Hoebel, 1974).

In the male rat, posterior hypothalamic self-stimulation is sometimes accompanied by emission of sperm in the absence of a female. The male's rate of hypothalamic stimulation decreases after castration and is restored by androgen replacement injections.

In some cases, castration and androgen had this effect on posterior hypothalamic self-stimulation but not lateral hypothalamic self-stimulation in the same rat. Conversely phenylpropanolamine, a common appetite suppressant drug, suppressed lateral hypothalamic self-stimulation but not posterior hypothalamic self-stimulation in the same rat. This has lead to a theory that the rewards of hypothalamic self-stimulation are related to natural rewards.

If this view is correct it means that one can tap into the neural processes that translate _homeostatic_ signals into behavioral action. This is the neural process that rewards feeding behavior when energy balance is low. On the other hand, when energy balance is high, then food-related signals are not rewarding, perhaps even aversive. Accordingly, it has been found that LH stimulation becomes aversive under these conditions. It is known that animals will press a lever to terminate hypothalamic stimulation. Even a self-stimulation electrode generates some aversion as measured by responses to obtain time-out from free, automatic stimulation. Rats will press about twice per minute to turn off continuous LH stimulation for 0.5 second. Clearly the stimulation is much more rewarding than aversive. Medial electrodes, however, tend to be more aversive than rewarding. The interesting finding from the point of view of homeostatic behavior is that not only did LH self-stimulation decrease after force feeding or obesity, but stimulation escape at the same electrode increased. This increase in escape occurred in spite of postmeal lethargy. Therefore the shift from self-stimulation toward stimulation escape—from reward toward aversion—seems to represent a change in the CNS mechanism controlling the reinforcement of feeding behavior. There is a shift from reward to aversion when the animal becomes very satiated.

It seems paradoxical that a rat will self-stimulate for the same LH stimulation which elicits feeding. There are several explanations. It may be that self-stimulation is like sham eating with an esophageal fistula. There are appetite-whetting cues to initiate the behavior and no postingestional cues to stop it. Not until the rats get full or fat does sham eating or LH self-stimulation become aversive. It is also possible that the LH stimulation elicits eating through activation that is not entirely the same as deprivation-induced hunger. A separation of the activation or "drive" inducing property of hypothalamic stimulation and the reward property has been accomplished by Gallistel (1973). Rats given free stimulation at the start of a runway for several minutes then display extra running speed to get to a lever for self-stimulation. This long lasting aftereffect is called _priming_. It is clear that one reason rats self-stimulate so vigorously is that each bout of stimulation both rewards them and also primes them to work for more. Any self-stimulation electrode will prime any other. The reward aspect, however, is more specific; when rats were given a choice they tended to prefer one self-stimulation electrode when thirsty and another when hungry.

Another question which often arises is how do we know that the stimulation is really rewarding in the sense of being pleasurable, and do we know that stimulation escape really means the neural activity is aversive or punishing? Anthropomorphism (attributing our own feelings to animals) is a very risky and often misleading practice. Strictly speaking, reward and aversion should denote nothing than their operational definitions in terms of bar presses to turn current on and off. Aversion has also been demonstrated by the strictest criterion, avoidance. A rat will learn to press a lever when a signal comes on and thereby avoid having to take a long 30 second train of LH stimulation. On the other hand, our own subjective feelings of reward and aversion must have something to do with brain self-stimulation and stimulation escape. People with chronic electrodes have reported pleasure and displeasure during stimulation of various sites. Unfortunately no one has ever had occasion to test the same site in humans before and after a big meal, for example, to see if a reward–aversion shift occurs.

Such a shift does occur in normal people who rate the taste of sucrose before and after a meal. The taste changed from "pleasant" to "unpleasant" (Cabanac, 1971). Perhaps brain stimulation at some sites has to do with what we call pleasure and displeasure. Monkeys laugh or scream depending on the location of the electrode during brain stimulation. Dogs wag their tails while self-stimulating. Rats must have their feelings too. A fly?

When people report pleasure, seek pleasure and avoid displeasure, it is called hedonism. When hedonism is geared to maintaining the person's energy balance, it is "homeostatic hedonism," or alliesthesia (allies=changed; esthesia=sensation). The essential idea is that the pleasure derived from stimuli is controlled by internal signals that relate to physiological balance. We saw the process in the behavior of the fly. We measured it in the CNS through self-stimulation and stimulation escape in the rat. We know it subjectively in the human. Someday we will know how the brain does it. It is already possible to record in the monkey brain from single cells that fire only when the monkey is given a preferred food, and the rate of firing is a function of the monkey's homeostatic need for food (Rolls, 1975).

IV. Summary

Drinking and feeding are motivated behaviors that are essential for the maintenance of metabolism. The essential feature of motivated behavior is its goal-directedness or selectivity: The behavior continues until certain conditions are satisfied. When body fluids are low we become thirsty and drink. When we have not eaten for some time we become hungry and we eat. Recent research on drinking and feeding has attempted to determine the physiological conditions and neuronal mechanisms responsible for the initiation, maintenance, and termination of these two types of motivated behavior.

Drinking is initiated by changes in blood salinity as well as blood volume and pressure produced by lowering of body fluids. We drink to maintain body water balance. Blood salinity appears to be sensed by receptors in the lateral preoptic area of the hypothalamus that respond to changes in cellular osmotic pressure. When blood salinity increases, these osmoreceptors activate brain processes that produce thirst and drinking. Drinking is also induced by changes in blood volume and pressure caused by loss of body fluids. When this occurs, renin is released from the kidneys and is converted to angiotensin II. This hormone acts on brain receptors to initiate drinking. Drinking is terminated when the fluid intake resulting from drinking rehydrates the cells (by reducing fluid salinity) and provides appropriate oral and gastric stimulation.

Feeding is also initiated by internal receptors. In the fly the process is relatively simple. Receptors on the fly's feet and proboscis are sensitive to salt, sugar and water. When food is encountered, the fly eats until the sensory receptors become adapted or until satiation is signaled by receptors activated by stomach distension. If the nerve from the stomach to the brain is cut the fly may continue eating until it bursts. Feeding is also determined by the fly's internal state. The acceptability of a substance depends upon whether the fly is satiated or deprived. Thus, the fly has a sliding threshold (or set point) for palatability which adjusts the fly's intake of certain types of foods. In mammals, the factors initiating and maintaining feeding are more complex. Taste, smell, temperature and texture are all involved and contribute toward developing "a taste preference" or conversely "a taste aversion." The effect of taste alone, however, is not critical for a taste preference. Animals display a taste preference even if taste receptors in the mouth are bypassed by an esophageal fistula. Moreover, rats regulate their intake without reference to taste, since rats fed directly through stomach fistula can regulate the amount of food intake. The regulatory factors are complex and there are many of them. In the brain, there are glucoreceptors in the hypothalamus which respond to glucose and insulin. These receptors monitor the ventricular fluid composition (glucose, hormone, etc.) which reflects the blood composition. The gut hormone cholecystokinin, for example, may affect feeding in this way. The ventral medial hypothalamus is conceived of as the satiety center. Lesions of the ventral medial hypothalamus cause overeating and obesity, underscoring the critical role of the area in feeding behavior. A lesion of this brain area upsets the metabolic and endocrine balance and the overall homeostasis of the animal. Animals with such lesions cannot stop eating. Overeating can also be produced by injecting 6-hydroxydopamine into the ventral noradrenergic bundle in the hypothalamus. Thus the reduction of hypothalamic norepinephrine may be involved in producing hyperphagia.

Lesions of the lateral hypothalamus cause undereating or hypophagia. After lateral hypothalamic lesions animals will acquire a new lower set point. The animals behave as though they think they are eating normally even though they are taking in an inadequate food supply. The basis of the lesion effect is not as yet understood. The effect might be due to interruption of dopamine pathways which pass through the lateral hypothalamus. This view is supported by evidence that impaired eating can also be produced by injecting 6-hydroxydopamine into the dopamine pathway.

Feeding can also be influenced by direct electrical stimulation of the brain. Direct electrical stimulation in the lateral hypothalamus causes eating which then stops when the current is off. This is called "stimulus-bound feeding." Animals can also be induced to self-stimulate, that is, to perform responses that will produce electrical stimulation of brain regions. However, the effect of the stimulation—whether rewarding or punishing—depends on the animal's internal state. If the animal is hungry the stimulation is usually rewarding, but if the animal is satiated, stimulation can be aversive.

Feeding or drinking is controlled by complex processes which are initiated by external and internal stimulation and which vary with our internal states. Thus external stimuli, and the state of the animal are both factors controlling feeding and drinking. Once the behavior is initiated, feeding and drinking involve enormously complex responses. We use the visual, auditory and motor systems to perceive and guide us to the food. We use previous memories for taste, skills in its preparation, and acts of dexterity in the process of eating. We stop when satiety centers signal that the internal state is adequate. In the experimental study of hunger and thirst we see the start of an exciting frontier—the integrative study of many aspects of complex behaviors that are essential to the maintenance of life.

Key Terms

Adipsia: No drinking.

Angiotensin: A peptide which is a powerful drinking stimulus. A blood plasma protein (angiotensinogen) is converted by renin to angiotensin I, a decapeptide. Angiotensin I, in turn, is converted to an octapeptide (angiotensin II), the most powerful drinking stimulus known. Angiotensin II acts on the brain to promote drinking.

Anorexia: Undereating.

Bait shyness: A learned taste aversion. An animal that samples a novel food and is made sick via some stimulus (X-irradiation, drugs, etc.) refuses to eat more of the food thereafter.

Cellular dehydration: Loss of water from cells.

Cellular thirst mechanism: A thirst mechanism in which the dehydration of certain brain cells produces thirst.

Cholecystokinin (CCK): A peptide hormone which aids in the digestion of food. In the body it appears to be produced in the intestines; it also appears to exist or be produced in nerve fibers in the brain.

Dietary obesity: Obesity caused by excessive eating of highly palatable foods. The overconsumption of these preferred foods leads to obesity.

Dual center theory: A theory which proposes that the medial hypothalamus acts as a "satiety center" and is inhibited by the lateral hypothalamus, a "feeding center."

Esophageal fistula: An experimental arrangement whereby a tubular bypass is placed in the throat which prevents food or drink from entering the stomach.

Extracellular thirst mechanism: A thirst mechanism stimulated by a reduction in extracellular volume.

Glucoreceptors: Receptors for glucose. They appear to be in the medial region of the hypothalamus as well as elsewhere in the body (e.g., liver).

Glucose utilization theory: A theory which states that, when blood glucose levels fall outside a certain level, glucoreceptors in the hypothalamus regulate feeding so as to restore the levels to normal. There tend to be dual, reciprocally related systems: Cells in the medial hypothalamus tend to increase their firing; those in the lateral hypothalamus tend to decrease their firing.

Homeostatic behavior: Actions (behaviors) that an animal exerts in order to maintain internal stability.

Hyperphagia: Overeating. Aphagia is the absence of eating.

Hypertonic: A solution more concentrated than physiological (isotonic) salt solutions.

Hypotonic: A solution less concentrated than a physiological salt solution.

Hypovolemia: A reduction of extracellular volume, particularly intravascular volume. It causes thirst and drinking.

Insulin: A polypeptide necessary for efficient transport of glucose across cell membranes.

Lateral hypothalamus: An area of the hypothalamus. Lesions of it block learning of taste aversions and produce the LH syndrome; electrical stimulation of it initiates feeding. It appears to be a critical integrative center for feeding. The lateral hypothalamus will support self-stimulation. Thus it appears to be related to internal reward circuitry.

Lateral hypothalamic syndrome (the LH syndrome): A series of stages a rat goes through in the process of recovering the ability to eat and drink in response to homeostatic requirements after lateral hypothalamic lesions. No eating or drinking is followed by selective undereating of hydrated foods and no drinking. This is followed by some eating and drinking (hydrated foods or sweet liquids) and finally, nearly complete recovery.

Lipostatic hypothesis: A hypothesis which states that there are satiety receptors which monitor fat availability.

Medial hypothalamus: An area of the hypothalamus. Lesions of it affect salt preference; it appears to be the primary location of satiety glucoreceptors. Electrical stimulation in the medial hypothalamus can inhibit feeding. According to the dual center theory the medial hypothalamus is an important integrative center for satiety.

Medicine preference effect: An ill animal that tastes a novel food and improves in health, later displays a learned preference for that taste. The medicine preference effect contrasts to bait shyness.

Osmoreceptor hypothesis of drinking: A hypothesis that when brain osmoreceptors detect an osmotic imbalance in brain fluids, they activate other brain systems which promote drinking behavior.

Osmoreceptors: Receptors in the brain which detect imbalances in the osmotic pressure of brain fluids.

Osmotic pressure: The relative tendency of dissolved substances to diffuse or move to regions of lower concentration.

Preference-aversion function: A plot of intake versus concentration of a taste which produces an inverted U-shaped curve.

Primary drinking: Drinking due to the actual loss of body fluids; it is promoted by the sensation of thirst.

Priming: A term used in the context of experiments on self-stimulation to emphasize the "drive" aspect of self-stimulation. Self-stimulation, at certain locations, primes animals to work for more stimulation in addition to rewarding them.

Renin: A proteolytic enzyme which is released from the kidneys due to manipulations influencing extracellular fluids; renin converts angiotensinogen to angiotensin II.

Secondary drinking: Drinking when the animal has a positive fluid balance; it is promoted by factors other than thirst.

Self-stimulation: Electrical stimulation of the brain which is controlled by the subjects. Most areas of the limbic system support self-stimulation. The consequences of self-stimulation depend, in part, on the state of the animal. Stimulation of the hypothalamus is more rewarding if the energy balance is low and more aversive if the energy balance is high.

Sensory enhancement: In feeding, a hyperresponsiveness to tastes. Animals which display sensory enhancement overeat palatable food and undereat unpalatable foods.

6-Hydroxydopamine: A toxic chemical which destroys adrenergic and noradrenergic neurons.

Stimulation-elicited (or induced) feeding: Feeding initiated by electrical stimulation of the brain, e.g., the lateral hypothalamus.

Thermostatic theory: A theory which maintains that total food intake and utilization (energy homeostasis) is temperature regulated.

General References

Epstein, A. N. (1971). The lateral hypothalamic syndrome: Its implications for the physiological psychology of hunger and thirst. *Prog. Physiol. Psychol.* **4**, 263–318.

Fitzsimons, J. T. (1972). Thirst. *Physiol. Rev.* **52**, 468–561.

Hoebel, B. G. (1971). Feeding: Neural control of intake. *Annu. Rev. Physiol.* **33**, 533–568.

Mogenson, G. J. (1976). Neural mechanisms of hunger: Current status and future prospects. *In* "Hunger: Basic Mechanisms and Clinical Implications" (D. Novin, W. Wyrwicka, and G. Bray, eds.) pp. 89–102. Raven, New York.

Myers, R. D. (1974). "Handbook of Drug and Chemical Stimulation of the Brain." Van Nostrand-Reinhold, New York.

Novin, D., Wyrwicka, W., and Bray, G. A., eds. (1976). "Hunger: Basic Mechanisms and Clinical Implications." Raven, New York.

Schacter, S. and Rodin, J. (1974). "Obese Humans and Rats." Erlbaum/Halsted Inc., Washington, D.C.

Teitelbaum, P. (1971). The encephalization of hunger. *Prog. Physiol. Psychol.* **4**, 263–318.

Wayner, M. J., and Oomura, Y., eds. (1975). "Central Neural Control of Eating and Obesity." Ankho International Inc., Phoenix, New York.

References

Adolph, E. F., Barker, J. P., and Hoy, P. A. (1954). Multiple factors in thirst. *Am. J. Physiol.* **178**, 538–562.

Ahlskog, J. E., Randall, P. K., and Hoebel, B. G. (1975). Hypothalamic hyperphagia: Dissociation from hyperphagia following destruction of noradrenergic neurons. *Science* **190**, 399–401.

Anand, B. K., and Brobeck, J. R. (1951). Hypothalamic control of food intake in rats and cats. *Yale J. Biol. Med.* **24**, 123–140.

Andersson, B. (1971). Thirst and brain control of water balance. *Am. Sci.* **59**, 408–415.

Blass, E. M. (1973). Cellular-dehydration thirst: Physiological, neurological, and behavioral correlates. *In* "The Neuropsychology of Thirst: New Findings and Advances in Concepts" (A. N. Epstein, H. R. Kissileff, and E. Stellar, eds.), pp. 37–72. Holt, New York.

Blass, E. M., and Epstein, A. N. (1971). A lateral preoptic osmosensitive zone for thirst in the rat. *J. Comp. Physiol. Psychol.* **76**, 378–394.

Blass, E. M., and Hall, W. G. (1976). Drinking termination: Interactions among hydrational, orogastric, and behavioral controls in rats. *Psychol. Rev.* **83**, 356–374.

Booth, D. A., Toates, F. M., and Platt, S. V. (1976). Control system for hunger and its implications in animals, and man. *In* Hunger: Basic Mechanisms and Clinical Implications" (D. Novin, W. Wyricka, and G. Bray, eds.), pp. 127–143. Raven, New York.

Borror, D. (1971). "An Introduction to the Study of Insects," 3rd ed. Holt, New York.

Boyle, P. C., and Keesey, R. E. (1975). Chronically reduced body weight in rats sustaining lesions of the lateral hypothalamus and maintained on palatable diets and drinking solutions. *J. Comp. Physiol. Psychol.* **88**, 218–223.

Buggy, J., Fisher, A. E., Hoffman, W. E., Johnson, A. K., and Phillips, M. (1975). Ventricular obstruction: Effect on drinking induced by intracranial injection of angiotensin. *Science* **190**, 72–74.

Cabanac, M. (1971). The physiological role of pleasure. *Science* **173**, 1103–1107.

Dethier, V. G. (1967a). Feeding and drinking behavior of invertebrates. *In* "Handbook of Physiology" (C. F. Code, ed.), Am. Physiol. Soc., Washington, D.C. Sect. 6, Vol. 1, pp. 79–96.

Dethier, V. G. (1967b). The hungry fly. *Psychol. Today* **1**, 64–72.

Dethier, V. G. (1968). Chemo-sensory input and taste discrimination in the blowfly. *Science* **161**, 389–391.

Dethier, V. G. (1976). "The Hungry Fly: A Physiological Study of the Behavior Associated with Feeding." Harvard Univ. Press, Cambridge, Massachusetts.

Dockray, G. J., Gregory, R. A., and Hutchison, J. B. (1978). Isolation, structure and biological activity of two cholecystokinin octapeptides from sheep brain. *Nature (London)* **274**, 711–713.

Epstein, A. N. (1967). Oropharyngeal factors in feeding and drinking. *In* "Handbook of Physiology" (C. F. Code, ed.), Sect. 6, Vol. I, pp. 197–218. Williams & Wilkins, Baltimore, Maryland.

Epstein, A. N. (1971). The lateral hypothalamic syndrome: Its implications for the physiological psychology of hunger and thirst. *Prog. Physiol. Psychol.* **4**, 263–318.

Epstein, A. N., and Teitelbaum, P. (1962). Regulation of food intake in the absence of taste, smell and other oropharyngeal sensations. *J. Comp. Physiol. Psychol.* **55**, 753–759.

Fitzsimons, J. T. (1961). Drinking by rats depleted of body fluid without increase in osmotic pressure. *J. Physiol. (London)* **159**, 297–309.

Fitzsimons, J. T. (1963). The effects of slow infusions of hypertonic solutions on drinking and drinking thresholds in rats. *J. Physiol. (London)* **167**, 344–354.

Gallistel, C. R. (1973). Self-stimulation: The neurophysiology of reward and motivation. *In* "The Physiological Basis of Memory" (J. A. Deutsch, ed.), pp. 175–267. Academic Press, New York.

Garcia, J., Hankins, W. G., and Rusiniak, K. W. (1974). Behavioral regulation of the milieu interne in man and rat. *Science* **185**, 824–831.

Gelperin, A. (1966). Investigations of a foregut receptor essential to taste threshold regulation in the blowfly. *J. Insect Physiol.* **12**, 829–841.

Gilman, A. (1937). The relation between blood osmotic pressure, fluid distribution, and voluntary water intake. *Am. J. Physiol.* **120**, 323–328

Gold, R. M. (1973). Hypothalamic obesity following knife cuts that minimize arterial damage. *Physiol. Behav.* **10**, 403–406.

Grossman, S. P. (1969). A neuropharmacological analysis of hypothalamic and extrahypothalamic mechanisms concerned with the regulation of food and water intake. *Ann. N.Y. Acad. Sci.* **157**, Artic. 2, 902–917.

Hall, W. G. (1973). A remote stomach clamp to evaluate oral and gastric controls of drinking in the rat. *Physiol. Behav.* **11**, 897–901.

Hess, W. R. (1957). "Functional Organization of the Diencephalon." Grune & Stratton, New York.

Hoebel, B. G. (1974). Brain reward and aversion systems in the control of feeding and sexual behavior. *In* "Nebraska Symposium on Motivation" (J. K. Cole and T. B. Sonderegger, eds.), pp. 49–112. Univ. of Nebraska Press, Lincoln.

Hoebel, B. G., and Teitelbaum, P. (1966). Weight regulation in normal and hypothalamic hyperphagic rats. *J. Comp. Physiol. Psychol.* **61**, 189–193.

Jordan, H. A. (1969). Voluntary intragastric feeding: Oral and gastric contributions to food intake and hunger in man. *J. Comp. Physiol. Psychol.* **68**, 498–506.

Keesey, R. E., Boyle, P. C., Kenmitz, J. W., and Mitchel, J. S. (1976). The role of the lateral hypothalamus in determining the body weight set point. *In* "Hunger: Basic Mechanisms and Clinical Implications" (D. Novin, W. Wyrwicka, and G. Bray, eds.), pp. 243–255. Raven, New York.

Kissileff, H. R. (1973). Nonhomeostatic controls of drinking. *In* "The Neuropsychology of Thirst: New Findings and Advances in Concepts" (A. N. Epstein, H. R. Kissileff, and E. Stellar, eds.), pp. 163–198. Holt, New York.

Lebowitz, S. F. (1972). Central adrenergic receptors and the regulation of hunger and thirst. *In* "Neurotransmitters," (Assoc. Res. Nerv. Ment. Dis., eds.) pp. 327–358. Williams & Wilkins, Baltimore, Maryland.

LeMagnen, J. (1976). Interactions of glucostatic and lipostatic mechanisms in the regulatory control of feeding. *In* "Hunger: Basic Mechanisms and Clinical Implications" (D. Novin, W. Wyrwicka, and G. Bray, eds.), pp. 89–101. Raven, New York.

McHugh, P. R., Moran, T. H., and Barton, G. N. (1975). Satiety; a graded behavioral phenomenon regulating caloric intake. *Science* **190**, 167–169.

Margules, D. L. (1970). Alpha adrenergic receptors in hypothalamus for the suppression of feeding behavior by satiety. *J. Comp. Physiol. Psychol.* **73**, 1–12.

Mook, D. G. (1963). Oral and postingestional determinants of the intake of various solutions in rats with esophageal fistulas. *J. Comp. Physiol. Psychol.* **56**, 645–659.

Novin, D. (1962). The relation between electrical conductivity of brain tissue and thirst in the rat. *J. Comp. Physiol. Psychol.* **55**, 145–154.

Olds, J. (1962). Hypothalamic substrates of reward. *Physiol. Rev.* **42**, 554–604.

Oomura, Y. (1976). Significance of glucose insulin and free fatty acid on the hypothalamic feeding and satiety neurons. *In* "Hunger: Basic Mechanisms and Clinical Implications" (D. Novin, W. Wyrwicka, and G. Bray, eds.), pp. 145–157. Raven, New York.

Peck, J. W., and Novin, D. (1971). Evidence that osmoreceptors mediating drinking in rabbits are in the lateral preoptic area. *J. Comp. Physiol. Psychol.* **74**, 134–147.

Powley, T. L., and Opsahl, C. A. (1976). Autonomic components of the hypothalamic feeding syndromes, *In* "Hunger Basic Mechanisms and Clinical Implications" (D. Novin, W. Wyrwicka & G. Bray, eds.), pp. 313–326. Raven, New York.

Richter, C. P., Holt, L. E., Jr., Barelace, B., Jr., and Hawkes, C. D. (1938). Changes in fat, carbohydrate and protein appetite in Vitamin B deficiency, *Am. J. Physiol.* **124**, 596–602.

Roberts, W. W. (1969). Are hypothalamic motivational mechanisms functionally and anatomically specific? *Brain Behav. Evol.* **2**, 317–342.

Rolls, E. T. (1975). "The Brain and Reward." Pergamon, Oxford.

Roth, S. R., Schwartz, M., and Teitelbaum, P. (1973). Failure of recovered lateral hypothalamic rats to learn specific food aversions. *J. Comp. Physiol. Psychol.* **83**, 184–197.

Rowland, N. E., and Antelman, S. M. (1976). Stress-induced hyperphagia and obesity in rats: a possible model for understanding human obesity. *Science* **191**, 310–312.

Rozin, P. (1967). Thiamine specific hunger. *In* "Handbook of Physiology" (C. F. Code, ed.), Sect. 6, Vol. I, pp. 411–431. Williams & Wilkins, Baltimore, Maryland.

Russek, M. (1970). Demonstration of the influence of an hepatic glucosensitive mechanism on food-intake. *Physiol. Behav.* **1**, 1205–1209.

Schacter, S., and Rodin, J. (1974). "Obese Humans and Rats." Erlbaum/Halsted Inc., Washington, D.C.

Schacter, S., and Singer, J. E. (1962). Cognitive, social and physiological determinants of emotional states. *Psychol. Rev.* **69**, 379–399.

Schwartz, M., and Teitelbaum, P. (1974). Dissociation between learning and remembering in rats with lesions in the lateral hypothalamus. *J. Comp. Physiol. Psychol.* **87**, 384–398.

Sclafani, A. (1976). Appetite and hunger in experimental obesity syndrome. *In* "Hunger: Basic Mechanisms and Clinical Implications" (D. Novin, W. Wyrwicka, and G. Bray, eds.), pp. 281–296. Raven, New York.

Sclafani, A., Berner, C. N., and Maul, G. (1975). Multiple knife cuts between the medial and lateral hypothalamus in the rat: A reevaluation of hypothalamic feeding circuitry. *J. Comp. Physiol. Psychol.* **88**, 210–217.

Smith, G. P., and Gibbs, J. (1976). Cholecystokinin and satiety: Theoretic and therapeutic implications. *In* "Hunger: Basic Mechanisms and Clinical Implications" (D. Novin, W. Wyrwicka, and G. Bray, eds.), pp. 349–355. Raven, New York.

Simpson, J. B., and Routtenberg, A. (1973). Subfornical organ: Site of drinking elicitation by angiotensin II. *Science* **181**, 1172–1174.

Stricker, E. M. (1966). Extracellular fluid volume and thirst. *Am. J. Physiol.* **211**, 232–238.

Stricker, E. M. (1968). Some physiological and motivational properties of the hypovolemic stimulus for thirst. *Physiol. Behav.* **3**, 379–385.

Stricker, E. M. (1969). Osmoregulation and volume regulation in rats: Inhibition of hypovolemic thirst by water. *Am. J. Physiol.* **217**, 98–105.

Stricker, E. M., and Zigmond, M. J. (1976). Recovery of function after damage to central catecholamine-containing neurons: A neurochemical model for the lateral hypothalamic syndrome. *Prog. Physiol. Psychol.* **6**, 121–187.

Stricker, E. M., Brodshaw, W. G., and McDonald, R. N., Jr. (1976). The reninoangiotensin system and thirst: A reevaluation. *Science* **194**, 1169–1171.

Teitelbaum, P. (1971). The encephalization of hunger. *Prog. Phsyiol. Psychol.* **4**, 263–318.

Thompson, R. F. (1975). "Introduction to Physiological Psychology." Harper, New York.

Ungerstedt, U. (1971). Stereotaxic mapping of the monoamine pathways in the rat brain. *Acta Physiol. Scand., Suppl.* **367,** 1–48.

Valenstein, E. S. (1973). "Brain Control: A Critical Examination of Brain Stimulation and Psychosurgery," pp. 1–48. Wiley, New York.

Wayner, M. J., and Oomura, Y., eds. (1975). "Central Neural Control of Eating and Obesity." Ankho International Inc., Phoenix, New York.

Woods, S. C., and Porte, D., Jr. (1976). Insulin and the set-point regulation of body weight. *In* "Hunger: Basic Mechanisms and Clinical Implications" (D. Novin, W. Wyrwicka, and G. Bray, eds.), pp. 273–280. Raven, New York.

World Book–Childcraft International, Inc. (1978). "The World Book Encyclopedia" Vol. 7. Field Enterprises Educational Corp., Chicago, Illinois.

Wyrwicka, W. (1976). The problem of motivation in feeding behavior. *In* "Hunger: Basic Mechanisms and Clinical Implications" (D. Novin, W. Wyrwicka, and G. Bray, eds.), pp. 203–213. Raven, New York.

Wyrwicka, W., and Dobrezecka, C. (1960). Relationship between feeding and satiation centers of the hypothalamus. *Science* **132,** 805– 806.

Ziegler, H. P. (1975). Oral satisfaction and obesity: The sensual feel of food. *Psychol. Today* **9,** 62–76.

14

Sleep and Activity Rhythms

We are asleep during one-third of our lifetimes. If we assume the Biblical lifetime of three score and ten, we can expect to sleep a total of 23 years! If time spent in an activity is used as a criterion of importance, then sleep is certainly highly important. Why is it that for every 2 hours of activity, 1 hour of sleep is extracted

(Kleitman, 1957)? The question, "Why do we sleep?" actually involves several issues. First in what way is sleep adaptive? Clearly, a sleeping animal is unable to fight or flee from predators. A sleeping person is useless. What physiological function is served by sleep? A common hypothesis is that sleep is restorative. According to this general view (Claparede, 1908; Coriat, 1912) waking activity either depletes some essential substance or causes an increase in some substance, and the function of sleep is to resupply the needed substance or eliminate the substance produced by the waking state. This view is popular in part because it fits well with our feelings about sleep. We feel fatigued and "need to sleep." After sleeping we feel "restored." The basis of fatigue and restoration is as yet not known. The simple view that sleep overcomes oxygen deficits (Wöhlisch, 1956) resulting from wakefulness is unsupported by evidence. Rate of cerebral oxygen consumption is similar during sleep and waking (Mangold et al., 1955).

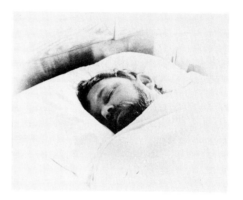

A second question concerns the mechanisms underlying sleep. Theories of sleep must explain why we go to sleep, why we remain asleep, why we awaken, and why the sleep–waking cycle is repeated every 24 hours. Historically, interest in sleep has been guided by biological concepts and technical concepts available at particular historical periods. The first recorded theory of sleep onset was proposed by a contemporary of Pythagoras in ancient Greece who suggested that sleep results from a retreat of blood away from the brain into the veins. This view of sleep was a forerunner of many theories attributing sleep to cerebral anemia.

A third question concerns the role of sleep as an influence on other processes. Sleep is accompanied by the release of hormones. Sleep affects learning and memory. These findings raise the question as to whether sleep plays a critical role in the regulation of bodily functions other than those directly involved in sleep and activity. We will consider evidence bearing on each of these questions.

In this chapter we summarize recent findings concerning the nature and neurobiological bases of sleep. Current research focuses on the comparative

14. SLEEP AND ACTIVITY RHYTHMS

analysis and ontogenetic development of sleep, the neural substrates of sleep and clinical abnormalities of sleep.

I. Electrophysiological Correlates of Sleep Stages

Major advances in understanding sleep have resulted from technical progress in neurophysiology. The development of techniques for measuring physiological events has provided means of characterizing the complex aspects of the states of sleep and waking activity.

The most important of these advances in technology was the development of *electroencephalography* which provided researchers with objective bioelectric correlates of changes in the states of consciousness. Later, the recording methods were extended by using a polygraph to include measures of eye movement, muscle tone, and somatic-visceral activity (Fig. 14-1). These developments led to the description of objectively defined states of wakefulness and sleep and prepared the way for the present intensive scientific assault upon the puzzle of sleep.

While the state of sleep is usually contrasted with wakefulness, it is important to note that the states of wakefulness and sleep are two ends of a continuum of level of alertness and *arousal*. At one end of the arousal continuum are states of high alertness, such as those that occur when we watch an exciting sports event or read a chilling mystery novel. Arousal may be based on sustained involvement,

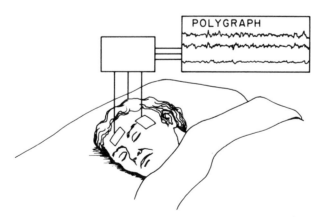

Fig. 14-1 Recording of bioelectric activity in a normal adult during sleep. Electrodes are attached to the subject's scalp for recording brain activity and to the skin at the corners of the eye to record eye movement. Leads are connected to a polygraph in another room. As the subject sleeps his brain waves and eye movements are recorded by pens of the instrument. In some experiments muscle tone, heart rate, and respiration are monitored in a similar way by polygraphic techniques.

such as that required by playing a game of chess. Arousal can, as we all know, also be elicited by a change in stimulation, such as seeing a flashing red light in a rearview mirror. States of alertness change with time, boredom, or fatigue into relaxed wakefulness, drowsiness, and states of sleep. As one goes to sleep, eye movements cease, body movements and muscle tone diminish, and there is a stabilization of many visceral functions, such as heart rate and respiration, to low but steady rates.

The pattern of electrical activity recorded from the brain changes rather dramatically with different stages of arousal and sleep. The beginning of sleep (Fig. 14-2) is associated with a shift from the waking alert pattern of low voltage, fast electroencephalographic (EEG) activity, often accompanied by rhythmic 8–12 Hz waves in the parietal–occipital region (*alpha waves*) to one of rhythmic 12–15 Hz bursts (*sigma rhythm* or sleep spindles) and eventually high voltage slow (2–4 Hz) waves. There are two quite different patterns of physiological organization that occur during sleep. Initially the EEG waves contain only spindled slow

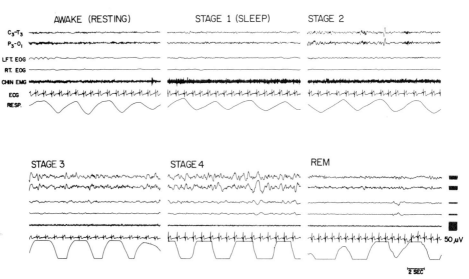

Fig. 14-2. Characteristic polygraphic patterns showing resting wakefulness and the stages of sleep in a normal adult. The sleep process proceeds from relaxed waking through four stages of quiet or slow-wave sleep, followed by an abrupt reversal and the emergence into the active or REM state pattern. During quiet sleep stages 2 and 4 are the most significant. This sleep cycle usually requires 90 minutes and is repeated four to six times throughout the night. Subsequent awakenings, if they occur, are brief, and stages 3 and 4 are replaced progressively by extended periods of stage 2 during quiet sleep. Note that stage 2 is characterized by bursts of rhythmic activity, called sleep spindles, which are diminished during stage 3 and obscured in stage 4 by the occurrence of large, continuous slow waves. Note also the similarity between stage 1 and REM sleep patterns. C_3-T_3, left central cortex; p_3-o_1, left parietal–occipital cortex; EOG, electrooculogram (eye movements); EMG, electromyogram; ECG, electrocardiogram; Resp., respiration. (From Sterman, 1972.)

14. SLEEP AND ACTIVITY RHYTHMS

waves. After about 1 hour of sleep a dramatic change occurs in the pattern of sleep. Heart rate and respiration increase (Snyder *et al.*, 1964), and the EEG appears to be almost like that recorded during wakefulness (Dement and Kleitman, 1957). We shall refer to this stage of sleep as *active sleep* (AS). This phase of sleep is accompanied by an almost complete relaxation of skeletal muscles and rapid eye movements (REM). Thus the state is often referred to as REM sleep. Because of the paradoxical occurrence of an awakelike EEG pattern in an obviously sleeping individual, this state of sleep is sometimes referred to as paradoxical sleep. Early research suggested a close association between this kind of sleep and dreaming. Individuals awakened during an active sleep episode often reported that they had been dreaming.

Although dream reports may be most rich and vivid if elicited during active sleep, it is now clear that mental activity during sleep is not limited merely to this particular stage of sleep. We now believe that the physiological organization that underlies the cyclic occurrence of active sleep also modulates emotional processes and memory functions. It is this organization that gives special qualities to the mental activity reported during the REM state (Hernández-Peón and Sterman, 1966). Thus, many researchers describe sleep in terms of its EEG characteristics as *quiet sleep* (QS), including stages 1–4, and active sleep (AS, or REM). In a normal night's sleep, these patterns alternate every 1 or 2 hours and form a QS–AS cycle that averages about 90 minutes in length in adults. This sort of sleep pattern can be seen in Fig. 14-3.

The obvious facts that arousal can be induced by stimulation and that drowsiness and sleep result when there is little change in stimulation clearly indicate that states of arousal are influenced by our sensory environment. However, variations in arousal and sleep states are not completely regulated by sensory events. We all sleep several hours within each 24 hour period, and we all eventually wake up each day even if we are not awakened by an alarm clock. Thus, variations in arousal depend both upon transient events and underlying endogenous cyclical changes. It is well known that arousal is produced by electrical stimulation of the brain, particularly in the brain stem reticular formation (Jouvet, 1967). Findings such as this suggest that aroused sleep might be regulated in part by reticular formation activity. It may well be, however, that the processes involved in transient alterations in arousal are different from those involved in the endogenous regulation of cyclical sleep–waking states.

II. Species Differences in Sleep

Polygraphic studies of sleep have been carried out in a wide variety of animals (Allison and van Twyver, 1970), and, with the exception of the very primitive

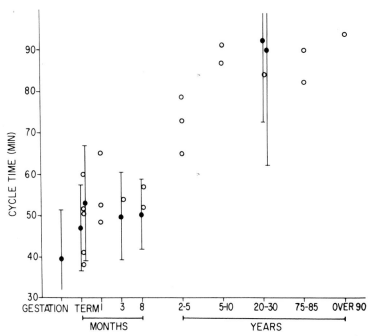

Fig. 14-3. Survey of the development of the human rest–activity, or REM state, cycle during ontogeny. Closed circles indicate reliable sample means for which adequate sample size and statistical description were available in the articles reviewed. Bars indicate standard deviation of these means. Open circles represent mean values derived from other data presented or merely stated without further statistical information. Collectively, these data indicate a slight trend toward lengthening of the cycle from the prenatal sample to 8 months of age. A clearly significant increase in cycle duration is evident by 20–30 years of age, which appears to be sustained into senescence. The precise period during which this shift occurs cannot be determined here, but the data suggest a transition between 2 and 10 years of age. (From Sterman, 1972.)

monotremes, all mammals show essentially similar physiological patterns of sleep, with alternating quiet sleep and active sleep activity. Cycles of sleep and waking are either *circadian* (about 24 hours, as in man) or *ultradian* (less than 24 hours, or polycyclic, as in rodents and carnivores). Species differ in the total amount of sleep during a 24 hour period. Opposums and bats sleep about 80% of the time, rats and cats about 60%, chimpanzees about 45%, donkeys and cows about 15% (Webb, 1973). Most primates are awake during the day and have one period of sleep during the night. Animals such as rats have 12 to 15 cycles of sleep and waking during a 24 hour period. During sleep the QS–AS cycle which is also ultradian, varies systematically with phylogeny, from approximately 12 minutes in rats and 20 minutes in cats, for example, to 60 minutes in nonhuman primates and 90 minutes in man. In most mammals studied, active sleep accounts for approximately 5–35% of total sleep time (Rojas-Ramírez and Drucker-Colín, 1977) (see

14. SLEEP AND ACTIVITY RHYTHMS

Table 14-1 Comparative percentages of total waking (W), slow wave sleep (SWS) and rapid eye movement (REM) sleep in some mammals[a]

| Subject | States | | |
	W	SWS	REM
Cat	42.3	42.2	15.5
Cow	82.6	15.8	1.6
Opossum	19.2	57.5	23.3
Echidna	64.2	35.9	0
Squirrel monkey	17.0	59.3	22.9
Man	60.6–76.3	16.6–28.5	6.6–10.6

[a] From Rojas-Ramírez and Drucker-Colín (1977).

Table 14-1). Of all mammals, only the echidna shows no active sleep phase in sleep (Allison *et al.*, 1972).

Species differences in sleep patterns are related to a number of physiological and ecological factors. Over a wide range of species, the amount of slow wave sleep (or QS) is inversely related to body weight. Amount of active sleep is inversely related to the degree to which the species must cope with predatory danger. Species vulnerable to predators tend to have little active sleep (Allison and Circhetti, 1976). This finding is not surprising, since animals are minimally responsive to external stimuli during active sleep. What is not clear is why animals subject to predators have any active sleep at all. Active sleep must serve some important function. The fact that large animals tend to sleep little is understandable, since the larger animals studied (elephant, cow, horse, donkey) must spend large amounts of time foraging for food.

Both active sleep and quiet sleep have also been demonstrated in birds, although the active sleep phase is very brief, and the longest duration of active sleep only reaches the very shortest values seen in mammals. Reptiles seem to show quiet sleep, but the presence of active sleep is still being debated, and conflicting evidence has been reported so far. Although amphibians and fish do appear to sleep (Tanber, 1974), more work needs to be done before we can draw any firm conclusions about the nature of various states of sleep in these animals. Generally more primitive animals show a rest–activity cycle that is similar to a QS–AS pattern in sleep (Kleitman, 1963).

Patterns of sleep change during development (Sterman, 1972). In animals that are mature at birth, such as the guinea pig, adultlike sleep periods are seen early. In slower developing animals, however, such as the cat and humans, the newborn period consists of undifferentiated quiet or stable periods, alternating with active sleep periods and interrupted by brief waking periods associated with feeding or discomfort. The primary features of postnatal development of sleep behavior in humans include: (a) the prolongation of waking periods as social behaviors begin to emerge, (b) the progressive shift to a circadian sleep–wake cycle, with sleep increasingly concentrated during the night, and (c) the appearance of EEG spindle and slow wave patterns characteristic of mature quiet sleep. Much of this development is complete by 3 or 4 months of age. The ultradian QS–AS cycle during this early period approximates 60 minutes, while the mature 90 minute cycle is firmly established only in early adulthood (see Fig. 14-3).

III. Neural Structures Affecting Sleep

These comparative and developmental observations provide clues which, taken together with many neurophysiological findings, constitute the basis for present theories of the neural substrates of sleep. Studies in cats have established that the lower brain stem (pons and medulla) is essential for the occurrence of active sleep (Jouvet, 1967). Animals with all brain tissues removed above the level of the pons show remarkably intact active sleep characteristics. The finding that higher brain areas are not necessary for active sleep is consistent with the idea that the REM pattern may represent a primitive state of arousal.

Localized lesions in the pons can eliminate the motor behavior during REM. This phenomenon is similar to a human sleep disorder called noctural myoclonas, or the *"restless-leg" syndrome*. Such involuntary movements often produce insomnia. It appears that the disorder may be caused by impairment of the brain stem mechanism that inhibits muscle tone during periods of active sleep. Treatment of this condition with antispasmodic or anticonvulsant drugs has been partially successful.

The localization of neural mechanisms associated with active sleep in the caudal brain stem has stimulated a neurophysiological search for the primary triggering substrate of this state. The earliest electrophysiological sign of impending active sleep is the appearance of *pontogeniculo-occipital* (PGO) waves in the EEG record. The PGO waves are spontaneous, intermittent high voltage sharp peaks that are seen more or less simultaneously in the pontine tegmentum, the lateral geniculate body, and in the occipital cortex (with transcortical electrodes). The PGO waves characteristically appear at these sites during the last few minutes of quiet sleep and continue into active sleep. Both electrophysiological studies (single neuron recordings) and neurochemical studies (histofluorescence and other transmitter labeling procedures) have exploited this phenomenon in an effort to identify the pontine structures involved in this phasic response, and also to map their central pathways. Attention in this regard has focused upon monoaminergic pathways involving norepinephrine or serotonin (Jouvet, 1974).

While one school of thought has attributed the organization of both active sleep and quiet sleep to monoaminergic neurons in the brain stem and their projections, other evidence suggests that the origin of quiet sleep is to be found in structures in the forebrain. Transection of the neuroaxis, separating caudal brainstem from forebrain, leaves the sleep–waking cycle intact in the forebrain, as indicated by both physiological and behavioral (ocular) indices, and the active sleep cycle intact in the brain stem. However, with time, these two cycles become totally dissociated (Villablanca, 1966; Sterman and Hoppenbrouwers, 1971). Stimulation and lesion studies in the cat and other mammals, as well as reports stemming from tumor pathology in humans, have focused the attention of many investigators on the possibility that a forebrain system may be involved in sleep. This system is believed to integrate both central and peripheral information and to initiate the appropriate physiological and behavioral adjustments leading to sleep onset.

IV. Chemical Substrates of Sleep

Since the beginning of this century, investigators have attempted to determine whether sleep is regulated by endogenous chemical substances. As early as 1913 Pieron and his associates found that cerebrospinal fluid (CSF) extracted from dogs deprived of sleep induced drowsiness and sleep in dogs that were not deprived of sleep. It seemed that toxins accumulated in the CSF during waking have sleep-inducing effects and that the toxins are eliminated during sleep. While similar effects were obtained in a few experiments conducted over the next several decades (Schnedorf and Ivy, 1939; Kroll, 1933), it is only in recent years that hormonal "sleep factors" have been the subject of intensive study.

What would happen to an awake animal if it was interconnected to another via the circulatory system? Would the awake animal be put to sleep by circulating factors? Monnier and his colleagues (1963) connected the jugular veins of two rabbits and then induced sleep in one of the rabbits by electrically stimulating a region of the thalamus (mediocentral intralaminary thalamus) with low frequencies (6 per second). The nonstimulated animal also went to sleep! These results suggested that some substance released into the blood of the stimulated animal was responsible for inducing sleep in the recipient animal. Subsequently, these investigators demonstrated that substances in the dialysate of cerebral venous blood taken from a sleeping rabbit induced sleep in awake rabbits (Monnier and Hatt, 1971). Recent analyses indicate that the dialysate contains a sleep-inducing substance consisting of a low molecular weight polypeptide containing at least seven amino acids.

In other recent experiments sleep has been induced in cats and rats by injecting cerebrospinal fluid (CSF) obtained from sleep-deprived goats directly into the brain. The sleep-inducing factor was determined to be a low molecular weight substance (Pappenheimer *et al.*, 1967; Fencl *et al.*, 1971). A sleep factor has also been obtained directly from the brains of animals. In several studies, brain perfusates were obtained by means of implanted cannulas using a push–pull technique. In these studies a Ringer's solution (a solution whose composition resembles the extracellular fluids of the brain) was slowly administered via one cannula and a perfusate withdrawn through an adjacent cannula. Simultaneously, EEG activity was recorded in order to determine the animal's sleep state. Perfusates obtained from the mesencephalic reticular formation (MRF) of sleeping cats induce sleep when perfused into the same brain region of awake cats. Opposite effects were obtained when perfusates from an awake donor were administered to sleeping cats (Drucker-Colín, 1972; Rojas-Ramírez, 1974).

Other recent evidence (Drucker-Colín *et al.*, 1975a, 1977) suggests that the content of brain perfusates differs with sleep states. In particular, the amount of protein in perfusates taken from the MRF of cats is greatest during active sleep. Further, the active sleep perfusate contains proteins not present in quiet sleep perfusates (Spanis *et al.*, 1976). These findings are consistent with other evidence suggesting that active sleep may involve protein systhesis. Active sleep is curtailed by antibiotic inhibitors of protein synthesis and active sleep deprivation causes decreases in brain protein synthesis (Bobillier *et al.*, 1974; Pegram *et al.*, 1973).

The role or roles of peptides and proteins in the onset and maintenance of stages of sleep remains to be determined. The low molecular weight factors isolated from CSF appear to influence sleep onset. The protein changes correlated with active sleep might be either consequences of or causes of changes in sleep state.

V. Hormones, Neurotransmitters and Sleep

There is considerable evidence that hormones are released during sleep. Growth hormone is released at the onset of sleep, during the quiet sleep stage (Takahashi *et al.*, 1974). This is particularly interesting in view of evidence that the decrease in active sleep produced by inhibition of protein systhesis is blocked by administration of growth hormone (Drucker-Colín *et al.*, 1975b). Other hormones secreted during sleep include prolactin, which in humans is secreted in increasing amounts throughout the night, and testosterone, which appears to be secreted during active sleep (Sassin, 1977). ACTH secretion is related to the basic circadian rhythm but is not closely related to the sleep–waking cycle. Hypophysectomy does not markedly affect sleep cycles. In general, while sleep is influenced by some changes in hormone levels and some hormones are released during sleep, hormonal factors do not appear to be involved in the normal regulation of the sleep–waking cycle (Jouvet, 1977). The fact that hormones released during sleep seem not to be involved in the control of sleep raises questions concerning the function of such hormonal release. It could be that such effects are merely the consequences of fundamental sleep mechanisms and have no physiological function. It seems more likely that hormones released during sleep are important in regulating other physiological processes. For example, there has been considerable speculation and some evidence suggesting that hormones released during sleep may influence memory by acting on biochemical processes involved in the consolidation of recent memory.

The involvement of neurotransmitters in sleep has been extensively investigated. Most of the research has concerned serotonin (5-HT) and norepinephrine (NE). There is much evidence suggesting that 5-HT is involved in the regulation of quiet sleep (Jouvet, 1977). Sleep is induced by administration of 5-HT or 5-hydroxytryptophan (5-HTP), the precursor of serotonin, directly to the brain. Administration of *p-chlorophenylalanine* (PCPA), which depletes 5-HT by inhibiting tryptophan hydroxylase, produces prolonged wakefulness in many species. Further, the insomnia produced by PCPA is overcome by 5-HTP. However, other recent studies have provided conflicting evidence concerning the role of 5-HTP in sleep. For example, animals given repeated injections of PCPA eventually recover normal sleep cycles even though serotonin levels remain low (Dement *et al.*, 1972). Further, in cats, lesions of the *raphé nuclei* that produce decreased levels of cerebral serotonin do not affect sleep–waking cycles (Jalowiec *et al.*, 1973). Thus it is not yet clear what role, if any, 5-HT plays in the regulation of sleep. Recent findings indicate that during quiet sleep the metabolism of 5-HT increases in the hippocampus and the metabolism of dopamine increases in the striatum and thalamus (Kovačević and Radulovački, 1976).

Early studies indicated that active sleep can be virtually eliminated by bilateral destruction of the nucleus locus coeruleus (Jouvet, 1969), which is the source of cell bodies of NE neurons projecting to the forebrain. However, subsequent studies show that lesions of the NE pathways to the forebrain do not produce consistent changes in sleep. Thus, it is not clear whether NE plays any specific role in the regulation of sleep.

There is some evidence that acetylcholine (ACh) is involved in sleep. In cats, sleep can be induced by microcrystals of ACh implanted in a number of brain regions. The effect is blocked by atropine. However, atropine is known to induce drowsiness and sleep in humans. ACh is released in the cortex during wakefulness and active sleep. Thus ACh may play some role in regulating cortical brain activity. Some studies have suggested that γ-aminobutyric acid (GABA) is involved in sleep. However, the evidence is, at best, conflicting. It is well known that sleep can be induced in many animals by γ-hydroxybutyrate (GHB), a metabolite of GABA. This is of interest because GHB is a constituent of some wines, and it has been speculated that GHB may be responsible for the soporific effect of wine.

The processes involved in regulation of sleep are not yet understood. Sleep can be influenced by numerous experimental treatments including ones influencing hormone release and neurotransmitter functioning. It appears unlikely that any of the hormones and transmitter substances studied so far have a specific role in regulation of sleep aside from their regular roles in regulating neuronal activity generally. Viewed from this perspective it seems likely that while many hormones and transmitters will be involved in the regulation of many aspects of behavior, it is unlikely that a particular hormone or transmitter will be uniquely associated with but one type of behavior.

VI. Sleep Disorders

The expanding physiological study of sleep in man has produced some surprising and important clinical developments (Dement *et al.*, 1975). The list of medical problems associated with sleep complaints, once limited to *narcolepsy*, a disorder characterized by the frequent need for short periods of sleep, and a poorly defined concept of *insomnia*, has today expanded to a long list of ailments and problems, some of which involve serious respiratory, cardiac, and central nervous system consequences. Estimates of the number of people complaining of significant sleep disturbances range from 15 to 50% of the population. People who report sleepiness during the day due to perceived disturbance of sleep at night are usually called *insomniacs*, whereas those who are sleepy during the day but do not associate this with sleep disturbance at night are termed *hypersomniacs*. Basic sleep disorder complaints can be classified into three major categories: (1) *daytime sleepiness* to a degree that impairs function or results in considerable discomfort; (2) night time *"episodes"* which generally cause someone other than the unaware patient to complain, and (3) *secondary* sleep disorders, stemming from problems not directly related to sleep. Complaints of excessive daytime sleepiness by far constitute the largest group in this classification.

In recent years polygraphic monitoring of severe hypersomniacs has disclosed two primary pathophysiological etiologies, occurring separately or together. One is the *narcolepsy–cataplexy syndrome*, involving attacks of generalized motor weakness and paralysis precipitated by strong emotion and excessive sleepiness. These patients often show sleep-onset REM, a configuration limited usually to infants and individuals forced into severe disruptions of normal sleep schedules and suggesting a basic disorder of sleep organization. The second is *upper airway sleep apnea*, a condition characterized by restricted airflow and increased respiratory effort during quiet sleep. This problem may be indicated by severe, episodic snoring, and can lead to serious cardiac damage due to progressively increasing pulmonary pressures during the night.

It is interesting to note that many patients who suffer from upper airway sleep apnea are quite unaware that they are aroused many times each night gasping for breath and complain only of excessive daytime tiredness. This points out an important, although often overlooked, feature of sleep. It seems to produce a kind of retrograde amnesia for events that occur shortly before sleep onset. Although patients that show upper airway sleep apnea are aroused each time, they suffer an oxygen deficit and gasp for breath with a loud snorelike sound; they then fall immediately back to sleep with apparently no recollection of the event. The same is true with other patients that suffer from excessive daytime sleepiness. However, daytime naps are not the worst problem that faces these people. A study of some 80 patients has shown that their greatest problems are related to a very abnormal state of consciousness that has been called *automatic behavior syndrome*.

Guilleminault and Dement (1977) have described the syndrome. First the patient feels drowsy and tries to fight it off by moving about, opening windows, and drinking coffee. Often this drowsiness occurs while driving and the driver will open the car windows and turn up the radio. Following these attempts to stave off drowsiness, the patient becomes less and less aware of his actions and performance deteriorates. Then for several minutes to several hours there is complete amnesia. A clinical report obtained from a taped interview can give us a good idea of the nature of this problem.

Clinical Case (40-Year-Old-Male)

I always needed more sleep than anybody else in the family when I was a child. During my early teens, I had a tendency to fall asleep during the 2:00 class, but it was not a real problem until I went to college. I had some irresistible sleep attacks at that time, particularly in the late morning and between 3 and 4 PM. I struggled through college and terminated with a masters degree in business. I learned to take a very short nap—10 minutes long, as a mean—during my lunch hour and have succeeded in my field. I am now the director of an important sales department.

About five years ago the clinical picture changed. First, I began to experience a sudden feeling of weakness throughout my body when I was surprised or laughing. Nobody really noticed anything but I experienced that feeling more and more frequently. I never fell asleep but about 2 years ago I began to experience a sudden drop of my head and my upper arms when I laughed or was under stress. During the same period I found myself in very embarrassing situations. I would be talking with someone and suddenly would burst out with a very inappropriate sentence. I would see a very surprised look on the faces of my companions but I would not remember what I said. Other times, I would not be able to remember anything about a conversation and when brought back to reality by an insistent question I would not know what the conversation (talk) was about.

Recently, I had two very frightening experiences. I took my car to go back home near 4 PM. I remember driving out and turning on the freeway. Then I had a complete amnesia. I found myself 70 minutes later somewhere in Oakland. I could not figure out where I was. The surroundings were entirely unfamiliar and I was completely lost. I could not and still cannot remember how I got there and what I did for more than an hour. I have no memory whatsoever of any event during that time. A similar episode occurred recently but the amnesic period lasted longer, about 100 minutes, and when I "came back" I was once again lost, with a complete feeling of disorientation. I had total amnesia of what happened during the last hour and a half and a complete loss of the notion of time (Guilleminault and Dement, 1977, p. 444).

Over the last several decades evidence that sleep facilitates memory has been reported, and those findings may have led to the notion that learning while asleep is possible. Much money has been spent by unwary people on expensive equipment that is purported to enable them to learn during sleep. However, there is relatively little solid research evidence that new information is readily learned during sleep. In fact, as we have seen, sleep often causes amnesia for those events that occur just before we go to sleep. This may explain why we usually have no recollection of falling asleep and why those dreams that are best remembered are those that aroused us from sleep.

VII.   Circadian Rhythms

It is an obvious fact of experience that we have recurring patterns of waking and sleeping each day. In addition to sleep and waking we, as well as animals, have many physiological processes that vary in a cyclical manner approximately every 24 hours. Our body temperature, blood sugar level, blood hormone levels and many other physiological states vary cyclically each day. Daily rhythms such as these are termed "circadian" which is from the Latin circa diem or about a day. Research concerned with mechanisms of sleep and waking has focused on factors that influence wakefulness within a 24 hour period. But the broader question of importance must be addressed. What processes regulate recurring patterns of activity? Why do we sleep a portion of each day? Why do we do so even if we do not have access to clocks and if we are not subjected to 24 hour cycles of light and dark? What mechanisms control patterns of biological processes that are so closely linked to a period of 24 hours?

We turn now to a discussion of circadian rhythms. Studies of the control of such time-locked patterns have begun to reveal mechanisms underlying this control and may provide clues to mechanisms of sleep and activity in humans.

Circadian rhythms, along with their related "circa-tidal" and "circa-lunar" rhythms, have characteristics which distinguish them from all other biological oscillations. The most obvious of these is that the rhythms are ordinarily linked with environmental cycles of days or tides. Most other biological rhythms (e.g., spontaneous spike discharge, heartbeat, and even some lifecycles) have no such temporal relationship with external cycles. This link with the environment has led to the almost certainly erroneous assumption that circadian rhythms are a direct response to, and consequence of, cyclical environment changes. For example, we generally sleep sometime after the sun sets and awaken sometime after the sun rises. However, it is clear that circadian rhythms are not directly regulated by light–dark cycles. The cycles are controlled by endogenous mechanisms. The proof that these cycles are due to endogenous timing mechanisms is provided in studies in which the light–dark cycle is eliminated, that is, the subjects are maintained in constant light (LL) or constant darkness (DD). When humans or animals live under such conditions, they maintain activity cycles that approximate 24 hours. Humans living in isolation from light cycles generally have circadian sleep–waking rhythms of a little over 24 hours. Interestingly, the rhythms for other biological processes, such as body temperature, may be slightly different from that of sleep and waking.

The important feature of such rhythms maintained under constant illumination is that they typically continue at periods which differ slightly, but consistently, from 24 hours. This is the strongest evidence that their timing is endogenous, and the result of a response to an underlying physiological "clock." If the rhythms continued at a period of exactly 24 hours it would not be possible to rule out the interpretation that the rhythms are controlled by other environmental features that vary with the earth's rotation, such as magnetic field or cosmic radiation, but under conditions of constant illumination circadian rhythms invariably drift relative to solar time, and it is thus clear that they can be temporally independent of such external controls.

This free-running drift away from solar time is characteristic of all endogenously timed daily rhythms. The term circadian should, strictly speaking, be applied only to free-running rhythms, or rhythms which are maintained under constant conditions. Because of this, the term carries with it a clear implication of endogenous physiological timing. Circadian rhythms have another feature that marks them off from other biological oscillators—they are stable at different temperatures. Unlike nearly all other physiological processes, circadian rhythms are relatively independent of changes in temperature, i.e., they exhibit Q_{10}'s (the rate change for a 10° elevation in temperature) which are typically close to unity. They are thus temperature compensated within normal biological limits.

VIII. Regulation of Circadian Rhythms: Locus of Oscillation

Circadian rhythms are a nearly universal aspect of the behavior of living organisms. Circadian rhythms exist in single cells as well as in organisms. There are currently two major sets of problems in the study of circadian rhythms. The first set concerns the nature of the pacemaker or oscillator that underlies the circadian rhythms that we can measure in many cells. Within this set are questions about the fundamental mechanism of the oscillator, its location within the cell, its genetic control, and its source of energy as well as the way in which the oscillator is influenced by environmental cycles of light and temperature. The second set of problems concerns the organization of the circadian system in complex multicellular organisms. Here we are primarily interested in questions on the nature and basis of coupling within the organism among the multiple circadian rhythmicities as well as the coupling of the whole circadian system with the natural environment. Even in the better known circadian systems, the hierarchy of circadian control mechanisms is far from understood, and the driving, coupling, and feedback relationships among the constituent oscillators can only be guessed at with the current information. It is these better known circadian systems that are the focus of this section.

A. Rhythms in Cells

The unicellular organism, *Acetabularia*, can sustain a clear circadian rhythm of photosynthesis in continuous dim light. Fragments of the cell are also capable of sustaining a circadian rhythm. The nucleus-free "stem" and "cap" was rhythmic for nearly 30 cycles. However, when one makes a classical *Acetabularia* chimera by grafting parts of two cells with rhythms 180° out of phase, the phase of the chimera is directed by the nucleated fragment. Thus, even in a single cell the control of oscillation is complex. Different parts of the same cell are equally capable of autonomous pacemaking activity although the nucleus has some sort of dominance in the system (Schweiger *et al.*, 1964).

B. Circadian Oscillation in Insects

In the cockroach locomotor activity is circadian. Surgical manipulations of the cockroach nervous system have been used to examine the role of the eyes, optic lobes, and midbrain in the locomotor circadian rhythm. The experimental results have clearly shown that the optic lobes are crucial elements in the circadian system and suggested that they might, in fact, be the site of the circadian pacemakers: removal of both lobes produces locomotor arrhythmia, whereas animals remained rhythmic following removal of either lobe alone. More extensive probing of the optic lobes with microelectrodes has shown that lesions in and around the second optic chiasma and lobula, especially those that damage cell bodies in this area, can disrupt the oscillating system that drives the circadian locomotion rhythm. Recent histological work has shown that neurons in one optic lobe send axonal projections directly to the opposite lobe. This pathway provides the anatomical basis for the functional coupling between the circadian pacemakers existing in each optic lobe. Unfortunately, the existing evidence does not allow one to conclude that any particular cell or group of cells in the optic lobe constitutes the circadian clock (Sokolove, 1975; Roth and Sokolove, 1975).

Although it is evident that the optic lobes are necessary for normal circadian timing in the cockroach, the optic lobes are clearly *not* involved in circadian timing in the silkmoth. Thus, while circadian rhythms are biologically important they need not be controlled by the same mechanisms in different species.

The transformation of a caterpillar into a silkmoth culminates with the emergence (*eclosion*) of the "pharate" moth from the old pupal casing. Eclosion occurs after biological development of the adult is completed but only during a particular time of day. This temporal gate is somehow controlled by the insect's circadian clock. Insects that achieve the appropriate developmental stage on a given day after the temporal "gate" has closed must wait for the appropriate time on the following day. Thus, the behavioral event of eclosion is not directly controlled by developmental processes.

The emergence behavior of *Pernyi* moths is very tightly coupled to the eclosion clock. Under regimen of 17 hours of light and 7 hours of dark, this species emerges during the last few hours of light. Stimulation of the moth approximately 10 hours before the opening of the gate does not produce emergence. Even if the pupal cuticle is completely removed, the moth is helpless and shows few adult motor patterns. With the subsequent arrival of the "gate," or appropriate time in the circadian cycle, these peeled moths first perform a pantomine eclosion before assuming the full adult repertoire of behavior. Emergence cannot be prematurely triggered by non-clock-related stimuli. At the prescribed time, the behavior is performed even if environmental conditions make it unnecessary.

It is known that the brain is involved in the gating of eclosion. If the brain of the silkmoth pupae is surgically removed, the brainless moths emerge without regard to time of day or night. However, this effect of brain extirpation can be completely reversed by implanting a brain into the abdomen of animals without brains. These moths with implanted brains showed the proper timing of emergence. Clearly the silkmoth brain has an important role in regulating the circadian timing and performance of the complex behavior acts that occur during emergence.

Under a regime of 17 hours of light and 7 hours of dark, *Cecropia* moths typically emerge during the first 6 hours of the day, with a peak after dawn, and *Pernyi* moths during the last 5 hours of the day; pupae transferred to constant darkness show subsequent emergence peaks at 22 hour intervals. If the brain is removed, the moths emerge randomly. If the brain is replaced, the emergence peaks approximate the above times. If the brain is transferred to debrained moths of the other species, the recipient moth adopts the donor's gate time (Fig. 14-4) but retains its own specific motor patterns. The brain is clearly responsible for the gating of eclosion. However, the detailed pattern of the behavior is coded elsewhere in the nervous system. The activation of the behavioral system by the brain systems must be based on hormones (Truman and Riddiford, 1970).

C. Circadian Oscillation in Birds

The findings of several studies indicate that, in vertebrates, endogenous oscillators that control circadian rhythms are located in the central nervous

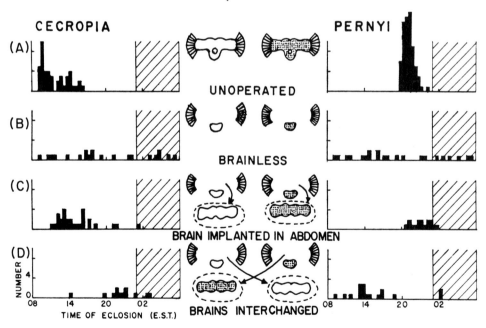

Fig. 14-4. (A) The eclosion of *Hyalophora cecropia* and *Antheraea pernyi* moths in a 17 hours light–7 hours dark (17L:7D) regimen showing the effects of brain removal (B), the transplantation of the brain to the abdomen (C), and the interchange of brains between the two species (D). (From Truman, 1971.)

system. Of particular relevance here are the findings that in birds removal of the pineal abolishes the free-running rhythm of locomotor activity, of body temperature, and of migratory restlessness. Transplantation of pineal explants from donor sparrows to recipient (and previously pinealectomized) sparrows produces transplanted rhythms as well. That is, pinealectomized (and arrhythmic) sparrows that receive a pineal explant from another sparrow will become rhythmic, with the circadian locomotion rhythm starting up at the precise phase (point on the oscillation) where it was just before the pineal was removed from the donor sparrow (Menaker, 1974). Thus, in birds, the pineal gland appears to be the locus of a self-sustained circadian pacemaker. However, there are marked species differences among vertebrates in the role of various neuroanatomical sites as circadian pacemakers (as there were among insects). Pinealectomies in mammals have repeatedly failed to eliminate normal free-running circadian rhythms.

D.   Circadian Oscillation in Mammals

For this reason, researchers have sought the locus of the driving oscillation for the whole system underlying circadian rhythms in mammals in other neuroanatomical areas. The hypothalamus has been studied as a possible locus of a circadian oscillator because of its known involvement in physiological processes that show circadian periodicities, such as endocrine functions, body temperature, drinking and feeding behavior. Also, the direct retinohypothalamic projections needed to account for the role of environmental lighting in the entrainment of these rhythms have been demonstrated. Direct projections from the retina to the _suprachiasmatic nucleus_ (SCN) of the hypothalamus (Fig. 14-5) exist for reporting environmental lighting to this area (Moore, 1974).

There is also direct evidence for the existence of circadian pacemakers in the hypothalamus of mammals. Lesions of the SCN block a variety of rhythms including the estrous cycle, the circadian rhythms in adrenal corticosterone secretion, pituitary ACTH secretion, pineal enzyme rhythms, and drinking behavior and locomotor activity (Stephan and Zucker, 1972; Stetson and Watson-Whitmyre, 1976). The SCN appears to be the locus of the driving oscillation for a number of circadian rhythms. Nevertheless, caution should be exercised in accepting this conclusion. As in the case of the cockroach optic lobes, the SCN of mammals may only be a necessary part of a more distributed pacemaking system. The SCN may not be a "primary" clock but rather a coupled oscillator in a two- or multioscillator system.

Early studies of endocrine involvement in circadian rhythms in mammals were concerned primarily with the localization of the clock within the various endocrine glands or within a cycle of nervous–endocrine–metabolic events.

From a series of experiments on blinded rats, it was concluded that free-running circadian activity rhythms were not impaired by any of the following forms of interference with the endocrine system: gonadectomy, adrenalectomy, hypophysectomy, hyper- and hypothyroidism, and pinealectomy (Richter, 1965). Apparently, the circadian clock driving the activity–rest cycle was not located in any of the glands involved.

The discovery that a rat adrenal gland cultured *in vitro* continues to produce corticosteroids in a circadian rhythmic fashion considerably modified existing views in the field concerning the regulating function of a localized clock (Andrews, 1971). Since at least one organ (and probably more) is capable of self-sustained oscillations, a centralized "clock" or "pacemaker" might serve to synchronize a number of peripheral oscillators rather than impose its rhythm on them. For instance, a circadian pacemaker apparently drives the rhythm of hypothalamic corticotropin releasing factor, which leads to a daily periodicity in adrenocorticotropic hormone (ACTH) production by the anterior pituitary. The self-sustained adrenal rhythm is entrained (synchronized) by the oscillating plasma (ACTH) concentration (Menaker, 1974). Recent findings place additional emphasis on the role of both neural and endocrine processes in the coupling of constituent oscillators of the circadian system of mammals (Moore-Ede, 1974). In

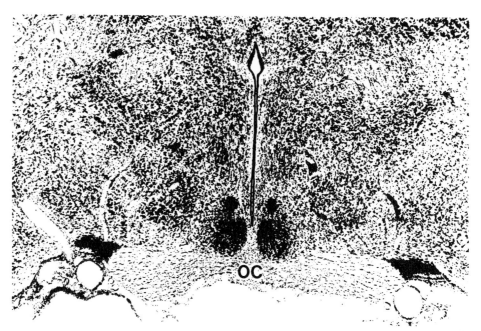

Fig. 14-5. Frontal section through the anterior hypothalamus of a rat showing the location of the suprachiasmatic nuclei with their characteristic closely compacted, small cells lying just above the optic chiasm (OC). (From Moore, 1974.)

adrenalectomized squirrel monkeys, the circadian rhythm in renal potassium excretion is free-running with respect to the environmental light–dark cycle. Furthermore, single pulses of cortisol delivered every 24 hours through intravenous catheters synchronize the potassium excretion rhythm in these adrenalectomized animals. It appears that the adrenals are required to couple this circadian oscillation in kidney function to the SCN pacemaker that receives light via the retinohypothalamic pathway and thus entrains the entire circadian system. The molecular events in the control of hormonal secretion are best understood in the pineal gland (see Chapter 5).

Some important beginning steps have been taken in an effort to understand how circadian rhythms are controlled by endogenous oscillators. In some species the general locus of oscillators in neural tissue has been discovered. However, as yet, little is known about how the oscillators are modulated by environmental events and how they act to synchronize the oscillation of the cells and organs of the body. Understanding the nature of the oscillators and the mechanisms by which they act to control our sleep and activity as well as other circadian rhythms constitutes an important and promising area for research.

IX. The Concept of Motivation

Psychologists have long been interested in a class of behaviors typically called "motivated." We have already discussed certain of these behaviors in previous sections. Motivated behaviors include feeding, drinking, predatory aggression and sexual behavior. Sleep is also similar in many ways. All these behaviors share common properties.

First, motivated behaviors are generally initiated when the animal is in an increased state of arousal; for example, as a result of food deprivation. Second, motivated behaviors share the property that they are directed in time and space to a specific goal-object. Finally, the achievement of the goal, called the consummatory act, typically results in a decrease in the animal's level of arousal, thus ensuring that the particular motivated behavior only occurs at the appropriate time. In general, we can define _motivation_ as a state that directs an organism in certain ways to seek particular goals. The concept of motivation has proved useful to researchers because it helps to explain some aspects of behavior more easily.

Our own experience tells us that when we are hungry, we show strong behavioral patterns that will allow us to find food and eat. In Chapter 13 (Thirst and Hunger) we saw that feeding behaviors depend on internal states, taste, post-ingestional factors as well as a variety of others. We saw that we can "tap" into the neural processes underlying feeding and that there are particular areas in the hypothalamus which, when stimulated, promote feeding behavior. However, we also saw that even with electrical stimulation, the state of the animal is critical. When an animal is satiated, for example, brain stimulation may actually be aversive and very high currents are needed to induce feeding. Thus, the composite internal state of the organism clearly directs the type of behavior—the results of peripheral and central stimulation depend on the overall state of the animal.

Sexual behavior, discussed in Chapter 12, also depends on external and internal conditions. We saw that the hypothalamus secretes releasing factors into the blood which reach the anterior pituitary gland and stimulate it to secrete in the female gonadotropic hormones that act on the ovary. Ovarian hormones are responsible for the estrous cycle and, as we shall see, the sexual characteristics of the animal. Females of certain species, particularly nonprimates, will accept the sexual advances of the male only during limited periods of the estrous cycle. Thus, under the influence of internal changes, the female rat is attracted by stimuli from the male. Contact is made and the female accepts the male, culminating the behavior and beginning reproduction.

Motivation may play a role in behaviors that are not strictly goal-directed, as well. Learning and memory, for example, are behavioral processes clearly dependent, in part, on the state of motivation of the animal. Learning ability may depend markedly on the relevance of that information to obtaining a particular goal, on its overall interest and usefulness, the time of day, the arousal level of the animal, etc. In many learning experiments it is usually the case that such factors are carefully controlled or defined. Animals are usually tested at a certain time of day, and in tasks where food or drink are a reward. The animals are usually deprived for a defined period of time prior to testing. Thus, as we have already mentioned in Chapter 8, complex behavioral processes such as learning and memory clearly depend on the motivational state.

While the concept of motivation has proved useful both at a behavioral and at a systems level of analysis, it has not proved as useful at a mechanistic level. Physiological analysis in search of the neural substrates of motivation have not, as yet, revealed a common process or even a system serving all aspects of motivation, although the limbic system and hypothalamus are generally involved. Aspects of motivated behaviors are critically dependent on the limbic system and nearly all feed in some way through the hypothalamus. However, the detailed pattern of involvements and interactions are complex.

Summary

Recent progress in understanding sleep resulted from development of electrophysiological techniques, such as the EEG and EMG, which provide objective measures of the complex states of sleep and waking activity. Sleep onset is accompanied by a shift in EEG activity from low voltage fast waves to high voltage slow waves. As one goes into the state of quiet sleep (QS) eye movements cease, body movements and muscle tone diminish and heart rate and respiration rates decrease. In a state of sleep occurring an hour or so after onset of quiet sleep, the EEG is like that in the waking state. This state is referred to as paradoxical sleep, REM sleep (because rapid eye movements occur), or active sleep. Dreams often occur during active sleep. There are marked species differences in the proportion of time spent in quiet sleep and active sleep as well as the number of cycles of sleep and activity each day. Over a wide range of species total amount of quiet sleep is inversely relative to body weight, and amount of active sleep is inversely related to degree of predatory danger facing the species. Patterns of sleep change with development. The features of development in humans include prolongation of waking periods and shift to a circadian cycle.

Active sleep appears to be regulated by structures in the lower brain stem. Quiet sleep may be regulated by forebrain systems. Several investigators have reported that sleep is regulated by endogenous chemical substances. Sleep can be induced in awake animals by administering substances obtained from the blood, cerebrospinal fluid, or mesencephalic reticular formation of sleeping animals. Studies of fluids taken from the mesencephalic reticular formation of sleeping cats indicate that samples taken during quiet sleep differ from those of active sleep in amount as well as type of protein. These findings considered together with evidence that active sleep is decreased by protein synthesis inhibitors suggests that protein synthesis is somehow involved in sleep.

A number of hormones, including growth hormone, testosterone and prolactin, are secreted during sleep. Removal of the pituitary does not markedly affect sleep cycles. In general, hormonal factors do not appear to regulate normal sleep patterns. While there is evidence that specific neurotransmitters are involved in regulating sleep, the evidence is conflicting. Sleep is induced by serotonin, and insomnia produced by drugs that inhibit the synthesis of serotonin. However, brain lesions of the raphé nuclei (which reduce cerebral serotonin) do not affect sleep, nor is sleep altered by lesions of norepinephrine pathways in the brain. Acetylcholine appears to be involved in regulating cortical brain activity. There is as yet no clear evidence for a role of γ-aminobutyric acid (GABA) in sleep and activity.

Disorders of sleep are commonly reported. The most common problems are excessive daytime sleepiness and insomnia. More severe disorders include the narcolepsy–cataplexy syndrome which consists of attacks of excessive sleepiness and sleep apnea which consists of restricted air flow and increased respiratory effort during quiet sleep.

Sleeping and waking are examples of circadian rhythms. Circadian rhythms are biological rhythms with a cycle of approximately 24 hours. Under conditions of constant illumination the rhythms "free-run" in 24-hour cycles. Thus, the rhythms are controlled by endogenous oscillators. Circadian rhythms are found in the biological activity of single cells as well as even fragments of cells. Thus, overall rhythms of organisms must be coordinated. In the cockroach, circadian locomotor rhythms are abolished by removal of the optic lobes. In moths, circadian rhythms appear to be controlled by brain hormones. In birds, circadian rhythms are controlled by the pineal gland. In mammals, a circadian oscillator appears to be located in the suprachiasmatic nucleus of the hypothalamus. Circadian activity rhythms in rats appear not to be controlled by hormones—at least hormones studied to date. However, hormones may play some role in synchronizing the oscillations of different organ systems.

In the past chapters we have discussed several behaviors which are typically called motivated. These include feeding, drinking, predatory agression, sexual behavior and, in some ways, sleep. Motivated behaviors are directed toward the fulfillment of particular goals. Motivated behaviors are often undertaken when an animal is in a high state of arousal and fulfillment of the goal will reduce the level of arousal.

Key Terms

Active sleep: A phase of sleep characterized by rapid eye movements (REM) and almost complete relaxation of skeletal muscles. The electroencephalogram appears desynchronized and similar to that seen when the subject is awake; most dreaming occurs during this sleep phase. Sometimes called REM sleep.

Alpha waves: A characteristic frequency pattern on an electroencephalogram (8–12 Hz), which is associated with relaxed wakefulness.

Arousal: A state of alertness characterized by desynchronization of the electroencephalogram and a high level of excitation or intensity of behavior.

Automatic behavior syndrome: A sleep disorder characterized by involuntary sleep. The patient continues existing activities but is unaware of his behavior.

p-**Chlorophenylalanine (PCPA):** A drug which depletes serotonin by inhibiting the synthesizing enzyme, tryptophan hydroxylase.

Circadian rhythms: Daily rhythms (from the Latin word, *circa diem*, about a day).

Eclosion: Emergence of a moth from the old pupal casing.

Electroencephalogram (EEG): A recording of the spontaneous electrical activity of the brain recorded from the scalp.

Electromyogram (EMG): A recording of the electrical activity of the muscle; it provides a simple means of monitoring muscle activity.

Hypersomnia: A disorder characterized by excessive sleep but otherwise normal behavior.

Insomnia: A prolonged and unusual inability to obtain adequate sleep.

Motivation: A physiological state that directs an organism in certain ways to seek particular goals.

Narcolepsy: A sleep disorder characterized by the frequent need for short periods of sleep.

Narcolepsy–cataplexy syndrome: A sleep disorder involving attacks of generalized motor weakness and paralysis precipitated by strong emotional situations and excessive sleepiness. Such persons are hypersomniacs.

Pontogeniculo-occipital waves: Spontaneous, intermittent, high voltage peaks that appear simultaneously in the pontine structures, the lateral geniculate, and occipital cortex. These waves are the earliest electrophysiological signals of impending active sleep.

Quiet sleep: Deep sleep in which the electroencephalogram is dominated by 2–4 Hz waves; sometimes called slow-wave sleep.

Raphé nuclei: A group of nuclei along the midline of the brain stem which contain serotonergic cell bodies.

"Restless-leg" syndrome: A human sleep disorder characterized by involuntary movements.

Sigma rhythm (or sleep spindles): A burst of rhythmic waves (12–15 Hz) on an encephalogram which are prevalent during light sleep.

Suprachiasmatic nucleus: A part of the hypothalamus involved in circadian rhythms.

Upper airway sleep apnea: A condition characterized by restricted airflow and increased respiratory effort during quiet sleep.

General References

Chase, T. N., ed. (1975). "The Nervous System," Vol. 2. Raven, New York.

Clemente, C. D., Purpura, D. P., and Mayer, F. E., eds. (1972). "Sleep and the Maturing Nervous System." Academic Press, New York.

Dement, W. C. (1974). "Some Must Watch While Some Must Sleep." Freeman, San Francisco, California.

Drucker-Colín, R. R., and McGaugh, J. L., eds. (1977). "Neurobiology of Sleep and Memory." Academic Press, New York.

Hartmann, E. L. (1973). "The Function of Sleep." Yale Univ. Press, New Haven, Connecticut.

Kales, A., ed. (1969). "Sleep, Physiology and Pathology." Lippincott, Philadelphia, Pennsylvania.

Kleitman, N., ed. (1963). "Sleep and Wakefulness." Univ. of Chicago Press, Chicago, Illinois (revised and enlarged edition).

Petre-Quadens, O., and Schlag, J. D., eds. (1974). "Basic Sleep Mechanisms." Academic Press, New York.

References

Allison, T., and Circhetti, D. V. (1976). Sleep in mammals: Ecological and constitutional correlates. *Science* **194**, 732–734.

Allison, T., and van Twyver, H. (1970). The evolution of sleep. *Nat. Hist.* (No. 4.) **79**, 56–65.

Allison, T., van Twyver, H., and Goff, W. R. (1972). Electrophysiological studies of the echidna *Tachyglossus aculeatus*. I. Waking and sleep. *Arch. Ital. Biol.* **110**, 145–184.

Andrews, R. V. (1971). Circadian rhythms in adrenal organ cultures. *Morphol. Jahrb.* **117**, 89–98.

Bobillier, P., Sakai, F., Seguin, S., and Jouvet, M. (1974). The effect of sleep deprivation upon the *in vivo* and *in vitro* incorporation of tritiated amino acids into brain proteins in the rat at three different age levels *J. Neurochem.* **22**, 23–31.

Claparede, E. (1908). Lafonchon du sommeil. *Rev. Sci.* **2**, 141–158.

Coriat, I. H. (1912). The nature of sleep. *J. Abnorm. Soc. Psychol.*, **6**, 329-367.

Dement, W. C., and Kleitman, N. (1957). Cyclic variations in EEG during sleep and their relation to eye movements, body motility and dreaming. *Electroencephalogr. Clin. Neurophysiol.* **9**, 673–690.

Dement, W. C., Mitler, M., and Henriksen, S. J. (1972). Sleep changes during chronic administration of *p*-chlorophenylalanine. *Rev. Can. Biol.* **31**, 239–246.

Dement, W. C., Guilleminault, C., and Zarcone, V. (1975). The pathologies of sleep: A case series approach. *In* "The Nervous System" (T. N. Chase, ed.), Vol. 2, pp. 501–518. Raven, New York.

Drucker-Colín, R. R. (1972). Transmisión neurohumoral en sueño: Efecto de un perfusado de la formación reticular. *Res. Congr. Nac. Cienc. Fisiol.* **15**, 8.

Drucker-Colín, R. R., Spanis, C. W., Cotman, C. W., and McGaugh, J. L. (1975a). Changes in protein levels in perfusates of freely moving cats: Relation to behavioral state. *Science* **187**, 963–965.

Drucker-Colín, R. R., Spanis, C. W., Hunyadi, J., Sassin, J., and McGaugh, J. L. (1975b). Growth hormone effects on sleep and wakefulness in the rat. *Neuroendocrinology* **18**, 1–8.

Drucker-Colín, R. R., Spanis, C. W., and Rojas-Ramírez, J. A. (1977). Investigation of the role of proteins in REM sleep. *In* "Neurobiology of Sleep and Memory" (R. R. Drucker-Colín and J. L. McGaugh, eds.), pp. 303–319. Academic Press, New York.

Fenel, V., Koski, G., and Pappenheimer, J. R. (1971). Factors in cerebrospinal fluid from goats that affect sleep and activity in rats. *J. Physiol.* (London) **216**, 565–589.

Guilleminault, C., and Dement, W. C. (1977). Amnesia and disorders of excessive daytime sleepiness. *In* "Neurobiology of Sleep and Memory" (R. R. Drucker-Colín and J. L. McGaugh, eds.), pp. 439–465. Academic Press, New York.

Hernández-Peón, R., and Sterman, M. B. (1966). Brain functions. *Annu. Rev. Psychol.* **17**, 363–394.

Jalowiec, J. E., Morgane, P. J., Stern, W. C., Zolovick, A. J., and Panksepp, J. (1973). Effects of midbrain tegmental lesions on sleep and regional brain serotonin and norepinephrine levels in cats. *Exp. Neurol.* **41**, 670–682.

Jouvet, M. (1967). Neurophysiology of the states of sleep. *In* "The Neurosciences" (G. C. Quarton, T. Melnechuk, and F. O. Schmitt, eds.), pp. 529–544. Rockefeller Univ. Press, New York.

Jouvet, M. (1969). Biogenic amines and the states of sleep. *Science* **163**, 32–41.

Jouvet, M. (1974). The role of monoaminergic neurons in the regulation and functions of sleep. *In* "Basic Sleep Mechanisms" (O. Petre-Quadens and J. D. Schlag, eds.), pp. 207–236. Academic Press, New York.

Jouvet, M. (1977). Neuropharmacology of the sleep-waking cycle. *In* "Handbook of Psychopharmacology" (L. L. Iverson, S. D. Iverson, and S. H. Snyder, eds.), Vol. 8, pp. 233–293. Plenum, New York.

Kleitman, N. (1957). Sleep, wakefulness and consciousness. *Psychol. Bull.* **54**, 354–359.

Kleitman, N. (1963). "Sleep and Wakefulness." Univ. of Chicago Press, Chicago, Illinois.

Kovačević, R., and Radulovački, M. (1976). Monoamine changes in the brain of cats during slow-wave sleep. *Science* **193**, 1025–1027.

Kroll, F. W. (1933). Veber das Vorkommen von ubertragbaren schlaferzeugenden stoffen im hirn schlafender tiere. Z. *Gesamte Neurol. Psychiatr.* **146**, 208–218.

Mangold, R., Sokoloff, L., Conner, E., Kleinerman, J., Therman, P. G., and Ketu, S. S. (1955). The effects of sleep and lack of sleep on the cerebral circulation and metabolism of normal young men. *J. Clin. Invest.* **34**, 1092–1100.

Menaker, M. (1974). Aspects of the physiology of circadian rhythmicity in the vertebrate central nervous system. *In* "The Neurosciences: Third Study Program" (F. O. Schmitt and F. G. Worden, eds.), pp.479–489. MIT Press, Cambridge, Massachusetts.

Monnier, M., and Hatt, A. M. (1971). Humoral transmission of sleep. V. New evidence from production of pure sleep hemodialysate. *Pfluegers Arch.* **329**, 231–243.

Monnier, M., Koller, T., and Graber, S. (1963). Humoral influences of induced sleep and arousal upon electrical brain activity of animals with crossed circulation. *Exp. Neurol.* **8**, 264–277.

Moore, R. Y. (1974). Visual pathways and the central neural control of diurnal rhythms. *In* "The Neurosciences: Third Study Program" (F. O. Schmitt and F. G. Worden, eds.) pp. 537–542. MIT Press, Cambridge, Massachusetts.

Moore-Ede, M. C. (1974). Control of circadian oscillations in renal potassium excretion in the squirrel monkey *(Saimiri scuireus)*. Doctoral Dissertation, Harvard University, Cambridge, Massachusetts.

Pappenheimer, J. R., Miller, J. B., and Goodrich, C. A. (1967). Sleep-promoting effects of cerebrospinal fluid from sleep-deprived goats. *Proc. Natl. Acad. Sci. U.S.A.* **58**, 513–517.

Pegram, V., Hammond, D., and Bridgers, W. (1973). The effect of protein synthesis inhibition on sleep in mice. *Behav. Biol.* **3**, 377–382.

Pieron, M. (1913). "Le problème physiologique du somneil." Masson, Paris.

Richter, C. P. (1965). "Biological Clocks in Medicine and Psychiatry." Thomas, Springfield, Illinois.

Rojas-Ramírez, J. A. (1974). Modificación de los estados de vigilia y de sueño mediante la técnica de perfusión cerebral localizado. *Res. Congr. Med.*, *30th Aniv.* pp. 292–293.

Rojas-Ramírez, J. A., and Drucker-Colín, R. R. (1977). Phylogenetic correlations between sleep and memory. *In* "Neurobiology of Sleep and Memory" (R. R. Drucker-Colín and J. L. McGaugh, eds.), pp. 57–74. Academic Press, New York.

Roth, R. L., and Sokolove, P. G. (1975). Histological evidence for direct connections between the optic lobes of the cockroach *Leucophaea* maderae, *Brain Res.* **87**, 23–39.

Sassin, J. F. (1977). Sleep-related hormones. *In* "Neurobiology of Sleep and Memory" (R. R. Drucker-Colín and J. L. McGaugh, eds.), pp. 361–372. Academic Press, New York.

Schnedorf, J. G., and Ivy, A. C. (1939). An examination of the hypnotoxin theory of sleep. *Am. J. Physiol.* **125**, 191–205.

Schweiger, E., Wallraff, H. C., and Schweiger, H. G. (1964). Endogenous circadian rhythm in cytoplasm of *Acetabularia:* Influence of the nucleus. *Science* **146**, 658–659.

Snyder, F., Hobson, J., Morrison, D., and Goldfrank, F. (1964). Changes in respiration, heart rate, and systolic blood pressure in human sleep. *J. Appl. Physiol.* **19**, 417–422.

Sokolove, P. G. (1975). Localization of the cockroach optic lobe circadian pacemaker with microlesions. *Brain Res.* **87**, 13–21.

Spanis, C. W., Carmen-Gutierrez, M., and Drucker-Colín, R. R. (1976). Neurohumoral correlates of sleep: Further biochemical and physiological characterization of sleep perfusates. *Pharmacol., Biochem. Behav.* **5**, 165–173.

Stephan, F. K., and Zucker, I. (1972). Circadian rhythms in drinking behavior and locomotor activity of rats are eliminated by hypothalamic lesions. *Proc. Natl. Acad. Sci. U.S.A.* **69**, 1583–1586.

Sterman, M. B. (1972). The basic rest-activity cycle and sleep: Developmental considerations in man and cats. *In* "Sleep and the Maturing Nervous System" (C. D. Clemente, D. P. Purpura, and F. E. Mayer, eds.), pp. 175–197. Academic Press, New York.

Sterman, M. B., and Hoppenbrouwers, T. (1971). The development of sleep–waking and rest–activity patterns from fetus to adult in man. *In* "Brain Development and Behavior" (M. B. Sterman, D. J. McGinty, and A. M. Adinolfi, eds.), pp. 203–227. Academic Press, New York.

Stetson, M. H., and Waston-Whitmyre, M. (1976). Nucleus suprachiasmaticus: The biological clock in the hamster? *Science* **191**, 197–199.

Takahashi, K., Takahashi, Y., Takahashi, S., and Honda, Y. (1974). Growth hormone and cortisol secretion during nocturnal sleep in narcoleptics and in dogs. *In* "Psychoneuroendocrinology" (N. Hadotani, ed.), pp. 67–76. Karger, Basel.

Tanber, E. S. (1974). Phylogeny of sleep. *In* "Advances in Sleep Research" (E. D. Weitman, ed.), Vol. l, pp. 133–172. Spectrum Publ., New York.

Truman, J. W. (1971). Circadian rhythms and physiology with special reference to neuroendocrine processes in insect. *Proc. Int. Symp. Circadian Rhythmicity* (Wageningen), pp. 111–135.

Truman, J. W. (1974). Circadian release of a prepatterned neural program in silkmoths. *In* "The Neurosciences: Third Study Program" (F. O. Schmitt and F. G. Worden, eds.), pp. 525–529. MIT Press, Cambridge, Massachusetts.

Truman, J. W., and Riddiford, L. M. (1970). Neuroendocrine control of ecdysis in silkmoths. *Science* **167**, 1624–1626.

Villablanca, J. (1966). Behavioral and polygraphic study of "sleep" and "wakefulness" in chronic decerebrate cats. *Electroencephalogr. Clin. Neurophysiol.* **21**, 562–577.

Webb, W. B. (1973). Sleep research past and present. *In* "Sleep: An Active Process" (W. B. Webb, ed.), pp. 1–10. Scott, Foresman Co., Glenview, Illinois.

Wöhlisch, E. (1956). Shlaf und Erholung als Probleme der Energetik und Gelassversorgung des Gehirns. *Klin. Wochenschr.* **34**, 720–729.

15

The Development, Remodeling and Aging of Neuronal Circuitry

I. Introduction

In previous chapters we have seen that the nervous system is precisely built to execute specific tasks. This, of course, does not just happen. The nervous system must be built; it must be modified; and it must be maintained. This chapter tells the story of the growth and changing of neuronal circuitry throughout life. It is a four-part story.

637

First we shall describe some of the general principles of neural development, focusing on the development of the cerebellar cortex. As we saw in Chapter 11, the cerebellum is a brain region involved in the smoothing of movement. It is particularly involved, for example, in dancing, gymnastics and handwriting. More important for our purposes, however, its cortex (in which its integrative work takes place) is a structure whose circuitry is simple and known in great detail. Thus, the development of this cortex can be studied with considerable fore-knowledge of what is being constructed. In describing the clear steps by which this construction takes place, we shall in effect "build" a small piece of cerebellar cortex, and this effort will be most worthwhile, because many (if not all) of the principles grasped through a study of cerebellar cortical development apply throughout the nervous system.

In Section III of this chapter we examine the trophic influences of nerves: how they act to maintain the integrity of the tissues of the body throughout its lifetime, as well as offering routes of communication and control to and from the CNS, respectively.

In Section IV we turn to the question of modifiability of circuitry during and after embryonic development. Can environmental, hormonal or other influences or pressures create changes in brain circuits? How is an experience ingrained indelibly into the tissues of the brain? We shall see that *basic* neural wiring is largely independent of external influences, but that certain extraneous events can indeed alter the fine detail of many connections. We saw some aspects of this plasticity previously in our study of the visual system (Chapter 10). Neuronal circuitry is mutable.

In Section V, we discuss some of the ways in which the structure of the brain is affected by aging. The brain is protected from abuse and much disease by its encasement by bone and its isolation from the blood by a barrier in its vessel walls, but there is no way it can escape old age.

II. Development of Neuronal Circuitry

The nervous system must be wired together properly if it is to work well. What does "proper wiring" mean when we are talking about the brain? At one level of analysis, the answer is simple: information must go to the right place, and there it must be received. Getting the information to the correct place is of course the job of the neuron's axon, which must therefore somehow find its way during de-velopment to the place or places (by means of branches) where meaningful connections can be made. The task of receiving the information, on the other hand, is accomplished by the dendrites of the target neuron. As we have seen, neurons themselves are tiny integrative and computational devices, and it is, therefore, the shape and size of the dendrites which largely determine how many axons the nerve cell can accommodate and, in fact, how these microprocessors of sundry information work.

Looking at neural development from an anatomical point of view then, we find ourselves with two main questions about neuronal connectivity: (1) How do axons "know" where to grow and what cells to innervate? (2) How do dendrites form the appropriate patterns of branches on which to receive these axons and integrate their many messages? Both of these issues have been important themes of research for many years, but they are only a part of a more general and truly profound question: How does the nervous system as a whole organize itself from a single sheet of undifferentiated cells in the embryo to the most complex structural organization in the body and, as far as we now know, in the universe?

Where do instructions for building a structure as complex as the human nervous system come from? Is this information only in the genes, or is it dependent on outside influences? And if both, in what combination?

The manner in which tissues arise and differentiate was defined decisively by Spemann in 1938, when he explored the origin of the nervous system in amphibian embryos. His experiments are milestones in the history of modern biology. The concepts he introduced are critical to our understanding of the function of the nervous system. The first of these concepts is *progressive determination*. Spemann conclusively disproved that the nervous system was preformed in some manner by demonstrating that it arises through the interaction of cells on the upper surface of the embryo with the underlying forerunners of axial body structures—the cells that form the backbone and its associated connective tissue and muscular investments. The nervous system is thus formed *de novo* from cells without intrinsic instructions. It seems instead that what these cells (or any cells) turn out to be is a result of many steps of extrinsic determination of outside influences: First a cell is only epidermal, and could as well form skin; then it becomes neural, and must join the neural plate; and later still, it finds itself in the cerebellar cortex and has to become a Purkinje cell. Spemann's famous analogy was that of a ball at the top of a furrowed hill. As the ball rolls down, it reaches many branch points between furrows, and, as "choices" are made, the possible future alternatives become fewer and fewer, until the ball ends up at some place at the bottom of the hill. But how are these courses determined, and how are these decisions made?

The factors that make a particular cell take one furrow or path and not another vary in the course of development. At the outset, the cues to the cell are largely internal, the consequence of what it has in its cytoplasm. Thus, at the beginning, many cells can be said to be self-determined as to their path of early differentiation, but if not, as is true for other cells, determination will usually occur later as determinant factors are passed to those undecided cells from elsewhere. This process is known as *induction*. In demonstrating the induction of the neural plate (the flattened sheet of surface cells that later curls into a trough and ultimately into the tube that is the early CNS), Spemann gave biology the second great embryological concept, the organizing principle behind development.

Many, if not most, of the steps in induction result from the influences of neighboring cells. These effects are mediated by the diffusion of substances (sometimes through specialized areas of cell-to-cell contact) which alter the course of a cell's development. While it was suspected in Spemann's time that inductive agents must often be chemicals, the techniques available then did not allow their recognition or isolation. Today, chemicals implicated in induction range from simple ions to large protein molecules, with possible sites of action all the way from the genome to the cytoplasmic organelles or cell membrane. When a cell assumes its characteristic form, cytology, and chemistry, it is said to have *differentiated*.

Initially, no neurons are recognizable in the early embryo, but through inductive interactions they soon take form, ultimately attaining the fully differentiated status of mature nerve cells with characteristic patterns of dendritic branching and axonal ramification. A central issue in development is to identify the nature of the interactions and to determine just how much information each step conveys toward later differentiation. Such problems, however, are in fact part of a larger, even more difficult issue: development does not end with completion of the embryo, nor with growth and eventual birth of the fetus. It continues into the neonatal period, into infancy, childhood, puberty, adolescence, youth and maturity—even into advancing age, where broader perspectives, experience and wisdom clearly demonstrate the never-ending growth of neural function. Indeed, senescence itself can be thought of as a kind of development, a life-long creative process winding down. Thus, we may be said to keep on developing through our entire lifetime. If we accept that idea, then our early upbringing and later experiences must have a great bearing on development.

All of us must have wondered at some time how much nurturing and subsequent history have to do with our abilities and personality. Are we strictly the result of our genetic makeup? Clearly, this cannot be. Most of us, as we seek to educate and improve ourselves, seem to feel that our abilities can always be enhanced, if not further developed. Just how far this enhancement can go, however, is a matter of great personal and social concern. In the last century the issue of the relative importance of heredity versus nurture on human maturation was largely a philosophical question, but today it has come down to a scientific one—one that can be addressed at many levels and with powerful techniques by the social and basic sciences.

So far as neural development goes, the question is approached in two ways: (1) How do particular environments influence the maturation of neural subsystems? Does rearing an animal in isolation away from other animals affect the final outcome—the definitive structure and function of the adult system? (2) How do interactions (inductive interplay) of cells within the developing brain itself influence the eventual structure and function of brain regions and areas? Which aspects of circuit construction are strictly genetic, according to "blueprint," and which are dependent on local cellular and substrate interactions?

By identifying modifiable and unmodifiable properties during maturation, today's investigators hope to find some which are particularly malleable. Tinkering with these will lead to understanding of local interactions during neurogenesis, which in turn almost certainly will enhance understanding of the more distant and perhaps even more puzzling environmental interactions.

In accord with this belief and hope, we shall now describe the development of the cerebellar cortex, emphasizing how young nerve cells just arriving in this structure from their birthplaces interact in various ways to bring about its construction. In the histogenesis of this highly organized piece of cortex, we find many illustrations of the critical balance between local interactions and genetic determinants. While some factors, such as cell-to-cell or axon-to-target recognition are not at all clear, other influences are quite straightforward—spatial and physical effects that "make sense" from a mechanistic point of view.

Before we proceed, we must recognize that there is no one explanation for neural development, no single key that unlocks the construction of the brain. In creating, shaping and wiring the immensely intricate entity of the CNS, the process of neurogenesis draws upon the widest imaginable range of determining factors, from ultramicroscopic molecular forces to easily discernible growth pressures of rapidly expanding cell populations upon organized substrates.

As the first step in our study of the development of the cerebellar cortex, we must take a quick look at its mature structure and cellular organization. Thus, we will know what we are working toward in our story.

The cellular organization of the mature cerebellar cortex is shown in Fig. 15-1. The cortex consists mainly of three kinds of neurons: _Purkinje_ cells (named after the Czech anatomist who described them), _granule_ cells (so tiny as to resemble grains of sand), and _basket_ cells (whose axons wrap about other cells in basketlike entanglements). These three types of cells are wired together in a definite and invariable manner (see Palay and Chan-Palay, 1974), as clear to a neuroanatomist as connections to a switch are to an electrician.

The Purkinje cells are the key elements. The largest and most impressive of the three types, they are the neurons through which all the output of the cortex will pass en route to the brain stem underneath. Like windbreaks of tall trees, they are arranged in neat rows with their flattened fanlike dendritic arborizations

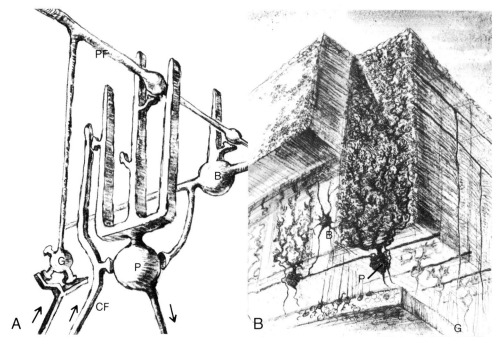

Fig. 15-1. Cellular organization of the mature cerebellum showing the major cell types. Purkinje cells (P); basket cells (B); and granule cells (G). (A) Purkinje cells receive connections from parallel fibers (PF) of the granule cells, basket cells and climbing fibers (CF). Right (B) General appearance of cellular architecture in the mature cerebellum.

carefully aligned in an outer cortical zone called the _molecular_ layer. The granule cells form an incredibly dense inner zone, the _granular_ layer, beneath the layer of Purkinje cell bodies. Millions of granule cells are found in even a cubic centimeter of this inner zone. Their axons pass straight up into the molecular layer, where they bifurcate and form an extremely orderly array of _parallel_ fibers that run in both directions from the branching points of the ascending fibers.

Parallel fibers intersect Purkinje cell dendrites at right angles, much as telephone lines intersect the crosspieces on the poles. Basket cells lie in the molecular layer, just above the Purkinje cell bodies and, therefore, also have their dendrites in this outer layer. Like the Purkinje cells, they too receive input from parallel fibers. The basket cell axons run along the row of Purkinje cell bodies over which they lie; this course takes them at right angles to the parallel fibers traveling above them. As each basket cell axon passes over a Purkinje cell body, it sends down a short branch that forms a complex terminal plexus or "basket" around that cell body. Purkinje cells, in their turn, send a side branch of their axons (which unlike those of the other cells are the only ones to leave the cortex) back to the neighboring basket cells, thus forming a recurrent loop (not shown in the figure).

Already we are beginning to get a picture of a brain region that has an extreme degree of internal organization—a formal geometry of nerve cells and fibers. We can see that there is opportunity here for the feedback modulation that we learned earlier is so important in regulating neuronal response, but there is more, while many other circuits exist in this cortex and could be described, the _climbing_ fibers are perhaps most worthy of mention. Each of these remarkable axons, which have come from a specialized region of the brain stem far below, singles out a particular Purkinje cell body, passes directly to it, and proceeds to wind its way upward over that cell body onto the principal dendrites (and then on along their finer branches like a clinging vine branching upon a trellis). Making multiple synapses on the main stems and branches of the Purkinje dendritic tree, the climbing fiber is probably the most powerful excitatory connection in the brain. Certainly it is the most thorough in making its connection; it synapses with the same target neuron over and over again!

Purkinje cells are always firing, and parallel fibers (especially if many are active) can further excite them. However, the climbing fibers exert a great intensifying influence upon Purkinje cell activity; one that always has some effect upon the frequency with which the latter is discharging at any moment. Thus, within this almost mathematically designed cerebellar cortex, inhibition and excitation continually flow around basket cell axons and climbing fibers (not to mention many other similar routes) with all the clarity and logic of a printed circuit in electronics. All modern vertebrates show more or less the same principal cell types and features of cortical organization that we have just described.

We shall deal primarily with construction of the cerebellar cortex of the rat. Among mammals alone, there is a great range in the time span of cerebellar development. The guinea pig's cerebellum is virtually complete at birth, while in the whale years may pass before it is finished. To almost the same extent, the same is true for man, as anyone who has watched children grow and acquire motor skills can appreciate. Almost certainly, the period required to build its cerebellum will have a strong effect upon the biological niche the young animal occupies, and this effect in turn will lead to others. One result is that the offspring of a species with a late-maturing cerebellar cortex must be reared by a parent or parents for a longer period of time. Such nurture could thereby offer a greater opportunity for social instruction of the relatively inexperienced (as well as help-less) young.

Rats, like most mammals (ourselves included), have a somewhat variable time of gestation, ranging from 21 to 24 days. In addition, the cerebellum itself shows a gradient of differentiation and growth, with some parts developing earlier and faster than others. We have tried to restrict our discussion to one area to standardize the timing of various events. This area is the *pyramis*, a pyramid-shaped set of parallel folds of cortex located in an ancient wormlike convolution (the vermis) that seems to inch along the midline of the cerebellum.

Keep in mind that developmental events are gradual, flowing and ebbing over a considerable period of time. They are like the slowly rising and falling themes of a symphony, not staccato statements of sudden new musical form and relationships, and, as when we listen to a symphony orchestra, many things are going on at once, almost too many for us to keep track of except in an overall way. It is not easy to watch or listen to multiple events taking place in parallel, let alone to imagine them. Therefore, we have selected certain times at which particular forms and relationships have been attained—"milestones" of developmental history. At these times we can check on the progress of all the parallel events in a systematic fashion.

This problem of description confronts us when we try to visualize the development of any tissue or organ, but it is most difficult when we come to the nervous system, where there are more *types* of cells to be put into place than there are kinds of cells in the rest of the body! For every part of the body, progressive determination, induction, local interaction, experience and whatever else may shape it occur over space and time. In embryology, therefore, we must study development at many artificially arrested stages. For the wonder of the developing brain, it is as if we were to watch the unfolding of a blossom in the successive frames of time-lapse cinematography.

A. Assembly of the Cerebellar Cortex—Stages in Its Development

1. THE PRENATAL PERIOD. After its primary induction by underlying skeletomuscular precursors, the neural plate deepens into a trough and then rolls itself into a tube by a process called *neurulation*. The neural tube sinks beneath the surface of the embryo from which it has formed, like a submerging submarine, and the skin closes over it smoothly to leave hardly a trace in the normal process of organogenesis. The neural tube then undergoes many further stages of development, expanding in some regions to form the primitive brain vesicles and also folding upon itself like a garden hose with prominent "kinks" in it at certain points. Our series of illustrations (Fig. 15-2) portrays the shaping of the human brain from seven weeks of gestation to birth.

At 5 weeks (Fig. 15-2A), the *hindbrain* (HB) shows little sign of a cerebellum, but by about 9 weeks (Fig. 15-2B) a distinct reverse curvature or kink has appeared within this lower chamber of the brain. The cerebellum may be seen as a modest thickening upon the uppermost of the two surfaces of the hindbrain approxi-

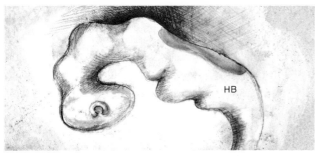

(A) Five weeks

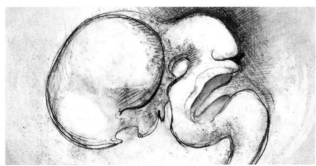

(B) Nine weeks

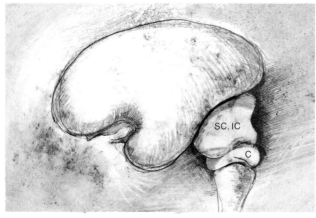

(C) Eleven weeks

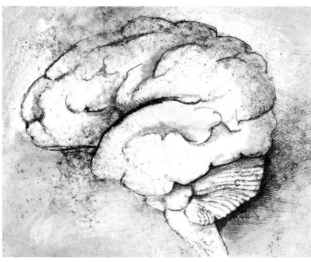

(D) Newborn

mated by this kink, right at the edge of these surfaces as they lie below and underneath the bulging midbrain roof or tectum. By 11 weeks (Fig. 15-2C), the cerebellum (C) is clearly visible as a small but wide nubbin behind the superior and inferior colliculi (SC and IC, respectively). In the newborn infant (Fig. 15-2D) the region has taken on its general shape and characteristically fissurated appearance, but it is only about one-twentieth its adult size. The great growth it will continue to show will be due in part to multiplication of a large number of cells upon its outer surface, but much more to the enhancement of dendrites and axons and all their branches inside it, with concomitant multiplication and enlargement of supportive cells, the neuroglia and vascular elements.

The development of the rat's cerebellum, with which we shall be concerned, is exactly the same as that of the human up to a certain point (somewhere between Figs. 15-2B and C). It just comes to an end sooner, without going on to reach the great size and pronounced fissuration we can see in the newborn child, but the basic principles appear similar, and actually more is known about the timing of nerve cell origin in experimental animals than we will probably ever know about these events in ourselves. [The reader interested in more detail about the general embryological stages of brain development as shown in Fig. 15-2 should consult Carpenter (1976) or most any embryology text.]

In the rat, the Purkinje cells come into being between the fifteenth and sixteenth days of gestation (Das and Nornes, 1972). They arise as daughter cells of parental cell types near the large internal cavity of the hollow hindbrain. Such germinal cells divide rapidly, by the familiar process of mitosis, in early embryonic stages. Many times, the daughter cells from these divisions stay where they are, and just keep on dividing, but at some point, certain cells that are destined to become neurons leave this intensely proliferative population of precursors. Such neurons are then said to "have been born." They will never return to their birthplace in the lining of the primitive brain vesicle, and they will never divide again. Like all newly born, neogenic or young neurons, they quickly migrate away from the zone of cell division to the brain area (in this case the cerebellar cortex) where they will differentiate and live out the rest of their lives as mature, active nerve cells.

The mechanism of neuron migration in the brain, at least in many of the regions in which it has been studied, is very different from that of motile cells elsewhere in the body. Normally we think of a long process emerging from one end of a cell, groping for and then sticking to some other cell or attractive place in some manner. From this anchor point, the cell pulls itself (its cell body) along for a distance, using contractile microfilaments inside for motive power. This procedure is repeated as necessary until the cell reaches its destination. How the cell "knows" it is there is still largely unknown. However, in the developing CNS, the cells that have been dividing have long processes already. These extend to the prospective surface of the brain, to the outer surface of the early neural tube. Thus, although the way in which a young neuron hauls itself along its own fiber may be quite similar to what we have just described, the way to go is already clear: just follow the fiber to its end! And the cell will know it has reached its destination when there is no more length of that fiber to go.

The discovery of this means of neuronal migration has been of great importance and excitement in the study of brain development. It explains not only how at least some young nerve cells know *how far* to go but also how they know *where* to go. The positions on the primitive brain's surface where the outer processes of the tall, spindly epithelial cells from which neurons take "birth" by mitosis terminate are the determinants, and the outer processes themselves guide the early neurocytes to these destinations. By the time the nerve cell bodies get to their predetermined final locations, pulling themselves up their outer processes like Hindu fakirs up so many rope ladders, these destinations will not be dots on the exterior surface of the hindbrain roof but specific distant places in the cerebellar cortex that is swelling forth from it. The developing brain is like an expanding universe: its parts are continually moving away from one another in a relative (as well as an absolute) sense. We know that if a "fix" can be attained on some nearby star (and there is no sideways motion), then the direction of that star will remain constant, even if it is receding with great velocity from the point of observation. Similarly, if a young neuron can get a fix (through its long outer process extending to the periphery of the immature CNS) on a nearby target, then its future direction of migration will present no major problem except that of time as it moves across the ever-widening space of the growing brain.

We emphasize that this sequence of events may not be true for all nerve cells, and, in fact, whether it holds for the cerebellar Purkinje cells is not firmly established. However they get there, Purkinje cells find themselves soon after birth of the rat pup in a little nubbin of brain that will become the cerebellar cortex. There they arrange their cell bodies in a diffuse layer three to four cells thick. For several days after the end of their "migration," not much appears to happen to them, at least as far as one can judge from routine cellular stains. The powerful climbing fibers may have arrived from the brain stem, but they also wait a few days before starting synaptogenesis (O'Leary *et al.*, 1971; West and Del Cerro, 1976). Apparently some inductive signal is needed for further progress, because at this point the Purkinje cells show little innate potential to grow into their adult forms.

It is possible, however, that activities of great importance are being carried out by these cells at this seemingly quiet time (in the form of axonal outgrowth). In the spinal cord, for example, motor neurons undergo a similar quiescent period during which they spin out their long axons to the muscles. The arrival of these axons causes the muscles to differentiate further. In this connection, it is interesting to note that not all motor neurons make contact with their distant targets. Those which do not [usually more than half (Jacobson, 1970)] die. The growth of axons to remote destinations is a more difficult challenge, perhaps more difficult than the migration of young neurons within the orderly scaffolding of processes in the developing brain. Such axons must follow other guidelines, such as the micro-orienting filaments of certain connective tissue proteins, in a manner not unlike the way in which they can follow the empty passageways of deceased axons in the regeneration of an injured or severed adult peripheral nerve. There again, many fibers fail to reach their destinations and are weeded out in atrophy and death.

As a safety factor in development (and perhaps for other reasons as well) overproliferation of neurons has been found not only with respect to motor nerve cells but in nearly every area of the brain studied. Cell death, along with cell origin, cell migration, and cell differentiation, is one of the major features of neurogenesis, as it is in the genesis of any organ or organ system. One indication that it occurs in the formation of the cerebellar cortex is the finding of a reduction in Purkinje cell number by 8% in the first few days after birth (Altman and Anderson, 1971). This reduction comes at what should be nearly the end of the suspected period of cell death, and may be only a whisper of the magnitude of the process. Whether this quiescent interval just before birth is really as peaceful as it appears awaits further investigation.

Nonetheless, by current measures the cerebellar cortex is lying in wait for the next inducing factors to come into play. While it waits, the source of many, if not most, of these factors is being assembled. This structure is the external granular layer.

2. BIRTH. At birth, or zero days (Fig. 15-3), the cerebellum is about one-

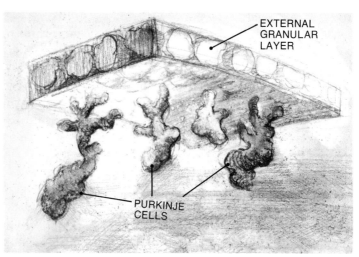

Fig. 15-3

twentieth its adult size. Purkinje cells are present, but are very small and undifferentiated. The surface of the cerebellum is covered by a zone of proliferating cells, the *external granular* layer, which is one to five cells deep (Addison, 1911). From this zone, a transient layer found only in development, the definitive granule cells and basket cells are being generated. The former will ultimately come to lie beneath the Purkinje cells in the mature internal granular layer, the latter just above the Purkinje cells in the molecular layer. When its germinal work is done, the external granular layer disappears. That it persists, however, for 2 years after birth of the human infant gives us some idea of the vast number of granule cells it produces. In many animals, in fact, such postnatal neurogenesis occurs in several brain regions, and undoubtedly is of special importance in certain areas related to learning and/or acquisition of motor skills.

3. FOUR DAYS. At 4 days (Fig. 15-4), many changes have occurred. The Purkinje cells have grown and arranged themselves in their characteristic monolayer. Many of the cells are somewhat conical, pointing upward toward the external granular layer. Their cell bodies are covered with spindly outgrowths, at the ends of which climbing fibers synapse. These are the first synapses established. The climbing fibers, by a procedure called *axon extension*, grow in from

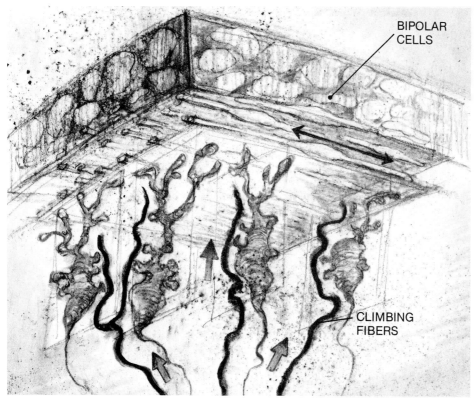

BIPOLAR CELLS

CLIMBING FIBERS

Fig. 15-4

the underlying brain stem, locate the Purkinje neurons, and form a few synapses on short dendritic processes extending outward all around the cell body. Initially they form synapses on more than one Purkinje cell, but later withdraw to only one. (This process is also seen, with less ultimate reduction, in the development of neuromuscular connections.)

The external granular layer has grown to almost 8 cells in depth, and its immature neurons are in various stages of differentiation according to their position within it. At the surface the actively mitotic germinal elements (derived from the cells lining the ventricle of the hindbrain that lies beneath) and the newborn granule cells are small, and round in shape. Under them is a zone of horizontal, rod-shaped cells oriented in the direction of the parallel fibers of the adult. At this stage of differentiation the young granule cells are called _bipolar cells_. As they sink deeper, toward the Purkinje cell layer, they become progressively more elongated, extruding from both ends long processes that will in time become the parallel fibers.

4. SEVEN DAYS. Although some precocious granule cells have migrated inward from the external granular layer at 4 days, their final home, the internal granular layer, only becomes recognizable a week after birth (Fig. 15-5). After

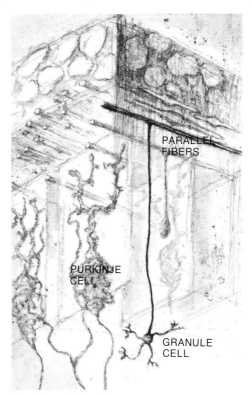

Fig. 15-5

extruding the bipolar processes that become the parallel fibers, the granule cells drop down beneath the Purkinje cells, leaving a vertical axon trailing behind. The unusual T-shaped axonal configuration characteristic of the cell results. This phenomenon is called *axon trailing*.

How does the granule cell body migrate to its final position? It does so by a procedure called *contact guidance* (Rakic, 1971; Rakic and Sidman, 1973). Certain early formed glial cells (not shown) are vertically oriented, and each of these elements forms a kind of rope upon which the granule cell slides down into its resting place. Contact guidance is a commonly used mechanism in development and has actually been known for many years in the development of peripheral nerves where fibers follow an oriented microstructure in the primitive connective tissues. Once a few cells or fibers have a particular organization, other elements can reach the same site by following the route of the pioneer. A striking example is seen in the development of the optic projection to the tectum in the freshwater flea, *Daphnia*. Here retinal axons track one along another, and the resultant ordered stack of fibers guides them to their correct targets in the central visual analyzer region (Lopresti *et al.*, 1973).

Hormones, such as those of the thyroid, appear to influence the normal development of granule cells from the external granular layer. Thus neural development seems to be tied in a subtle way to the growing and pervasive function of the endocrine system. Thyroid hormone plays an important role in the timing, rate and quantity of cell proliferation and growth (Lauder, 1977); such effects extend to the growth of axons and formation of connections. In the cerebellar cortex, hypothyroidism results in permanently shorter parallel fibers, whereas hyperthyroidism accelerates parallel fiber growth and elongates them by as much as 1.5 mm. It would appear that one of the ways that brain maturation is related to the environment of the surrounding body is through hormonal systems. Such *peripheral rebound* effects are numerous, however, and are by no means confined to endocrine influences from the maturing ductless glands. Influences from innervated muscle and skin are also very important in determining the ultimate size and intrinsic features of related parts of the CNS.

The proliferation of basket cells is coming to a close at 7 days. These cells, unlike the granule cells, do not migrate far but differentiate essentially at the level where they were born. They are produced by the external granular layer near the beginning of a stacking sequence of parallel fibers. As the stack of such fibers grows (in the manner indicated earlier when we described the inward settling of granule cells), basket cells are entrapped near the tops of the Purkinje cell bodies. The latter have by this time amassed most of their cytoplasm in the conical caps as described. At this stage, coincident with the appearance of the internal granular layer, the molecular layer becomes apparent as the relatively cell-free zone left behind after granule cell translocation.

5.   TEN DAYS.   By 10 days Purkinje cells have lost their somatic (cell body) spines, and basket cell axons have begun synaptogenesis, articulating with the Purkinje cell bodies (Fig. 15-6). The Purkinje caps have given rise to an apical dendrite and some secondary dendritic branches, upon which climbing fibers now synapse. In the external granular layer cell division is slowing to a halt, while cell migration is now in full swing. The later-descending granule cells stack up upon those which first established the internal granular layer. The result is that the earliest granule cells sit at the bottom of the layer, sending their axons up into the lower reaches of the overlying molecular layer, while the succeeding granule cells stack both their cell bodies and their axons upon their predecessors in roughly the order of their time of formation (Alman, 1972a,b).

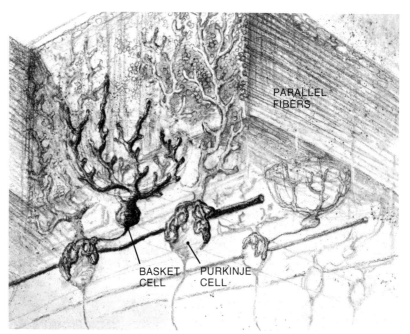

Fig. 15-6

In the rat, the granule cells find themselves in the same limbo after migration as did the Purkinje cells, awaiting a signal to begin the next phase of differentiation. In humans and in whales, however, both of which possess extremely large cerebella which require an extended period of development, events take a somewhat different course. In these animals the major input to the cerebellar cortex, the _mossy fibers_ (so named because of mosslike excrescences at their tips), arrive before their target neurons, the granule cells, have migrated. They form a transient clear layer beneath the cell bodies of the Purkinje cells that corresponds in location to the future internal granular layer (Rakic and Sidman, 1970). There they await arrival of the granule cells from up above. Normally, one would expect that such axons, having grown to a destination remote from the brain stem in which they arise, would either degenerate or else continue to grow up into the cortex until the specified contacts are made. That neither of these two courses is followed suggests that the mossy fibers may be receiving some factor that prevents their deterioration. In man, they are in such a suspended state for 10 weeks; the situation in the whales is not known, but may be even longer.

6. FIFTEEN DAYS. Parallel fibers and Purkinje cells are now ready to connect. Beginning on about the tenth day and in full force by 15 days the granule cells' axons commence outgrowth and initiate a wave of synaptogenesis with the dendrites of Purkinje, basket and stellate cells (a later forming, smaller variety of basket cell). As shown in Fig. 15-7, there is a corresponding initiation of rapid dendritic growth in all these cellular targets, and, along with this growth, there is a rapid establishment of a variety of other intrinsic synaptic connections between

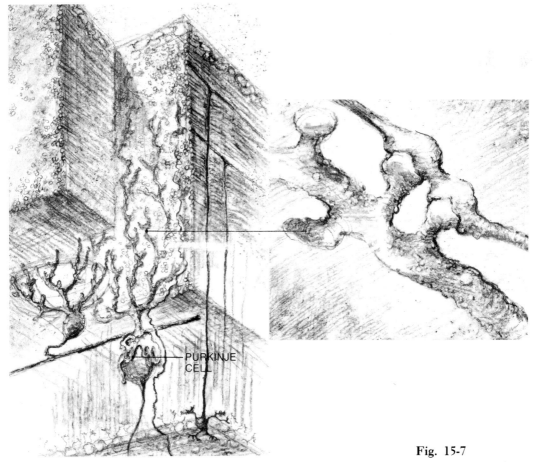

PURKINJE
CELL

Fig. 15-7

the variety of cerebellar interneurons. The basket cell axons make contact with the inner regions of the Purkinje cell dendritic tree, and even with a region near the origin of the Purkinje axon, while the stellate cells (which as a consequence of later formation lie more superficially) synapse upon more distal segments of the Purkinje dendrites. Meanwhile, down in the internal granular layer, the mossy fibers are forming their characteristically swollen (or glomerular) contacts with the granule cells and also with Golgi type II cells, a kind of input-modulating neuron we have not described in the interest of simplicity.

Events are happening at all levels. The stages involving the actual formation of a synapse are illustrated in Fig. 15-8.

Fig.15-8. A close look at the process of synaptogenesis. Synaptogenesis (the birth of a synapse) is the critical event in the ordering of neuronal circuitry. Axons must reach the correct targets and form the appropriate synapses. In order to study these two events in detail many investigators have resorted to the use of tissue culture. Dissociated neurons or small aggregates of neurons when provided with appropriate nutrients will grow in small dishes and form their correct synapses. This figure highlights some of the major events and show how explants of embryonic rat thoracic spinal cord, grown in culture, contact individual isolated neurons of the superior cervical ganglion (Rees *et al.*, 1976). Most likely the same events transpire in the growing cerebellum. (A) Axon extension. Fine undulating processes extend from the growing axonal tip in all directions. In motion pictures taken of this process, the processes appear to be searching the environment to determine which way to proceed. The tip seems to pull itself forward in one direction spinning out the newly formed axon behind it. The distal specialized portion of the elongating axon shown in this picture is called a *growth cone*. Typically the growth cone consists of a bolus expansion called a varicosity from which the fine filapodia (F) extend in all directions. These filapodia extend either as numerous cylindrical projections (microspikes) or less commonly as single sheetlike projections of filapodia. Many extend 10–20 μm in 60 seconds, wait for a period, say 5 minutes, and then advance or retract. A growing process must recognize its appropriate target as, for example, in the construction of the correct circuitry of the cerebellum. Processes may bypass competent targets, so there is specificity inherent in the interaction between growing afferent and target. Recognition often appears to be due to a selective adhesion or chemoaffinity between cell membrane surfaces (see Barondes, 1976). (B) Contact. Synapse localization is determined when the transient contact becomes a permanent site of synaptic adhesion and the membranes differentiate to form a synapse. In the next stage growth cone filapodia become extensively applied to the target cell and show numerous punctate areas on the postsynaptic plasma membrane. (C) Synaptogenesis. A characteristic electron dense matrix begins to develop between the membranes, and the Golgi apparatus (Go) of the target neuron hypertrophies and produces numerous coated vesicles (CV). These fuzzy coated vesicles find their way to the target site, insert into the membrane and form the postsynaptic density. Synaptic vesicles gradually become clustered opposite the postsynaptic density. (D) The final outcome: the synapse. As the synapse matures synaptic vesicles increase in number, the cleft widens and the postsynaptic density expands as coated vesicles continue to insert into the postsynaptic membrane. The enzymes for the biosynthesis of the transmitter and the receptors responsible for the particular activating characteristics of the postsynaptic membrane are produced. The synapse becomes operative.

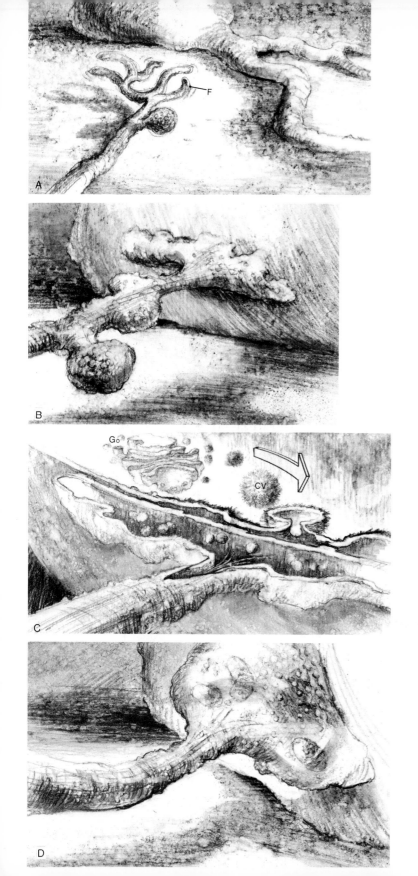

The main point is that by the fifteenth day the basic neuronal circuitry of the cerebellar cortex is complete in its essentials. The continuation of development postnatally results in its elaboration and refinement. With the widespread onset of parallel fiber synaptogenesis, the Purkinje dendrites start to branch extensively, while continuing their upward growth. At about 20 days in the rat, the last cells of the external granular layer migrate, and the tips of the Purkinje dendrites at last touch the overlying vascular membrane, the pia mater. These already impressive dendrites keep on branching and refining themselves, however, for a long period—beyond 90 days of age.

7. ADULT. Construction is now complete (Fig. 15-9). Each Purkinje cell has acquired some 80,000 parallel fiber synapses, received one climbing fiber, many basket and stellate cell contacts, and developed an elaborate dendritic fan. As is evident from our series of illustrations, the assembly of the cerebellar cortex is no less ordered than the final result. Also apparent is that the cerebellum is to a large degree self-assembling in its development. Many of the keys to the mysteries of its highly organized cellular architecture are to be found within its meticulous and progressive histogenesis.

What interactions result in the formation of the Purkinje cell dendritic tree? As seen from the foregoing description, dendritic growth occurs at nearly all stages of development. What *initiates* such outgrowth is not yet clearly resolved, but most evidence suggests it is an "intrinsic" neuronal property, induced or determined previously and differentiating in the absence of further interactions (Privat, 1975). On the other hand; it is now clear that for the most part the *shape* of the dendritic tree is under the control of the afferent fibers. It is the billions of parallel fibers which have the final say about the luxuriant form of the Purkinje dendritic fan.

Proof that this is so comes from experiments with X irradiation. With this powerful mode of developmental intervention, the external granular layer may be prevented from forming granule cells for a brief period. This hiatus results in a gap in the formation of parallel fibers, and their vacant zone is filled up largely by neuroglia (Altman and Anderson, 1973; Altman, 1973). In this situation, the Purkinje dendrites assume a characteristic "weeping willow" form, with many dendrites growing downward instead of upward (Altman, 1973; Altman and Anderson, 1973; Bradley and Berry, 1976) (Fig. 15-10). Three-dimensional analysis of these abnormal dendrites demonstrates that they are generated in the normal manner, but also that their unusual configuration results from the changed demands of parallel fibers, which are missing at certain levels and present at others (Bradley and Berry, 1976).

Although the final shaping of the Purkinje dendritic fan is under the control of the parallel fibers, responsibility for the total amount of growth is shared with

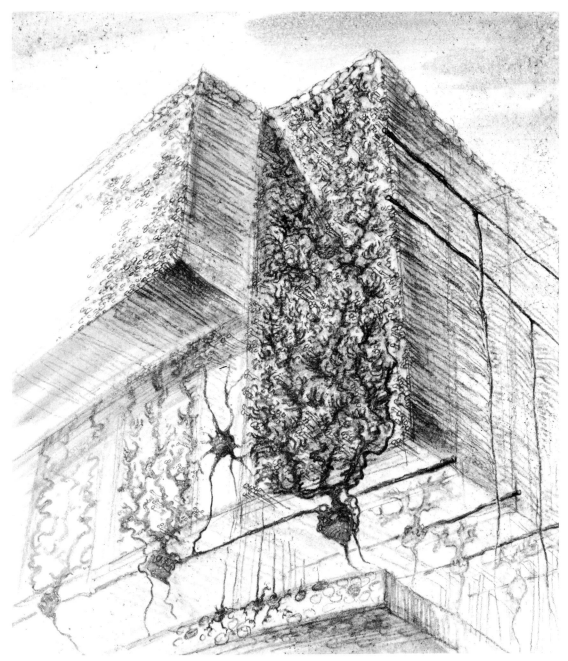

Fig. 15-9. The mature cerebellum.

the climbing fibers. If the Purkinje cells are deprived of climbing fibers early in development (by severing the connection over which they arrive), the dendrites grow only half as much as normally (Bradley and Berry, 1976) (Fig. 15-10). This effect in itself is remarkable and attests to powerful influences by this afferent fiber in development as well as in adult cerebellar cortical function.

Thus nearly all aspects of Purkinje dendritic development, from the formation of dendritic spines to the overall shape and size of the tree, can be demonstrated to be under the control of the afferent fibers, rather than an intrinsic property of the Purkinje cell itself. It is possible, however, that the manner in which the Purkinje cell reacts to the inductive influences of the afferents is intrinsic at some level.

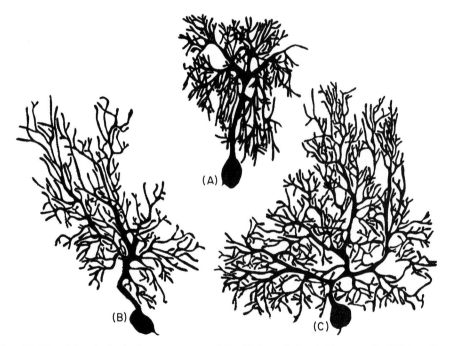

Fig. 15-10. Morphological appearance of Purkinje cell dendritic trees in (A) irradiated cerebella (B) climbing fiber deficient cerebella, and (C) normal cerebella. Representative drawings based on camera lucida tracings. (From Bradley and Berry, 1976.)

B. Summary of Cerebellar Cortical Development

At the beginning of this chapter, we raised the issue of the relative importance of local interactions versus genetic determinants. Our knowledge of cerebellar cortical development is not yet complete, particularly at the molecular level where the final answers must ultimately come. Nonetheless, we see that most aspects of the development of neural circuitry are not self-determined, but are rather influenced and molded by interactions with other cells and other events. A cell, like Spemann's ball at the top of that furrowed hill, must make many choices in the course of its development. Inductive interactions bring out particular gene expressions, which in turn prepare the cell for other interactions and so forth. A cell must be at the right place at the right time with the right capability in order to develop properly. A neuron is a neuron very early in embryogenesis, but its subsequent developmental history and that of its partners (other neurons or muscles) depend on good interactions.

Genetic factors, of course, are critically important. The information must be present in order to be induced, and this information must be correct in every detail, or the final product will not work well, or perhaps last as long. However, it is now clear that the development of the nervous system is to a large extent the calling forth—singly and in combination—of the right events at the right times from the archives of the genes.

Other brain areas develop in accordance with many of the same principles displayed in the genesis of the cerebellum. Each area, however, utilizes a slightly different set of principles, tailored in a slightly different way to meet unique constructional problems. In the visual system, for example, it appears as if the formation of specific retinal fields in the colliculus of some animals depends on a selective affinity or matching of cell membrane surfaces (see Jacobson, 1970). In this model, called the _chemoaffinity model_ (Sperry, 1963), retinal fibers are specifically coded to recognize their specific target sites in the colliculus. Recent studies support this model and indicate that membrane molecules isolated from retina (which probably contain carbohydrates) will combine with specific cells in the colliculus in a manner which mimics the topographical organization of the retinal input (see Barondes, 1976). Moreover, tissue culture studies of a retina explanted near a colliculus will form to a degree at least the appropriate connections (Smalheiser and Crain, 1978). Thus local _in situ_ cues are not essential for the formation of the correct connections. At present it is not clear whether chemoaffinity is involved in the specification of synapses in the cerebellum.

We have seen how in the cerebellar cortex the complexity of the final product is greatly reduced if we examine the straightforward and logical stages of the progressive assembly mechanisms. Such step-by-step construction seems to be a general principle of development: each single simple step is an essential prerequisite to the next. Only when the end is reached, and the steps forgotten (or never witnessed), does the product appear excessively complicated.

For example, we have witnessed how the external granular layer, which forms a transient veil over the surface of the developing cerebellar cortex, solves the problem of the T-shaped axonal configuration of the granule cell which (emitting opposed processes) descends from it by axon trailing. We have also seen how the velvety saillike Purkinje dendritic tree, which is able to catch so many afferent fibers in its wide expanse, is actually brought into being by the cues and proddings of these very inputs. The great beauty in the development of the nervous system is not only the magnificence of the finished structure, but also the simplicity of the ultimate underlying mechanisms in building it.

III. Trophic Influences of Nerves—A Lasting Partnership between Neurons and Their Target Cells

Nerves not only develop in concert with other structures (other nerves, skin or muscle), but once developed, that interdependence persists. Neurons exert a lasting *trophic influence* upon the targets to which they connect. A partnership develops. As we saw in the cerebellar cortex, the climbing fibers exert a trophic influence on cerebellar development, as do the parallel fibers.

Such trophic interactions are displayed at all levels of the nervous system. An excellent example of the partnership between nerve fibers and their target cells is seen in the neuromuscular junction.

Some muscles (so-called "fast" ones) contract rapidly, while others ("slow" muscles) contract slowly. The differences in speed of shortening are due to distinct molecular properties in the muscles themselves. But when a fast muscle is experimentally transposed with a slow one, a surprising thing happens: the contraction of the fast muscle becomes slower and that of the slow muscle becomes faster (Buller *et al.*, 1960). Apparently the motor nerves dictate certain properties of the muscles, so that the enzymatic and protein contents of the muscle fibers are transformed. As a result, the slow muscles develop intrinsic components characteristic of fast muscles and vice versa (Close, 1972).

Denervation of a muscle also illustrates the trophic dependency: the nerveless muscle rapidly shows a lessened resting potential and, therefore, is closer to the point of contracting (Albuquerque *et al.*, 1971). Further, the entire surface of the muscle, not just the normally responsive neuromuscular junction, becomes sensitive to the neurotransmitter acetylcholine (Axelsson and Thesleff, 1959). This increase in muscle irritability is called *denervation supersensitivity*.

All these findings clearly show that the normal properties of a muscle depend on the presence of a nerve. The nature of this transsynaptic influence, however, is not straightforward or clear (see Purves, 1976).

One school maintains that activity on the part of the target cells is all that is required. Thus, for example, programmed electrical stimulation of a muscle in the absence of a nerve can simulate, to a degree, the influence of neural input

(Drachman and Witzke, 1972; Lømo and Rosenthal, 1972; Lømo and Westgaard, 1975). But another school holds that nerves secrete trophic substances which nourish and regulate the properties of the target cells. In accord with this nutrient concept, the denervation syndrome mentioned above occurs sooner when the nerve is transected near the muscle than when it is cut farther away (Deshpande *et al.*, 1976). Presumably there is more nutrient to draw upon, for a while at least, in the latter instance, or as another example, young muscle cells grown in a tissue culture mature only to an early stage unless innervated or supplied with trophic substances from a neural extract (Oh, 1975; Oh *et al.*, 1972).

What could be happening that might resolve the two opposing points of view is that artificially induced activities similar to those evoked by nerve stimulation could cause the muscle cells to secrete or otherwise generate substances which mimic the trophic materials of the nerve. In line with this idea, the nerve itself usually has a more pronounced effect than that which follows simulated nerve activity.

In the CNS, trophic interactions can be so important that the loss of such essential input leads to the death of the target cell or cells. Thus there are two broad categories of signals passing continually between neurons and their targets. Some signals carry reports of information (of neural business that must be processed), while others seem to regulate cellular metabolism so as to meet new functional needs. We can see how the latter class of signals are in reality a way of perpetuating the kind of cellular interactions that are central to the construction of the nervous system in the first place—an expression of the life-long process of development.

IV. Remodeling of Neuronal Circuitry

Brain function, like the function of an electronic device, depends on correct circuitry. Unlike an electronic device, however, the brain does not always do the same thing under a given set of circumstances. How is it that the response to the same stimulus can vary so widely?

One answer, of course, is that neural activity is routed and integrated along different circuits from one moment to the next. Another explanation, however, is that the connections may be changed and the circuits rewired from time to time.

At the turn of the century, neuroanatomists first proposed that synaptic connections may be modified, even in the adult, by experience. Such changes, however, were not found, and for the next 50 or so years the brain was regarded as "hard-wired." However, we now know that the brain, like the ultimate in computer-serviced electronic equipment of the space age, can change its structure with experience and even repair itself to some degree when damaged. In this section, we shall discuss the many ways in which the nervous system can be induced to alter its circuitry during growth and maturation.

A. Influences of the Environment on Neuronal Circuitry

Until recently, very little research supported the notion that the brain's anatomy could be affected by experience. The turning point came in the 1960's, stimulated first by the work of David Krech and co-workers at Berkeley, and then by others. These studies showed that variations in the social and sensory qualities of the environment of the organism during development could affect both the gross and fine structure of the brain (Greenough, 1975; Greenough et al., 1976; Diamond, 1978).

If neural circuitry is to be modified, the two most commonly proposed ways of bringing such changes about are the selective strengthening and/or weakening of existing synaptic connections among nerve cells, or the formation of new connections and/or decay of old ones. Accordingly, measurements of possible changes in the brain have fallen into three general classes.

1. Changes in the overall dimensions of brain structures, or in the numbers and dimensions of nerve and glial cell bodies. Such alterations would reflect general growth or metabolic changes in the CNS.

2. Changes in the structure of individual synapses, such as size of the terminals or features of the synaptic interfaces. Such alterations would reflect strengthening or weakening of circuits.

3. Changes in the number of synapses in a given amount of brain tissue. Such alterations in the density of connectivity would reflect the formation or loss of synapses.

Early work by Hebb at Montreal and others had indicated that rats reared in complex environments were better maze learners than were laboratory-reared animals. Subsequently Rosenzweig at Berkeley and contemporaries developed what they called "enriched" rearing by bringing up young rats in groups in a large cage with various "toys" such as shown in Fig. 15-11. The toys were changed regularly, and in some experiments the immature rats were also trained on mazes. For comparison with this enriched nurturing procedure, other rats from the same litters (thereby minimizing effects of genetic and prior environmental differences) were raised either individually or in small groups in standard laboratory cages.

Examination of the brains of these animals revealed that certain regions of the cerebral cortex were thicker in the "enriched" rats than in those reared in isolation or in small groups. This difference was evident either when small areas

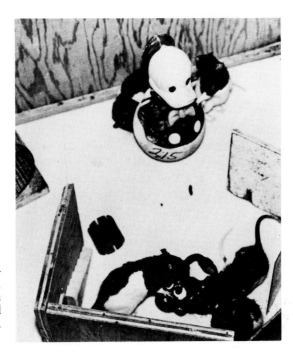

Fig. 15-11. Example of an "enriched" environment. (From Greenough, Wolkmar and Fleischman, "Behavior Control and Modification of Physiological Activity." Reprinted by permission of Prentice-Hall, Inc., Englewood Cliffs, New Jersey.)

of cortex were removed and weighed or when the depth of the cortex was measured microscopically. The effects were greatest (about 6% difference in weight) in the occipital (visual) region, although lesser differences were noted in other cortical areas, including somatosensory cortex. The differences in depth appeared to reflect true brain growth, rather than increased fluid content or some other swelling process. Evidence for such growth came from tissue analysis of enzyme activity and levels of RNA. The branching pattern of dendrites depends on the environment (Fig. 15-12). Synaptic connections are also remodeled, increasing and decreasing in highly specific ways. These findings showed that pronounced metabolic and structural effects could result from early experience.

It should be emphasized that "enriched" is a relative term. It is used relative to the standard laboratory situation. Wild rats probably lead quite considerably "richer" lives than their laboratory cousins could ever achieve, even in artificially enhanced environments. The constant changes in scene and threats to survival are matters that cannot be duplicated in a well-controlled animal room. Not surprisingly, therefore, rats reared in seminatural outdoor environments showed even greater brain effects than those in the enriched situation (Rosenzweig *et al.*, 1972).

These environmental effects, moreover, are not restricted to the newborn. Further chemical and anatomical studies have shown that such plasticity of the

IV. REMODELING OF NEURONAL CIRCUITRY   663

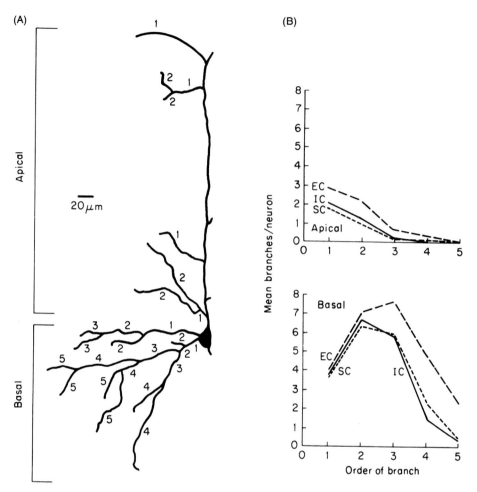

Fig. 15-12. Changes in the branching pattern of pyramidal neurons in rats reared in isolation (IC), in enriched (EC), or social (SC) environments. (A) shows half of the neuron with the order of branches away from the cell body designated. 1 is a primary branch, 2 a secondary branch, and so on. (B) indicates the number of these branches in layer V pyramidal neurons raised in the different environments. (Adapted from Greenough, 1975.)

cortex can occur at any age to varying degrees. The most dramatic changes are seen during development, but similar changes may also occur in adults. It has been found that the size of the cortex can decrease, as well as increase, at any age studied, even in rats 500 days old (Rosenzweig *et al.*, 1972; Cummins *et al.*, 1973). [These effects may have occurred against a decreasing baseline (see Feldman and Dowd, 1975; Vaughn, 1977; Diamond *et al.*, 1975).]

Thus it appears that environmental influences can rapidly change brain structure by modifying existing synapses, stimulating the formation (or loss) of others, altering neuronal size, or adjusting the number of glial cells. Such adjustments in response to the environment might reasonably be expected to serve an adaptive function. In Chapter 10 we have already described how specific changes in visual environment can change the visual system. We can now conclude that a multitude of environmental situations—sensory to social—can influence brain structure.

The brain is also sensitive to another environmental factor—diet. Although the adult brain is resistant to nutritional restrictions, the developing brain is not. Even mild undernutrition can produce widespread structural and functional modification at certain critical periods (Dobbing, 1968). In rat pups, for example, if the daily time of suckling is limited so that the pups are deprived of their normal milk supply, weight gain is retarded and development of the cerebellum (and perhaps other brain areas) permanently distorted. The overall size of the cerebellum is about 30% less, and microscopically there are fewer granule cells, while Purkinje cells have fewer and shorter dendritic segments (Fig. 15-13). The total

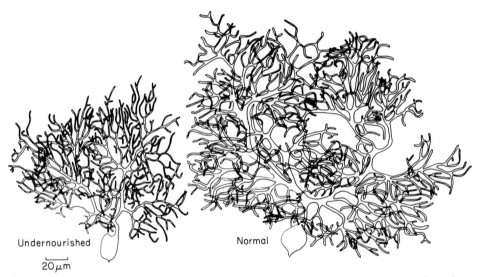

Undernourished   Normal

20 μm

Fig. 15-13. Effect of undernutrition on the development of Purkinje cell dendritic form (From McConnell and Berry, 1978.)

length of the Purkinje dendritic network, in fact, is reduced by 37%—a serious curtailment of the receptive properties of these key cerebellar cortical neurons (McConnell and Berry, 1978).

Such undernutrition probably alters RNA–DNA ratios and protein synthesis so that cells do not develop properly. The late-forming granule cells are particularly susceptible, but one must remember what we learned above: effects on one component during development can have repercussions on other components. The effects on Purkinje cell dendrites are due to loss of granule cells, as well as to direct effects upon Purkinje cell metabolism (McConnell and Berry, 1978).

Since the human brain continues to develop postnatally (and is supplied with copious additional numbers of granule cells and probably other small neurons at that time), similar changes may occur if infants do not receive adequate nourishment. The quality, as well as the quantity, of milk is important, particularly when infant formulas are substituted for breast milk. Many formulas are deficient in amino acids such as taurine. While no direct information is available to confirm or reject the rodent findings in humans, studies on animals and infants show that the amount of some bloodborne amino acids is lower, especially in premature offspring, with certain formulas. This may put the nervous system at a disadvantage (Rassin and Gaull, 1978).

B.   Axon Sprouting and Reactive Synaptogenesis

Another instance where neuronal circuitry is actively reorganized is after partial damage to the CNS. When a fraction of an input to a neuron or group of neurons is lost (the X in Fig. 15-14), the axons of the residual undamaged inputs often sprout and form new connections in place of those lost (the dashed line in Fig. 15-14). This phenomenon, _axon sprouting_, was first clearly identified in the 1950's in the peripheral nervous system. Following transection of a few motor fibers, those remaining sprouted new side branches and reinnervated the muscle (Edds, 1953; Hoffman, 1950). Subsequently this process was observed in autonomic ganglia (Murray and Thompson, 1957), spinal cord (Liu and Chambers, 1958), and brain (Raisman, 1969). It is now apparent that such synaptic replacement is widespread, occurring in both the peripheral and central nervous systems.

Studies on the reorganization of neuronal circuitry in response to damage are important for two reasons. First, they tell us how the brain may repair itself after injury. This ability has obvious clinical significance, but is also relevant to physiological psychology, where lesions are used to investigate the roles of brain areas in behavior. After such lesions, the rewiring of residual circuitry must be taken into account. Second, studies on neural plasticity tell us about the fundamental capacities of the brain to grow new synapses and adjust its circuitry. Perhaps such responses are restricted to repair, but possibly they can be induced in other ways.

We shall refer to this process of reorganization as _reactive synaptogenesis_ (Cotman and Lynch, 1976; Cotman and Nadler, 1978), to emphasize that it is a reaction to some stimulus—not a part of the normal course of neural development. Reactive synaptogenesis may involve axon sprouting, but the use of the latter term can lead to inappropriate or premature mechanistic inferences. In many cases, we cannot be sure what is happening. For example, the axons may not sprout new fibers, but only new terminals instead. Or the undamaged fibers may simply develop new swellings or varicosities.

Up to now practically all studies on reactive synaptogenesis have made use of lesions to investigate this phenomenon and its underlying mechanisms. Doubtless other stimuli are also effective in triggering it. Ultimately, these studies are expected to clarify the processes involved in the recovery of function after brain or spinal cord damage and the capacities of the normal CNS to respond to a wide variety of stimuli with new synaptic growth.

Reactive synaptogenesis is a highly selective process. Which fibers grow or in some way form new synapses? Which neurons are reinnervated, and at what age does it occur? To illustrate the basic findings we shall briefly consider what happens after partial interruption of the inputs to the *dentate gyrus*, a part of the region of the cerebral cortex known as the *hippocampus* (Cotman and Nadler, 1978) (see Fig. 15-14). The dentate gyrus is an associative area where a few inputs

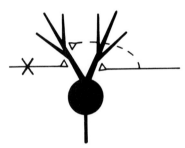

Fig. 15-14. Axon sprouting. Damage to a nerve fiber (X) causes the distal end to die. In response a nearby undamaged fiber sprouts new collaterals (dashed line) to replace the lost synapses.

converge on a single cell type—the granule cells, which like granule cells in the cerebellar cortex are extremely small. These inputs are arranged in a highly ordered manner, as shown in Fig. 15-15. In studying anything in the CNS, where so much complexity abounds, it is critically important to select a well-defined and relatively simple system. The dentate gyrus provides such a system.

Consider the events which follow removal of the entorhinal cortex in adult rats. This region provides 85% of the input to the outer three-quarters of the granule cell dendrites. The incoming fibers stay largely on the same side of the brain, so that the opposite side serves as a control and comparisons can be made in the same animal. Initially, loss of this key input leaves the granule cells with less than half their synapses (Fig. 15-16A). Such massive loss is transient, however; as shown, over a period of a few weeks new synapses grow and replace those lost.

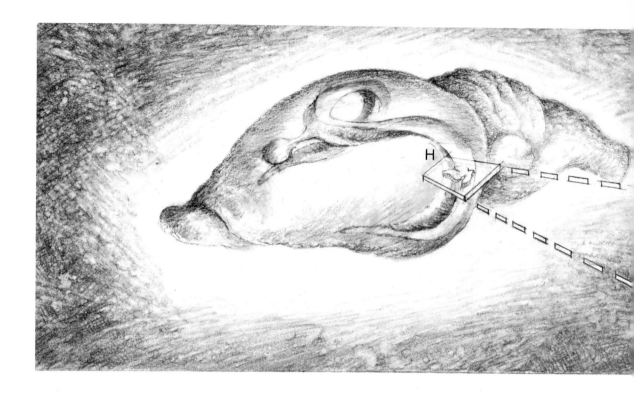

What fibers are responsible for the repopulation of synapses? Regeneration of the original entorhinal input is impossible, since these cells have been destroyed. The most straightforward restoration might be if the minor input from the opposite, the intact entorhinal cortex could proliferate new endings and recapture all the territory lost by the original, same-sided input. In fact, some such fibers do arrive and form functional contacts (Steward *et al.*, 1976), but cannot gain back all the old ground (Cotman *et al.*, 1977). Most of the new synapses come from septal inputs (from the region near the septum pellucidum) that are already there and from other crossed or associative fibers (the commissural–associational system) that normally make their synapses in the inner half of the dendritic tree. The latter system expands up the tree by about 140% and then, for unknown reasons, stops and forms a new boundary (Fig. 15-16B). Thus the granule cells receive a new arrangement of inputs built up from elements of the original circuitry.

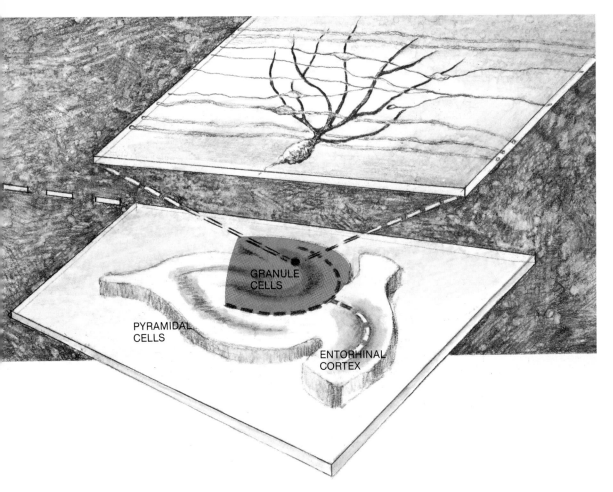

GRANULE
CELLS

PYRAMIDAL
CELLS

ENTORHINAL
CORTEX

THE HIPPOCAMPUS

Fig. 15-15. Diagram showing the position of the hippocampal formation in the rat brain and the organization of the major cell types. The hippocampus (H) appears as a bilaterally symmetrical curved structure underlying the cerebral cortex. The dentate gyrus (shaded area) is part of the hippocampal formation. The granule cells are the major cell type in the dentate gyrus. Their major projection is from the entorhinal cortex which overlies the dentate gyrus.

Changes in synapses after an entorhinal lesion

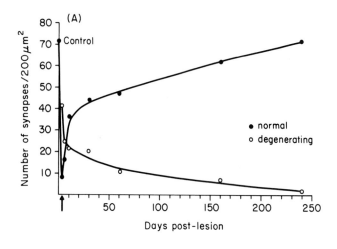

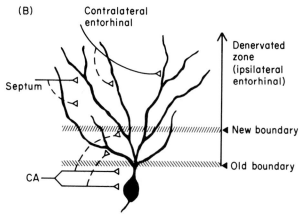

Fig. 15-16. Reactive synaptogenesis in the dentate gyrus. (A) Graph showing the disappearance (open circles) and reappearance (closed circles) of synapses over time following an entorhinal lesion. The number of synapses per unit area were counted from electron micrographs taken from the granule cell's dendritic field. (From Cotman and Nadler, 1978.) (B) Diagram illustrating the arrangement of the primary inputs to the granule cells before an entorhinal lesion and after reactive synaptogenesis is complete. The organization prior to the operation is shown by the solid lines. The commissural–associational (CA) projection is restricted to the inner one-quarter of the granule cell dendritic field. The primary projection to the outer three-quarters of the dendritic field is from the entorhinal cortex on the same side as that half of the hippocampus (i.e., the ipsilateral entorhinal cortex). There are also a few fibers from the septum and opposite (contralateral) entorhinal cortex. After destruction of the ipsilateral entorhinal cortex residual fibers proliferate (dashed lines) and establish a new organization. The CA projection, for example, grows outside its old boundary to establish a new one (see hatched lines).

1. MECHANISMS OF REACTIVE SYNAPTOGENESIS.   These can be summarized
in terms of five stages (Fig. 15-17).

a. Normal.   Normally, in the dentate gyrus and in most other brain regions, synapses form terminals as they pass by the dendritic spines. These terminals are called *boutons en passant*.

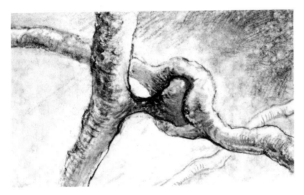

Fig. 15-17A

b. Degeneration.   Disconnection of the incoming axon from the parent
cell body (which has been destroyed by the experimental removal of the source of
the input) causes the axon and its boutons to degenerate. The earliest signs of this
breakdown are seen within a few hours, and by 2 days degenerating terminals (as
studied under the electron microscope) are extremely electron-dense and
shriveled up.

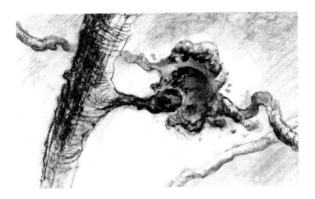

Fig. 15-17B

c. Glial reaction.   The few scattered neuroglial cells in the normal welter
of cells and fibers (*neuropil*) proliferate and extend their processes into the denervated zone. These cells remove degeneration products, stabilize the extracellular environment and perhaps give off signals which regulate neuronal
growth. Thus they prepare the neuropil for a rapid transition into the next stage.

IV. REMODELING OF NEURONAL CIRCUITRY

Figure 15-17C shows a glial cell removing a dying terminal, which it engulfs and digests. Sometimes, in its thoroughness, it ingests the spine and postsynaptic density of the target neuron as well as the moribund presynaptic element!

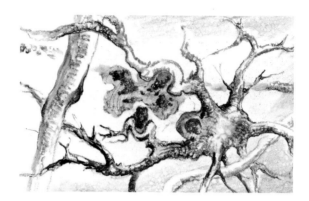

d. Sprouting. The remaining undamaged axons, stimulated by the loss of terminals, sprout new processes, and these go in search of a dendritic region that has a reduced number of synapses. In some cases the afferent fiber will locate an old, vacated synaptic site and reuse it. In other cases, a totally new synapse can form, including the construction of a new spine.

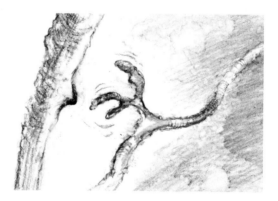

e. Synaptogenesis. The new synapses become functional in about 9 days. The ending can release transmitter, and that substance will successfully elicit a postsynaptic response. Many new synapses will continue to form until the normal complement is restored.

What allows some incoming fibers to grow and connect to specific parts of target neurons? The answer seems to lie in two fundamental mechanisms: the selective initiation of growth and the specification of synapse position.

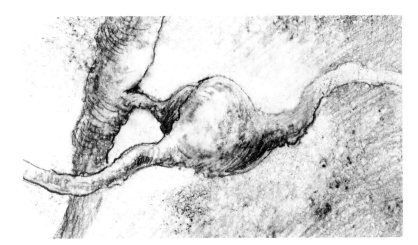

Fig. 15-17E

In the early literature (on axon sprouting in the peripheral nervous system) initiation of growth was thought to be catalyzed by diffusible substances (Hoffman and Springell, 1951). Furthermore, there are indications that growth-promoting factors that act upon other parts of the body may catalyze growth in the CNS as well (Björklund and Stenevi, 1972). In addition, however, active suppression as opposed to induction may regulate the growth of sprouts (Diamond *et al.*, 1976). Experiments carried out in the dentate gyrus of the hippocampus (Goldowitz and Cotman, 1977) and in the hindlimb of the salamander (Diamond *et al.* (1976)) support the *active suppression model*. It has been reasoned that perhaps axons normally release a substance which prevents the growth of other fibers into the zone of that axon. If this is the case, then a temporary block of the flow of that substance should allow collateral growth (growth of side branches) into the zone. To test this idea, colchicine, a substance which blocks axonal transport (flow of substances within a nerve fiber), was applied to a nerve with the hope of impeding the flow of presumed growth-suppressing substance. It was shown that colchicine transiently prevented transport of materials down the axon, but did not suppress electrical activity—nerve damage, therefore, was negligible. A few days after colchicine application, the neighboring incoming fibers were examined to see if they had formed sprouts and invaded the territory of the blocked axons (Fig. 15-18). Indeed, neighboring fibers had sprouted and formed new functional connections there.

Thus, experimental denervation usually serves as an important stimulus for

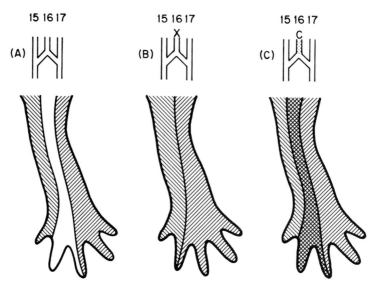

Fig. 15-18. Nerve territories in the dorsal skin of the salamander hindlimb. (A) Control limb in which the nerves of 15 and 17 do not meet. (B) Experimental limb in which nerve 16 has been cut showing enlargement of the fields of nerves 15 and 17. (C) Experimental limb in which nerve 16 has been treated with colchicine (C). Nerves 15 and 17 increased their populations of receptors. (After Diamond *et al.*, 1976. Copyright 1976 by the American Association for the Advancement of Science.)

fiber growth. But denervation per se is not a necessary prerequisite for reactive synaptogenesis. The foregoing experiments show that it can simply be a matter of blocking the flow of some critical substance down the axon. Denervation is especially effective, because the damaged input no longer releases suppressant factors that may tonically restrain fiber growth in the normal nervous system. Thus *damage* is central to the first mechanism.

At present we know very little about the second fundamental mechanism (about what specifies the position of synapses on denervated cells) compared to what we have learned about the first. Some type of recognition process must take place, but its nature is unknown.

2.   PRINCIPLES AND SIGNIFICANCE OF REACTIVE SYNAPTOGENESIS.   From the studies on the dentate gyrus described above and similar studies on other parts of the CNS, it is possible to derive a few general principles of reactive synaptogenesis in the brain (Cotman and Nadler, 1978). We need such rules to predict the events following natural or experimental damage to the nervous system and to elucidate underlying mechanisms.

1. The onset of functional recovery at physiological and behavioral levels usually coincides with the onset of reactive synaptogenesis.

2. The number of synapses formed on a given cell is determined primarily by

the cell itself, and reactive synaptogenesis can restore this value to normal.

3. Growth is initiated by factors released from the degenerating elements (the afferent fibers and their terminals) or from the denervated cells. These factors may be opposed by growth-retarding substances.

4. Reactive synaptogenesis is selective in that it results only in an increase in inputs already present on a neuron. No new pathways are created.

5. Fibers homologous to those removed do not always have the advantage in reinnervation. Other fiber systems, even those which employ other transmitters, may react.

6. Proximity to a denervated zone is a necessary, but insufficient, condition for reactive growth. Some potentially reactive fibers may not send sprouts or new terminals into an adjacent denervated zone, even if it is upon the very same neuron.

What is the significance of reactive synaptogenesis? In all systems that have been studied, a clearly aberrant pattern of connections is formed, and in some cases this produces abnormal behavior (McCouch *et al.*, 1958; Schneider, 1973). In other cases, however, the regrowth of new connections aids in the recovery from damage (Guth and Bernstein, 1961; Goldberger and Murray, 1978; Rsukahara, 1978). Each system has to be dealt with in the context of its own changes. Whatever the outcome of the particular changes in circuitry, it is clear that the adult brain has the capacity to dynamically reorganize its circuitry, and after brain damage this plasticity must be taken into account. For example, in physiological psychology lesions are often used to identify the brain structures that are necessary for certain behaviors. In interpreting the results of such selective destruction of brain components, one cannot assume that the only consequence has been the removal of those components. It must be kept in mind that after a period of time the residual circuitry may have been reorganized.

Studies on reactive synaptogenesis clearly demonstrate that the adult brain has an innate capacity to form new synapses in a highly selective manner. It would be surprising if this extraordinary ability were used only for the purpose of repair. Indeed, the finding that synaptogenesis can be induced in the absence of denervation supports the contention that neuronal circuitry continuously remodels itself (Sotelo and Palay, 1971), perhaps according to the balance of trophic materials in the environment. It seems that denervation studies bring out the extreme expression of the inherent plastic properties of the adult brain.

Thus reactive synaptogenesis, as the term implies, provides insights into the types of changes which can occur in the wiring of the brain, the mechanisms which underlie these changes, and the perturbations, both normal and pathological, which will elicit them. The challenge of the future is to narrow the gap between environmentally induced changes and those induced internally by denervation—by "snipping wires."

IV. REMODELING OF NEURONAL CIRCUITRY

C. Axonal Regeneration

The best way to restore lost function after nerve damage is to promote the regeneration of the lost connections. Note that regeneration is distinct and different from axon sprouting. In the former the damaged axons grow and reestablish their original connections (Fig. 15-19); whereas in the latter the nearby undamaged fibers grow and form new connections in place of those lost. _Axonal regeneration_ is common in the peripheral nervous system. After a severe cut, for example, we lose sensation in the tissue distal to the cut, but as the severed nerve fibers regenerate feelings return. Cutaneous fibers in particular can regenerate to very close to their original targets (Burgess and Horch, 1973).

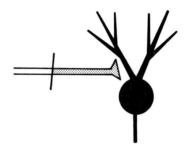

Fig. 15-19. Regeneration. In the strict sense regeneration can be said to occur when an axon is severed (line) and regrows to its original target (shaded area).

In the CNS the situation is quite different. The great neurohistologist Ramón y Cajal (1968), for example, transected the spinal cord of small mammals and observed that nerve fibers begin to regenerate across the cut surfaces but that within about 2 weeks the regenerating fibers succumb and die back. Growth then ceases, and consequently functional restitution cannot occur.

This general observation has been confirmed many times in mammals. Some regeneration takes place, but in no case is there definitive evidence for complete recovery of function after severance of the spinal cord (Bernstein *et al.*, 1978). Curiously, however, mammals seem to be different—perhaps unique—among vertebrates in their inability to regenerate spinal connections. If the spinal cord is transected in a teleost fish, for example, the cord regenerates and soon the fish swims as well as before.

Recently, research on regeneration in the CNS is being reevaluated: certain axons in mammalian brain and spinal cord *will* regenerate under certain circumstances, specifically ones in which artificial targets are held out to them. If a piece of extraneural tissue is implanted into the brain, the cut brain fibers near the implant will sometimes show a regenerative-like growth into it. For example, the medial forebrain bundle (a fiber bundle interconnecting the hypothalamus and the septum) was severed in a rat and an iris of the eye from a donor animal implanted into the transected area. A histochemical technique for noradrenergic fibers showed that the damaged fibers (in keeping with our definitions, see above) had grown into the implant (Björklund and Stenevi, 1971). In other cases, where other types of target tissues are implanted, cholinergic and possibly GABA-nergic fibers will "regenerate" (see Moore *et al.*, 1974) and in some cases functional synapses may be established (Björklund *et al.*, 1975).

These studies are not only significant, they are highly exciting. They show that regeneration (growth of *damaged* axons) can occur in the CNS, that it is specific, and that the CNS is a suitable medium to support such regrowth after all. At this time, however, it is not known whether central fibers can regenerate to their own natural targets, form working synapses and thus restore function. Moreover, regeneration seems (as far as is known) to be confined to only certain classes of fibers, such as local ones of small caliber. There has been no clear demonstration of the regeneration of long myelinated axons. Here is the greatest challenge, for it is the loss of these far-reaching fibers that is so devastating to integrated central neural function and behavior.

Implants have not been restricted to foreign nonneural or neural tissues. Prenatal brain tissue can be reimplanted into adult brain. As an example, the locus coeruleus (a cluster of noradrenergic cell bodies in the brain stem) was removed from a prenatal brain and reimplanted near the hippocampus of an adult rat (Björklund *et al.*, 1976). Remarkably, the implant remained viable. In fact, it formed an extensive net of fibers which grew down into the outer layer of the hippocampal dentate gyrus and formed there an extensive fiber plexus like that of the normal noradrenergic innervation from the locus (Fig. 15-20). In the normal brain, this innervation arrives from a great distance—from far down the brain stem.

The key factor underlying the success of this remarkable implant as a fiber source appears to be whether or not a vascular bed forms to nourish it. It is not known whether its outgoing fibers form functional synapses in the hippocampal region or whether it receives functional connections from other central areas. It must be remembered that the implant is embryonic tissue; no success has been reported to date on transplanting adult brain tissue into adult brain.

Finally, there is some evidence that regeneration and sprouting are incompatible and that sprouting can interfere with successful regeneration. In an autonomic (sympathetic) ganglion, for example, local sprouting reduces the number of fibers that can regenerate effectively and form functional connections (Roper, 1978). It would appear that, in some cases at least, target neurons can take on only a given number of inputs. Thus the sprouts, which grow faster, fare better than the slowly progressing regenerating fibers. It is quite possible that sprouting suppresses regeneration in the CNS as well (Raisman, 1969).

IV. REMODELING OF NEURONAL CIRCUITRY

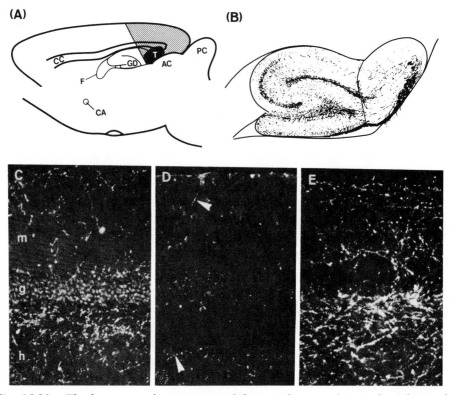

Fig. 15-20. The locus coeruleus is removed from embryos and transplanted into the entorhinal area after removal of the entorhinal area. Animals were subjected to an intracranial sympathectomy and were given 6-hydroxydopamine in order to destroy intrinsic norepinephrine fibers. This aids in the visualization of the regenerating fibers from the implant. (A) Relationship of the implant in the entorhinal cortex (T) to the hippocampus (GD) in the animal. (B) A norepinephrine transplant after 3 months survival. Fibers from the neural transplant have grown towards the hippocampus and formed an extensive fiber meshwork throughout it. (C), (D), and (E) show in detail the dorsal part of the dentate gyrus in normal (C), 6-hydroxydopamine treated (D), and implanted rats (E). (From Bjorklund *et al.*, 1976.)

In summary, despite the encouraging recent developments in the field of CNS regeneration, it is clear that the capacity of the brain and spinal cord to regenerate is much less than that of the peripheral nerves. Nevertheless, all CNS regeneration is not abortive, as once thought. Catecholaminergic and cholinergic fibers certainly will regenerate. It may be that growth and reestablishment of such fibers reflect a normal process which takes place from birth to death as these neurotransmitter subsystems alter their functional circuitry. The great unsolved mysteries are: Why do myelinated axons not regenerate and reestablish lasting functional connections with their original targets, and, more importantly, how can these stern restrictions be overcome?

V. Aging of Neuronal Circuitry

What changes, if any, take place in the nervous system of the aged? We all recognize the symptoms of aging: selective impairment of memory, increased failure in problem solving, mental fatigue and difficulties in perceiving certain stimuli. There are many general notions on aging, but none directed toward explaining specific deficits, such as those in learning. These, of course, cannot come until the mechanisms of such mental functions are elucidated.

One well-known correlate of aging is that certain neurons die. In the substantia nigra of the midbrain, for example, there is a progressive loss of those dopaminergic neurons that send their axons up to the basal ganglia (McGeer *et al.*, 1977). These are the neurons which, if they fail to provide sufficient transmitter, play such a critical role in Parkinson's disease (see Chapter 6). The nigra of a 25-year-old person contains about 400,000 dopamine neurons (Fig. 15-21), yet an 80-year-old person has only half this number—a mighty loss. Such cell death leads to a loss of synaptic connections and a reduction in the normal redundancy of neuronal circuitry.

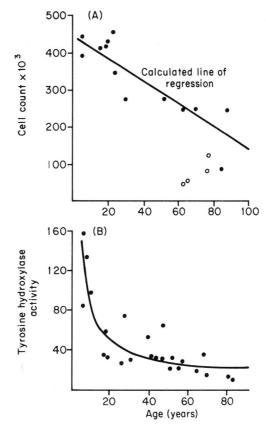

Fig. 15-21. (A) Cell counts in substantia nigra of humans plotted against age. (B) Tyrosine hydroxylase (TH) activities as function of age in basal ganglia of humans dying without neurological illness. Individual values also shown for TH. Measurements for TH in nanomoles per hour per 100 mg of protein (Data from McGeer *et al.*, 1977. Copyright 1977 by the American Medical Association.)

The decrement in number of terminals can be examined by measuring one of the enzymes involved in the synthesis of dopamine—tyrosine hydroxylase. Other nigral neurons do not synthesize dopamine or related molecules, so that they do not have this enzyme. As shown in Fig. 15-21, tyrosine hydroxylase also decreases with age. Aging of this connection from the substantia nigra to the basal ganglia (the nigrostriatal tract) appears to be a general feature of the mammalian brain, since it occurs in laboratory animals as well as humans (Finch, 1973; Jonec and Finch, 1975).

Selective nerve cell loss, however, is not the only correlate of aging. There is also reduced blood flow, and this can be almost as severe a limitation to neural activity, if not more so. Blood flow in the human CNS can be studied by injecting radioactive substances (such as xenon-133) into the internal carotid artery (which directly supplies the head) and charting its passage through the brain. The pattern of brain radioactivity is analyzed by a computer and displayed on an oscilloscope screen. In an aged person, brain blood flow is markedly reduced, as is the utilization of oxygen, which is only three-quarters of that in younger persons (Sokoloff, 1976).

Other changes implicated in aging are reductions in sensory receptors. In the ear they degenerate and impair hearing, for example. Accumulation of enzyme molecules lacking in activity and decreased rates of metabolic processes involved in stimulus response are also described (Adelman, 1970; Adelman and Freeman, 1972), and even reactive synaptogenesis, which still can occur, is slower in the aged (Cotman and Scheff, 1978). Finally, it has been suggested that there are changes of gene expression in the old brain, but this has not been confirmed experimentally.

Aging in mammals seems to result from a constellation of causes. It is not unlike the operation of an old automobile. When the car is driven at top speed, or raced up to speed from a standstill, its age shows, and it is more prone to problems—signs of which show up when stressed. In the entire body, including the CNS, the fine tuning and balance are worn.

Some other animals, however, grow old and die in peculiar ways—sometimes without aging. Take the octopus, for example. Curiously, it dies in its prime. The female dies soon after her eggs hatch, and the male lives only a few months past sexual maturity. There are no old-age problems, social security or despair for the octopus! In them, it appears that death is programmed; they have a "self-destruct" system. Secretions from a pair of endocrine bodies (the optic glands) seem to set the time of death. When these glands are removed, both males and females live longer (Wodinsky, 1977).

How some humans, through exercise, diet, the power of positive thinking or whatever, are able to forestall aging and prolong vitality is outside the scope of this chapter, if not our understanding. But it is now clear that normal aging is distinctly different from senility. Senility is a disease; in fact, it is generally known as *Alzheimer's disease*, an affliction of great frequency affecting upward of 6% of the total population (Selkoe, 1978). Those afflicted show deficits in problem solving, learning, remembering and speaking. What is worse, they experience a progressive disorganization and deterioration of personality. As the disease progresses there is often a severe failure to recognize people and objects. For example, a physician showed a man who had Alzheimer's disease a photograph of a voluptuous red-headed woman in a bikini. The patient did not recognize the image as that of a woman. At other times, however, such recognitions can be made, often when least expected. Moments of great clarity may come and go, like patches of youth amid the heavy burden of the disease.

What is the basis of this disease? As is the case with normal aging, there seem to be many aspects to Alzheimer's disease. One of the hallmarks to the neuropathologist is the presence of numerous *plaques* and tangles in the senile brain (Fig. 15-22). The healthy aged brain, in contrast, shows few such plaques. These distinctive structures, interspersed among the brain's nerve cells, consist of crystalline-like deposits of protein. In addition, the cytoplasm of the neurons themselves commonly contains abnormal twisted tubular structures: proteins related to the normal cytoskeletal network which have become tangled. These tubular or fibrillar structures are so prominent in silver-impregnated pieces of brain tissue as seen in the light microscope that the disease historically has been known as Alzheimer's neurofibrillary cell change. Despite its striking microscopic pathology, the molecular cause of this widespread disorder is still unknown (Selkoe, 1978). Various factors (from the accumulation of trace metals such as aluminum to disease of the body's autoimmune system) have been suggested, but no clear cause has been identified, nor has prevention of the disease or reduction of its terrible consequences for human beings been found.

VI. The Saga of Neuronal Circuitry: Summary and Conclusions

In the beginning, the nervous system is only a membrane—a layer of cells. But by birth these cells have proliferated, organized themselves and begun to connect into what will become the most complex organization in the universe. We have witnessed, in the cerebellar cortex, many of the basic principles of construction and viewed the growth and modeling of this beautiful cellular assembly. The structures formed in this cortex may be highly stereotyped, but they can be molded by environmental stimuli, hormones in the awakening body and perhaps other influences. It is as if the brain builds small but important modifications into

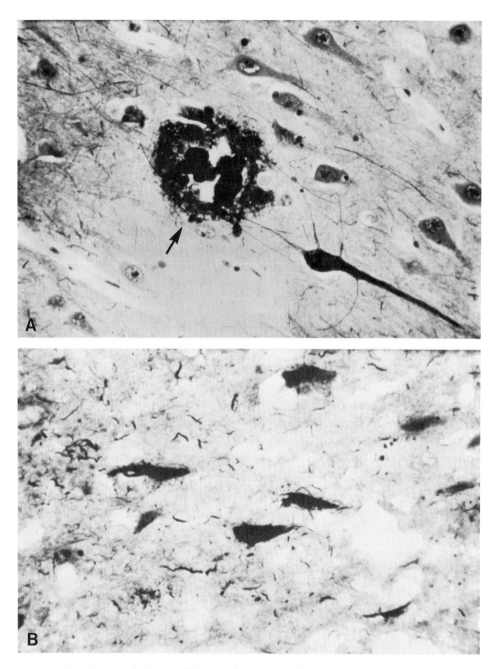

Fig. 15-22. Neuronal abnormalities in the temporal cortex in a patient who died from senile dementia as revealed by the Bielschowsky stain. Affected neurons or tangles of neurofibrillary degeneration stain very darkly. (A) A large extracellular senile plaque (arrow). A degenerating neuron (stained dark) has processes which contribute to the senile plaque. Normal neurons (small arrow) do not pick up the stain. (B) Darkly stained neurons indicating the cells contain neurofibrillary tangles. (Courtesy of Dr. D. Selkoe.)

its circuitry in accordance with the challenges to it as it develops. The brain meets these challenges with subtle changes in design, but it does meet them.

Such modifications are most readily seen in development, but the adult nervous system also seems amenable to remodeling, even though many constraints have by now been placed upon it from without and within. In reactive synaptogenesis and selective regeneration of severed connections, we get some insight into its capabilities for plasticity, into its repertoire of ways to repair lost functions—into its yearnings, as it were, to meet all the challenges that come its way during our lifetime.

This tale does not end in adult mammals, but runs its full course in the aged. In old animals, and in old people, neurons die at a tremendous, truly frightening, rate, and function progressively deteriorates along with crumbling circuitry. The story of the nervous system, then, can only be called a saga. The brain is born in a flash of majesty, it lives in an ever-changing, subtle and mysterious way, and it decays in some cases with tragedy.

Key Terms

Active suppression model of synaptogenesis: A model in which new synapse formation in the mature nervous system is restrained by the presence of suppression factors released from intact nerve fibers.

Alzheimer's disease: An affliction which produces senility. The brain of a person with the disease shows the presence of numerous plaques and tangles (neurofibrillary tangles).

Axonal regeneration: The regrowth of damaged axons and the reestablishment of their original connections.

Axon extension: The process by which axons extend from the cell body and grow toward their point of termination.

Axon sprouting: Growth of new axonal branches in reaction to denervation or similar stimuli; a specific type of reactive synaptogenesis.

Axon trailing: A process by which the cell body migrates and leaves its axon behind.

Basket cells: Small, local-circuit neurons which drop basket-like entanglements of synapses over Purkinje cell bodies.

Bipolar cells: A cell with two processes. In the development of the cerebellum, young granule cells, as they form from the external granular layer, are called bipolar cells.

Chemoaffinity model: A mechanism for the formation of specific connections; appropriate recognition depends on a selective affinity, or matching, of cell membrane surfaces.

Climbing fibers: One of the major excitatory inputs to the cerebellum; climbing fibers synapse on the main dendritic shafts of Purkinje cells.

Contact guidance: A type of mechanism in which a growing process uses another already developed structure as a guide to reach its final destination.

Denervation supersensitivity: An increase in responsiveness to transmitter as a result of loss of nerve input. At a neuromuscular junction, muscle becomes sensitive to transmitter along its entire length.

Dentate gyrus: A part of the hippocampus.

Differentiation: The developmental process by which a cell assumes its characteristic form, cytology and chemistry.

External granular layer: A thin layer of proliferating cells covering the surface of the cerebellum which give rise to granule cells and basket cells.

Granular layer: The layer containing the granule cells.

Granule cells: Small cells found in the cerebellum which give rise to the parallel fibers.

Induction: In embryology, the process by which factors cause undifferentiated cells to differentiate.

Molecular layer: The outer, cortical zone of the cerebellum consisting primarily of Purkinje cell dendrites and parallel fibers.

Mossy fibers: The name of major input to the granule cells in the cerebellum; so-named because of mosslike boutons at their tips.

Neurulation: The process by which the neural plate dips into a trough and then rolls itself into a tube.

Parallel fibers: The axons of the granule cells; they provide the major input to the Purkinje cells.

Plaques: A crystallinelike deposit of protein interspersed among the brain's nerve cells in people with Alzheimer's disease.

Progressive determination: The concept that the final destiny of a cell is established by a series of choices made in the course of its development.

Purkinje cells: The large output cells of the cerebellum which have planar, fanlike dendritic arborizations.

Reactive synaptogenesis: Synapse formation which is not a normal part of neural development initiated in reaction to a stimulus (denervation, for example).

Trophic interactions: The influence a nerve has on its targets other than by direct electrical communication; a nutritive effect necessary for the target to maintain its normal properties.

General References

Altman, J. (1967). Postnatal growth and differentiation of the mammalian brain, with implications for a morphological theory of memory. *In* "The Neurosciences: A Study Program" (G. C. Quarton, T. Melnechuk, and F. O. Schmitt, eds.), pp. 723–743. Rockefeller Univ. Press, New York.

Carpenter, M. B. (1976). "Human Neuroanatomy," 7th ed. Williams & Wilkins, Baltimore, Maryland.

Cotman, C. W., ed. (1978). "Neuronal Plasticity." Raven, New York.

Cotman, C. W., and Banker, G. (1974). The making of a synapse. *In* "Reviews of Neuroscience" (S. Ehrenpreis and I. Kopin, eds.), Vol. 1, pp. 1–62. Raven, New York.

Diamond, M. C. (1978). The aging brain: Some enlighting and optimistic results. *Am. Sci.* **66**, 66–71.

Finch, C. E. (1976). The regulation of physiological changes during mammalian aging. *Q. Rev. Biol.* **51**, 49–83.

Greenough, W. T. (1975). Experiential modification of the developing brain. *Am. Sci.* **63**, 37–46.

Jacobson, M. (1970). "Developmental Neurobiology." Holt, New York.

Palay, S. L., and Chan-Palay, V. (1974). "Cerebellar Cortex: Cytology and Organization." Springer-Verlag, Berlin and New York.

Sidman, R. L. (1974). Cell-cell recognition in the developing central nervous system. *In* "The Neurosciences: Third Study Program" (F. O. Schmitt and F. G. Worden, eds.), pp. 743–758. MIT Press, Cambridge, Massachusetts.

References

Addison, W. H. F. (1911). The development of the Purkinje cells and of the cortical layers in the cerebellum of the albino rat. *J. Comp. Neurol.* **21**, 459–485.

Adelman, R. C. (1970). An age-dependent modification of enzyme regulation. *J. Biol. Chem.* **245**, 1032–1035.

Adelman, R. C., and Freeman, C. (1972). Age-dependent regulation of glucokinase and tyrosine aminotransferase activities of rat liver *in vivo* by adrenal, pancreatic and pituitary hormones. *Endocrinology* **90**, 1551–1560.

Albuquerque, E. X., Schuh, F. T., and Kauffman, F. C. (1971). Early membrane depolarization of the fast mammalian muscle after denervation. *Pfluegers Arch.* **328**, 36–50.

Altman, J. (1972a). Postnatal development of the cerebellar cortex in the rat. II. Phases in the maturation of Purkinje cells and of the molecular layer. *J. Comp. Neurol.* **145**, 399–464.

Altman, J. (1972b). Postnatal development of the cerebellar cortex in the rat. III. Maturation of the components of the granular layer, *J. Comp. Neurol.* **145**, 465–514.

Altman, J. (1973). Experimental reorganization of the cerebellar cortex III. Regeneration of the external germinal layer and granule cell ectopia. *J. Comp. Neurol.* **149**, 153–179.

Altman, J., and Anderson, W. J. (1971). Irradiation of the cerebellum in infant rats with low-level X-ray: Histological and cytological effects during infancy and adulthood. *Exp. Neurol.* **30**, 492–509.

Altman, J., and Anderson, W. J. (1973). Experimental reorganization of the cerebellar cortex. II. Effects of elimination of most microneurons with prolonged X-irradiation started at four days. *J. Comp. Neurol.* **149**, 123–152.

Axelsson, J., and Thesleff, S. (1959). A study of supersensitivity in denervated mammalian skeletal muscle. *J. Physiol. (London)* **147**, 178–193.

Barondes, S. A. (1976). "Neuronal Recognition." Raven, New York.

Bernstein, J. J., Wells, M. R., and Bernstein, M. E. (1978). Spinal cord regeneration: Synaptic renewal and neurochemistry. *In* "Neuronal Plasticity" (C. Cotman, ed.), pp. 49–71. Raven, New York.

Björklund, A., and Stenevi, U. (1971). Growth of central catecholamine neurons into smooth muscle grafts in the rat mesencephalon. *Brain Res.* **31**, 1–20.

Björklund, A., Johansson, B., Stenevi, U., and Svendgaard, N.-Aa. (1975). Reestablishment of functional connections by regenerating central adrenergic and cholinergic axons. *Nature (London)* **253**, 446–448.

Björklund, A., Stenevi, U., and Svendgaard, N.-Aa. (1976). Growth of transplanted monoaminergic neurones into the adult hippocampus along the perforant path. *Nature (London)* **262**, 787–790.

Bradley, P., and Berry, M. (1976). The effects of reduced climbing and parallel fibre input on purkinje cell dendritic growth. *Brain Res.* **109**, 133–151.

Buller, A. J., Eccles, J. C., and Eccles, R. M. (1960). Interactions between motoneurones and muscles in respect of the characteristic speeds of their responses. *J. Physiol. (London)* **150**, 417–439.

Burgess, P. R., and Horch, K. W. (1973). Specific regeneration of cutaneous fibers in the cat. *J. Neurophysiol.* **36**, 101–114.

Carpenter, M. B. (1976). "Human Neuroanatomy," 7th ed. Williams & Wilkins, Baltimore, Maryland.

Close, R. I. (1972). Dynamic properties of mammalian skeletal muscles. *Physiol. Rev.* **52**, 129–197.

Cotman, C., Gentry, C., and Steward, O. (1977). Synaptic replacement in the dentate gyrus after unilateral entorhinal lesion: Electron microscopic analysis of the extent of replacement of synapses by the remaining entorhinal cortex. *J. Neurocytol.* **6**, 455–464.

Cotman, C. W., and Lynch, G. S. (1976). Reactive synaptogenesis in the adult nervous system: The effects of partial deafferentation on new synapse formation. *In* "Neuronal Recognition" (S. Barondes, ed.), pp. 69–108. Plenum, New York.

Cotman, C. W., and Nadler, J. V. (1978). Reactive synaptogenesis in the hippocampus. *In* "Neuronal Plasticity" (C. W. Cotman, ed.). pp. 227–272. Raven, New York.

Cotman, C. W., and Scheff, S. W. (1978). Compensatory synapse growth in aged animals after neuronal death. *In* "Mechanisms of Ageing and Development" (B. L. Strehler, ed.) pp. 103–117. Elsevier, Amsterdam.

Cummins, R. A., Walsh, R. N., Budtz-Olsen, O. E., Konstantinos, T., and Horsfall, C. R. (1973). Environmentally-induced changes in the brains of elderly rats. *Nature (London)* **243**, 516–518.

Das, G. D., and Nornes, H. C. (1972). Neurogenesis in the cerebellum of the rat: An autoradiographic study. *Z. Anat. Entwicklungs gesch.* **138**, 155–165.

Deshpande, S. S., Albuquerque, E. X., and Guth, L. (1976). Neurotrophic regulation of prejunctional and postjunctional membrane at the mammalian motor endplate. *Exp. Neurol.* **53**, 151–165.

Diamond, J., Cooper, E., Turner, C., and Macintyre, L. (1976). Trophic regulation of nerve sprouting. *Science* **193**, 371–377.

Diamond, M. C. (1978). The aging brain: Some enlighting and optimistic results. *Am. Sci.* **66**, 66–71.

Diamond, M. C., Johnson, R. E., and Ingham, C. A. (1975). Morphological changes in the young, adult and aging rat cerebral cortex, hippocampus and diencephalon. *Behav. Biol.* **14**, 163–174.

Dobbing, J. (1968). Vulnerable periods in developing brain. *In* "Applied Neurochemistry" (A. N. Davison and J. Dobbing, eds.), pp. 287–316. Davis, Philadelphia, Pennsylvania.

Drachman, D. B., and Witzke, F. (1972). Trophic regulation of acetylcholine sensitivity of muscle: Effect of electrical stimulation. *Science* **176**, 514–516.

Edds, M. V., Jr. (1953). Collateral nerve regeneration. *Q. Rev. Biol.* **28**, 260–276.

Feldman, M. L., and Dowd, C. (1975). Loss of dendritic spines in aging cerebral cortex. *Anat. Embryol.* **148**, 279–301.

Finch, C. E. (1973). Catecholamine metabolism in the brains of ageing male mice. *Brain Res.* **52**, 261–276.

Goldberger, M. E., and Murray, M. (1974). Restitution of function and collateral sprouting in the cat spinal cord: The deafferented animal. *J. Comp. Neurol.* **158**, 37–54.

Goldowitz, D., and Cotman, C. W. (1977). Does neurotrophic material control synapse formation in the adult rat brain? *Neurosci. Abstr. (Soc. Neurosci.)* **3**, 534.

Greenough, W. T. (1975). Experiential modification of the developing brain. *Am. Sci.* **63**, 37–46.

Greenough, W. T., Wolkmar, F. R., and Fleischman, T. B. (1976). Environmental effects on brain connectivitiy and behavior. *In* "Behavior Control and Modification of Physiological Activity" (D. I. Mostofsky, ed.), pp. 220–245. Prentice-Hall, Englewood Cliffs, New Jersey.

Guth, L., and Bernstein, J. J. (1961). Selectivity in the re-establishment of synapses in the superior cervical sympathetic ganglion of the cat. *Exp. Neurol.* **4**, 59–69.

Hoffman, H. (1950). Local reinnervation in partially denervated muscle: A histophysiological study. *Aust. J. Exp. Biol. Med. Sci.* **28**, 383–397.

Hoffman, H., and Springell, P. H. (1951). An attempt at the chemical identification of "neurocletin" (the substance evoking axon sprouting). *Aust. J. Exp. Biol. Med. Sci.* **29**, 417–424.

Jacobson, M. (1970). "Developmental Neurobiology." Holt, New York.

Jonec, V., and Finch, C. E. (1975). Ageing and dopamine uptake by subcellular fractions of the C57BL/6J male mouse brain. *Brain Res.* **91**, 197–215.

Lauder, J. M. (1977). Effects of thyroid state on development of rat cerebellar cortex. *In* "Thyroid Hormones and Brain Development" (G. D. Grave, ed.), pp. 235–252. Raven, New York.

Liu, C. N., and Chambers, W. W. (1958). Intraspinal sprouting of dorsal root axons: Development of new collaterals and preterminals following partial denervation of the spinal cord in the cat. *AMA Arch. Neurol. Psychiatry* **79**, 46–61.

Lømo, T., and Rosenthal, J. (1972). Control of ACh sensitivity by muscle activity in the rat. *J. Physiol. (London)* **221**, 493–513.

Lømo, T., and Westgaard, R. H. (1975). Further studies on the control of ACh sensitivity by muscle activity in the rat. *J. Physiol. (London)* **252**, 603–626.

Lopresti, V., Macagno, E. R., and Levinthal, C. (1973). Structure and development of neuronal connections in isogenic organisms: Cellular interactions in the development of the optic lamina of *Daphnia*. *Proc. Natl. Acad. Sci. U.S.A.* **70**, 433–437.

McConnell, P., and Berry, M. (1978). The effects of undernutrition on Purkinje cell dendritic growth in the rat. *J. Comp. Neurol.* **177**, 159–171.

McCouch, G. P., Austin, G. M., Liu, C. N., and Liu, C. Y. (1958). Sprouting as a cause of spasticity. *J. Neurophysiol.* **21**, 205–216.

McGeer, P. L., McGeer, E. G., and Suzuki, J. S. (1977). Aging and extrapyramidal function. *Arch. Neurol. (Chicago)* **34**, 33–35.

Moore, R. Y., Björklund, A., and Stenevi, U. (1974). Growth and plasticity of adrenergic neurons. *In* "The Neurosciences: Third Study Program" (F. O. Schmitt and F. G. Worden, eds.), pp. 961–978. MIT Press, Cambridge, Massachusetts.

Murray, J. G., and Thompson, J. W. (1957). The occurrence and function of collateral sprouting in the sympathetic nervous system of the cat. *J. Physiol. (London)* **135**, 133–162.

Oh, T. H. (1975). Neurotrophic effects: Characterization of the nerve extract that stimulates muscle development in culture. *Exp. Neurol.* **46**, 432–438.

Oh, T. H., Johnson, D. D., and Kim, S. U. (1972). Neurotrophic effect on isolated chick embryo muscle in culture. *Science* **178**, 1298–1300.

O'Leary, J. L., Inukai, J., and Smith, J. M. (1971). Histogenesis of the cerebellar climbing fiber in the rat. *J. Comp. Neurol.* **142**, 377–392.

Palay, S. L., and Chan-Palay, V. (1974). "Cerebellar Cortex: Cytology and Organization." Springer-Verlag, Berlin and New York.

Privat, A. (1975). Dendritic growth *in vitro*. *Adv. Neurol.* **12**, 201–216.

Purves, D. (1976). Long-term regulation in the vertebrate peripheral nervous system. *Int. Rev. Physiol.* **10**, 125–177.

Raisman, G. (1969). Neuronal plasticity in the septal nuclei of the adult rat. *Brain Res.* **14**, 25–48.

Rakic, P. (1971). Neuron-glia relationship during granule cell migration in developing cerebellar cortex. A golgi and electronmicroscopic study in *Macacus rhesus*. *J. Comp. Neurol.* **141**, 283–312.

Rakic, P., and Sidman, R. L. (1970). Histogenesis of cortical layers in human cerebellum, particularly the lamina dessicans. *J. Comp. Neurol.* **139**, 473–500.

Rakic, P., and Sidman, R. L. (1973). Sequence of developmental abnormalities leading to granule cell deficit in cerebellar cortex of weaver mutant mice. *J. Comp. Neurol.* **152**, 103–132.

Ramón y Cajal, S. (1968). "Degeneration and Regeneration of the Nervous System" (transl. by R. M. May). Hafner, New York.

Rassin, D. K., and Gaull, G. E. (1977). Protein requirements and the development of amino acid metabolism in the preterm infant. *In* "AMA Clinical Nutrition Update: Amino Acids" (H. L. Greene, M. A. Holiday, H. N. Munro, eds.), pp. 84–97. Am. Med. Assn., Chicago, Illinois.

Rees, R. P., Bunge, M. B., and Bunge, R. P. (1976). Morphological changes in the neuritic growth cone and target neuron during synaptic junction development in culture. *J. Cell Biol.* **68**, 240–263.

Roper, S. (1978). Synaptic remodelling in the partially denervated parasympathetic ganglion in the heart of the frog. *In* "Neuronal Plasticity" (C. W. Cotman, ed.). pp. 1–26. Raven, New York.

Rosenzweig, M. R., and Bennett, E. L. (1976). Enriched environments: Facts, factors, and fantasies. *In* "Knowing, Thinking, and Believing" (L. Petrinovich and J. L. McGaugh, eds.), pp. 179–213. Plenum, New York.

Rosenzweig, M. R., Bennett, E. L., and Diamond, M. C. (1972). Brain changes in response to experience. *Sci. Press* **226**, 22–29.

Schneider, G. E. (1973). Early lesions of superior colliculus: Factors affecting the formation of abnormal retinal projections. *Brain, Behav. Evol.* **8**, 73–109.

Selkoe, D. J. (1978). Cerebral aging and dementia. *In* "Current Neurology" (H. R. Tyler and D. M. Dawson, eds.) pp. 360–387. Houghton, Boston, Massachusetts.

Smalheiser, N. R., and Crain, S. M. (1978). Formation of functional retinotectal connections in co-cultures of fetal mouse explants. *Brain Res.* **148**, 484–492.

Sokoloff, L. (1976). Circulation and energy metabolism of the brain. *In* "Basic Neurochemistry" (G. J. Siegel *et al.*, eds.), 2nd ed., pp. 388–413. Little, Brown, Boston, Massachusetts.

Sotelo, C., and Palay, S. L. (1971). Altered axons and axon terminals in the lateral vestibular nucleus of the rat. *Lab. Invest.* **25**, 653–671.

Spemann, H. (1938). "Embryonic Development and Induction." Yale Univ. Press, New Haven, Connecticut.

Sperry, R. W. (1963). Chemoaffinity in the orderly growth of nerve fiber patterns and connections. *Proc. Natl. Acad. Sci. U.S.A.* **50**, 703–710.

Steward, O., Cotman, C., and Lynch, G. (1976). A quantitative autoradiographic and electrophysiological study of the reinnervation of the dentate gyrus by the contralateral entorhinal cortex following ipsilateral entorhinal lesions. *Brain Res.* **114**, 181–200.

Tsukahara, N. (1978). Synaptic plasticity in the red nucleus. *In* "Neuronal Plasticity" (C. W. Cotman, ed.) pp. 113–130. Raven, New York.

Vaughn, D. W. (1977). Age-related deterioration of pyramidal cell basal dendrites in rat auditory cortex. *J. Comp. Neurol.* **171**, 501–516.

West, M. J., and Del Cerro, M. (1976). Early formation of synapses in the molecular layer of the fetal rat cerebellum. *J. Comp. Neurol.* **165**, 137–160.

Wodinsky, J. (1977). Hormonal inhibition of feeding and death in octopus: Control by optic gland secretion. *Science* **198**, 948–951.

16

Development of Behavior

The nervous system continues to develop and change throughout an individual's lifetime. It is obvious from experience that behavior also continues to develop and change. Different species of animals develop different behaviors, and the behavior of animals of a particular species changes with age. The behavior of a cat is obviously different from that of a bird, and so is the behavior of a kitten and a newly hatched bird different from that of their parents. Further, although cats behave like cats and birds like birds, there are, at all ages, large individual differences in behavior of animals of the same species.

The development of the nervous system and the resulting behavior is, as is emphasized throughout this book, subject to many influences. The initial influence is, of course, genetic. From the moment of conception an individual's genetic makeup initiates and regulates development and sets ultimate morphological and behavioral constraints. However, influences other than genes also begin to influence development from the moment of conception. While individuals of the same species have similar genetic makeup and environments, no two individuals experience the same environment, and except for monozygotic twins and clones no two individuals are alike genetically. Differences in genetic makeup and environmental influences lead to different patterns of neural and behavioral development. The result is not a simple summation of genetic and environmental influences. An environmental influence may have markedly different effects on individuals with different genetic makeup. Thus, throughout life the genes and environment work together to create variety in the midst of similarities.

In this chapter, we consider some of the processes that influence the development of behavior. We begin with a discussion of genetic and hormonal influences and then consider the role of environmental influences.

I. Single Gene Influences on Behavior

There is considerable evidence that individual differences in the nervous system and behavior can result from differences in a single gene. In humans, for example, the ability to taste the substance phenylthiocarbamide and the ability to distinguish the complementary colors red and green are known to be based on differences in single _genes_, or, more precisely, on the different versions of a gene, called _alleles_, at a single genetic locus. Classical Mendelian genetic techniques are used to determine the number of genes involved in a trait, which alleles of the gene are dominant or recessive, and whether the genes are on the sex-determining (X or Y) _chromosomes_. In humans, the analyses are based on studies of relatives. In primates, the analyses are generally based on systematic breeding studies.

Such mating experiments were used to investigate the genetic control of _"hygienic behavior"_ in bees. Rothenbuhler (1964) observed that some colonies of bees controlled disease by uncapping the cells of diseased larvae and removing the larvae from the hive. A genetic analyses revealed that this highly complex behavior is controlled by just two genes, one controlling uncapping and one controlling removal of the larvae. The complete behavior is carried out only by bees that have two _recessive_ alleles (recessive _homozygotes_) for each of the two genes. Bees that have one dominant allele for each gene (_heterozygotes_) are completely nonhygienic. Bees that have a dominant allele for one gene and recessive alleles for the other gene will either uncap the cells or remove the larvae, depending

690

upon the gene in which a dominant allele suppresses the behavior. They will not do both. Thus the complete behavior requires a sequence of behavior which is based on two separate genes.

Another approach for studying single genes and behavior is to compare the behavior of animals carrying a mutant allele of a gene with the behavior of animals that have the normal, or wild-type, allele. An albino condition is based on a single gene. Albino animals are different from normal animals in behavior and anatomy as well as appearance. Albino mice, for example, are less active, more emotional (as assessed by defecation in novel situations), slower to learn a conditioned avoidance response, and less inclined to drink alcohol than normally pigmented mice of the same strain (McClearn and DeFries, 1973). Albinism in cats, including tigers, reduces the bifurcation of the optic tract, causing relatively little information from each eye to reach the contralateral hemisphere of the brain and hence altering visually guided behavior (Guillery, 1974).

Single gene analysis of behavior is particularly important because it provides a means of investigating the physiological or biochemical basis for the behavior. The genetic change responsible for producing the different behavior may ultimately be traceable to a single altered protein. Understanding the biochemical mechanisms that mediate the effects of genes on neural and behavioral development can also suggest strategies for correcting genetic diseases. One example of this approach involves a recessive neurological mutation, called *pallid*, in mice. Mice that inherit two copies of the mutant *pallid* allele (recessive homozygotes) have difficulty maintaining equilibrium. This mutation has been correlated with deficiencies in manganese transport (Erway *et al.*, 1966). The decreased concentration of manganese weakens bone development and partially or completely destroys the otoliths, small granules in the inner ears that provide information about gravity. The *pallid* allele also retards the mouse's ability to transport L-dopa and L-tryptophan into the brain (Cotzias *et al.*, 1972). It is not known whether defects in the transport of these amino acids are direct effects of the *pallid* allele or secondary (pleiotropic) effects of the manganese deficiency. It has been shown, though, that the deleterious behavioral effects can be prevented during development by feeding the gestating mother large supplements of manganese.

This example illustrates how understanding the physiological pathway of gene action on behavior can suggest successful remedies. Appropriate changes, such as a change in diet, can sometimes prevent the individual's genetic makeup, or genotype, from being expressed in the behavior, or phenotype. Such a situation exists for at least one human mutation that affects behavior. *Phenylketonuria*, or PKU, produces severe mental retardation in individuals with two recessive alleles. The gene involved is carried on one of the *autosomes* (chromosomes other than the X or Y *sex chromosomes*), so either sex may be affected. The mental defect results from an accumulation of phenylpyruvic acid and other phenylalanine byproducts that build up because the individual cannot metabolize phenylalanine to tyrosine. The required enzyme, _phenylalanine hydroxylase_, is missing. Fortunately, understanding PKU at the biochemical level produced a rational therapy. Today newborns are tested for PKU (by law in most states) and affected children are placed on a low phenylalanine diet. Mental development is greatly improved if this diet is started early, but delayed treatment cannot reverse the progress of the disease.

The biochemical bases of other genetic forms of mental retardation, such as Lesch–Nyhan syndrome or Tay–Sachs disease, are also known (Okada and O'Brien, 1969; Omenn, 1976). _Lesch–Nyhan syndrome_ is caused by a recessive allele of a gene carried on the X chromosome and occurs only in males. Boys with Lesch–Nyhan syndrome exhibit cerebral palsy, involuntary movements of limbs, hands, feet, and facial muscles; mental retardation; and aggressiveness. Some also mutilate themselves by compulsively biting their fingers and lips. The Lesch–Nyhan syndrome appears to result from reduced activity of an enzyme (hypoxanthine-guanine phosphoribosyltransferase) involved in purine synthesis. This enzyme deficiency causes extreme overproduction of uric acid. Patients displaying self-mutilation also have elevated levels of dopamine β-hydroxylase (the enzyme that converts dopamine to norepinephrine) in their plasma and do not show a pressor response (increased blood pressure) to cold. Thus, disturbed adrenergic mechanisms may be involved in this peculiar pathology (Rockson _et al._, 1974).

Tay–Sachs disease, also known as infantile amaurotic idiocy, is one of several enzymatic disorders causing accumulation of lipids in nerve cells. Like PKU, it results from inheritance of two recessive alleles of a gene carried on one of the autosomes. Children affected by Tay–Sachs disease produce a defective version of the enzyme β-D-N-acetylgalactosaminidase (hexosaminidase A). The behavioral problems begin with spasmodic eye movements and progress to blindness, paralysis, idiocy and death, usually before the child is 2 years old. No cure has been developed yet for either Tay–Sachs disease or Lesch–Nyhan syndrome. However, as a result of understanding the enzymatic defects involved, both diseases can be diagnosed prenatally by sampling the amniotic fluid that surrounds the developing fetus (a procedure known as amniocentesis).

A. Polygenes and Behavior

Unfortunately, straightforward Mendelian analyses cannot always be used to study the role of genes in development of the nervous system and behavior. When a dramatic change in development occurs, as in the examples given above, it is relatively easy to determine that genetic factors are involved by studying the pattern of inheritance of the distinctive character or disorder. Yet for many interesting traits, individuals cannot be neatly sorted into the distinctive categories (such as color-blind versus not color-blind or afflicted by PKU versus not afflicted) needed for Mendelian analyses. A simple example of a trait that defies such categorization is height. Individuals are not simply tall, average or short. Rather, they come in a range of heights. Many behaviors, such as activity, temperament, and performance on IQ tests, present the same problem. Such traits are said to vary quantitatively and are presumably influenced by the combined action of many genes (*polygenes*) as well as by the environment. To study polygenetic influences on neural or behavioral development, one must obtain measurements or scores on many individuals and compare the average scores, and the variability of the scores, for different groups or populations of individuals. One could compare, for example, the temperaments of genetically different breeds of dogs. If the differences in temperament persist when the dogs are reared in identical, or nearly identical, environments, this would suggest that genetic differences between the breeds influence the dog's temperaments.

Usually, though, genetic research is done using highly *inbred strains* of animals. Such strains are developed by mating individuals with their close relatives (inbreeding), for example by mating brothers and sisters, for many generations. Because the brother–sister parents often possess and pass on identical alleles for their genes, the offspring become more genetically alike with each generation. Eventually, all the members of one strain come to share a nearly common genetic makeup (*genotype*), and differ genetically from all other inbred strains. Such inbred strains differ from each other in essentially every behavior that has been studied, including activity, emotionality, aggressiveness, preference for alcohol, relative brain weight, activities of various enzymes, susceptibility to sound-induced seizures, conduction speed in nerves and learning abilities. This suggests that genetic differences between individuals may contribute to the individual differences in behavior observed when populations of genetically variable mice are studied.

Inbred strains are also useful for studying environmental influences on behavior because studies of animals within the same strain are not complicated by genotypic variation. Similarly, the complex ways in which the genotype and environment interact can be highlighted by testing two or more strains in each of several environments. The effects of social stress on alcohol consumption by mice have been studied this way (Thiessen, 1972). When mice of the C57/Bl strain are caged individually, they prefer 10% alcohol to plain tapwater. In fact, they consume 90% of their daily fluids from the alcohol bottle. In contrast, isolated mice of the RIII strain are moderate drinkers. When stressed by being caged in groups, C57/B1 mice drink less alcohol than they do when they live alone. This stress does not affect the drinking habits of the RIII mice. Thus stress has distinctly different effects on alcohol consumption depending on the genotype of the animal.

Another technique used in genetic studies is _selective breeding_. Simply put, animals displaying extreme behavior of some sort are mated, and the procedure is continued for a number of generations. If such procedures produce differences in behavior of the offspring, the behavior is influenced in part by genetic differences.

A number of experiments have shown, for example, that rats can be selectively bred for maze learning ability. In the most well known of such experiments, Tryon (1942) trained rats on a complex maze and mated "maze-dull" males with compatible females and "maze-bright" males with compatible females. This process was continued for many generations. After eight generations the maze performance of the two genetic lines was markedly different. Further studies of the "maze-bright" and "maze-dull" strains indicated that the two strains did not differ consistently on other types of learning tasks. Such studies do not, by themselves, shed much light on the basis of the strain differences. The difference in maze performance might be due to genetic differences in a number of processes, including learning mechanisms, motivation, and sensory processes. Other experiments and other approaches are needed to determine the bases of the strain difference in behavior.

Like inbred strains, selected lines can be used to study how environmental changes affect the development of behavior in animals with different genotypes. An interesting example is the effect of "enriched" versus "impoverished" environments on learning ability in the "bright" and "dull" rats discussed above. Offspring from each of these selected lines were raised either alone (impoverished condition), in groups of three (normal condition), or in larger groups with toys available (enriched condition). As adults, they were tested for learning ability. The results obtained are illustrated in Fig. 16-1. Rats from both selected lines performed very well when raised under enriched conditions and performed very poorly when raised in an impoverished environment. Differences between the lines were restricted to the normally raised rats; these, of course, were the conditions that prevailed during selection. Clearly it does not make sense to classify one of these lines as consistently better than the other at learning mazes. Also, it does not make sense to speak in general terms about the effects of environmental changes on learning in this case, except to compare the extreme conditions of enriched versus impoverished environments. The advantages of a normal environment over an impoverished one existed only for the "bright" rats. In contrast, the advantage of an enriched environment over a normal environment existed only for the "dull" rats. Neither the genotype nor the environment alone can account for the behavioral _phenotype_. Clearly, the two interact.

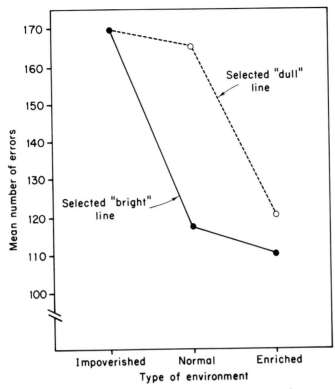

Fig. 16-1. Genetic and environmental factors interact in complex ways to influence behavioral development. Two genetically different groups of rats raised in a normal laboratory environment may show distinct differences in a behavior such as maze learning ability (as assessed by the number of errors made while learning the maze). When such selected lines of rats are raised under different environmental conditions, the behavioral differences may disappear. The data shown here indicate that rats selected to make many errors when raised normally actually make relatively few errors when raised in an enriched environment. In contrast, rats selected to make few errors when raised normally actually make many errors if raised in an impoverished condition. Thus the behavioral performance is not determined by either genetic or environmental influences alone but by their interaction. (After Cooper and Zubek, 1958.)

B. Chromosomes and Behavior

An analysis of chromosomes can be useful in investigating the genetic bases of behavior in humans. Some individuals are born with more or less than the normal complement of 46 chromosomes. Such chromosomal anomalies represent natural experiments since the chromosomal excess or loss may have behavioral consequences.

1. DOWN SYNDROME. In humans with *Down syndrome*, for example, men-

tal development is severely retarded. Among institutionalized cases, IQ scores generally fall below 50 with an average of about 25, although children raised at home may score somewhat higher. The disorder results from a chromosomal excess. Most people with Down syndrome have three copies (termed *trisomy*) of chromosome 21 because the paired chromosomes did not separate during sperm or egg formation. However, a few people with this disorder have only an extra segment of chromosome 21 fused to another chromosome (usually chromosome 13, 14, or 15). Individuals with this latter type of Down syndrome have slightly better mental abilities. Fortunately, it is possible to reduce greatly the number of individuals with Down syndrome because the extra chromosome can be detected during pregnancy by amniocentesis. Since more than half of Down syndrome babies are born to women over 35, expectant mothers in this age group often seek such genetic tests and counseling.

Anomalies related to the <u>*sex chromosomes*</u> (X and Y) can also affect behavior. Normally at fertilization the egg, which contains an X sex chromosome, is invaded by a sperm, which contains either an X or a Y sex chromosome (see Fig. 16-2). Under normal developmental conditions, a fertilized egg containing an XX chromosome complement will develop into a female offspring, while a fertilized egg containing an XY chromosome complement will develop into a male. In this brief description the words "normal" and "normally" were used deliberately because errors do occur, both in chromosome pairing and in the later stages of the sexual differentiation process. In the production of the gametes, genetic errors can occur. For example, in some cases a sperm may contain two X chromosomes, or both an X and a <u>*Y chromosome*</u>, instead of *either* an X or a Y chromosome. When this happens the fertilized egg will contain an XXX or an XXY chromo-

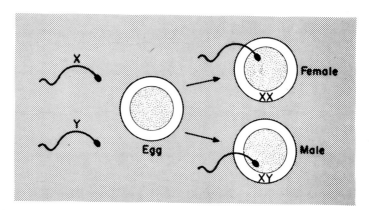

Fig. 16-2. Genes determine the basic male and female characteristics. Each egg contains an X chromosome. A sperm may contain either an X or a Y chromosome. If the egg is fertilized by a sperm carrying an X chromosome, a female develops. If the egg is fertilized by a sperm carrying a Y chromosome, a male develops.

16. DEVELOPMENT OF BEHAVIOR

some complement. Errors in pairing of sex chromosomes result in the development of abnormal morphology, physiology and behavior.

2.   KLEINFELTER SYNDROME.   This syndrome occurs when there is one extra X chromosome in an otherwise normal male (XXY pattern). Individuals with this syndrome have a masculine body form but show atrophy of the reproductive duct system and impaired testicular function. The syndrome is found in approximately 0.2% of newborn males.

3.   TURNER SYNDROME.   This syndrome results when one sex chromosome is missing (XO pattern). These individuals have a female body form but the ovaries fail to develop. Its incidence is approximately 0.03% of female births. Affected women have essentially normal IQ scores, but often show a distinctive difficulty with perceptual problems (Alexander *et al.*, 1966). Figure 16-3 illustrates this deficit, which has been termed "space-form blindness." The girls tested viewed the figures on the left side of the figure and then attempted to draw them from memory. Below each girl's drawing is her age, plus her verbal, perceptual and full IQ scores. Apparently the perceptual defect does not involve memory failure, since the girls performed just as poorly when they were allowed to copy designs (see Fig. 16-4). Figure 16-5 shows what the Turner syndrome girls drew when asked to "draw a person." Chromosomally normal children of this age

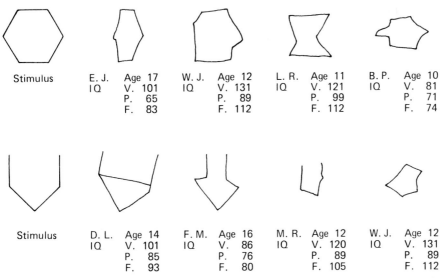

| Stimulus | E. J.
IQ | Age 17
V. 101
P. 65
F. 83 | W. J.
IQ | Age 12
V. 131
P. 89
F. 112 | L. R.
IQ | Age 11
V. 121
P. 99
F. 112 | B. P.
IQ | Age 10
V. 81
P. 71
F. 74 |

| Stimulus | D. L.
IQ | Age 14
V. 101
P. 85
F. 93 | F. M.
IQ | Age 16
V. 86
P. 76
F. 80 | M. R.
IQ | Age 12
V. 120
P. 89
F. 105 | W. J.
IQ | Age 12
V. 131
P. 89
F. 112 |

Fig. 16-3.   Human females that have Turner syndrome obtain essentially normal IQ scores; however, they have distinctive problems with spatial perception. This problem has been called "space-form blindness." The figures on the far left of each row were shown to girls with Turner syndrome. Then the girls were asked to draw the figure from memory. The girls' drawings are shown to the right of each stimulus figure. Below each girl's drawing is her age plus her verbal, performance, and full IQ scores. (From Alexander *et al.*, 1966.)

I. SINGLE GENE INFLUENCES ON BEHAVIOR   697

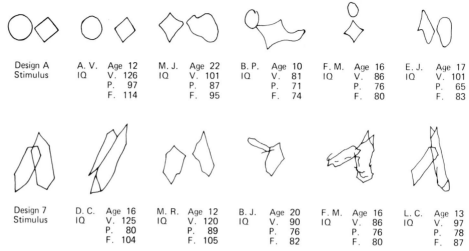

Design A Stimulus	A. V. IQ	Age 12 V. 126 P. 97 F. 114	M. J. IQ	Age 22 V. 101 P. 87 F. 95	B. P. IQ	Age 10 V. 81 P. 71 F. 74	F. M. IQ	Age 16 V. 86 P. 76 F. 80	E. J. IQ	Age 17 V. 101 P. 65 F. 83

Design 7 Stimulus	D. C. IQ	Age 16 V. 125 P. 80 F. 104	M. R. IQ	Age 12 V. 120 P. 89 F. 105	B. J. IQ	Age 20 V. 90 P. 76 F. 82	F. M. IQ	Age 16 V. 86 P. 76 F. 80	L. C. IQ	Age 13 V. 97 P. 78 F. 87

Fig. 16-4. The problems that the Turner syndrome girls had in drawing the stimulus figures shown in Fig. 16-3 apparently did not result from memory problems. As shown here, the Turner syndrome girls had similar problems even if they could see the stimulus figure (again on the left) while they tried to draw it. (From Alexander *et al.*, 1966.)

M. J. IQ	Age 12 V. 134 P. 99 F. 119	W. J. IQ	Age 12 V. 131 P. 89 F. 112	F. M. IQ	Age 16 V. 86 P. 76 F. 80	M. R. IQ	Age 12 V. 120 P. 89 F. 105

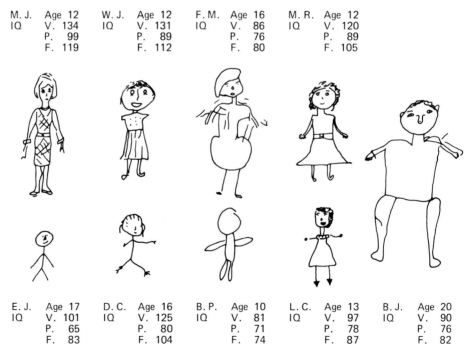

E. J. IQ	Age 17 V. 101 P. 65 F. 83	D. C. IQ	Age 16 V. 125 P. 80 F. 104	B. P. IQ	Age 10 V. 81 P. 71 F. 74	L. C. IQ	Age 13 V. 97 P. 78 F. 87	B. J. IQ	Age 20 V. 90 P. 76 F. 82

Fig. 16-5. The "space-form blindness" that occurs in girls with Turner syndrome is also obvious when they try to draw a person. Obviously, though, there are considerable differences among the affected individuals. (From Alexander *et al.*, 1966.)

usually draw a person of their own sex. Where the sex of the figure drawn can be determined, Turner girls drew females, suggesting that their sexual identity is female. These "draw-a-person" figures also reveal the variation in this syndrome. One girl (H. J.) drew quite well, whereas others had considerable difficulty. Note, for instance, the frequent erasures around the arms in the drawings by F.M. and B.J.

4. TRIPLE-X SYNDROME. The triple-X syndrome is the result of an extra X chromosome in an otherwise normal female. These individuals have a female phenotype, are usually fertile, but may have early menopause. The syndrome occurs in about 0.14% of the newborn population and is often accompanied by mental retardation.

5. THE XYY SYNDROME. This syndrome (Hook, 1973; Kessler and Moos, 1970; Jarvik *et al.*, 1973) occurs in approximately 0.1% of males. Males with this disorder have an additional Y, or male-determining, chromosome. Until 1965, only twelve such cases were known. Then nine more cases were detected among 315 men in a maximum security hospital in Britain. This meant that nearly 3% of the patients were affected. Soon more surveys of mental–penal institutions uncovered more XYY males, and newspapers began reporting that an extra Y chromosome predisposes men to criminal behavior. More cautious researchers stressed the need to know the incidence of XYY males in the general population before the risk of criminal behavior in XYY men could be specified. Table 16-1 summarizes such survey data. It indicates that men with an extra X chromosome (Kleinfelter syndrome) and men with an extra Y chromosome occur equally often in newborns and normal adults. Both anomalies are detected more often in mental patients and criminals than in other men, but among criminals the frequency of XYY males exceeds the frequency of XXY males. Although these data support the suggestion that XYY males run a higher risk than normal males

Table 16-1   The numbers and percentage of XYY and XXY males detected in chromosome surveys on newborns, normal adults, mental patients and criminals[a]

Type of males	Number surveyed	Number of XYY	Percentage of XYY	Number of XXY	Percentage of XXY
Newborns	9904	13	0.13%	14	0.14%
Normal adults	2021	4	0.20%	7	0.35%
	4127	4	0.10%	Not studied	
Mental patients	597	6	1.00%	6	1.00%
	260	0	0	Not studied	
Criminals	4293	61	1.42%	37	0.86%
	773	37	4.79%	Not studied	

[a] From Jarvik *et al.* (1973).

I. SINGLE GENE INFLUENCES ON BEHAVIOR

of imprisonment, several important facts should be remembered: (1) XYY males constitute a small fraction of criminal offenders; (2) XYY prisoners are no more aggressive toward people than other prisoners are and are often less so; (3) most XYY males are never institutionalized for any reason and presumably lead normal lives.

II. Development of Sex-Related Behavior: Genetic and Hormonal Influences

Chromosomal errors are not the only type of genetic errors that occur in sexual development. Some individuals possess an XY chromosome complement, yet fail to develop in the masculine direction.

These individuals with a normal male chromosome pattern are insensitive to their own male hormones, the _androgens_ which are secreted by the testes. Because they are insensitive to their own androgens, these individuals develop in a female fashion; at birth, their external genitalia are similar in morphology to those of normal XX females. The reason for this femalelike appearance is that the chromosomes do not entirely determine the development and differentiation of the reproductive organs and genitalia. Early in the developmental process both genetic males and females possess the same primordial reproductive duct systems, the _Wolffian_ and _Mullerian duct_ systems, as well as sexually undifferentiated gonads. At an appropriate stage of development, the undifferentiated gonads develop either into testes or into ovaries as shown in Fig. 16-6. If the gonads develop into ovaries, they remain functionally quiescent during development. However, if the gonads develop into testes, the testes begin to produce and secrete androgens, _testosterone_ and androstenedione primarily, as well as a locally active "differentiating substance." The androgens are carried by the blood to various targets, such as the genital sinus, where they induce the development of the penis and scrotum. In the absence of androgenic stimulation, as in normal females or in androgen-insensitive males, the sinus tissues develop into the clitoris, labia and vaginal opening. Normally in males the secretions of the testes (androgens and the differentiating substance) facilitate the sexual differentiation of the Wolffian duct system into the masculine duct system, the vas deferens and seminal vesicles, and inhibit the Mullerian system. In females, in the absence of hormonal stimulation, the Mullerian system develops into the uterus, fallopian tubes and vagina, while the Wolffian system regresses.

Thus, the differentiation of the reproductive apparatus in males and females is under the control of chromosomes, genes and hormonal stimulation during development. The important question is whether the genetic and hormonal

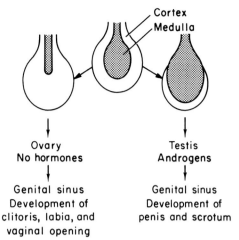

Cortex
Medulla

Ovary
No hormones

Testis
Androgens

Genital sinus
Development of
clitoris, labia, and
vaginal opening

Genital sinus
Development of
penis and scrotum

Fig. 16-6. Undifferentiated Gonad. Early in development, both males and females possess indifferent or bipotential gonads. At the appropriate stage of development, these gonads differentiate into ovaries or testes. If the inner part, or medulla, of the indifferent gonad develops, it forms a testis. If the outer part, or cortex, of the gonad develops, it forms an ovary. The differentiated gonads then influence, via their secretions, the sexual differentiation of the reproductive duct systems and the genitalia. Both sexes begin with the same duct systems (Wolffian and Mullerian systems). The tissues that form the genitalia have the potential to develop in either the male or female direction. If the gonads develop into testes and secrete androgen hormones, the Wolffian system develops into the masculine duct system (vas deferens, seminal vesicles), and the genital sinus develops into the penis and scrotum. Since the testes also secrete an as yet unidentified Mullerian inhibiting substance, the absence of androgens allows the Mullerian system to develop into the uterus, fallopian tubes and vagina, and the genital sinus to develop into the clitoris, labia and vaginal opening. The absence of testes also causes regression of the Wolffian system.

processes outlined here have implications for the development of behavior. The answer appears to be yes.

Some genetic females are stimulated by androgenic hormones during fetal development. This occurs when, for genetic reasons, the adrenal gland of the female fetus fails to secrete normal levels of the hormone cortisol. This defect results in the adrenal gland secreting high levels of androgens, hormones which are closely related biochemically to cortisol. The androgens produced by the adrenals cause the genital sinus to develop in a malelike fashion with, in extreme cases, the clitoris developing into a penis and the labia fusing to produce a scrotum-like structure. This condition is termed the *adrenogenital syndrome* and is estimated to occur as often as 1 in 5000 births. Similar masculinizing effects have been produced when pregnant women were administered testosterone or one of a variety of progesterone-like compounds which have androgenic activity. The changes caused by these drugs are usually recognized at birth, and the external genitalia are surgically corrected to conform to the female pattern. With appropriate therapy, these girls develop normal reproductive function (although puberty may be delayed), and they are capable of bearing children. Although these girls are identified as female at birth and are raised as females, they do develop some behavioral patterns characteristic of males in our society. According to Money and Ehrhardt (1972) these girls display "tomboyish" behavior as adolescents as indicated both by self-report and parental description. These girls tend to engage in vigorous, outdoor, large muscle activities which are usually more characteristic of age-mate males. These girls also show less rehearsal of maternalism, although there is no evidence that they are more aggressive than matched "control" girls.

In comparison, genetic males with the *androgen-insensitivity syndrome* fail to develop normal male genitalia. Rather, they develop labia and a vagina, which may be indistinguishable from that of normal girls at birth. These individuals are usually identified as female at birth and are raised as girls. At puberty these individuals develop breasts and the hip structure of women under the influence of estrogens secreted by the undescended testes. Psychosexually, these people develop as women in our culture, and although infertile, since they lack ovaries and a uterus, may marry as women.

These two examples, the adrenogenital syndrome and the androgen insensitivity syndrome, are particularly interesting because in one case the individuals involved have XX chromosomes and in the other XY chromosomes; in one case the individuals were stimulated by androgens early in development, but not in the other case; and in both instances the individuals are identified and reared as females in our culture. Yet, in the androgenized individual with female chromosomes, behavior patterns develop that are more typical of males, while in non-androgenized individuals with male chromosomes typically female patterns of behavior emerge. Although assigned gender is constant, some behavior differs and appears to reflect the type of hormonal stimulation. This, of course, does not mean that the hormonal environment totally determines gender development. Money *et al.* (1955) reported on the gender role and sexual orientation of hermaphroditic children who were reared as males or females even though some of their sexual characteristics, such as chromosomes, hormones, internal reproductive organs or external genitalia, were not appropriate for the sex of rearing. They found that the sex of assignment, that is, how the child was reared, was the best predictor of the child's sexual orientation. For example, genetic girls with the adrenogenital syndrome, who had sexually ambiguous genitalia at birth and who were raised as boys, developed a masculine gender role. Those with the same syndrome who were raised as girls developed a feminine gender role. The most dramatic case reported to date (Money, 1975) concerns a girl who was born a normal boy (one of two identical twin boys) but who lost his penis during circumcision. By surgery, a vagina was constructed for the child and she is being reared as a girl. Her genetically identical twin is being raised as a boy. According to Money, the girl's behavior and sexual identity at 9 years of age are those of a normally active girl and are quite different from that of her male twin. Clearly, while hormones may play a role in the development of behavior in humans, experiential influences can override these biological effects.

The genetic errors which occur in humans are natural experiments which give us insights into potential relationships between genes or hormones and the development of behavior. These natural experiments cannot, however, provide us with precise information. For example, individuals with the adrenogenital syndrome are genitally masculinized at birth, yet we do not know when the hormonal stimulation began or how intense it was. Partially masculinized genitalia could reflect an early onset of low levels of hormonal stimulation or a late onset of high levels of stimulation. To obtain precise information about the parameters of hormonal stimulation and the development of behavior, one must turn to animal studies where a variety of factors can be controlled. Since 1959 a large number of such studies have provided relevant information.

In 1959, Phoenix and his associates reported that the female offspring of guinea pigs that were administered testosterone during pregnancy were less likely than offspring of normal females to show female sexual behavior as adults, but were more likely to show male-type sexual behavior in adulthood. Subsequent studies from that laboratory showed that these effects occurred only if the testosterone was given during a particular period of fetal development. These findings were interpreted to mean that the presence of hormones during sensitive periods of development could permanently alter brain function, although the brain had not been studied directly. However, many experiments had shown that the brain is intimately involved in the control of male and female sexual behavior. For example, lesions of specific parts of the brain were known to disrupt mating behavior. The placement of small amounts of hormones in particular brain regions was also known to reinstate mating responses in animals whose gonads had been removed. Because of these earlier findings, it was reasonable to postulate that early hormone stimulation in some way altered brain function in a masculine direction. Their studies also showed that the prenatal hormone stimulation would masculinize the external genitalia in a way similar to that seen in people with the adrenogenital syndrome.

Since 1969, literally hundreds of experiments have explored the relationship between hormonal stimulation during development and the later display of behaviors which show sex differences, such as mating behavior, aggressive behavior, exploratory behavior and ingestive behavior. Typically, these studies involve the administration of exogenous hormone by injection or the removal of endogenous hormones by gonadectomy at various developmental stages. When the animals are mature, they are administered sex-typical hormones (e.g., testosterone to males) or sex-atypical hormones (e.g., testosterone to females). Then they are observed for display of masculine and feminine patterns of behavior. Using this approach, studies of rats have shown that exposure to testosterone during the first few days after birth inhibits the animal's ability to respond to _estrogen_ or to estrogen and progesterone in adulthood. In untreated female rats, these hormones elicit the display of sexual receptivity in adulthood (Whalen and Edwards, 1967). Female rats treated postnatally with androgen do not show a large enhancement of masculine behavior. However, it appears that in the rat prenatal stimulation by androgen does enhance masculine behavior. Clemens (1973), for example, showed that the probability that a female rat would show male-type mounting behavior when administered testosterone depended upon the sex of adjacent littermates in the uterus prior to her birth. If only females were in the litter, they rarely showed male behavior. However, if a female was between two males in the uterus, she readily showed male behavior when administered testosterone as an adult.

Thus, the hormone-induced enhancement of the potential to show masculine behavior occurs at a different time during development than does androgen-induced inhibition of the potential for feminine behavior. This indicated that _"masculinization"_ and _"defeminization"_ are independent developmental processes. This phenomenon has been clearly demonstrated in hamsters and dogs. If a normal adult female hamster is administered estrogen and progesterone, she will display receptive behavior. If she is administered testosterone, she does not show any signs of masculine (mounting) behavior. Thus, following normal maturational conditions, the female hamster develops the potential to show feminine, but not masculine, behavior. However, if the female hamster is administered as little as 1 μg of testosterone on the day of birth, she develops the potential to show both masculine and feminine behavior. Such an animal will, as an adult, display receptivity when given estrogen and will display mounting behavior when given testosterone. The neonatal hormone treatment therefore masculinized, but did not defeminize her. If, however, the female hamster is given 100 μg of testosterone at birth she can, as an adult, display masculine behavior, but even large doses of estrogen and progesterone will fail to elicit receptive behavior. The high dose of testosterone in infancy, therefore, both masculinized and defeminized the animal (DeBold and Whalen, 1975). Figure 16-7 summarizes some of these concepts.

Beach and his colleagues (1973) have found that the normal adult female dog will respond to estrogen by displaying female sexual behavior, but will not respond to testosterone with mounting behavior. The normal male dog will show masculine sexual behavior when given testosterone, but will not respond to estrogen. Female dogs given testosterone shortly after birth will display neither masculine nor feminine sexual behavior when given hormones in adulthood—this treatment

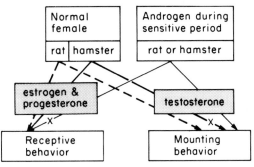

Fig. 16-7. Adult male and female rats and hamsters differ in their behavioral responses to hormones as a result of their exposure to hormones early in development. Normal female rats and hamsters are not exposed to androgens immediately after birth. As a result, they show receptive behavior in adulthood when given estrogen and progesterone. If they are exposed to androgen during the sensitive period of sexual differentiation, they will not display receptive behavior when treated with estrogen and progesterone in adulthood. Early exposure to androgen will cause female hamsters to show mounting behavior when they are given testosterone in adulthood, although they do not do this if they develop normally, without androgenic stimulation. Female rats, in contrast, show mounting behavior as adults in response to testosterone whether or not they were given androgens shortly after birth. The behavioral sensitivity of female rats to testosterone in adulthood does vary, though, depending on their positions in the uterus relative to their brothers. Exposure to androgens secreted by their brothers in the uterus may contribute to the behavioral responsiveness of female rats to testosterone in adulthood.

defeminizes, but does not masculinize. However, females given testosterone both before and shortly after birth are both masculinized and defeminized.

These studies show that it is possible to change, quite independently, the potential of the animal to show masculine and feminine responses in adulthood by manipulating hormone levels during early development. These studies also suggest that testosterone masculinizes the animal at an earlier stage of development than it defeminizes the animal. The studies of the rat and hamster also suggest that a lower dose of testosterone is needed to masculinize than is needed to defeminize. These findings might be related to the human adrenogenital syndrome where the excess of androgen seems to masculinize the girl partially without inhibiting her potential to show feminine behavior.

One other important point that can be derived from these studies of the guinea pig, rat and hamster is that the sensitive period when hormones can effect permanent changes in later behavior reflects some important maturational stage that is quite independent of birth. In the guinea pig, where gestation is long (68 days) masculinization and defeminization can occur prior to birth but not after birth. In the rat, where gestation is 21 days, masculinization can occur prior to birth, while defeminization can be brought about only by hormone stimulation after birth. In the hamster, both masculinization and defeminization can occur only after birth. Treatment of the hamster with hormones prior to birth has no effect upon later sexual behavior.

To illustrate the general finding that these developmental effects of hormones are not limited to the organization of sexual patterns, we might briefly consider the hormonal control of *aggressive behavior*. If male and female mice are reared together from birth, one finds relatively little fighting behavior in the colony. However, if adult mice are isolated for 3 weeks and then paired, males show a great deal of fighting behavior, while females rarely fight. This fighting occurs only if the males possess their testes at the time of testing. If the males are castrated before being isolated and are then paired, fighting does not occur. If, then, both the male and female mice are given testosterone therapy, the males, but not the females, will fight. Edwards (1969) has shown that if the female mice are administered testosterone at birth they, like the males, will fight when given testosterone in adulthood. If testosterone treatment of the females is delayed until they are 10 days of age, the hormone has little effect upon later fighting behavior. Thus, exposure to testosterone shortly after birth masculinizes in the sense of enhancing the mouse's potential to show typically masculine fighting behavior. These findings are illustrated in Fig. 16-8.

The studies discussed above indicate that the presence of testosterone during sensitive periods of development can masculinize and/or defeminize. One might ask about the development of the potential to show female-typical behavior. The studies of persons with the androgen-insensitivity syndrome would suggest that in the absence of effective androgenic stimulation during development both morphological and behavioral development proceeds along female-typical lines. A similar pattern emerges from animal studies. Spontaneously agonadal animals develop female body form and behavior. Similarly, male animals which are gonadectomized early during development (or which are treated with anti-androgenic compounds at the appropriate time) develop the potential to respond to ovarian hormones in adulthood. Thus, if one examines, in adulthood, the receptive behavior of male rats castrated on the day of birth, females ovariectomized on the day of birth, and females ovariectomized in adulthood, one finds no difference in their behavioral response to estrogen or to estrogen and progesterone (Whalen and Edwards, 1967). If male rats are castrated 1 week after birth, they do not respond to estrogen in adulthood, indicating that testicular secretions during the first few days after birth permanently defeminize the animal. Interestingly, female rats administered large doses of either testosterone or estrogen at birth are also permanently defeminized. These findings indicate that the ovaries of the female probably do not contribute to the development of female behavior. The absence rather than the presence of hormones seems critical for the potential for female sexual behavior to develop. These findings are summarized in Table 16-2.

16. DEVELOPMENT OF BEHAVIOR

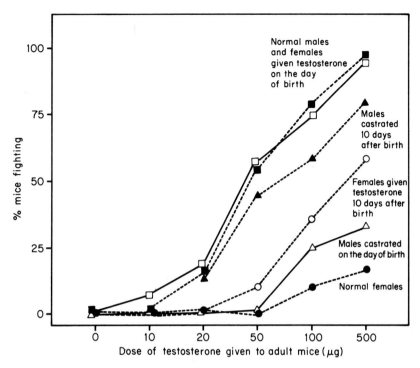

Fig. 16-8. Exposure to androgens during early development can also influence the ability of testosterone to stimulate aggressive behavior in adult mice. Normally, female mice are not as aggressive as male mice even if the females are given testosterone in adulthood. If female mice are exposed to testosterone during the first few days after birth, they become behaviorally sensitive to testosterone as adults. (After Edwards, 1969.)

Table 16-2   Effects of hormonal stimulation before and after birth on the development of the potential to show masculine and feminine behavior in adulthood

| | Male behavior | | Female behavior |
	Partial pattern	Full pattern	
Hormone before and after birth	+ +	+ +	− −
Hormone before birth	+ +	− −	+ +
Hormone after birth	?	?	− −

Edwards (1969) has shown that a similar process occurs for aggressive behavior. Male mice which are castrated at birth are unlikely to show fighting behavior even when administered large doses of testosterone in adulthood (see Fig. 16-8).

III. Mechanism of Hormone Action in Sexual Development

The generalization which has emerged from studies of both animal and human behavior is that early during development genetic males and females pass through an undifferentiated state during which they are sensitive to hormonal stimulation. If such stimulation is absent, the individual develops in a female-typical direction, that is, the individual develops female, but not male potential. If gonadal hormones are present, and if the individual is responsive to those hormones, differentiation occurs which is characterized as an enhancement of the potential to show male-typical behaviors and an inhibition of the potential to show female-typical behavior.

In recent years, there have been a number of studies directed toward understanding the biological bases of hormonally controlled sex differences in behavior. These studies have been of behaviors, such as mating and aggression, which appear to be mediated by the action of hormones in the central nervous system. For example, as mentioned earlier adult female, but not male, rats display behavior characteristic of sexual receptivity when they are administered estrogen systemically. These behaviors can also be induced in the females when minute amounts of estrogen are implanted in limited regions of the medial basal diencephalon. Implants in other brain regions are ineffective. These findings suggest that certain neurons of females, but not of males, respond to estrogen and mediate receptive behavior. The assumption is made that it is these neurons which are altered in the male by hormonal stimulation early in development.

Based on the logic that hypothalamic neurons of males and females respond differently to estrogen, investigators have studied the cellular and subcellular response of hypothalamic neurons to estrogen. These studies employ radioactive hormones as tracers. Although there has been some controversy in this area, several studies have shown that the hypothalamic tissue of males as well as females accumulates and retains estrogen following the administration of radioactive estrogen. Cerebral cortical tissue from both males and females accumulates rather little estrogen. Thus, looked at in a relatively gross way the brains of males and females do not differ in their response to estrogen.

Current theory as described in Chapter 12 states that hormones such as estrogen enter cells of target tissues where they are selectively bound to *"receptor"* *proteins* in the cytoplasm of the cell. The hormone–receptor complex is then transported to the cell nucleus where the complex binds to the nuclear chromatin material which is composed of DNA, histones and nonhistone proteins. There is some evidence to suggest that the hormone–receptor complex binds selectively to the nonhistone (acidic) proteins in such a way as to free the DNA for genetic transcription and the production of messenger RNA, which then migrates to the cytoplasm where new proteins are synthesized. This model of hormone action is diagrammed in Fig. 16-9.

In terms of sex differences in responsiveness to estrogen, it seemed possible that males do not possess the cytoplasmic protein receptors characteristic of the

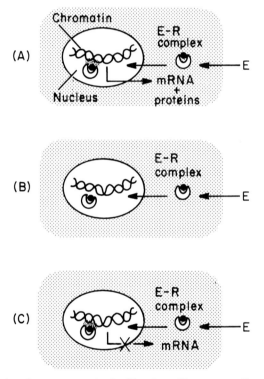

Fig. 16-9. In females, free estrogen in the blood readily enters cells in the hypothalamus. Once in the cytoplasm, the estrogen (E) combines with a protein receptor (R). The estrogen–receptor (E–R) complex then enters the cell nucleus where it binds to the nuclear chromatin. Presumably this interaction stimulates messenger RNA and protein synthesis which regulates cell function. This model is shown in (A). The failure of normal males to show receptive behavior when given estrogen is not due to failure of the hormone to enter hypothalamic cells. In fact males, like females, have protein receptors in hypothalamic cells that bind estrogen and transport it to the nucleus (B). The inability of males to respond to estrogen may be due to an inability of the estrogen–receptor complex to stimulate messenger RNA (mRNA) synthesis in males. This hypothesis is shown in (C).

female or that the estrogen–receptor complex fails to interact properly with the cell nucleus. The first of these hypotheses has proved to be incorrect. If the cytoplasm of hypothalamic cells is isolated from males and females and analyzed for its ability to bind estrogen selectively, one finds no sex difference in this ability. Cytoplasm from cortical cells binds very little estrogen regardless of the sex of the animal. Thus, both males and females possess estrogen receptors in the cytoplasm of their hypothalamic cells.

Males and females do, however, differ in the degree of binding of estrogen by hypothalamic nuclei. If one administers radioactive estrogen to male and female rats or hamsters and then removes the hypothalamus and isolates the hypothalamic nuclei, one finds that nuclei from males accumulate less estrogen than nuclei from females. The nuclei from males are also less able to retain estrogen for long periods of time (see Fig. 16-10).

Thus, it may be the case that the critical difference between the sexes in their ability to respond to estrogen is localized in the nuclei of hypothalamic cells. Possibly, in males, estrogen is unable to free the DNA and allow the production of RNA and proteins that are critical for the neurons to change their pattern of firing in such a way as to permit the display of mating behavior. Exposure to hormones early in development might therefore alter the ability of the nuclei of

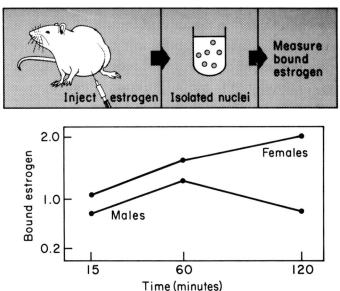

Fig. 16-10. Males and females differ in the degree to which their hypothalamic neurons bind and retain estrogen. Rats were injected with radioactive estrogen. At various times after injection, the animals were sacrificed and the nuclei of the hypothalamic cells were isolated. Then the amount of radioactive estrogen bound by the nuclei was measured. Nuclei from hypothalamic cells of females retain estrogen longer than the nuclei of male hypothalamic cells do. (After Whalen and Massicci, 1975.)

hypothalamic cells to respond to hormones later in life. This conclusion has yet to be established firmly, but could well be correct.

Hormone-induced changes in brain cell function are not the only way hormones act during development. Indeed, early hormone stimulation alters the way in which neurons make synaptic connections. Raisman and Field (1973) have shown that within the preoptic area of males, fibers of nonamygdaloid origin form synapses upon the *shafts* of dendrites. In females, fibers of the same origin synapse to a much greater degree upon dendritic *spines* (see Fig. 16-11). These workers have further shown that these patterns of synaptic connections are the result of early gonadal hormone stimulation. Male rats castrated at birth develop the female pattern, while females administered testosterone at birth develop the male pattern of synaptic connections. Thus, males and females differ in their behavioral response to hormones, in the biochemical responses of their hypothalamic nuclei, and in the morphology of their synaptic connections in the diencephalon.

In the past decade, a great deal has been learned about sex differences in behavior and how these differences are controlled by the presence or absence of hormones during sensitive periods of perinatal development. In the past few years, it has been found that there are sex differences in brain anatomy and in brain cell function, differences which are also controlled by hormonal stimulation during development. In the next decade the relationships between sex differences in anatomy, biochemistry and behavior should be more fully elucidated.

IV. Environmental Influences on the Development of Behavior

As the findings discussed in section III indicate, the development of behavior is not simply a matter of unfolding a preprogrammed pattern. The effects of genes

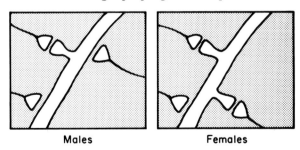

Males   Females

Fig. 16-11. The pattern of synaptic connections in the preoptic nucleus of the hypothalamus are different in male versus female rats. In males *nonamygdala* fibers make more connections on dendritic shafts while the same fibers in females form synaptic connections more frequently on dendritic spines. This difference in neural circuitry depends on early hormonal stimulation. At present the functional significance of this difference is unclear.

depend upon other regulating influences. A major source of regulation is environmental stimulation. As is discussed in Chapters 10 and 15, the development of neural systems underlying perception is strongly influenced by experience, particularly experience occurring early in life. Experiences can produce changes in the nervous system and behavior that alter the course of development throughout the lifetime of an individual. Recent studies of the development of singing in birds illustrate the complex interplay of genetic, hormonal, and environmental factors influencing the development of behavior (e.g., Marler, 1970; Nottebohm, 1975). Numerous studies investigated the development of the song of the male white-crowned sparrow (*Zonotrichia leucophrys*), a bird common to much of North America. The research has concentrated on a nonmigratory subspecies (*Nuttalli*) found in the San Francisco Bay area. These birds are monogamous and establish well-defined breeding territories in the late winter. After establishing the territory, the male patrols it, stridently singing, until he attracts a mate. The song of the adult male lasts 2 seconds and seems to serve several functions. It advertises the fact that he is in breeding condition, thus attracting prospective mates. Simultaneously, it signals to other males that the territorial boundaries are being patrolled. The song also identifies the singer as a white-crowned sparrow, though there are regional differences in the ordering of the elements of the song (Marler and Tamura, 1964). The regional differences in the ordering of the elements are referred to as *dialects* and identify the singer as belonging to a given region of the Bay area, since they are stable from year to year (Baptista, 1976). The difference in song dialects is illustrated in Fig. 16-12. The song also identifies the individual singer, since each individual's song is slightly different. These differences allow the different breeding males to recognize one another.

Thus the song has several potential functions. It identifies the species, the regional location, and the particular individual. Since the song also signals the reproductive condition of the male, it attracts females seeking a mate, warns away males seeking a territory, and establishes territorial boundaries between the singing male and his neighbors who are also patrolling their territorial boundaries.

The song of the white-crowned sparrow is quite stereotyped. Each male usually has only one song. Every male develops the species-characteristic song as it reaches adulthood in the spring of its first year of life. This genetically programmed developmental sequence is influenced, however, by the specific songs to which the developing birds are exposed during a *sensitive period* in their development.

The sensitive period for song learning occurs between the ages of 10 and 50 days (Marler, 1970). Typically, the young bird hears the song of its parent male most prominently, since the male parent remains actively singing on the home

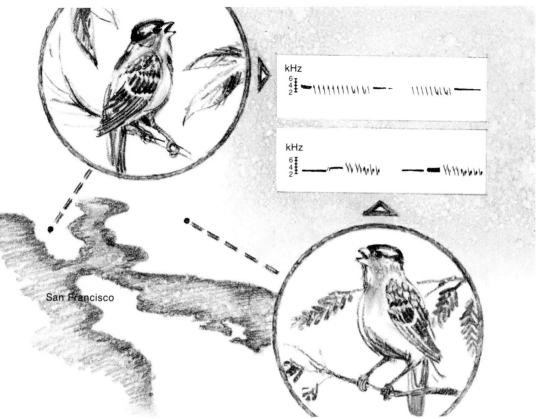

Fig. 16-12. Male white-crowned sparrows living in different parts of the San Francisco Bay area sing slightly different songs. These regional dialects can be easily distinguished using sonograms which show the change in sound frequency (in kilohertz, kHz) over time as the males sing. The dialects are stable over many years.

territory and assists the female in the care and feeding of the young, but what happens if the newly hatched bird does not hear the male parent's song during the sensitive period? If the young are removed from the nest and placed in acoustic isolation before the sensitive period, they develop a song at the appropriate time—when they are 200–250 days old. This song, however, will not have the detailed characteristics of the normal adult song. It will lack the characteristic complex trill notes, the rapid buzz, and other niceties. Rather, the song will consist of modulated whistle notes only. (Compare the song shown in Fig. 16-13B with the normal song shown in Fig. 16-13A.) When the tape-recorded song of a bird raised in acoustic isolation is played to territorial birds in the field, the territorial birds do not respond aggressively to the recording, as they do to a

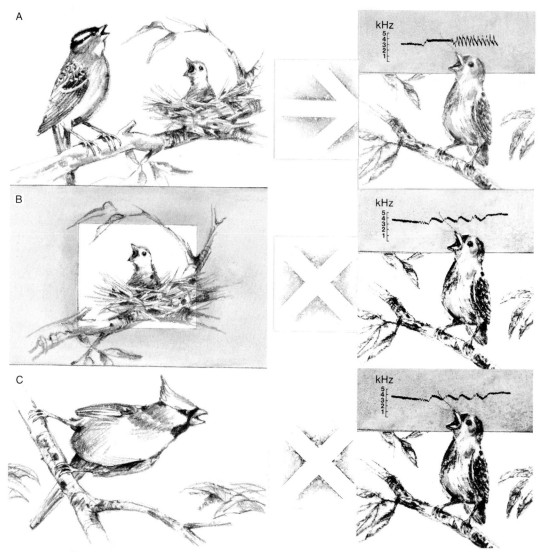

Fig. 16-13. In order to develop a normal song in adulthood, a young male white-crowned sparrow must hear adult males singing (A). If he is raised without such stimulation, his song will be abnormal (B). If he is exposed only to the song of a different species, such as a Mexican junco, during development, he will develop as if he heard no song (C). He will not accept any song except a white-crowned sparrow song as a model for his own song development.

recording of the normal adult song. Thus, the songs of isolated males do not seem to communicate the fact that the singer is a male white-crowned sparrow in breeding condition.

If a young bird is taken from the nest before the sensitive period and is tutored with the song of an adult from either his own or a different dialect group, it will learn the training song, and recordings of those songs will be responded to in a normal aggressive manner when it is played to territorial birds in the field.

If the song to which the isolated bird is exposed is that of an alien species, such as a song sparrow (*Melospiza melodia*) or a Mexican junco (*Junco phaenotus*), it will not learn the song. It will develop a song that is the same as that of an acoustically isolated bird who had heard no song at all (see Fig. 16-13C). Territorial birds to whom the songs of either the song sparrow or the Mexican junco are played do not respond to them.

These findings lead to several general principles of development. The first is the principle of a *sensitive period*, a time in the developmental history of an organism during which it is maximally receptive to certain classes of stimuli. For the white-crowned sparrow, that period is 10–50 days after hatching. If stimulation with certain specified characteristics is experienced during the sensitive period, development will proceed. These effective stimuli are sometimes referred to as *releasing stimuli*. For white-crowned sparrows, the sound stimulation must have the characteristics of the male white-crowned sparrow song. The specific sufficient physical characteristics that the adequate song must possess have not been determined yet. If the adequate stimulus is not experienced during the sensitive period, it will not affect development at other times. Apparently the developmental process, either neural or hormonal, does not permit utilization of the stimulation at later ages. The process has moved into a phase where the organism can no longer utilize the stimulation, or the developmental sequence has taken an alternate path and the once appropriate stimulation is no longer effective. This sequence of events has been identified in several species of birds. This phenomenon is called *imprinting*, since once the adequate stimulus has been experienced, its effects become "stamped in" and are usually irreversible. In developmental sequences of this type, the appropriate stimuli are those which the developing young will almost always experience in the normal course of events.

On the basis of the findings with white-crowned sparrows, it is argued that the birds acquire a sensory "template" of the appropriate song pattern during the sensitive period. This template is then remembered or "held" for a period of 5 or 6 months, at which time the levels of reproductive hormones rise and the bird develops the full song represented by the template. If the template is not established during the sensitive period, the characteristics of local dialects are lacking and the full song is an abnormal one. Thus, there is a stage during which sensory inputs of a rather specific nature establish a permanent copy of the full song, and this copy is held in the developing bird's memory. The birds will imitate only a limited range of auditory inputs: inputs that resemble quite closely the song of their species. Beyond this species specificity, there is some flexibility, since regional dialects are developed and are transmitted from male adults to their offspring.

A comment should be made regarding the rather remarkable *memory mechanism* involved in the process of song development. It appears that a very small number of repetitions of the song are sufficient to store the sensory template in some species. Since the birds store a memory trace of an input which has certain specific stimulus characteristics, there seems to be either a rather finely tuned sensory gating mechanism or a motor mechanism which is activated by only a narrow range of inputs. As mentioned earlier, this sensory template is held for several months. Then, when reproductive hormone levels rise in the spring, the male begins to sing the full song it heard several months before. It seems unlikely that the bird rehearses the song in this interval, since it does little singing during the time between "storage" and "retrieval." The singing that it does do is qualitatively quite different from the full song. The possibility that this trace system is rehearsed seems even more unlikely because female birds, which normally do not sing, will sing if administered the male hormone, testosterone. As is the case with males, the resulting song is the dialect to which they were exposed prior to the hormone administration.

This memory mechanism is quite unusual, since the storage of the memory trace is temporally very distant from its subsequent retrieval. It seems reasonable that memory mechanisms involved in such natural, species-typical behaviors as song development might be more analogous to those involved in the development of natural languages in other species, such as humans, than are the species-general memory mechanisms, such as those discussed in Chapter 8.

Other research (Konishi, 1965) has shown that if a white-crowned sparrow male is deafened after its song is fully developed, it will continue to sing the song quite well for 2 or 3 years. The deleterious effects of deafening on the development of the full song are greater the earlier the deafening occurs in the process of song development. If a white-crowned sparrow is exposed to adult song during the sensitive period and is then deafened, its song is abnormal and resembles the song of birds that are deafened before exposure to any song—the song is that of an acoustically isolated sparrow, as shown in Fig. 16-14. Thus it seems that the bird must hear its own vocal reproductions to match its vocal motor output to its memory template. This auditory feedback is necessary if full song is to develop. The effects of deafening on the song are quite analogous to those observed in humans, and the implications of these findings for human language are of considerable interest.

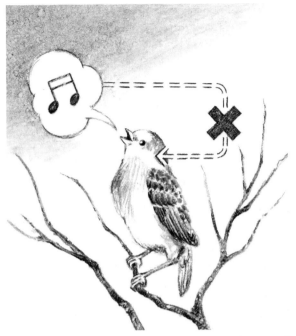

Fig. 16-14. When male white-crowned sparrows become mature, they begin singing. Gradually they match the song they sing to the model provided by songs they heard during development. In order for the song to develop properly, though, the male must be able to hear himself sing. If he is deafened, he will not develop a normal song.

V. Development of Language in Humans

One advantage of research with natural systems is that it deals with processes which have proved to be satisfactory in meeting the demands of environmental adjustment for the particular species under consideration. The class of such satisfactory adjustments must be finite, especially if we confine ourselves to the study of organisms which are adapted to a restricted range of ecological niches. It can be argued, for example, that vocalization in both birds and humans developed in response to similar selection pressures and that both are subject to similar general principles and mechanisms guiding adaptation and survival. If human and avian vocalizations can be considered to have similar ecological significance, then the development of both human and avian vocalizations might be expected to obey the same kinds of biological principles. Understanding the biological mechanisms of one system might provide insight into the biological mechanisms governing the other.

Before we consider the possible analogies between developmental systems such as those found in white-crowned sparrows and in humans, a *caveat* should be issued. The system which has been described to typify the development of song in the white-crowned sparrow does not typify the development of avian song in general. Almost every conceivable kind of developmental system exists in terms of the necessary and sufficient conditions which lead to the development of normal vocalizations in birds. Species exist which develop normal vocalizations even though the young are deafened shortly after hatching (domestic chicks, ring doves, and turkeys). Other species require only intact hearing to develop normal song in isolation (song sparrows). Still other species require not only intact hearing but must also have peers present during their mutual development (Oregon juncos). Some require not only intact hearing but exposure to adult song of their own species during a sensitive period (chaffinch and white-crowned sparrow). Thus, caution must be exercised when attempting to extrapolate from findings on one avian species to another. This diverse state of affairs provides as many advantages as it does disadvantages. Such a range of diversity allows one to employ the comparative method at its strongest. Do the patterns of differences and of similarities correspond to the ecological demands with which the organisms are faced? Do similar environmental demands result in similar functional solutions? What range of different solutions are possible given similar ecological demands? How are the functional solutions demanded by the ecology attained, given biological structures which arise from different phylogenetic origins? These questions are among the most interesting and exciting ones facing ethologists, psychobiologists, and sociobiologists at the present time (Wilson, 1975).

What is the nature of the development of human language? Can we find any compelling parallels between the developmental story for humans and the one for birds which we have recounted above?

First of all, we know that all normal young humans will, without any specialized training, develop into speakers of the language to which they are exposed. Studies of the pattern of normal speech development and the effects of deafness on development show that there is a sensitive period for normal vocal development (Petrinovich, 1972). There appears to be a regularity in the development of an infant's speech sounds from vocalic utterances to articulations in which the greatest possible phonemic distinctions are made with further developments occurring gradually as finer and finer movements of the articulatory apparatus are mastered. Velten (1943) maintains that the process of development from the greatest possible phonemic distinctions to smaller and smaller differentiations is the same for children of all linguistic communities. The number of sounds a child uses as it babbles gradually increases until at 30 months of age almost all vowels are present as well as two-thirds of the consonants. This increase probably is due to both neural maturation and to exposure to the particular sound community of the culture.

The importance of the maturational factors alone can be appreciated when the development of babbling in the deaf is considered. Children who are born deaf babble at about the normal age. Babbling continues for some time, but at a later stage, when auditory feedback would begin to assume some importance, babbling fades in the deaf child unless it can see people responding to its vocalizations. If the deaf child is provided with a hearing aid (assuming that there is some small amount of residual hearing), the babbling continues its normal course instead of fading out. In cases where the diagnosis of deafness takes place a short time after the normal babbling stage, the child begins to babble spontaneously some time after the introduction of a hearing aid.

Whitnall and Fry (1964) have found that after the age of 3 years the ability to learn to recognize new sounds diminishes, so that by the age of 5, it is difficult to teach a child using auditory inputs if there has been no previous training. By the age of 7, it is almost impossible to develop speech if training has not already begun. If sudden deafness occurs after an individual has learned to speak, there is no immediate loss of, nor any great modification in, the ability to speak. The changes that occur are very gradual, such as would occur as a function of a gradual drift in control due to the lack of sensory feedback.

It appears that there is a sensitive period during which the child can transform its babbling into the articulations that constitute its language. If the deaf child does not receive this sensory feedback from babbling, the babbling fades and normal language does not develop. If this sensitive period is passed, then the presentation of feedback (by way of a hearing aid) does not result in normal language.

The evidence on the development of song in deaf birds reveals a similar pattern to that observed with deaf children. Konishi (1965) has found that deafened white-crowned sparrows develop calls that are relatively normal both in number and in type. They also develop a normal subsong. The full songs, however, are composed of irregular "syllables" that have more frequency inflections than do normal syllables. Deafened white-crowned sparrows do not develop home dialects. Instead the song is made up of short, irregular notes and of fluctuating tones.

The picture for these birds, then, is similar to that for deaf children. The onset of babbling (and subsong) occurs whether or not the child (or bird) hears. However, if there is no auditory feedback during a sensitive period, normal speech (or full song) cannot develop. Babbling and the elements of subsong seem to be genetically determined, since both appear in deaf and in isolated organisms.

There is also an interesting parallel between the neural systems involved in human language and in the control of bird song. It is well known that, for right-handed individuals, the left side of the cerebral cortex subsumes language function. Damage to the left cortex results in a variety of language deficits such as a loss in the ability to recognize verbal utterances, an inability to relate verbal material to that presented to other sensory modalities, and great difficulties in producing utterances. Strong lateralization of complex functions has not been demonstrated for species other than man. Recently, however, Nottebohm (1975, 1977) has reported that the effects of denervation of the vocal apparatus of birds, the *syrinx*, are lateralized. If the right branch of the hypoglossal nerve, which controls the muscles of the right side of the syrinx, is sectioned, there is little loss of normal vocalizations. However, if the left branch of the hypoglossal nerve is sectioned, most of the components of calls, subsong, and song are lost. Nottebohm has demonstrated this effect in chaffinches, canaries, and white-crowned sparrows. In chaffinches the effects are irreversible in adults. If denervation is produced before song learning has occurred, however, the right hypoglossal nerve can take over and vocal functioning is not greatly impaired. The same pattern occurs in humans: if damage to the left cerebral hemisphere occurs in a child before the language function has been developed, the right hemisphere will take over and language will develop normally. However, if the lesion occurs after the child has acquired language, the marked abnormalities noted above are found, and they are almost always irreversible. Thus, the pattern both for vocal birds and for vocal humans is one in which both sides of the neural substratum have the potential to support complex vocal functions. However, after function has been assumed by one side, this equipotentiality is lost and the other side can no longer take over after damage to the dominant side. Karl Lashley demonstrated many years ago that this same principle of equipotentiality was necessary to account for the sparing and loss of learned habits in the laboratory rat as a function of lesions to various parts of the brain (Lashley, 1929).

It can be assumed that vocal functioning has a high priority in development. There seems to be a favored neural location in most individuals (the left hemisphere for right-handed individuals), and it is this location which subserves language in most individuals. If this location is damaged before functioning is established, the other side is utilized. Once language functions are established in the favored site, the neural tissue of the other side does not remain passively unused. It is utilized for other functions, such as visual symbolic functioning in humans, and is no longer available to assume the control of language. The pattern appears to be the same in the birds considered here, although it should be emphasized that in birds we are speaking only of control of motor functioning.

It can be argued that there are enough points of correspondence between the development of babbling in normal and deaf infants and the development of song dialects in normal, deaf, and acoustically isolated passerine birds to suggest that the analogy between the different language systems is a good one. Further, there are some suggestive parallels between the organization of the neural systems which control the two language systems. It appears, then, that the biological mechanisms involved in the development of the two systems are quite similar and that an understanding of one system might suggest useful approaches to an understanding of the other system. Since it is possible to manipulate experimentally the crucial environmental and organismic variables in birds, such experimentation might yield further insights into some of the biological mechanisms involved in the development of human language—mechanisms that cannot be directly explored in the developing human organism.

VI. Summary

The development of behavior is influenced by a complex interaction of genetic, hormonal and environmental factors. In some cases, a single gene is responsible for a major change in behavioral development. This allows the physiological mechanism of the genetic influence to be analyzed and can, in turn, suggest strategies for correcting genetically based behavioral disorders by changing the environment. For example, the severe mental retardation associated with phenylketonuria is caused by a single gene defect in phenylalanine metabolism. The retardation can be largely prevented if the disease is detected early and the child is placed on a low phenylalanine diet.

Most individual differences in behavioral development, though, reflect the interaction between many genes and environmental influences. Comparisons of inbred strains and development of selected lines are two ways in which the contribution of polygenes to behavioral development can be examined.

Chromosomal abnormalities can also cause changes in behavioral development. In Down syndrome, for example, mental retardation occurs as a result of an extra autosomal chromosome or chromosome segment. Behavioral changes are also associated with an abnormal complement of the sex chromosomes.

Development of sexual morphology and behavior are influenced by hormones, particularly androgens, during early development. In humans and other mammals, sexual differentiation of the reproductive tract and genitalia proceeds in the female direction in both genetic males and females unless the reproductive structures are stimulated by the secretions of the testes. Similarly, development in the male direction can occur in either genetic sex if the individual is exposed to male hormones during certain critical stages of development. This has been shown experimentally in animals. For humans, evidence for this conclusion is based on genetic disorders that affect either hormone secretion or the ability to respond to hormones. For example, genetic males that display the androgen-insensitivity syndrome develop as females because they are not able to respond to the masculinizing influences of their own testicular hormones. Genetic females with the adrenogenital syndrome are born with masculinized genitalia as a result of excessive secretion of androgens from their adrenal glands.

Sexual differentiation of behavior is also influenced by exposure to male hormones during early development. Genetically female animals exposed to androgens during critical periods of development can be both masculinized and defeminized in their adult behavior patterns. Similarly, genetic male animals that are not exposed to androgens during critical stages of development will be neither masculinized nor defeminized in their adult behavior patterns. The critical periods for masculinization and defeminization are different, though, which indicates that these two processes are independent. Masculinization here refers to the ability to respond to androgens with male behavior patterns in adulthood. Defeminization refers to the inability to respond to estrogen and progesterone with receptive behavior in adulthood. Such early developmental influences of androgens may also exist in humans, but environmental influences can override them.

Research on the cellular mechanisms underlying sexual differentiation of behavior has focused on sex differences in hypothalamic neurons, particularly on their responses to estrogen. Hypothalamic neurons of both sexes accumulate estrogen from the blood and retain it in their nuclei; however, the hypothalamic nuclei in males do not retain estrogen as long as the nuclei of females do. This biochemical difference between the sexes may be related to sex differences in behavioral responses to estrogen. Hormone-sensitive sex differences have also been observed in the patterns of synaptic connections with the preoptic area, which is adjacent to the hypothalamus.

Environmental stimulation during critical periods of development may also have profound effects on behavioral development. The process of song learning in male white-crowned sparrows illustrates this. Singing is stimulated in males by androgens secreted by the testes at sexual maturity. Yet in order to sing a song that is recognized as a white-crowned sparrow song, the male needs additional stimulation. He must be able to hear himself singing. Without such auditory feedback, his song will not develop properly. Equally important, he must be exposed when young to the songs of adult male white-crowned sparrows. Although he himself will not begin singing for months, he must hear the songs during a critical period of development in order to use them as models later. If he does not hear them when young, he will sing an abnormal song as an adult even if he does hear white-crowned sparrow songs in adulthood. The song to which the young male is exposed must be a white-crowned sparrow song in order to serve effectively as a model. Songs of other species will not be copied. Thus, while environmental stimulation is necessary for singing to develop normally, there are constraints on which stimuli will be accepted and on the ages at which they will be effective.

Some interesting parallels exist between the development of song in white-crowned sparrows and the development of language in humans. A child needs auditory feedback to change from babbling to articulating the sounds of its language. Moreover, this feedback must be provided during a restricted period of early development. The neural systems controlling singing in birds and language in humans are also similar in that both are controlled primarily by the left side of the nervous system. Language is controlled by the left hemisphere of the brain in most humans and singing is controlled by the left branch of the hypoglossal nerve to the vocal apparatus in birds. In both species, the right side can take over the functions of the left side if the left side is damaged before singing or language develop. However, if the left side is damaged in adulthood the effects are irreversible because the right side can no longer take over these functions.

Key Terms

Adrenogenital syndrome: A syndrome in which genetic females develop malelike genitalia; the adrenal gland secretes high levels of androgen and causes the genital sinus to develop in a malelike fashion.

Alleles: One of two or more alternative forms of a gene.

Androgens: Male hormones; a class of hormones (19-carbon steroids) secreted by the testis, e.g., testosterone.

Androgen-insensitivity syndrome: A syndrome in which genetic males fail to develop normal male genitals because they are not stimulated by testosterone; they develop as females except they lack ovaries and a uterus.

Autosome: A chromosome other than a sex chromosome.

Chromosome: One of the rod-shaped structures into which the chromatin of a cell nucleus resolves itself prior to cell division; chromosomes carry the genes.

Defeminization: The inability to respond to estrogen and progesterone with receptive behavior in adulthood.

Dialects: In bird song, regional differences in the ordering of the elements of the song.

Down syndrome: A genetic disorder whereby mental development is severely retarded; it results from a chromosomal excess.

Estrogen: A generic term for hormones which produce estrus; specifically, the female steroid hormone (a derivative of cholesterol). Estrogen is secreted by the ovaries, adrenal gland and placenta. It promotes the development of female sexual characteristics and behaviors.

Gene: The fundamental unit of heredity that consists of a certain sequence of DNA.

Genotype: The genetic makeup of an individual or cell.

Heterozygous: Different alleles at a given locus.

Homozygous: Identical alleles at a given locus.

Hygienic behavior: A behavior displayed by bees in which they uncap the cells of diseased larvae and remove them from the hive.

Imprinting: The process whereby once an adequate stimulus is experienced it becomes fixed into the individual's behavioral characteristics.

Inbred strain: A population with specific characteristics obtained by repeated mating of individuals closely related to each other.

Kleinfelter syndrome: A syndrome in which individuals have a masculine body but show atrophy of the reproductive tube system and impaired testicular function; it is a result of one extra X chromosome in an otherwise normal male.

Lesch–Nyhan syndrome: A male genetic disorder which results in cerebral palsy, involuntary movements, mental retardation and aggressiveness; it is due to a deficiency of an enzyme in purine synthesis resulting in excess uric acid.

Masculinization: The ability to respond to androgens with male behavior patterns in adulthood.

Mullerian duct: The female part of the primordial sexual structures of the developing embryo.

Pallid: A recessive neurological mutation in mice which results in difficulty in maintaining equilibrium.

Phenotype: A visible trait or characteristic common to a group as determined by their genetic makeup or environment.

Phenylalanine hydroxylase: The enzyme which converts phenylalanine to tyrosine; severe deficiencies produce phenylketonuria.

Phenylketonuria: A human mutation that produces severe mental retardation; the amino acid, phenylalanine, is improperly metabolized owing to the absence of phenylalanine hydroxylase.

Polygenic: Determined by many different genes whose action on the phenotype is additive.

Progesterone: A 21-carbon steroid produced by the ovary and adrenal cortex that acts on the uterus to maintain pregnancy.

Receptor proteins: In endocrinology, specific protein(s) contained in the cytoplasm of target cells which bind hormones. The hormone–receptor complex is then translocated to the nucleus where it activates the genes and stimulates the production of specific messenger RNAs.

Recessive: A gene not expressed in the phenotype due to the existence of another dominant form of the gene.

Releasing stimuli: In imprinting, stimuli with certain specified characteristics which, if experienced during the sensitive period, allow normal development.

Selective breeding: Mating of individuals who are phenotypically more similar (with respect to behavior or other characteristics) than other individuals in a population.

Sensitive period: In bird development, the time period when the development of song is influenced by the songs it hears; the time in the developmental history of an organism during which it is maximally receptive to certain classes of stimuli.

Sex chromosome: Chromosomes involved in sex determination; there are two such chromosomes designated by the letters X and Y. The Y chromosome carries male-determining properties.

Tay–Sachs disease: A genetic disorder resulting in progressive blindness, paralysis, idiocy and death; it is due to a deficiency in an enzyme of carbohydrate metabolism.

Testosterone: An androgen; a male steroid hormone. It is the primary hormone secreted by the testes and responsible for the development of male sex characteristics.

Triple-X syndrome: Individuals have a female phenotype and are usually fertile but may have an early menopause; it is a result of an extra X chromosome in an otherwise normal female.

Turner syndrome: Individuals have a female body form but the ovaries fail to develop; one sex chromosome is missing (XO pattern).

Wolffian duct: The masculine part of the primordial sexual structures of the developing embryo.

XYY syndrome: Males with this disorder have an additional Y, or the male-determining chromosome.

Y chromosome: The male determining chromosome.

General References

Jarvik, L. F., Klodin, V., and Matsuyama, S. S. (1973). Human aggression and the extra Y chromosome. *Am. Psychol.* **28,** 674–682.

McClearn, G. E., and DeFries, J. C. (1973). "Behavioral Genetics." Freeman, San Francisco, California.

Money, J., and Ehrhardt, A. A. (1972). "Man and Woman, Boy and Girl." Johns Hopkins Univ. Press, Baltimore, Maryland.

Montagna, W., and Sadler, W., eds. (1973). "Reproductive Behavior." Plenum, New York.

Nottebohm, F. (1972). The origins of vocal learning. *Am. Nat.* **106,** 116–140.

Nottebohm, F. (1975). A zoologist's view of some language phenomena with particular emphasis on vocal learning. *In* "Foundations of Language Development" (E. H. Lenneberg and E. Lenneberg, eds.), Vol. 1, pp. 61–103. Academic Press, New York.

Omenn, G. S. (1976). Inborn errors of metabolism: Clues to understanding human behavioral disorders. *Behav. Genet.* **6**, 263–284.

Petrinovich, L. (1972). Psychobiological mechanisms in language development. *Adv. Psychobiol.* **1**, 259–285.

Thiessen, D. D. (1972). "Gene Organization and Behavior." Random House, New York.

References

Alexander, D., Ehrhardt, A. A., and Money, J. (1966). Defective figure drawing, geometric and human, in Turner's syndrome. *J. Nerv. Ment. Dis.* **142**, 161–167.

Baptista, L. F. (1976). Song dialects and demes in sedentary populations of the White-crowned Sparrow (*Zonotrichia leucophrys Nuttalli*). *Univ. Calif., Berkeley, Publ. Zool.* **105**, 1–52 (monogr.).

Beach, F. A., Keuhn, R. E., Sprague, R. H., and Anisko, J. J. (1973). Coital behavior in dogs. XI. Effects of androgenic stimulation during development on masculine mating responses in females. *Horm. Behav.* **3**, 143–168.

Clemens, L. G. Neurohormonal control of male sexual behavior. *In* "Reproductive Behavior" (W. Montagna and W. Sadler, eds.), pp. 23–53. Plenum, New York.

Cooper, R. M., and Zubek, J. P. (1958). Effects of enriched and restricted early environment on the learning ability of bright and dull rats. *Can. J. Psychol.* **2**, 159–164.

Cotzias, G. D., Tang, L. C., Miller, T., Sladic-Simic, D., and Hurley, L. S. (1972). A mutation influencing the transportation of manganese, L-dopa, and L-tryptophan. *Science* **176**, 410–412.

DeBold, J. F., and Whalen, R. E. (1975). Differential sensitivity of mounting and lordosis control systems to early androgen treatment in male and female hamsters. *Horm. Behav.* **6**, 197–209.

Edwards, D. A. (1969). Early androgen stimulation and aggressive behavior in male and female mice. *Physiol. Behav.* **4**, 333–338.

Erway, L., Hurley, L. S., and Fraser, A. (1966). Neurological defect: Manganese in phenocopy and prevention of a genetic abnormality of inner ear. *Science* **152**, 1766–1768.

Guillery, R. W. (1974). Visual pathways in albinos. *Sci. Am.* **230**, 44–54.

Hook, E. B. (1973). Behavioral implications of the human XYY genotype. *Science* **179**, 139–150.

Jarvik, L. F., Klodin, V., and Matsuyama, S. S. (1973). Human aggression and the extra Y chromosome. *Am. Psychol.* **28**, 674–682.

Kessler, S., and Moos, R. H. (1970). The XYY karyotype and criminality: A review. *J. Psychiatr. Res.* **7**, 153–170.

Konishi, M. (1965). The role of auditory feedback in the control of vocalization in the White-crowned Sparrow. *Z. Tierpsychol.* **22**, 770–783.

Lashley, K. (1929). "Brain Mechanisms and Intelligence." Univ. of Chicago Press, Chicago, Illinois.

McClearn, G. E., and DeFries, J. C. (1973). "Behavioral Genetics." Freeman, San Francisco, California.

Marler, P. (1970). A comparative approach to vocal learning: Song development in White-crowned Sparrows. *J. Comp. Physiol. Psychol.* **71**, 1–25. (monogr.)

Marler, P., and Tamura, M. (1964). Culturally transmitted patterns of vocal behavior in sparrows. *Science* **146**, 1483–1486.

Money, J. (1975). Ablatio penis: Normal male infant sex-reassigned as a girl. *Arch. Sex. Behav.* **4**, 65–71.

Money, J., and Ehrhardt, A. A. (1972). "Man and Woman, Boy and Girl." Johns Hopkins Univ. Press, Baltimore, Maryland.

Money, J., Hampson, H. J., and Hampson, J. L. (1955). Examination of some basic sexual concepts: The evidence of hermaphroditism. *Bull. Johns Hopkins Hosp.* **97**, 301–319.

Nottebohm, F. (1975). A zoologist's view of some language phenomena with particular emphasis on vocal learning. *In* "Foundations of Language Development." (E. H. Lenneberg and E. Lenneberg, eds.), Vol. 1, pp. 61–103. Academic Press, New York.

Nottebohm, F. (1977). Asymmetries in neural control of vocalization in the canary. In "Lateralization in the Nervous System" (S. Harnad, ed.), pp. 23–44. Academic Press, New York.

Okada, S., and O'Brien, J. S. (1969). Tay-Sachs disease: Generalized absence of a β-D-N-acetylhexaminidase component. *Science* **165**, 698–700.

Omenn, G. S. (1976). Inborn errors of metabolism: Clues to understanding human behavioral disorders. *Behav. Genet.* **6**, 263–284.

Petrinovich, L. (1972). Psychobiological mechanisms in language development. *Adv. Psychobiol.* **1**, 259–285.

Phoenix, C. H., Goy, R. W., Gerall, A. A., and Young, W. C. (1959). Organizing action of prenatally administered testosterone propionate on the tissues mediating mating behavior in the female guinea pig. *Endocrinology* **65**, 369–382.

Raisman, G., and Field, P. M. (1973). Sexual dimorphism in the neuropil of the preoptic area of the rat and its dependence on neonatal androgen. *Brain Res.* **54**, 1–29.

Rockson, S., Stone, R., van der Weyden, M., and Kelly, W. N. (1974). Lesch-Nyhan syndrome: Evidence for abnormal adrenergic function. *Science* **186**, 934–935.

Rothenbuhler, W. C. (1964). Behaviour genetics of nest cleaning in honey bees. I. Responses of four inbred lines to disease-killed brood. *Anim. Behav.* **12**, 578–583.

Thiessen, D. D. (1972). "Gene Organization and Behavior." Random House, New York.

Tryon, R. C. (1942). Individual differences. In "Comparative Psychology" (F. A. Moss, ed.), pp. 330–365. Prentice-Hall, Englewood Cliffs, New Jersey.

Velten, H. V. (1943). The growth of phonemic and lexical patterns in infant language. *Language* **19**, 281–292.

Whalen, R. E., and Edwards, D. A. (1967). Hormonal determinants of the development of masculine and feminine behavior in male and female rats. *Anat. Rec.* **157**, 173–180.

Whalen, R. E., and Massicci, J. (1975). Subcellular analysis of the accumulation of estrogen by the brain of male and female rats. *Brain Res.* **89**, 255–264.

Whitnall, E., and Fry, D. B. (1964). "The Deaf Child." Heinemann, London.

Wilson, E. O. (1975). "Sociobiology: The New Synthesis." Harvard Univ. Press, Cambridge, Massachusetts.

17

Behavioral Disorders

I. Introduction

Disorders of the nervous system can ruin the lives of individuals and are of such a magnitude that they create many of our greatest social problems. People become mentally ill, insane or psychotic, and a few such individuals in a society can destroy its fabric. People can become addicted to drugs. They can ruin their lives, and their habits create an underworld willing and able to exploit them. Some people become alcoholics. In this chapter we will explore these behavioral disorders. What are their characteristics, and what are their biological origins? By understanding these behavioral disorders we can help those affected understand themselves, help others understand them and devise cures.

II. Schizophrenia

In the fifteenth century, the mentally ill were considered madmen. They were persecuted, tortured and burned alive. They were all thought to be possessed by evil spirits. Even into the 1800's the insane were not understood by society. They

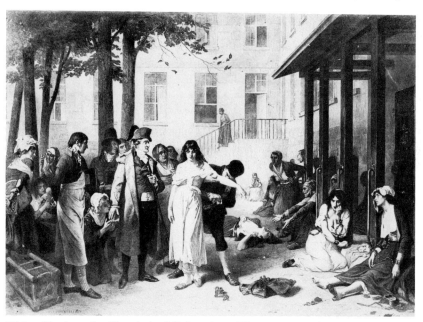

Fig. 17-1. Pinel at the Hospital of Salpetriere. This painting shows the general sorry state of an early women's mental institution. Pinel was one of the first to reform these institutions. He believed that mental illness was a disease like other diseases and patients could be rehabilitated and better cared for in other ways. He is shown here releasing patients. (Courtesy of Culver Pictures.)

17. BEHAVIORAL DISORDERS

were put away, chained in rows and treated inhumanely (Fig. 17-1). Today we realize, through modern research, that most mental disease is a biochemical dysfunction of the brain which can be treated in many cases.

There is no universally accepted definition of schizophrenia, and, in fact, it remains unclear as to whether schizophrenia is a single disorder or a heterogeneous group of disorders. Schizophrenia may be a clinical syndrome with multiple causes. It is, however, also possible that the diversity of symptoms associated with schizophrenia results from various modifying factors that influence the expression of a specific defect. The question of single versus multiple causes is a critical one which bears directly on the strategies of research used to identify biological variables that might be related to schizophrenia as well as on the choice of appropriate treatment procedures.

A. Clinical Description and Treatment

The primary characteristic of schizophrenia is the impairment of logical thought processes. Speech is often bizarre and confused, reflecting a disturbed mind. Thoughts that are usually only remotely connected emerge together in speech (loose associations), and in extreme cases speech may be completely incomprehensible. It comes out, as some have said, like "word salad."

Schizophrenic patients often present flattened or completely inappropriate emotional responses. Other symptoms include autism, ambivalence, stereotypy, as well as delusions and hallucinations.

We can see many of these characteristics from first person accounts written by schizophrenics.

Thinking is disorganized.

My concentration is very poor. I jump from one thing to another. If I am talking to someone, they only need to cross their legs or scratch their heads and I am distracted and forget what I was saying.

Half the time I am talking about things and thinking about half a dozen other things at the same time. I must look queer to people when I laugh about something that has got nothing to do with what I am talking about, but they don't know what's going on inside and how much of it is running around in my head. You see I might be talking about something quite serious to you and other things come into my head at the same time that are funny and this makes me laugh. If I could only concentrate on one thing at the one time I wouldn't look half so silly.

My thoughts get all jumbled up. . . . People listening to me get more lost than I do (from "Schizophrenia: Is There an Answer?," 1972).

Emotions are extreme.

I felt all this tumult of madness—all this stark, lonely living which is worse than death—and the pain, futility and hopelessness of it all—and the endlessness, the eternity (from "Schizophrenia: Is There an Answer?," 1972).

Speech is obscure.

The seabeach gathering homestead building upon the site of the bear mountains. Time placed of the dunce to the recovery of the setting sun, upon the stream, poling paddleboat, Mickey, Rooney, Bill. Proceeded of, to the onlivenment. Placed upon the assiduous laboriousness of keeping aloof, yet alive to the forest stream. Haunting the distance of the held possession, requiring means of liberty of sociability . . . (Lehmann, 1967, p. 627).

Schizophrenia is often divided into subtypes on the basis of the pattern of symptoms. However, individuals can be included in several different subtypes during the course of their illness because the predominant clinical signs may change over time.

The major advances made in the treatment of schizophrenia over the last several decades have been attributed primarily to the development of several classes of drugs called neuroleptics. *Neuroleptics* are defined generally as any medication with antipsychotic properties. This class includes the *phenothiazines* such as chlorpromazine (Thorazine), thioxanthenes such as thiothixene (Navane), and butyrophenones such as haloperidol (Haldol). These drugs have specific antipsychotic properties unlike the minor tranquilizers or sedatives (Klein and Davis, 1969).

The availability of drugs for the treatment of mental disease had tremendous impact on psychiatric patient care practices (Ban, 1969; DiMascio and Shader, 1970; Hollister, 1973). Before the major classes of antipsychotic and antidepressant medications were introduced during the 1950's, mental patients were being hospitalized in alarmingly increasing numbers. Approximately 50% of all hospital beds in the United States were occupied by psychiatric patients! This trend has been reversed by the discovery of effective pharmacological therapies, so that over the last 15 years hospital occupancy has been reduced by as much as 75%. The drug therapy is so effective that severely disabled patients regain relatively normal functioning in a very large number of cases. How did this triumph of modern medicine come about?

Interestingly, discovery of the psychotherapeutic drugs came about in the course of research on seemingly unrelated topics. Thus, *chlorpromazine,* the prototypic antipsychotic phenothiazine, was originally synthesized in an effort to develop more effective antihistamines. In 1951, when chlorpromazine was used as part of an anesthetic "lytic cocktail," its potential antipsychotic properties were recognized, and in 1952 it was tested in schizophrenics. In the early 1950's, iproniazid, the prototypic monoamine oxidase inhibitor, was found to produce euphoric effects in patients with tuberculosis, and by 1957 it was used clinically as an antidepressant agent. Curiously, the initial clinical trials of lithium—an important drug for the treatment of mania—were prompted by the observation that lithium produced a state of lethargy in guinea pigs.

The therapeutic efficacy of each of these drugs has been discovered more or less by chance. It is generally agreed that the rational development of psychotherapeutic agents must await a more complete understanding of the etiologies of the psychiatric disorders. A number of models currently exist which have generated considerable research directed at determining the pathogenesis of schizophrenia and affective disorders.

B. Hypotheses on the Molecular Basis of Schizophrenia

Research on the causes of schizophrenia is very difficult because of the complex nature of the disease and the absence of animal models. How does one create and measure schizophrenia in a rat, if indeed rats become schizophrenic? It would seem that researchers would be confined to the analysis of blood and occasional biopsy samples of patients. Such studies have been tried and rarely yield satisfactory results because of small and heterogeneous groups as well as complications due to the medication the patients receive. The main approach used to identify the molecular malfunctions in schizophrenics has been to study the mechanisms of action of neuroleptic drugs in experimental animals. If certain drugs alleviate schizophrenia, identifying their common mechanisms of action should reveal the basic causes. Such a strategy has yielded good, if not amazing, progress.

C. Dopamine Hypothesis

According to the dopamine hypothesis, schizophrenia results from overactivity of dopaminergic systems in the brain (Mathysse and Lipinski, 1975; Snyder, 1976). Dopaminergic systems overstimulate brain cells and in some way upset the delicate balance necessary for normal brain function. Prior to discussing the evidence behind this idea, consider for a moment its implications. If true, the dopamine hypothesis means that normal thought and emotional processes can become bizarre due to malfunctions in one chemical system of the brain.

The initial breakthrough came from the observation that phenothiazines produce an elevation in dopamine (DA) metabolites in experimental animals. It was suggested that this is a reflection of a compensatory increase in DA neuron activity in response to the drug-related receptor blockade. The increase in DA metabolites caused by drugs closely parallels their antipsychotic potencies. For example, promethazine (Phenergan), which is ineffective as an antischizophrenic agent, does not produce an increase in the level of DA metabolites.

Perhaps, then, the therapeutic effect of phenothiazines is related to their effectiveness as DA receptor antagonists. Dopamine receptors can be studied, as we previously saw (see Chapter 5), by analyzing the binding of DA receptor antagonists to brain synaptic membranes. Synaptic membranes are isolated, and the relative ability of antischizophrenic drugs to displace a radioactive dopamine antagonist is analyzed. Using this technique, startling parallels emerge between receptor affinity and antischizophrenic efficacy for both the phenothiazines and butyrophenones (Burt *et al.*, 1975; Creese *et al.*, 1976a,b) (Fig. 17-2). It appears that the affinity of phenothiazines for the DA receptor is determined by their relative ability to assume a DA-like conformation. Electrophysiological studies

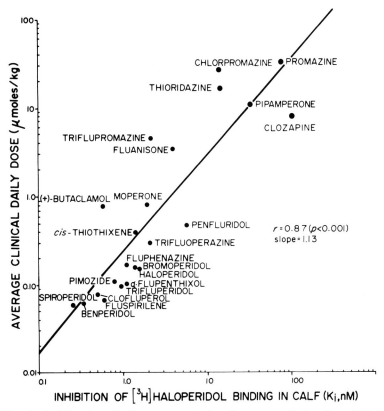

Fig. 17-2. Antischizophrenic drugs: correlation between affinity for [³H]haloperidol binding and clinical potency. (From Creese *et al.*, 1976. Copyright by the American Association for the Advancement of Science.)

also show that phenothiazines block the effects of locally applied DA on DA receptors (Aghajanian and Bunney, 1974).

Additional biochemical evidence implicating DA receptor blockade in the therapeutic effects of the phenothiazines has involved the use of *adenylate cyclase* activity as an index of receptor sensitivity. Recall that one of the consequences of dopamine's action on postsynaptic receptors is to stimulate adenylate cyclase activity (Fig. 17-3). In brain regions relatively selective in their response to DA, phenothiazines block the DA-induced stimulation of the cAMP generating system, and this is proportional to their clinical efficacy (Clement-Cormier *et al.*, 1974; Miller *et al.*, 1974; Lippmann *et al.*, 1975). The phenothiazines will also act presynaptically to inhibit DA release (Seeman and Lee, 1975); however, their primary locus of action appears to be on postsynaptic receptors (Iversen *et al.*, 1976).

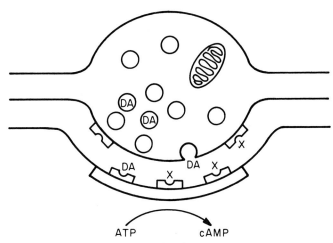

Fig. 17-3. Phenothiazines (X) antagonize the action of dopamine (DA) on dopamine receptors. They block the receptors and prevent the DA-induced stimulation of adenylate cyclase which synthesizes cAMP from ATP. Phenothiazines also appear to act on presynaptic receptors and reduce DA release.

Further evidence implicating DA in schizophrenia comes from research with amphetamine. Amphetamine produces a paranoid psychosis in nonpsychotic individuals, especially when administered at chronic high doses (Connell, 1958; Angrist and Gershon, 1970). An association between amphetamine psychosis and schizophrenia is suggested by the fact that neuroleptics appear to be the best antidotes for these amphetamine-induced behavioral states. In addition, many of the behavioral effects produced by amphetamines have been attributed to an increase in extracellular DA (Groves and Rebec, 1976).

Thus schizophrenia may be caused by DA hyperactivity in certain brain DA pathways. The particular pathway(s) involved in schizophrenia are unclear, but the mesolimbic pathway is frequently mentioned in this regard. Hyperactivity of dopaminergic systems in schizophrenia could result from excess synthesis or release of DA, its impaired metabolism or inactivation, or DA receptor hypersensitivity (Matthysse and Lipinski, 1975; Snyder, 1976). The next chapter of the story must await measurements on tissue from schizophrenia patients.

D. The Transmethylation Hypothesis

Over the last two decades a considerable amount of research has been generated within the context of the transmethylation hypothesis (Wyatt *et al.*, 1971). This hypothesis was originally based on the structural similarities between hallucinogenic compounds (such as mescaline and N,N-dimethyltryptamine) and norepinephrine and serotonin (Fig. 17-4). Since many of the hallucinogens are

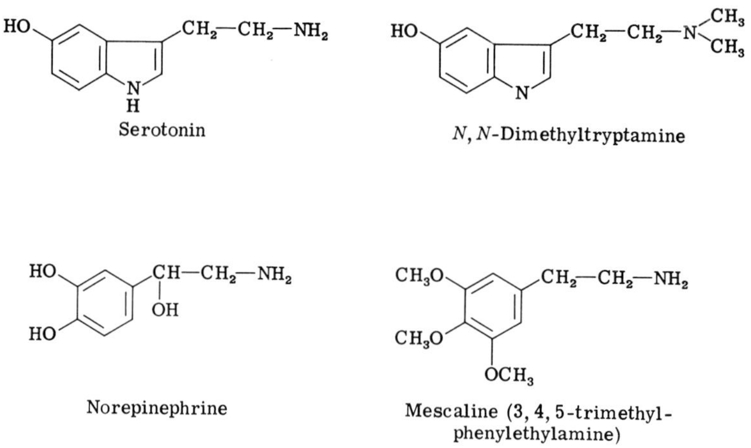

Fig. 17-4. Chemical structures of serotonin, N,N-dimethyltryptamine, norepinephrine, and mescaline.

essentially methylated analogues of the catecholamine (CA) and indoleamine neurotransmitters, it may be that under some circumstances a "schizotoxin" might be naturally formed that, if accumulated in sufficient concentrations, produces psychotic behavior. In other words, perhaps the brain makes its own hallucinogens (Osmond and Smythies, 1952). Although much of the research generated by this model has yielded conflicting results, it has continued to have heuristic value. One line of research which has recently received renewed attention involves the possible role of dimethyltryptamine in the pathophysiology of schizophrenia (Gillin *et al.*, 1976). In support of this possibility is the finding that the means for synthesizing this compound, including the presence of amine methylating enzymes, exist in humans. Moreover, there is evidence that neuroleptics may inhibit the activity of N-methyltransferase, the enzyme thought to mediate the formation of dimethyltryptamine from tryptamine. These findings are certainly provocative, and as further research is carried out it will be exciting to see if the brain does, in fact, contain endogenous "schizotoxins."

E. Norepinephrine Reward Pathways and Schizophrenia

According to this hypothesis progressive damage to the norepinephrine reward pathways underlies schizophrenia (Stein and Wise, 1971). It was shown that in rats a significant reduction in intracranial self-stimulation is, in fact, produced by 6-hydroxydopamine, a drug which under certain circumstances appears to be relatively selective in its destruction of norepinephrine (NE) neurons in the brain. Since the effects of this neurotoxin on self-stimulation are blocked by chlorpromazine, it was proposed that the therapeutic action of neuroleptics may be related to their inhibition of cellular mechanisms responsible for the accumulation of 6-hydroxydopamine. Perhaps 6-hydroxydopamine accumulates during schizophrenia and NE pathways are progressively destroyed. In support of this hypothesis, some evidence shows that NE pathways may be damaged in schizophrenia patients (Wise and Stein, 1973); however, subsequent research has not confirmed these findings (Wyatt *et al.*, 1975).

F. Endorphin Theory

As discussed in Chapter 6, *endorphins* are a class of peptides found in brain which have opiatelike activities, i.e., they have a powerful analgesic action. However, their influence does not appear restricted to analgesia. One particularly curious effect suggests a possible relation to schizophrenia. Small quantities of β-endorphin (a specific endorphin) were injected directly into the brain of rats. Within 10 minutes animals showed general depressed motor activity, by 15 minutes they displayed a profound analgesia, and by 30 minutes they showed a striking catatonic state. A catatonic state is generally defined as one characterized by muscular rigidity and immobility. Such animals were "stiff as a board" and could be placed across metal bookends which were in contact only at the upper neck and base of the tail (Fig. 17-5). Animals remained in this state for a couple of hours at which time they rapidly and completely recovered. All actions of β-endorphin were reversed by *naloxone* (a relatively specific endogenous opiate antagonist), and endorphins other than β-endorphin were ineffective. The concentration of

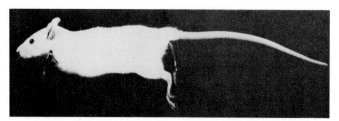

Fig. 17-5. Thirty minutes after the intracisternal injection of β-endorphin (14.9 nmoles) this rat exhibited sufficient rigid immobility to remain totally self-supporting when placed across metal bookends which are in contact only at the upper neck and base of the tail. Note the erect ears and tail. (From Bloom *et al.*, 1976. Copyright by the American Association for the Advancement of Science.)

β-endorphins required were 1/100 those at which Met[5]-enkephalin inhibited responses to noxious agents (Bloom *et al.*, 1976).

Schizophrenics often show catatonic states. It was, therefore, suggested that β-endorphin induces a "catatonic state in rats reminiscent of some aspects of schizophrenia" (Bloom *et al.*, 1976). Other findings in animals as well suggest a relationship of endorphins to various psychotic states (McMillan, 1971; Holtzman, 1974; Cox *et al.*, 1976; deWied, 1979).

Are endorphins involved in the etiology of schizophrenia in humans? Perhaps schizophrenics have elevated levels of endorphins. If so naloxone should reduce the symptoms of schizophrenia. Initial reports indicated that some schizophrenics had abnormally high levels of endorphins in their cerebrospinal fluid (Terenius *et al.*, 1976) and that naloxone rapidly abolished hallucinations (Gunne *et al.*, 1977). However, other studies have failed to find that naloxone has rapidly occurring antipsychotic effects in schizophrenics (see Volanka *et al.*, 1977; Janowsky *et al.*, 1977). Studies on patients are complex indeed. Schizophrenia is a complex disease, and it may be that subgroups not yet consistently identified and tested may be assisted by naloxone therapy. Also the fact that patients tested are most often on other drugs, may complicate the results.

We can conclude that endorphins have actions in animals which suggest a possible relationship to schizophrenia in humans. The results on patients, however, while suggestive are certainly not definitive. More work is necessary.

III. Affective Disorders

We all experience a range of emotions. However, some extremes of mood may be so disabling as to be considered an illness. An individual severely *depressed* may be so overwrought by feelings of loneliness, guilt, and worthlessness that suicide may seem to be the only avenue of escape. At the other extreme, *mania* may be associated with overoptimism, grandiosity, and unrealistic self-confidence that results in pronounced social dysfunction. Such disorders of mood are termed *affective disorders*. These disorders differ from schizophrenia in that thought processes are not markedly changed and patients do not tend to behave in a bizarre manner.

A.   Clinical Description and Treatment

Depression is diagnosed as being either primarily endogenous or exogenous. The endogenous form of depression refers to severe depression which occurs in the absence of any identifiable external source; the exogenous form of depression results from external stresses. Endogenous depression is associated with a greater number of somatic symptoms and is more responsive to drug and electroconvulsive therapies.

Another approach to classification involves the differentiation between primary and secondary affective disorders. The primary form refers to those disorders which occur without the coexistence of other psychiatric disturbances. Secondary affective disorders occur in the wake of some other psychiatric disorder.

One category widely used in the United States is manic-depressive psychosis. Individuals diagnosed as manic-depressive frequently have a family history of affective disease. They may exhibit either depressive or manic periods (unipolar) or both (bipolar) during the cyclical course of this illness.

Drugs or electroconvulsive therapy are usually required for the treatment of severe affective disorders. The *tricyclic antidepressants* such as *imipramine* (Tofranil) are most frequently used for treating depression. For some reason as yet not understood, usually 2–3 weeks of treatment are necessary before noticeable improvement.

Electroconvulsive therapy has been demonstrated to be an extremely effective and relatively safe method for treating severe depression; 80–90% of patients improve as compared to 70–80% for the tricyclics. As with drug treatment, significant alleviation of symptoms with electroconvulsive therapy is not immediately apparent after the initiation of treatment.

Manic patients are usually treated with neuroleptics (see Section II), especially for acute relief of symptoms. However, *lithium* appears better for the long-term treatment of mania. Improvement in about 70% of manic patients is observed after 5–10 days of treatment. Accumulating evidence also indicates that in bipolar patients—patients sometimes manic and sometimes depressive—lithium may also have protective qualities for the treatment of both manic and depressive episodes.

B. Molecular Basis of Depression and Mania: Catecholamine Hypothesis of Affective Disorders

The catecholamine hypothesis of affective disorders is a landmark in biological psychiatry. Since its conception in 1965, it has served the purposes a good hypothesis should: it has stood the test of time fairly well, it has promoted vast amounts of research both clinical and experimental, and it has generated many new insights into brain function. It is straightforward, reasonable and testable. As Schildkraut stated in his original paper:

> During the past decade there has been a gradual accumulation of evidence suggesting a possible link between the affective disorders (depressions and elations) and changes in central nervous system catecholamine metabolism. Most of this evidence is indirect, deriving from pharmacological studies with drugs such as reserpine, amphetamine and the monoamine oxidase inhibitor antidepressants which produce affective changes in man.
>
> These studies have shown a fairly consistent relationship between drug effects on catecholamines, especially norepinephrine, and affective or behavioral states. Those drugs which cause depletion and inactivation of norepinephrine centrally produce sedation or depression, while drugs which increase or potentiate brain norepinephrine are associated with behavioral stimulation or excitement and generally exert an antidepressant effect in man.
>
> The "catecholamine hypothesis of affective disorders" proposes that some, if not all, depressions are associated with an absolute or relative decrease in catecholamines, particularly norepinephrine, available at central adrenergic receptor sites. Elation, conversely, may be associated with an excess of such amines (Schildkraut, 1965).

Since the early formulation of this hypothesis, as might be expected, a more complicated picture has evolved regarding both the mechanisms of action of therapeutic drugs and the possible etiology of affective disease. In a recent review

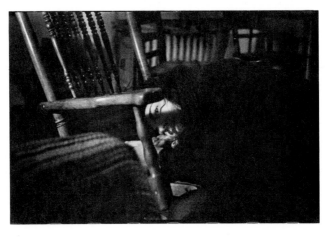

it was concluded that the available evidence is "more compatible with a catecholamine (CA) hypothesis of mania than one of depression" (Bunney, 1975). Thus, all the drugs which are effective in the treatment of mania reduce central CA's. Phenothiazines and butyrophenones appear to block CA receptors, and lithium is reported to prevent NE release and facilitate its uptake inactivation. *α-Methyl-p-tyrosine* (an inhibitor of CA biosynthesis) has also been reported to alleviate mania in some patients. Furthermore, a number of agents alleged to facilitate CA transmission, including L-dopa, amphetamine, tricyclics, and cocaine, precipitate severe manic or hypermanic episodes. These relationships are summarized in Fig. 17-6.

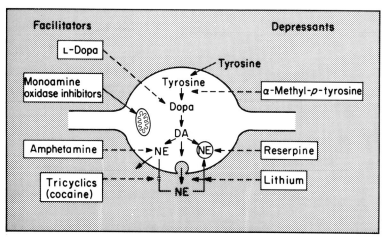

Fig. 17-6. Summary of the mechanism of action of drugs which have pronounced effects on depression and mania. In general, drugs which facilitate the amount of CA available to receptors precipitate mania. L-Dopa and monoamine oxidase inhibitors increase CA stores making more available for release; amphetamines stimulate release and tricyclics and cocaine block reuptake inactivation. Those drugs which reduce CA availability to receptors are effective in its treatment. α-Methyl-p-tyrosine inhibits tyrosine hydroxylase, reserpine depletes CA stores, and lithium facilitates reuptake and reduces release.

The strategy of amino acid loading has been used to examine more directly the role of CA's in the pathogenesis of depression. Since it is the precursor of the CA's (NE and DA do not readily cross the blood–brain barrier), L-dopa would be expected to be an effective antidepressant. Furthermore, L-dopa has been shown to reverse the lethargy produced in animals by *reserpine*. However, clinical studies show that L-dopa is beneficial in only certain types of depression, indicating that depression may be a heterogeneous group of disorders with different neurochemical systems being implicated in the various subtypes (Goodwin *et al.*, 1970).

One aspect of therapeutic drug action, which until quite recently has not received sufficient attention, involves the delay in clinical improvement following the initiation of antidepressant drug treatment. In fact, most studies have evaluated the mechanism of antidepressant drug action after acute administration. However, recent clinical results, using urinary CA metabolites as a measure of central CA activity, indicate that in contrast to the acute action of antidepressant drugs, chronic administration may reduce CA activity (Beckmann and Goodwin, 1975). This finding is consistent with the decrease in tyrosine hydroxylase (the rate-limiting enzyme in CA biosynthesis) that results from chronic administration of tricyclic drugs to experimental animals (Segal et al., 1974). Therefore, it is conceivable that depression results from an excess rather than a deficiency in central CA activity.

C.   Serotonin (5-HT) Hypothesis

Many of the pharmacological agents effective in the treatment of the affective disorders or capable of producing behavioral syndromes which resemble affective disorders alter serotonin as well as CA mechanisms. Thus, reserpine reduces serotonin levels and lithium, at least initially, appears to enhance serotonin activity. _Monoamine oxidase inhibitors_ block serotonin degradation, thus producing an elevation of serotonin levels. Some _tricyclic antidepressants_ are potent serotonin reuptake blockers.

One strategy, which would reveal the relative contribution of the various biogenic amines in the therapeutic action of the tricyclic antidepressants, is to compare their clinical potency with their effectiveness in blocking NE and serotonin reuptake (Carlsson, 1976). In general, tricyclics that have a greater effect on blocking serotonin reuptake are more effective antidepressants than the tricyclics that block NE uptake. Such structure–function relationships indicate that the serotonin systems may play a very prominent, if not preeminent, role in the mood-elevating action of the tricyclic antidepressants. This preeminence is further indicated by the observation that inhibition of serotonin, but not CA, synthesis reverses the therapeutic effects of imipramine.

Additional evidence supporting a role for serotonin stems from clinical studies which report reduced levels of 5-hydroxyindolacetic acid (5-HIAA), the metabolite of serotonin, in the cerebrospinal fluid of some depressed patients and of both serotonin and 5-HIAA in the autopsied brains of individuals who had committed suicide (Coppen, 1972). On the basis of these and other converging results, it has been postulated that at least some forms of depression may be caused by a reduction in central serotonergic activity.

As with the CA hypothesis, the precursor load strategy has also been used to test the role of indoleamine systems in affective disorders. Some clinical studies have reported positive results with respect to the effects of L-_tryptophan_, the

742

amino acid precursor of 5-HT. Some clinical investigators have also suggested that L-tryptophan may have antimanic properties. However, in contrast to the many positive results, some clinical investigators report that most depressed patients who do not respond to L-tryptophan show improvement with other treatments and that, at best, only a specific subgroup of bipolar patients show any improvement (Murphy *et al.*, 1973; Farkas *et al.*, 1976).

It is apparent that the whole range of affective abnormalities cannot be explained solely on the basis of a defect in either CA or serotonin functioning. It does appear, however, that these monoamines are implicated in the pathogenesis of at least some types of mania and depression, and, in fact, that various abnormalities in the balance between these and other neurochemical systems may be responsible for different forms of affective disease. Furthermore, it appears that, as with schizophrenia, depression may be a biochemically heterogeneous group of disorders, each requiring different treatment procedures to achieve maximal therapeutic effects.

IV. Summary and Conclusions

We have indeed come a long way. Schizophrenia is a treatable disorder, and it is becoming more and more understandable at both a clinical and biological level. Phenothiazines, the main drug class used to relieve the symptoms of schizophrenia, block DA receptors and correct the hyperactivity of dopamine systems in brain.

The maintenance of normal mood is dependent on a delicate balance in the brain's chemistry. Mania appears to result from an excess of norepinephrine in the brain; it is treated with lithium or neuroleptics. Depression is probably a result of deficiency of serotonin and perhaps NE; it is treated with tricyclic antidepressants or electroconvulsive therapy. Tricyclics block norepinephrine and serotonin reuptake and thus elevate the levels available to receptors.

Perhaps less extreme changes in brain chemistry underlie most normal mood changes. Whether such swings in mood are directed by swings in brain chemistry of the type described for affective disorders is still unknown, but it is certainly a possibility.

V. Behavioral Disorders Created by Drug Abuse

Repeated or even occasional use of narcotics, alcohol, sleeping pills, stimulants and hallucinogens can lead to markedly abnormal behavior and in some cases addiction to the drug. The nature of the behavioral response and the effect of repeated use varies with the drug. In this section, we will describe the effects of repeated usage on the user and discuss the current state of information on addiction to narcotic drugs.

We emphasize at the outset, however, that the factors underlying drug dependence are complex and have pharmacological and psychosocial bases. The intensity of any drug effect in a person is dependent on dose, potency, frequency of administration, and sensitivity of the individual. For example, a lot of caffeine can be more harmful than a bit of a narcotic. Quantitative aspects are critical. However, the development of drug dependence is dictated by many factors other than the pharmacological effect the drug produces. Psychological facets and the setting in which a person takes the drug also play a large part in the behavioral effects produced and in determining whether a person will use a drug to a compulsive and detrimental degree. Availability of the drug, socioeconomic status, the context in which the drug is taken and prevailing attitudes about that particular drug can all be decisive. Attitudes, socioeconomic influences and drug markets all change and can, with time, alter the pattern of drug use and the magnitude of drug dependence.

VI. Drug Types

Drugs that are subject to abuse can conveniently be classified according to their effect on the central nervous system into four main groups: *narcotics*, *general depressants*, *stimulants*, and *hallucinogens*. While drugs have multiple effects, and generalizations tend to oversimplify them, each of the four categories has a pharmacological profile that is characteristic and fairly easy to recognize. All drugs of abuse have in common the property of providing escape to the user, either by lifting him or her to a new psychological high or by relieving anxiety and tension.

There are some agents that affect the brain but do not appear to relieve anxiety or produce sufficiently pleasurable effects to make their abuse a serious problem. The major tranquilizers (the antipsychotics) appear to have few inherent properties of their own to promote drug dependence. However, some types of antipsychotics enhance the effects of the narcotics and the general depressants. Among the many antipsychotic agents that have low potential for abuse are the phenothiazines, such as chlorpromazine, and the reserpine alkaloids. The antihistamines also have little addictive potential, although Pyribenzamine is sometimes used to enhance morphine effects (Blue Velvet). The atropinelike alkaloids have been experimented with sporadically by different generations of youth, but the hallucinogenic effects are not pleasant enough to make these agents popular.

Two important factors that contribute to the abuse potential of some drugs are related to the development of tolerance and dependence. *Tolerance* develops when a substance becomes less effective with repeated administration; larger and larger doses are required to achieve the desired effect. The development of tolerance appears to cause more serious drug dependence. Prime examples of drugs that produce tolerance from each of the four groups include the narcotic, heroin; the general depressant, secobarbital (red birds); the stimulant, methamphetamine (speed, crystals); and the hallucinogen, LSD (acid).

In addition to causing tolerance, repeated administration of drugs induces a state of physical and psychic dependence in many cases. *Physical dependence* is defined as a state in which bodily processes become modified so that continued administration of the drug is required to prevent uncomfortable withdrawal symptoms. The importance of physical dependence as a reinforcing factor that promotes drug dependence varies with the drug groups. The term *withdrawal syndrome* (or abstinence syndrome) is used to describe the symptoms associated with removal of the drug once it has produced physical dependence. *Psychic dependence* is defined as a compulsion that requires periodic or continuous administration of a drug to produce pleasure or avoid discomfort. This compulsion is the most powerful factor in chronic intoxication with psychotropic drugs, and with certain types of drugs may be the only factor involved in the perpetuation of abuse even in the case of most intense craving (Isbell and Chruściel, 1970).

A.   Narcotics

The major pharmacologic effect of *morphine*, *heroin*, or other narcotics such as Dilaudid, meperidine and methadone is selective depression of the central nervous system. The classic effects include analgesia, changes in mood, drowsiness, and respiratory depression. In subjects with pain, fatigue, worry, tension, or anxiety, the euphoric effects of morphine afford considerable relief. While morphine is not generally used therapeutically for mood alteration because of the high probability of physical dependence, it is a most effective tranquilizer. The subject with anxieties loses feelings of insecurity and inferiority while on morphine. Since the morphine user no longer cares, everything looks rosy and in harmony until the pleasurable drug effects wear off and it is necessary to restore confidence with another dose.

The abuse potential of narcotic drugs is greatly enhanced by the rapid development of both tolerance and physical dependence. After frequent repeated administration of heroin for 2–3 weeks, a tenfold tolerance can easily develop. The development of tolerance is also accompanied by the development of physical dependence and this encourages the user to rationalize his need for continuing to take the drug. Failure to repeat the administration of heroin results in an acute *withdrawal syndrome* that becomes increasingly apparent several hours after the last injection, reaching a peak in 2 or 3 days, and lasting about 1 week. The signs of heroin abstinence are highly characteristic and include tearing, nasal discharge, yawning, chills, fever, vomiting, muscular aches, and diarrhea. The heroin withdrawal syndrome is quite acute, very discomforting, extraordinarily unpleasant, and may be almost immediately terminated by an injection of a narcotic.

In contrast to the gradual development of abstinence symptoms in the addict after discontinuance of a narcotic, an explosive withdrawal syndrome is precipitated within minutes when a specific narcotic antagonist such as naloxone is administered to a dependent subject. The induced signs are similar to those noted after natural withdrawal, but are more severe and last only about 1 hour. The physical dependence liability of heroin, while important, has been overemphasized. Today it is well recognized that the fear of withdrawal provides the abuser with a basis for rationalizing his emotional dependence on drugs.

Cure of physical dependence is a relatively simple medical problem; cure of psychic dependence is another matter. Narcotic drugs promote escape by producing pleasurable effects (euphoria) and by relieving anxiety or tension. Time and time again, the heroin-dependent personality may be freed of physical dependence by medical treatment, but each time, shortly after detoxification and discharge, he relapses because of an inability to cope with the emotional dependence. The patient continues to take the drug in spite of conscious admission that it causes harm to his health and social and family status.

The context of a situation plays a marked role in the extent of psychic dependence. Hospital patients given opiates, for example, develop physical dependence and tolerance and when drug administration is withdrawn show abstinence symptoms. Significantly, however, only a very small percent continue to crave the drug (Wilder, 1977). The contextual cues of self-administration are a very important determinate of dependence.

Good health and productive work are not necessarily incompatible with dependence on narcotics. Many addicts have worked productively for years while physically dependent on heroin or methadone. The point to emphasize is that the ill health, social irresponsibility, and crime that often accompany narcotic abuse result not from the direct pharmacologic effects of the agent, but from the addict's need to satisfy his compulsion when the drug is not easily available.

B.   General Depressants

In this class there are a variety of drugs, which differ markedly in their physicochemical properties but which have the common characteristic of causing generalized depression of the central nervous system. The agents that are abused are those that are used for their effects on anxiety and tension. Far and away the agent most widely used and abused is ethyl alcohol, although many are not aware that it belongs in this category of general CNS depressants, and it does not always cause depression. The drugs most people readily recognize as members of this group are the sedative-hypnotics such as the *barbiturate* sleeping pills; Seconal, Nembutal, and Tuinal are some of the better-known ones. The nonbarbiturates Doriden and Quaalude also create problems, as do the so-called minor tranquilizers such as meprobamate, known also as Miltown or Equanil, and the popular antianxiety drugs Valium and Librium. Two older agents, chloral hydrate and paraldehyde, anesthetic agents such as ether, as well as various glue solvents may also be placed in this drug grouping. All of these agents have differences in their pharmacologic actions and may differ also with respect to onset and duration of effects, but they have in common that in high doses they produce motor incoordination (ataxia), stupor in which arousal is difficult, and severe respiratory depression. At lower doses, they may produce a "lift" by disinhibition, i.e., by depressing brain sites that are concerned with controlling our responsible acts. In essence, disinhibition is mood alteration produced by taking the foot off the brakes rather than by stepping on the gas. The behavior at ether frolics, glue sniffings, and the convivial cocktail hour exemplifies this effect.

Psychic dependence on sedative-hypnotic drugs develops rather insidiously. Physical dependence on these agents is more difficult to produce than with narcotics. Although it may require high doses over several months to produce overt abstinence signs upon withdrawal, once physical dependence is established, the syndrome is difficult to arrest and far more severe and dangerous to life than the abstinence symptoms produced by withdrawal from narcotics. There are quantitative differences with respect to the potential hazards of abused drugs in this class. The more serious abuse generally occurs with the short-acting barbiturates. Longer acting barbiturates such as phenobarbital and barbital present less of a hazard, as do the newer diazepam types used as antianxiety drugs.

The signs and symptoms of withdrawal from sedative-hypnotics generally include restlessness, agitation, unpleasant hallucinations, tremors, and, in the more severe cases, convulsions. To minimize these effects, it is necessary to withdraw the compound gradually by decreasing the daily intake in small increments. The cross-tolerance property of agents in this group is useful for mitigating the withdrawal signs and symptoms of other agents in this class. The *delirium tremens* (d.t.'s) of the heavy alcohol user is a form of acute drug withdrawal which can be alleviated by any general depressant that exhibits cross-tolerance to alcohol. *Cross-tolerance* is defined as the state in which tolerance to one drug has the effect of causing tolerance to another. Drugs such as meprobamate (Miltown and Equanil), chlordiazepoxide (Librium), diazepam (Valium), and paraldehyde, all used to "treat" alcoholism, act primarily as substitutes for alcohol.

C. Stimulants

The principal agents of abuse in this group are *cocaine* and the *amphetamines*. The latter compounds are used for CNS stimulation, to combat fatigue, and to suppress appetite in the treatment of obesity. Examples of the amphetamine type are Benzedrine, Dexedrine, methamphetamine (Desoxyn), phenmetrazine (Preludin). The terms "speed" and "crystals" have been used for this group, but generally these terms are reserved for methamphetamine, abuse of which is the most serious. Synthesis of methamphetamine is relatively easy, and consequently it is available at a price within reach of many users.

Whatever the reason, a person can easily slip into drug abuse. Some take amphetamines as diet pills, others as stimulants to stay awake. Johnny Cash, the country western singer, describes his experience.

> With all the traveling I had to do, and upon reaching a city tired and weary, those pills could pep me up and make me really feel like doing a show. I got a handful of the little white ones from Gordon.
>
> Those white pills were just one of a variety of a dozen or more shapes and sizes. Truck drivers used them as did people with the problem of being overweight. They called them amphetamines, Dexedrine, Benzedrine, and Dexamyl. They had a whole bunch of nice little names for them to dress them up, and they came in all colors. If you didn't like green, you could get orange. If you didn't like orange, you could get red. And if you really wanted to act like you were going to get weird, you could get black. Those black ones would take you all the way to California and back in a '53 Cadillac with no sleep.
>
> Inside that bottle of white pills, which only cost eight or ten dollars for a hundred, came at no extra cost a demon called Deception. . . .
>
> Before I really got hooked, I would realize what was happening and I'd think, "What am I doing to myself?" I think back now to interviews where questions would be coming, and I couldn't think of the answers. Or, I'd be answering a question, and then all of a sudden right in the middle of it I'd forget what the question was. And I'd realize it was the pills. They regulated my mind and began to take control.
>
> Everyone noticed the change the pills brought about in me. My friends made a joke out of my "nervousness." I had a twitch in the neck, the back, the face. My eyes dilated. I couldn't stand still. I twisted, turned, contorted, and popped my neck bones. It often felt like someone had a fist between my shoulder blades, twisting the muscle and bones, stretching my nerves, torturing them to the breaking point (Cash, 1975, pp. 82–83).

Intravenous abuse of methamphetamine has become an established and extensive form of drug abuse, although its usage has lessened somewhat because its availability has been decreased by legislative sanctions. The user begins with a 10 mg dose that is repeated at 1–2 hour intervals. Tolerance develops rapidly, and the continuous use necessitates the injection of 100–200 mg to perpetuate the effects. The initial "flash" is likened to an intense sexual orgasm, and there is a sensation of extreme mental and physical power. However, as the dose is increased, the subject develops an extreme psychotoxic syndrome with unpleasant hallucinations, becomes paranoid and disorganized, and may become transfixed—carrying out a nonsensical task for hours ("hung up"). At this stage some abusers may be using as much as 1 gm of the dissolved crystals at 1–2 hour intervals. The development of severe tremors, pain in muscles and joints, and utter exhaustion necessitate termination of the injections. On discontinuance, the

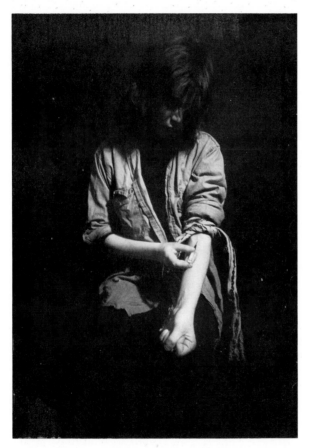

subject falls into a prolonged semicomatose state. Upon awakening the user feels lethargic, depressed, and compelled to resume the drug, and begins another series of injections that may last for several days. It appears likely that the continuance of these bouts leads to both physical and mental impairment.

Physical dependence on the amphetamines is not a major factor in promoting abuse, as it is with heroin. Despite this, its addiction and relapse potential is comparable to that of heroin, and the damage it produces is greater. The intravenous form of methamphetamine abuse is extremely disabling from both a social and psychological viewpoint. These considerations clearly indicate the fallacy of placing too great an emphasis on physical dependence as the causal factor in drug abuse.

In order to come down off of amphetamines people often resort to barbiturates. The combination is extremely serious as is the withdrawal, as Cash said.

If people actually knew the terrors of coming off drugs—understand, I was what people like to call "habituated" to amphetamines and barbiturates. That sounds nicer than "addicted." I sometimes took as many as twenty a day of five and ten-milligram amphetamines. It took that many barbiturates, Equanil or meprobamate, a few at a time over two or three hours, to bring me down enough to doze off and get a little sleep. Then six or eight more amphetamines the next day to get me going. The amphetamines were tough to kick, but the barbiturates were what caused the real terror . . .

It was the same nightmare every night, and it affected my stomach—I suppose because the stomach was where the pills had landed, exploded, and done their work. I'd be lying in bed on my back or curled up on my side. The cramps would come and go, and I'd roll over, doze off, and go to sleep.

Then all of a sudden a glass ball would begin to expand in my stomach. My eyes were closed, but I could see it. It would grow to the size of a baseball, a volleyball, then a basketball. And about the time I felt that ball was twice the size of a basketball, it lifted me up off the bed.

I was in a strange state of half-asleep and half-awake. I couldn't open my eyes, and I couldn't close them. It lifted me off the bed to the ceiling, and when it would go through the roof, the glass ball would explode and tiny, infinitesimal slivers of glass would go out into my bloodstream from my stomach. I could feel the pieces of glass being pumped through my heart into the veins of my arms, my legs, my feet, my neck, and my brain, and some of them would come out the pores of my skin. Then I'd float back down through the ceiling onto my bed and wake up. I'd turn over on my side for awhile, unable to sleep. Then I'd lie on my back, doze off, get almost asleep—and the same nightmare would come again.

I never imagined a hole in the roof. I just went right through it without an opening. Sometimes in addition to glass coming out of my skin and the corners of my eyes, I would be pulling splinters of wood and briars and thorns out of my flesh, and sometimes worms. I wanted to scream, but I couldn't (Cash, 1975, pp. 130–131).

Abuse of amphetamines and barbiturates is serious business and all do not come out intact, as Cash eventually did.

D. Hallucinogens

Agents in this group can be further categorized into subgroups exemplified by four prototypes: LSD, marijuana, atropine, and nalorphine. The last two types yield hallucinogenic effects that are generally unpleasant and for this reason will probably not become major drug abuse problems.

The LSD type of hallucinogen may include, besides LSD, its related derivatives and also other agents that give pharmacologic effects fairly similar to LSD. These drugs also exhibit cross-tolerance to LSD. Two examples, present in plants indigenous to Mexico and the southwestern United States, are mescaline (from the peyote cactus plant) and psilocybin (from the Aztec mushroom). Of the agents in this group, LSD has been studied most extensively, and the scientific papers number in the thousands.

The effects of LSD have been described in detail by professionals and nonprofessionals. LSD causes marked changes in mood, judgment, and perception; 0.1 mg usually suffices to cause hallucinations. The more pleasurable hallucinogenic experiences are associated with visual changes that occur in color and form perception. With higher doses and in predisposed persons, however, acute, severe psychotic episodes are often produced lasting from 8 to 10 hours. In addition, suicide and prolonged psychotic behavior have been precipitated by the drug. Abuse of the drug is more likely to be periodic rather than continuous, mainly because tolerance develops very rapidly; however, physical dependence does not occur. Tolerance develops after daily usage for 3 or 4 days, but is lost after an equal period of abstinence. Data on long-term chronic effects of LSD are meager and controversial. The therapeutic claims with respect to treatment of alcoholism, schizophrenia, sexual disorders, mental retardation and as a psychological aid to dying patients are, by and large, unconvincing. Despite the numerous articles about LSD, there remains a need for well-controlled pharmacologic, sociologic, and epidemiologic studies.

Marijuana is a plant (*Cannabis sativa*) found growing mostly in Jamaica, Mexico, Africa, India, and the Middle East but also in the United States. The active constituents of marijuana (cannabinols) are concentrated in the resin at the flowering tops. The principal psychoactive compound is l-Δ^9-tetrahydrocannabinol, more commonly called THC. The potency of marijuana varies with the plant strain and the growing conditions; a preparation containing 2% THC is considered to be good. Hashish is an extract of marijuana containing THC concentrated about two- to tenfold.

In anecdotal reports describing the effects of marijuana, most users report that the drug induces a dreamy, euphoric state of altered consciousness, with feelings of detachment, gaiety, and a preoccupation with simple and familiar things. Drowsiness and sleep may occur if the smoker is alone, but in the company of others, there is a tendency toward laughter and loquaciousness. Users are sometimes recognized by the characteristic hilarity of their laughter which may become prolonged and uncontrolled. Perceptual distortion of space and time is regularly reported; distances may be judged inaccurately, and the passage of time may be overestimated.

There may be an unusually vivid remembrance or reliving of experiences or mood states of the past. On the other hand, there may be loss in short-term memory. Libido is variably affected. Since sexual desire may be enhanced, marijuana has gained a reputation as an aphrodisiac. However, there is little concrete evidence that sexual performance is improved, and, indeed, with high doses it is likely to be impaired. Increased appetite and appreciation of the flavor of food are usually claimed, and although weight gain may accompany regular smoking, demonstration that this effect is due to marijuana is not conclusive.

A *paranoid* state is sometimes reported in which the smoker is keenly sensitive of others watching him. Some users forsake marijuana for this reason. However, antisocial behavior under the influence of marijuana appears to be rare; the user ordinarily withdraws from company that he finds unpleasant.

Regular use of marijuana may result in a pervasive feeling of apathy, the so-called "amotivational syndrome" without development of physical dependence. This development may be especially damaging to the psychological maturation of the adolescent. Such a syndrome may be caused by many factors, but in many adolescents undergoing psychotherapy, its development has been observed to coincide temporally with regular use of marijuana. On the other hand, it has also been reported that no such syndrome is detectable in a general population of heavy, long-term users.

While the description of the effects of marijuana appears also to fit the LSD type of drug, there are distinct differences between these two agents, and experienced drug takers can generally distinguish the effects of the two drug types. The LSD type generally causes wakefulness, whereas marijuana tends to produce sedation. Unlike LSD, marijuana does not dilate the pupils nor materially raise blood pressure and body temperature; on the other hand, marijuana is more likely to increase pulse rate. Marijuana is milder than LSD, and its effects are more predictable. Also, since marijuana acts almost immediately when smoked, it can be titrated better than LSD to obtain the desired "high" without the likelihood of a bad trip.

An argument frequently advanced by law enforcement against legalizing marijuana is that its usage leads to more addicting drugs such as heroin. However, there are many heroin addicts who have never used marijuana. Moreover, although many heroin addicts may have a prior history of marijuana smoking, such individuals usually also smoked cigarettes and drank beer before using marijuana. The argument could be equally misapplied that these habits led to heroin use. The problem lies not in the fact that one drug causes the use of another but rather that the drug user is likely to experiment with many drugs particularly under peer pressure. It should be pointed out, however, that a possible exception to these generalizations is that the user of a stimulant drug (uppers) sometimes feels the need of a depressant drug (downers) to overcome the toxic effects of the stimulant. Sustained repeated use of the depressant could lead to the development of physical dependence.

VII. Mechanisms of Narcotic Dependence and Tolerance

What are the mechanisms underlying physical dependence and tolerance and why are withdrawal symptoms so severe?

As described previously, physical dependence refers to a modified physiological condition produced by the chronic administration of a drug which necessitates its continued administration to prevent the appearance of withdrawal signs and symptoms. The best known example of drug dependence is that caused by the narcotic drugs, in particular, heroin. The heroin withdrawal syndrome is easily identifiable by a number of characteristic signs that reflect autonomic nervous system hyperactivity (tearing, yawning, sweating, goose pimples, chills, dilated pupils, nausea and vomiting). In general terms, dependence appears to be a part of body defenses to the continued effect of the drug. Withdrawal phenomena involve an exaggerated rebound or overshoot of some functions that are overly depressed. Thus, the abnormal contraction of the pupils, respiratory depression, decreased body temperature, sedation and analgesia resulting from acute morphine inhibition become dilation of the pupils, labored respiration, increased body temperature, excitability and hyperalgesia during withdrawal. A most remarkable change of behaviors.

The discovery of the naturally occurring opiatelike peptides, the endorphins and enkephalins, has revolutionized our understanding of the brain's response to opiates and led to exciting new insights into their mechanism of action. Let us begin the story with the endorphins and enkephalins. Like morphine, β-endorphin and the enkephalins have their own analgesic properties (see Chapter 6). The critical question is: Do animals become dependent on them?

When *enkephalin* is continuously infused for 72 hours into the ventricles of rats, and they are then injected with the opiate antagonist naloxone to precipitate withdrawal, the animals have immediate withdrawal symptoms including teeth chattering, wet-dog shakes, desire to escape and diarrhea (Table 17-1). These signs clearly indicate a dependence on the enkephalin. Similar signs are observed when animals are given β-endorphin instead of enkephalin. Moreover, repeated injections result in an increase in the amount of the peptide required to elicit the same degree of analgesia. Tolerance develops. Endorphin tolerance appears to be by a mechanism similar to morphine tolerance, since animals tolerant to

Table 17-1 Continuous infusion of opiatelike peptides into the periaqueductal gray of the rat brain and the development of physical dependence[a]

Chemical	Concentration of chemical in infusion (μg/μl)	Total estimated dose delivered in 72 hours[c] (μmole)	N	Animals showing withdrawal sign (%)		
				Teeth chattering	Escape responses	Wet shakes
Distilled water			4	0	0	0
Morphine sulfate	1.64	0.481	8	100	100	37
Met-Enkephalin[b]	9.00	1.537	7	100	86	14
β-Endorphin	0.67	0.019	7	100	86	0

[a] From Wei and Loh (1976).
[b] Met, methionine.
[c] Minipump flow rates of 1.40 ± 0.04 μl/hour.

β-endorphin also require higher morphine levels to produce analgesia. Conversely, animals implanted with morphine pellets are also tolerant to β-endorphin. The development of tolerance is also observed at the single neuronal level. Both enkephalin and β-endorphin fail to inhibit the firing of single neurons at the cortex or spinal cord when the animal has been implanted with morphine. Tolerance to these peptides is observed in the CNS and at the myenteric plexus of the guinea pig ileum.

What is the probable role of endorphins or enkephalins in analgesia, and how does dependence develop? One prominent model is the presynaptic model. In the presynaptic model (Fig. 17-7) (Snyder, 1977) enkephalins or endorphins bind to

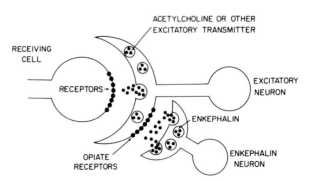

Fig. 17.7. Possible mechanisms of enkephalin action.

the nerve terminals of the excitatory neurons and inhibit the release of the excitatory transmitters by partially depolarizing the excitatory terminals. Since the amount of any transmitter released is determined by the net depolarization, partial depolarization reduces the amount of excitatory transmitter released. Such inhibition of neuronal firing in the ascending pain pathways in the spinal cord and brain stem might be the mechanism of analgesia. Dependence and tolerance might develop as follows. After a period of time the receptors, overloaded by the opiate drugs, send a message via a hypothetical feedback loop to enkephalin neurons to stop firing and releasing enkephalin. With the decrease in the output of the enkephalin at the synaptic sites, more and more opiate is required to produce the same degree of inhibitory action and hence the development of tolerance. The abrupt removal of the opiates from these sites will leave the excitatory inputs unmodulated because both exogenous and endogenous opioid materials are absent. Such an absence of modulation will lead to the excitatory withdrawal symptoms.

An exciting and key insight into molecular mechanisms has come from studies of cancerous hybrid nerve cells (glial neuroblastoma hybrids) grown in tissue culture (Sharma *et al.*, 1975). These cells thrive in culture, where the media conditions can be carefully controlled, so they provide a valuable model system for studies on brain mechanisms. Addition of morphine to the cell media causes a rapid drop in the basal level and the prostaglandin-stimulated level of adenylate cyclase. This response to morphine is stereo-specific and is blocked by the opiate antagonist, naloxone. This indicates that the action of morphine and its agonists is mediated through opiate receptors. After exposure to morphine for a long period of time (about 72 hours) these hybrid cell cultures develop a tolerance response (Fig. 17-8). Although morphine initially inhibits activity of adenylate cyclase in these cells, prolonged exposure to the opiate increases the activity of adenylate cyclase in order to compensate for the effect of the narcotic. As a result, higher concentrations of opiate are required to inhibit the production of *cyclic adenosine monophosphate* (cAMP) to the same degree. The cells adapt to chronic morphine exposure. Thus, when morphine is removed from the media, the level of cAMP markedly rises because there is more adenylate cyclase in the cell and the inhibitory effect of morphine is gone. This excessive production of cAMP by the hybrid cells may be the biochemical event of withdrawal symptoms. The number of receptors does not change, so the receptor per se is probably not the fundamental locus of change. Identical changes are seen with enkephalins.

In the mouse, the development of physical dependence and tolerance to morphine can be inhibited by administration of the protein synthesis inhibitor cycloheximide along with morphine (Loh *et al.*, 1969). It was found that the inhibiting effect of cycloheximide on tolerance development was independent of the analgesic response. Repeated injection of morphine resulted in considerable

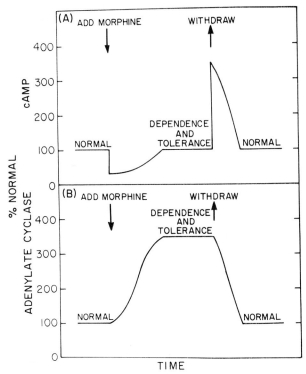

Fig. 17-8. A model of the role of adenylate cyclase regulation in the development of morphine tolerance and dependence. (A) shows the effects of morphine upon cAMP levels, and (B) shows the effects of the opiate upon adenylate cyclase activity as a function of time. (From Sharma *et al.*, 1975.)

tolerance development: the dose of morphine required to produce analgesia in this group increased several fold. The administration of cycloheximide along with morphine did not result in an elevation of the morphine analgesia. Moreover, treatment with cycloheximide prevented the development of physical dependence (Fig. 17-9). These findings indicate that a protein is involved in tolerance and/or physical dependence. Probably adenylate cyclase is one of the proteins. Whatever the molecule is, it must have a rapid turnover.

In order to account for the intense behavioral changes tied to opiate use, it seems reasonable that there must be many changes in the brain. A number of pharmacological tools have been used to affect, as selectively as possible, the synthesis, storage, release, or degradation of acetylcholine, dopamine, norepinephrine, and serotonin. Based on such studies, it appears that acetylcholine, norepinephrine, and dopamine may all participate in the mediation of acute pharmacologic responses to morphine as well as in certain withdrawal signs from

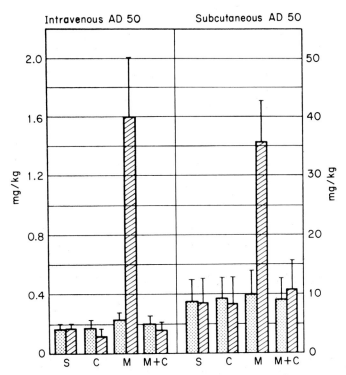

Fig. 17-9. Cycloheximide inhibition of morphine tolerance development as measured by the analgesic response to morphine before (stippled bars) and after (hatched bars) repeated daily treatment for 21 days with saline (S), cycloheximide (C), morphine (M), and morphine and cycloheximide (M+C). AD 50 is the dose required to reduce the effect 50%. The rules denote S.E. (From Loh *et al.*, 1969.)

the dependent state. However, these neurotransmitters seem less directly concerned with the development of tolerance and physical dependence.

On the other hand, serotonin does seem to be involved in the development of morphine tolerance and dependence (Way *et al.*, 1974). Its precise role in the two syndromes is unclear, but a relationship is suggested by the fact that a reduction in serotonin function results in an inhibition of tolerance and dependence development. Conversely, stimulation of serotonin synthesis by loading with its precursor tryptophan causes an enhancement of tolerance and dependence development. Serotonergic fibers from the raphé to the spinal cord, as you may recall, participate in analgesia (see Chapter 12). Therefore, it is not too surprising they are involved here as well.

In view of the fact that a case can be made for a participatory role for many neurotransmitters in the acute morphine response, it would appear that the effect of morphine is mediated by some basic mechanism common to neuronal function in general. There is increasing evidence that morphine can inhibit the release of various neurotransmitters, including acetylcholine, dopamine and norepinephrine. It appears that this acute inhibition is due to a decrease in Ca^{2+} influx into synaptic endings (Harris *et al.*, 1976).

There is some evidence that the development of tolerance may be dependent on environmental cues and be related to classical conditioning. It was, in fact, Pavlov (1927) who first suggested the possibility that the administration of a drug might serve as a conditioning trial. Unique environmental cues at the time of drug administration would serve as the conditional stimulus (CS), and the drug stimulus as the unconditional stimulus (UCS). If morphine, for example, is given to rats in the presence of environmental cues that have previously been paired with morphine administration, the response, such as the degree of analgesia, is decreased. That is, only when tested in the environment in which they experienced morphine did the rats show the high pain sensitivity which characterized analgesic tolerance. Clearly, the environmental context plays a role, and an association between environmental cues and the systemic effects can influence, in part at least, the development of tolerance. It is believed that as the CS and UCS are paired more and more times the compensatory conditional responses become more pronounced so that the effect of the drug is less (tolerance). The animal learns a behavioral strategy to compensate for the drug-induced impairments. Associative factors in tolerance development appear established, but have not gone unchallenged (see Hayes and Mayer, 1978; Siegel, 1978).

Brain Sites of Naloxone-Precipitated Withdrawal

Dependence on morphine can develop in many places in the CNS, although the degree of sensitivity to morphine and its effects may vary (Way *et al.*, 1974). Leaping attempts to escape from a jar and wet shakes are distinctive abstinence behaviors in rats, and they indicate a high degree of physical dependence. Their neuroanatomical correlates have been investigated in morphine-dependent rats by stereotaxically introducing crystalline naloxone hydrochloride to discrete areas of the brain. Areas in the brain in which the withdrawal symptoms are most easily evoked by naloxone are in and around the medial mesodiencephalon. Application of naloxone to lateral thalamic nuclei, neocortical, or hippocampal areas does not precipitate withdrawal. Areas surrounding the floor of the fourth ventricle are even more sensitive sites for precipitating withdrawal. The medial mesodiencephalic regions of the brain are involved in the integration of thermosensory information and the regulation of body temperature. Body temperature fluctuates widely during withdrawal from morphine in experimental animals; some of the symptoms of abstinence in man also reflect disruption of thermoregulation.

During withdrawal from morphine such signs as teeth chattering, wet shakes, and a huddled posture may indicate that the animal is trying to conserve heat. Other signs, including salivation and escape behavior, may also be signs of heat loss mechanisms. Escape jumping, precipitated by naloxone, is markedly enhanced in a hot environment, but wet shakes behavior is completely suppressed. In a cold environment, on the other hand, the frequency of wet shakes is enhanced but no change in escape frequency is noted.

The neural elements underlying shaking behavior in normal rats in a cold environment appear similar to those associated with morphine withdrawal. Lesions in the midbrain block the ability of the animals to shake both in response to cold and in response to morphine withdrawal. Moreover, morphine completely blocks the wet shake response elicited by immersion of the animal in ice water, and tolerance to the morphine block could be induced by implantation of a morphine pellet for 72 hours. It appears, therefore, that some withdrawal signs resemble a disruption of central thermoregulatory mechanisms. Escape behavior and wet shakes may thus be viewed as behavioral events triggered by the sudden occurrence of an error signal in the thermosensory or thermal control system: compensatory heat gain and heat loss mechanisms are then activated to return the set point to normality.

VIII.   Summary and Conclusions

Drugs acting on the nervous system may be classified as narcotics, general depressants, stimulants and hallucinogens. Narcotics create a state of euphoria, and their continued use produces physical and psychic dependence. The body and mind come to need the drug in order to avoid the powerful and wicked withdrawal symptoms. Tolerance always develops along with physical dependence. The severity of psychic dependence depends on contextual cues. Among the depressant drugs are the sedative-hypnotic drugs, such as barbiturates and some of the minor tranquilizers. Psychic dependence develops easily. Physical dependence develops slowly, but once it sets in it is even more hazardous than psychic dependence on narcotics. Stimulant drugs consist primarily of cocaine and amphetamine. Tolerance to amphetamines develops quickly, so large amounts are necessary to sustain the "high." Extensive and long term use is extremely disabling and can lead to physical and mental impairment. Hallucinogens (LSD, marijuana, atropine) do not result in physical dependence, but tolerance does develop. The effects are not easily predicted. Therapeutic effects of these drugs seem to be minimal.

The development of physical dependence and tolerance appear to reflect an exaggeration of normal physiologic attempts to maintain homeostasis. Withdrawal is a rebound of overly depressed functions. The endorphins and enkephalins appear centrally involved in narcotic addiction. Animals given endorphin develop physical dependence and tolerance and display withdrawal signs. Diencephalic areas are closely associated with addictiveness. At a molecular level, endorphins and morphine appear to change cAMP and adenylate cyclase levels. Initially opiates (or opioid peptides) reduce cAMP levels, but with prolonged exposure additional adenylate cyclase is synthesized restoring cAMP levels to normal. Upon removal of the enkephalin or morphine, the cAMP levels shoot up due to the extra enzyme now present.

IX. Alcoholism

The effects of alcoholic beverages on individuals and our culture are nothing short of remarkable (Table 17-2). From grain and hops comes beer; from corn, whiskey; from sugarcane, rum; from potatoes, vodka. Alcohol is produced in beverages when yeast in the absence of air ferments sugar into carbon dioxide and ethanol (alcohol). The reaction stops when the alcohol concentration reaches 12–15% (as in wine). Production of more concentrated beverages requires processing.

Behavioral responses to alcohol differ widely between individuals (Goodwin, 1977). Some can consume massive quantities and little seems to happen. Others

Table 17-2 Effects of alcoholic beverages on individuals and our culture[a]

1. Over 25,000 alcohol-related traffic fatalities occur annually
2. The alcoholic's life span is shortened on the average by over 10 years
3. Suicide is over 50 times more common among alcoholics than among nonalcoholics
4. Excessive use of alcohol increases by over 20 times the probability of cirrhosis of the liver
5. Alcoholics have significantly higher rates of hypertension, ulcers, and cerebrovascular disease than nonalcoholics
6. Almost half of all arrests are alcohol-related
7. Alcoholism is a major element in divorce rates and broken homes
8. For men over 25, alcohol-related disorders are the most common diagnoses among those in mental hospitals; among women over 25, they are among the most common
9. Two million arrests for public drunkenness occur annually
10. The lives of nearly 40 million Americans are directly affected by alcohol problems

[a] From Sarason (1976).

develop headaches, dizziness and illness from only a small amount of alcohol. The response to alcohol is usually influenced by one's expectations. If people feel good, alcohol will probably make them feel better. If they feel sleepy, alcohol will make them even sleepier. If they feel sexy, alcohol will make them feel sexier. Excessive alcohol, of course, leads to drunkenness. Unlike any other drug, alcohol can cause amnesia or blackout. The person may not remember what happened the next day. In general people feel much better getting drunk than sobering up.

Some individuals and animals become alcoholics and develop physical dependence, tolerance and withdrawal symptoms. Tolerance for alcohol is less than that for narcotics. A seasoned alcoholic may be able to drink only twice as much as a normal person of similar age and health, whereas a person tolerant to narcotics can take a dose many times that tolerated by a normal person. An alcoholic's behavior is very diverse, ranging from near normal to complete loss of control. Withdrawal symptoms are extremely severe. Alcoholics suffer the _delirium tremens_ (the d.t.'s). The following excerpt from "Huckleberry Finn" vividly describes the d.t.'s:

> I don't know how long I was asleep, but all of a sudden there was an awful scream and I was up. There was Pap looking wild, and skipping around every which way and yelling about snakes. He said they was crawling up his legs; and then he would give a jump and scream, and say one had bit him on the cheek—but I couldn't see no snakes. He started round and round the cabin, hollering, "Take him off, take him off; he's biting me on the neck!" I never see a man look so wild in the eyes. Pretty soon he was all fagged out, and fell down panting; then he rolled over and over wonderful fast, kicking things every which way, and striking and grabbing at the air with his hands, and screaming and saying there was devils a-hold of him. He wore out by and by, and laid still awhile, moaning. Then he laid stiller, and didn't make a sound. I could hear the owls and wolves away off in the woods, and it seemed terrible still. He was lying over by the corner. By and by he raised up part way and listened, with his head to one side. He says, very low: "Tramp—tramp—tramp; that's the dead; tramp—tramp—tramp; they're coming after me but I won't go. Oh, they're here! don't touch me—don't! hands off—they're cold; let go. Oh let a poor devil alone." Then he went down on all fours and crawled off, begging them to let him alone, and he rolled himself up in his blanket and wallowed in under the old pine table, still a-begging; and then he went to crying. I could hear him through the blanket (Clemens, 1923).

A. The Fate of Alcohol in the Body

What happens to alcohol when you drink it? The answer is simple and direct. It turns to vinegar (acetic acid), just as it does when you do not drink it!

The enzymes responsible for this reaction are alcohol dehydrogenase and aldehyde dehydrogenase.

$$C_2H_5OH \quad + \quad DPN \xrightarrow{\text{alcohol dehydrogenase}} CH_3CHO \quad + \quad DPNH$$

| (Ethanol) | (Diphosphopyridine nucleotide) | | (Acetaldehyde) | (Reduced diphosphopyridine nucleotide) |

$$CH_3CHO \quad + \quad DPN \xrightarrow[\text{dehydrogenase}]{\text{aldehyde}} CH_3COOH \quad + \quad DPNH$$

| (Acetaldehyde) | (Diphosphopyridine nucleotide) | | (Acetic acid) | (Reduced diphosphopyridine nucleotide) |

Alcohol dehydrogenase converts alcohol to acetaldehyde. The enzyme is localized primarily in the liver and apparently does nothing other than metabolize alcohol. It can use up 86 proof (43%) distilled spirits at a rate of one ounce per hour. Acetaldehyde is toxic, however, and must be further metabolized. Aldehyde dehydrogenase in the liver and throughout the body converts acetaldehyde into acetic acid, which is harmless. Nearly all alcohol is completely oxidized in the liver. Small amounts are excreted in the breath, urine and sweat.

B.   Mechanisms of Physical Dependence, Tolerance and Withdrawal

What causes alcoholism? This is obviously a highly significant and important question. In 1970 Davis and Walsh presented an idea that shook up existing theories of alcoholism and initiated research that has provided some exciting new concepts on alcoholism. They argued that alcohol in the brain promotes the formation of compounds having opiatelike properties. When dopamine is metabolized, it goes to dopaldehyde, and dopaldehyde requires aldehyde dehydrogenase to degrade it further. Now aldehyde dehydrogenase is also required by acetaldehyde, the first metabolic product of alchol. In the body, the enzyme prefers acetaldehyde leaving some of the dopaldehyde unmetabolized. Dopaldehyde, when present in high concentrations, then condenses to form *tetrahydropapaveroline*, a benzyl tetrahydroisoquinoline alkaloid derivative of dopamine. Tetrahydropapaveroline is a precursor of opium alkaloids in the poppy (Fig. 17-10)! Very interesting!

It may be that the brain makes its own tetrahydropapaveroline and related condensation products and that alcoholism and opiate addiction are closely related through common biochemical pathways. This theory stirred quite a controversy and *Science* magazine featured one of the rebuttals (Seevers *et al.*, 1970). However, shortly after the theory appeared it was shown that perfusion of cow adrenal glands with acetaldehyde resulted in the formation of *tetrahydro*

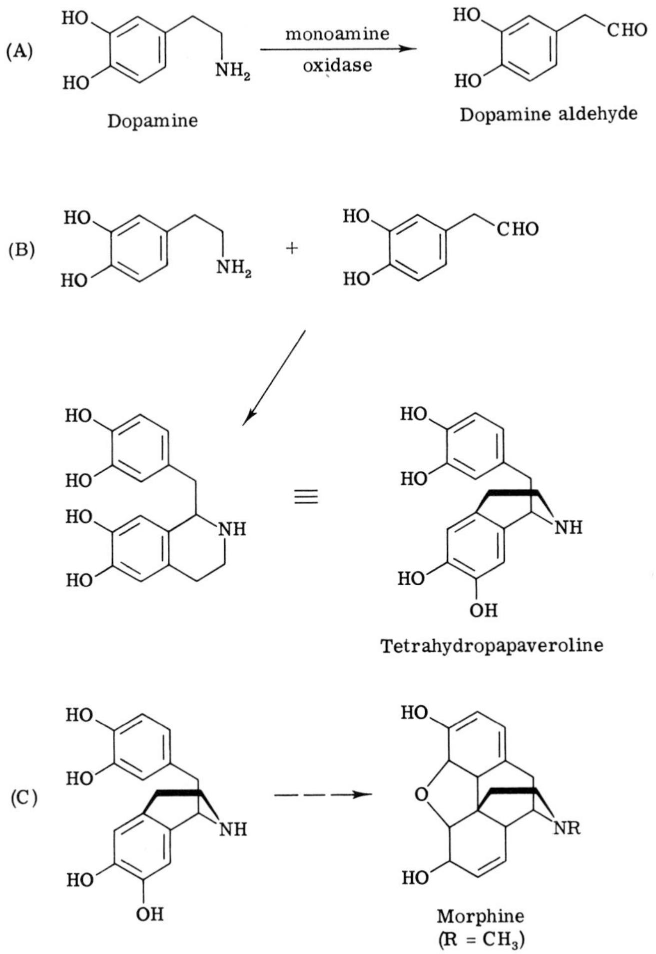

Fig. 17-10. A biochemical hypothesis for alcohol addiction. Condensation reactions of monoamines such as dopamine result in the synthesis of opiatelike alkaloids. (A) Dopamine or other monoamines are oxidized to aromatic aldehydes. These aromatic aldehydes accumulate in tissues rich in them because they must compete with acetaldehyde, a metabolite of alcohol, for aldehyde dehydrogenase, the enzyme which normally degrades the aromatic aldehyde derivations of monoamines. (B) The aldehyde derivative of monoamines are very reactive and easily condense with the parent compound. Condensation reactions of dopamine and the dopamine aldehyde derivative generate tetrahydropapaveroline. (The formula on the left is equivalent to that on the right only drawn differently.) (C) Tetrahydropapaveroline is a precursor of morphine in the opium poppy. (After Davis *et al.*, 1970.)

isoquinoline alkaloids* (Cohen and Collins, 1970). This at least lent support to the notion.

If tetrahydroisoquinolines are involved in alcoholism, it should be possible to

* Tetrahydroisoquinoline is the name used to refer to the class of alkaloid conjugates derived from biogenic amines.

introduce them into the brain and promote addictive processes. Myers and co-workers at Purdue have implanted cannulas into brains of a strain of rats that do not normally drink alcohol at all, and infused them around the clock with tetrahydropapaveroline (Myers and Melchior, 1977a; Melchior and Myers, 1977). The rats are given a free choice between water and alcohol solutions of various concentrations (e.g., 3 to 30%). After 3–6 days of alkaloid treatment they become raging alcoholics! They hit the "hard stuff" (30% alcohol or 60 proof) and drink excessively (Fig. 17-11). They show withdrawal symptoms (Fig. 17-12) and even have a preference for alcohol over water days after the infusion is stopped. A number of tetrahydroisoquinoline derivatives have similar effects (Myers and Melchior, 1977b). The quantities of alkaloids needed to produce these effects are minuscule (less than 1 μg per day).

But are such compounds actually formed in brain? Direct measurements are

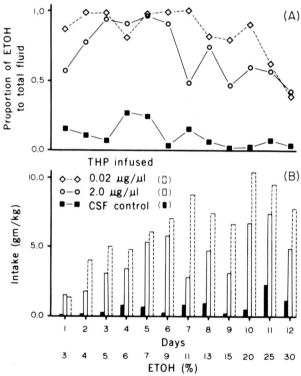

Fig. 17-11. (A) Proportion of alcohol (ETOH) to total fluid intake for each concentration of alcohol offered (see abscissa) on each day of the 12-day test sequence. Rats were infused every 15 minutes during these 12 days with tetrahydropapaveroline (THP) at a rate of 0.02 μg/μl, or 2.0 μg/μl, or with cerebrospinal fluid (CSF). (B) Corresponding mean amount of alcohol (expressed as grams per kilogram of body weight) consumed by these groups on each day of the alcohol test sequence. (From Myers and Melchior, 1977a. Copyright by the American Association for the Advancement of Science.)

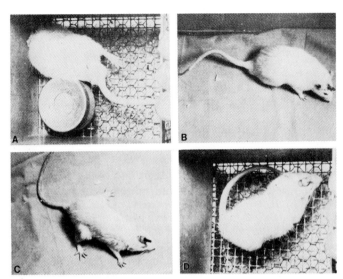

Fig. 17-12. Representative patterns of "withdrawal-like" behavior exhibited in rats after an alkaloid conjugate was infused intraventricularly once a day for 12 days. (A) Hindlimb catalepsy. (B) Stiffness of the tail. (C) Broad-based gait. (D) Preconvulsive squirming with a stiffly arched tail. (From Myers and Oblinger, 1977.)

necessary. The search began using sensitive analytical procedures since very little is probably there. Rats were given ethanol and dopamine degradation was blocked in order to increase the likelihood of finding the alkaloids. Most remarkably the results clearly show the presence of tetrahydroisoquinolines in the brain (Collins and Bigdeli, 1975).

If alcoholism and opiate addiction share common biochemical mechanisms, an opiate antagonist should inhibit the development of physical dependence on ethanol. Physical dependence on ethanol can be induced in mice by housing them in air-tight chambers and exposing them to a slow stream of air–ethanol vapors for 3 days. What happens if one group of mice receive naloxone every 6 hours during the experimental period and another group do not? It turns out that the naloxone-treated animals' withdrawal symptoms are much less severe than those of untreated controls. Brain Ca^{2+} levels are also changed. Naloxone, which by itself has no effect on the Ca^{2+} levels, prevents the ethanol-induced depletion of brain Ca^{2+} (Blum et al., 1977).

C. Summary and Conclusions

We can conclude from the available evidence that ethanol and opiates share common biochemical mechanisms. Condensation products of dopamine or other monoamines produce metabolites (tetrahydroisoquinoline alkaloids) which act on brain to induce a craving for alcohol, and over time, alcoholism results. Just how far the analogy between opiates and alcohol can be carried remains a challenge for the future.

Why do some individuals become alcoholics, while others can drink and drink and never become alcoholics? There is no clear answer at present, but recent work suggests a few possibilities (Myers, 1978; Schuckit and Rayses, 1979). It may be that some individuals are genetically predisposed toward becoming alcoholics, or it may be that environmental factors interact with a predisposed individual in some manner to create malfunctions in brain chemistry. More metabolites may be synthesized in some individuals. Metabolites produced in the body may gain greater entry into the brain. Maybe excessive drinking promotes the development of a leaky blood–brain barrier. Brain chemistry in certain persons may be unable to degrade metabolites. Alcoholics may be particularly disposed toward changes in monoamine systems, in amino acids, and in Ca^{2+} metabolism, as mediated by the tetrahydroisoquinolines. The encouraging news is that we now know enough to formulate such possibilities and that these can be tested. In the near future we can be hopeful that much new understanding will come, and with knowledge perhaps new ways to treat this behavioral disorder will become available.

Key Terms

Abstinence syndrome: The symptoms associated with removal of a drug after it has produced physical dependence. The term "withdrawal syndrome" is often used in place of abstinence syndrome.

Adenylate cyclase: The enzyme which synthesizes cAMP from ATP. Its activity can be modulated by various transmitters and drugs.

Affective disorders: Severe emotional disturbances involving depression or mania.

α-Methyl-*p*-tyrosine: An inhibitor of catecholamine biosynthesis. It appears to compete with the precursor tyrosine.

Amphetamine: A stimulant drug which appears to promote the release of catecholamines from their nerve endings.

Barbiturate: A class of drugs which induces sedation or sleep.

Catecholamine hypothesis of affective disorders: Mania is a result of excess norepinephrine in the brain; depression is a result of a deficiency of serotonin and, perhaps, norepinephrine.

Chlorpromazine: A phenothiazine which can act as a dopamine receptor antagonist. It is an antipsychotic drug and major tranquilizer.

Cocaine: A stimulant drug which is believed to act by inhibiting the reuptake of catecholamines.

Cross-tolerance: The state in which tolerance to one drug has the effect of causing tolerance to another.

Cyclic adenosine monophosphate (cAMP): The "second messenger": A molecule whose intracellular levels are regulated by hormones, transmitters, etc., and which acts to mediate intracellular changes in metabolism. cAMP is synthesized from ATP by adenylate cyclase.

Delirium tremens (the d.t.'s): A brain condition produced by long periods of alcohol intake. It is characterized by delirium, tremors and visual hallucinations that usually result in a state of terror.

Depression: Extreme sadness or feeling of worthlessness.

Dopamine hypothesis of schizophrenia: Schizophrenia results from an overactivity of the dopaminergic system in the brain.

Electroconvulsive therapy: A treatment sometimes used for severe depression. It involves the electrical stimulation of the brain and production of a controlled convulsion.

Endorphins: The generic term used to describe any endogenous compound which has opiatelike action. β-Endorphin is a specifiic endorphin.

Endorphin theory of schizophrenia: Schizophrenia is due to an overstimulation of endorphin receptors which causes schizophrenic behaviors.

Enkephalins: Pentapeptides (Leu-enkephalin or Met-enkephalin) which have opiatelike actions.

Imipramine: One of the class of tricyclic antidepressants. It acts in part to block the reuptake of norepinephrine into presynaptic terminals.

Lithium: A metallic element. Lithium salts are effective in treatment of mania. One of its actions is that it blocks the reuptake of catecholamines.

L-Tryptophan: An amino acid which, among other roles, serves as a biosynthetic precursor of serotonin.

Mania: Excessive excitement.

Monoamine oxidase: An intracellular enzyme which degrades monoamines.

Monoamine oxidase inhibitors: Drugs which inhibit the enzyme monoamine oxidase. As a result relatively large quantities of intraneuronal monoamines accumulate and are available for release.

Naloxone: A relatively specific opiate antagonist.

Neuroleptic drugs: Any medication with antipsychotic properties.

Norepinephrine reward pathway theory of schizophrenia: Schizophrenia is caused by the progressive destruction of norepinephrine reward pathways. This theory is generally discounted.

Paranoia: Delusions of persecution or grandeur.

Phenothiazines: A class of drugs used in the treatment of schizophrenia. Chlorpromazine is a prototypic one. Phenothiazines appear to act by blocking dopamine receptors and reducing dopamine release.

Physical dependence: The state in which a drug modifies bodily processes so that continued administration is required to prevent withdrawal symptoms.

Psychic dependence: A state of compulsion in which continual administration of a drug is necessary to avoid discomfort or produce pleasure.

Psychosis: A severe mental disturbance in which a person is out of touch with reality.

Reserpine: A drug which prevents the storage of catecholamines in their secretory granules; it is used as a tranquilizer and antihypertensive agent.

Tetrahydroisoquinoline: The name used to refer to the class of alkaloid conjugates derived from biogenic amines.

Tetrahydropapaveroline (THP): A benzyl tetrahydroisoquinoline alkaloid derivative of dopamine. It is structurally related to morphine. Intraventricular administration of THP will cause rats to develop the characteristics of alcoholism.

Tolerance: The state in which a drug becomes less effective with repeated administration and larger doses are required to achieve the desired effect.

Tricyclic antidepressants: Drugs used for treatment of depression. They act primarily by blocking serotonin and norepinephrine reuptake making more transmitter available to the receptors.

Transmethylation hypothesis of schizophrenia: Schizophrenia is caused by the production of methylated derivatives (a $-CH_3$ group is added) of various catecholamines and/or indoleamines which, if accumulated in sufficient quantities, produce psychotic behavior.

Withdrawal syndrome: *see* Abstinence syndrome.

General References

Goodwin, D. W. (1977). Alcohol. *In* "Psychopharmacology in the Practice of Medicine" (M.E. Jarvik, ed.), pp. 407–416. Appleton, New York.

Kosterlitz, H. W., ed. (1976). "Opiates and Endogenous Opioid Peptides." North-Holland Publ., Amsterdam.

Meyers, F. H., Jawetz, E., and Goldfien, A. (1976). "Review of Medical Pharmacology," 5th ed. Lange Med. Publ., Los Altos, California.

Mulé, S. J., and Brill, H., eds. (1972). "Chemical and Biological Aspects of Drug Dependence." CRC Press, Cleveland, Ohio.

Myers, R. D. (1978). Psychopharmacology of alcohol. *Annu. Rev. Pharmacol. Toxicol.* **18,** 125–144.

Myers, R. D. (1978). Tetrahydroisoquinolines in the brain: The basis of an animal model of alcoholism. *Alcohol Clin. Exp. Res.* **2,** 145–154.

Snyder, S. H. (1977). Opiate receptors and internal opiates. *Sci. Am.* **236,** 44–56.

Wilder, A. (1977). Characteristics of opioid addiction. *In* "Psychopharmacology in the Practice of Medicine" (M. E. Jarvick, ed.), pp. 419–432. Appleton, New York.

References

Aghajanian, G. K., and Bunney, B. S. (1974). Central dopamine neurons: Neurophysiological identification and responses to drugs. *In* "Frontiers in Catecholamine Research" (E. Usdin and S. H. Snyder, eds.), pp. 643–648. Pergamon, Oxford.

Angrist, B. M. and Gershon, S. (1970). The phenomenology of experimentally induced amphetamine psychosis: Preliminary observations. *Biol. Psychiatry* **2**, 95–107.

Ban, T. A. (1969). "Psychopharmacology." Williams & Wilkins, Baltimore, Maryland.

Beckmann, H., and Goodwin, F. K. (1975). Antidepressant response to tricyclics and urinary MHPG in unipolar patients. Clinical responses to imipramine or amitriptyline. *Arch. Gen. Psychiatry* **32**, 17–21.

Bloom, F., Segal, D., Ling, N., and Guillemin, R. (1976). Endorphins: Profound behavioral effects in rats suggest new etiological factors in mental illness. *Science* **194**, 630–632.

Blum, K., Futterman, S., Wallace, J. E., and Schwertner, H. A. (1977). Naloxone-induced inhibition of ethanol dependence in mice. *Nature (London)* **265**, 49–51.

Bunney, W. E., Jr. (1975). The current status of research in the catecholamine theories of affective disorders. *Psychopharmacol. Commun.* **1**, 599–609.

Burt, D. R., Enna, S. J., Creese, I., and Snyder, S. (1975). Dopamine receptor binding in the corpus striatum of mammalian brain. *Proc. Natl. Acad. Sci. U.S.A.* **72**, 4655–4659.

Carlsson, A. (1976). The contribution of drug research to investigating the nature of endogenous depression. *Pharmakopsychiatrie Neuro-Psychopharmakol.* **9**, 2–10.

Cash, J. (1975). "Man in Black." Zondervan, Grand Rapids, Michigan.

Clemens, S. L. (1923). "Huckleberry Finn." Harper, New York.

Clement-Cormier, Y. C., Kebabian, J. W., Petzold, G. L., and Greengard, P. (1974). Dopamine-sensitive adenylate cyclase in mammalian brain: A possible site of action of antipsychotic drugs. *Proc. Natl. Acad. Sci. U.S.A.* **71**, 1113–1117.

Cohen, G., and Collins, M. (1970). Alkaloids from catecholamines in adrenal tissue: Possible role in alcoholism. *Science* **167**, 1749–1751.

Collins, M. A., and Bigdeli, M. G. (1975). Tetrahydroisoquinolines *in vivo*. I. Rat brain formation of salsolinol, a condensation product of dopamine and acetaldehyde, under certain conditions during ethanol intoxication. *Life Sci.* **16**, 585–602.

Connell, P. H. (1958). "Amphetamine Psychosis." Chapman & Hall, London.

Coppen, A. (1972). Indoleamines and affective disorders. *J. Psychiat. Res.* **9**, 163–171.

Cox, B., Ary, M., and Lomax, P. (1976). Changes in sensitivity to apomorphine during morphine dependence and withdrawal in rats. *J. Pharmacol. Exp. Ther.* **196**, 637–641.

Creese, I., Burt, D. R., and Snyder, S. H. (1976a). Dopamine receptor binding predicts clinical and pharmacological potencies of anti-schizophrenic drugs. *Science* **192**, 481–483.

Creese, I., Burt, D. R., and Snyder, S. H. (1976b). Dopamine receptors and average clinical doses. *Science* **194**, 546.

Davis, V. E., and Walsh, M. J. (1970). Alcohol, amines and alkaloids: A possible biochemical basis for alcohol addiction. *Science* **167**, 1005–1007.

Davis, V. E., Walsh, M. J., Yamanaka, Y. (1970). Augmentation of alkaloid formation from dopamine by alcohol and acetaldehyde *in vitro*. *J. Pharmacol. Exp. Ther.* **174**, 401–412.

deWied, D. (1979). Schizophrenia as an inborn error in the degradation of β-endorphin—a hypothesis. *Trends Neurosci.* **2**, 79–82.

DiMascio, A., and Shader, R. I., eds. (1970). "Clinical Handbook of Psychopharmacology." Science House, New York.

Farkas, T., Dunner, D. L., and Fieve, R. R. (1976). L-Tryptophan in depression. *Biol. Psychiatry* **11**, 295–302.

Gillin, J. C., Kaplan, J., Stillman, R., & Wyatt, R. J. (1976). The psychedelic model of schizophrenia: The case of N,N-dimethyltryptamine. *Am. J. Psychiatry* **133**, 203–208.

Goodwin D. W. (1977). Alcohol. *In* "Psychopharmacology in the Practice of Medicine" (M. E. Jarvik, ed.), pp. 407–416. Appleton, New York.

Goodwin, F. K., Murphy, D. L., Brodie, H. K. H., and Bunney, W. E., Jr. (1970). L-DOPA, catecholamines, and behavior: A clinical and biochemical study in depressed patients. *Biol. Psychiatry* **2**, 314–366.

Groves, P. M., and Rebec, G. V. (1976). Biochemistry and behavior: Some central actions of amphetamine and antipsychotic drugs. *Annu. Rev. Psychol.* **27**, 91–127.

Gunne, L. M., Lindstrom, L., and Terenius, L. (1977). Naloxone-induced reversal of schizophrenic hallucinations. *J. Neural Transm.* **40**, 13–19.

Harris, R. A., Yamamoto, H., Loh, H. H., and Way, E. L. (1976). Alterations in brain calcium localization during the development of morphine tolerance and dependence. *In* "Opiates and Endogenous Opioid Peptides" (H. Kosterlitz, ed.), pp. 361–368. North-Holland Publ., New York.

Hayes, R. L., and Mayer, D. J. (1978). Morphine tolerance: Is there evidence for a conditioning model? *Science* **200**, 343–344.

Hollister, L. E. (1973). "Clinical Use of Psychotherapeutic Drugs." Thomas, Springfield, Illinois.

Holtzman, S. G. (1974). Behavioral effects of separate and combined administration of naloxone and d-amphetamine. *J. Pharmacol. Exp. Ther.* **189**, 51–60.

Isbell, H., and Chruściel, T. L. (1970). Dependence liability of "non-narcotic" drugs. *Bull. W.H.O.* **43**, Suppl., 1–111.

Iversen, L. L., Rogawski, M. A., and Miller, R. J. (1976). Comparison of the effects of neuroleptic drugs on pre- and postsynaptic dopaminergic mechanisms in the rat striatum. *Mol. Pharmacol.* **12**, 251–262.

Janowsky, D. S., Segal, D. S., Abrams, A., Bloom, R., and Guillemin, R. (1977). Negative naloxone effects in schizophrenic patients. *Psychopharmacology* **53**, 295–297.

Klein, D. F., and Davis, J. M. (1969). "Diagnosis and Drug Treatment of Psychiatric Disorders." Williams & Wilkins, Baltimore, Maryland.

Lehmann, H. E. (1967). Schizophrenia. IV. Clinical features. *In* "Comprehensive textbook of Psychiatry" (A. M. Freedman and H. I. Kaplan, eds.), pp. 621–648. Williams & Wilkins, Baltimore, Maryland.

Lippmann, W., Pugsely, T., and Merker, J. (1975). Effect of butaclamol and its enantiomers upon striatal homovanillic acid and adenyl cyclase on olfactory tubercle in rats. *Life Sci.* **16**, 213–224.

Loh, H. H., Shen, F. H., and Way, E. L. (1969). Inhibition of morphine tolerance and physical dependence development and brain serotonin synthesis by cyclohexamide. *Biochem. Pharmacol.* **18**, 2711–2721.

McMillan, D. E. (1971). Interactions between naloxone and chlorpromazine on behavior under schedule control. *Psychopharmacologia* **19**, 128–133.

Mathysse, S., and Lipinski, J. (1975). Biochemical aspects of schizophrenia. *Annu. Rev. Med.* **26**, 551–565.

Melchior, C. L., and Myers, R. D. (1977). Preference for alcohol evoked by tetrahydropapaveroline (THP) chronically infused in the cerebral ventricle of the rat. *Pharmacol., Biochem. Behav.* **7**, 19–35.

Miller, R. J., Horn, A. S., and Iversen, L. L. (1974). The action of neuroleptic drugs on dopamine-stimulated adenosine 3′,5′-monophosphate production in rat neostriatum and limbic forebrain. *Mol. Pharmacol.* **10**, 759–766.

Murphy, D. L., Baker, M., Kotin, J., and Bunney, W. E., Jr. (1973). Behavioral and metabolic effects of L-tryptophan in unipolar depressed patients. In "Serotonin and Behavior" (J. Barcus and E. Usdin, eds.), pp. 529–537. Academic Press, New York.

Myers, R. D. (1978). Tetrahydroisoquinolines in the brain: The basis of an animal model of alcoholism. *Alcohol Clin. Exp. Res.* **2**(2), 145–154.

17. BEHAVIORAL DISORDERS

Myers, R. D., and Melchior, C. L. (1977a). Alcohol drinking: Abnormal intake caused by tetrahy-dropapaveroline in the brain. *Science* **196**, 554–556.

Myers, R. D., and Melchior, C. L. (1977b). Differential actions on voluntary alcohol intake of tetrahydroisoquinolines or a β-carboline infused chronically in the ventricle of the rat. *Pharmacol., Biochem. Behav.* **7**, 381–392.

Myers, R. D., and Oblinger, M. M. (1977). Alcohol drinking in the rat induced by acute intra-cerebral infusion of two tetrahydroisoquinolines and a β-carboline. *Drug Alcohol Depend.* **2**, 469–483.

Osmond, H., and Smythies, J. (1952). Schizophrenia: A new approach. *J. Ment. Sci.* **98**, 309–315.

Pavlov, I. P. (1927). "Conditioned Reflexes," pp. 35–37. Oxford Univ. Press, London and New York.

Sarason, I. G. (1976). "Abnormal Psychology. The Problem of Maladaptive Behavior," 2nd ed. Prentice-Hall, Englewood Cliffs, New Jersey.

Schildkraut, J. J. (1965). The catecholamine hypothesis of affective disorders: A review of supporting evidence. *Am. J. Psychiatry* **122**, 509–522.

Schuckit, M. A., and Rayses, V. (1979). Ethanol ingestion: Differences in blood acetaldehyde concentrations in relatives of alcoholics and controls. *Science* **203**, 54–55.

"Schizophrenia: Is There an Answer?" (1972). National Institute of Mental Health, Washington, D.C.

Seeman, P., and Lee, T. (1975). Antipsychotic drugs: Direct correlation between clinical potency and presynaptic actions on dopamine neurons. *Science* **188**, 1217–1219.

Seevers, M. H., Davis, V. E., and Walsh, M. J. (1970). Morphine and ethanol physical dependence: A critique of a hypothesis. *Science* **170**, 1113–1114.

Segal, D. S., Kuczenski, R., and Mandell, A. J. (1974). Theoretical implications of drug-induced adaptive regulation for a biogenic amine hypothesis of affective disorder. *Biol. Psychiatry* **9**, 147–159.

Sharma, S. K., Klee, W. A., and Nirenberg, M. (1975). Dual regulation of adenylate cyclase accounts for narcotic dependence and tolerance. *Proc. Natl. Acad. Sci. U.S.A.* **72**, 3092–3096.

Siegel, S. (1978). Morphine tolerance: Is there evidence for a conditioning model? *Science* **200**, 344–345.

Snyder, S. H. (1976). The dopamine hypothesis of schizophrenia: Focus on the dopamine receptor. *Am. J. Psychiatry* **133**, 197–202.

Snyder, S. H. (1977). Opiate receptors and internal opiates. *Sci. Am.* **236**, 44–56.

Stein, L., and Wise, C. D. (1971). Possible etiology of schizophrenia: Progressive damage to the noradrenergic reward system by 6-hydroxydopamine. *Science* **171**, 1032–1036.

Terenius, L. A., Wahlström, A., Lindström, L., and Widerlov, E. (1976). Increased CSF levels of endorphins in chronic psychosis. *Neurosci. Lett.* **3**, 157–162.

Volanka, J. A., Mallyer, A., Barg, S., and Perez-Cruet, J. (1977). Naloxone in chronic schizophrenia. *Arch. Gen. Psychiatry* **34**, 1227–1228.

Way, E. L., Ho, I. K., and Loh, H. H. (1974). Brain 5-hydroxytryptamine and cyclic AMP in morphine tolerance and dependence. *Adv. Biochem. Psychopharmacol.* **10**, 219–231.

Wei, E., and Loh, H. H. (1976). Physical dependence on opiate-like peptides. *Science* **193**, 1262–1263.

Wilder, A. (1977). Characteristics of opioid addiction. *In* "Psychopharmacology in the Practice of Medicine" (M. E. Jarvick, ed.), pp. 419–432. Appleton, New York.

Wise, C. D., and Stein, L, (1973). Dopamine-β-hydroxylase deficits in the brains of schizophrenic patients. *Science* **181**, 344–347.

Wyatt, R. J., Termini, B. A., and Davis, J. (1971). Biochemical and sleep studies of schizophrenia: A review of the literature, 1960–1970. *Schizophr. Bull.* **4**, 10–66.

Wyatt, R. J., Schwartz, M. A., Erdelyi, E., and Barchas, J. D. (1975). Dopamine-β-hydroxylase activity in brains of chronic schizophrenic patients. *Science* **187**, 368–370.

18

Why Am I What I Am?

I. Introduction

In the previous chapters we have discussed hearing and seeing, learning and memory, and goal-directed behaviors such as feeding and drinking. We have considered how internal body state and circadian rhythms can influence certain behaviors, and we have described how the body responds by motion under neuronal command. In real life it is rare to see one of these facets of behavior isolated from the influences of others. Behavior is a blend, a brilliant mix, in which the nervous system integrates external and internal influences, focuses them and directs a response through its effector systems. The main result may be movement, but movement may be accompanied by the creation of a memory of the experience and a change in feelings and subjective state. Imagine, for a moment, a dinner engagement with a very special friend. Candle light, quiet music, excellent food create contentment and fond memories. All stimuli, internal and external, play together, blend together into an intricate and elaborate weave producing rich, exciting and personal experiences.

This chapter will focus on man and the aspects of the human nervous system which make man unique among all living creatures. First, we will describe the subdivisions and specialized functions of the human cerebral cortex, the most advanced and sophisticated cerebral cortex. In Chapter 2 we noted that the cortex synthesizes patterns and consists of many subdivisions. In Chapter 10 we described the particular ways the cortex extracts features and reassembles stimuli. Cortical function, though, goes far beyond the processing of sensory stimuli; it creates a higher and more global mix of many stimuli and provides the computational machinery to produce language, spoken and written, a unique attribute of man. Finally, we shall wrestle with the problem of consciousness. Consciousness gives to us an impression of self, "I," providing unity and reality to perceptions. It is "focal mind" at its ultimate. As Sherrington wrote, "Each waking day is a stage dominated for good or ill in comedy, farce, or tragedy by a *dramatis persona* the 'self' and so it will be until the curtain drops" (1947).

II. Organization of the Human Cerebral Cortex

In man the cerebral cortex is much more developed and complex than in other animals such as chimpanzees, rats and tree shrews (Fig. 18-1). Man, in particular, has large areas of cortex that are uncommitted at birth which with development, we might say, become programmed for serving the subjective self and speech (Penfield, 1975). The large areas of the cerebral cortex that man possesses above and beyond other animals are concentrated in the parietal lobe, temporal lobe and frontal lobe (see Fig. 18-2). In this section we shall discuss the functions of some of these highly integrative cortical areas.

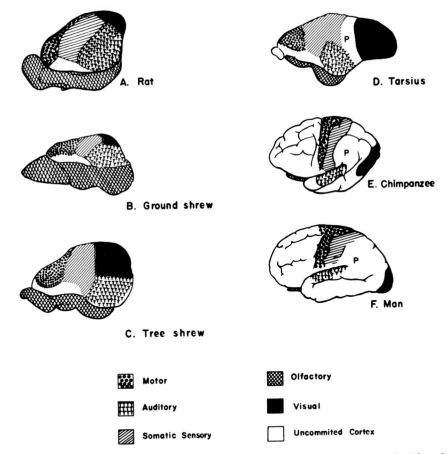

Fig. 18-1. The general organization of the cerebral cortex of some mammals. The white areas suggest the areas of gray matter uncommitted to sensory function at birth. (From Penfield, 1975.)

A. The Parietal Lobe—Mapping the Body, Blending the Senses, Knowing

The somesthetic cortex analyzes and combines sensations from the skin and deeper regions of the body, including its joints, where angles bespeak position and movement. Other regions of the parietal lobe blend all these sensations with others, the sights and sounds evaluated by the nearby occipital and temporal lobes. In the parietal lobe (see Fig. 18-2) afferent input from many systems, particularly the somatosensory, visual, and vestibular, is integrated. The result is a bigger, more meaningful picture in which one's *self* begins to take form amidst its environment.

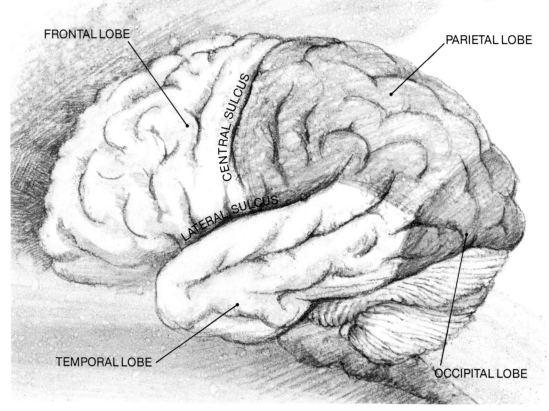

Fig. 18-2. Various lobes of the human brain.

We should remember that such a weave of sensory impressions is necessary if we are to *know* what sights, sounds and other sensations mean. For example, a metallic click takes on added significance if we see someone pointing a camera at us. Contact with something in the dark would acquire very different meanings if accompanied by a bump, or by heavy breathing not our own! From such combinations we arrive, moment by moment, at a knowledge of what is going on around us. Only if we have that knowledge can we decide what, if anything, to do and begin to carry our responses out.

Obviously, such syntheses may take place before speech is possible. However, even more serious deficits than loss of speech may result from damage to the parietal lobe. Such losses are in knowledge, or awareness, of the significance of things, and are called _agnosias_ ("not knowings"). There may be inability to localize sensations or recognize the meaning of palpated objects. Or there may be loss or failure to heed visual and auditory cues, even though sight and hearing remain intact ("psychic blindness and deafness"). In extreme cases, where the

18. WHY AM I WHAT I AM?

hemisphere (usually the right) necessary to appreciate spatial relationships has been damaged, awareness and acceptance of an entire half of the personal, as well as extrapersonal, space is lost. The afflicted person may fail to dress or undress the left side of the body or attend to its cosmetic care—and even complain about the strange unwanted presence that seems to be in bed. Figure 18-3 further illustrates the nature of the syndrome. A patient with unilateral parietal lobe damage was

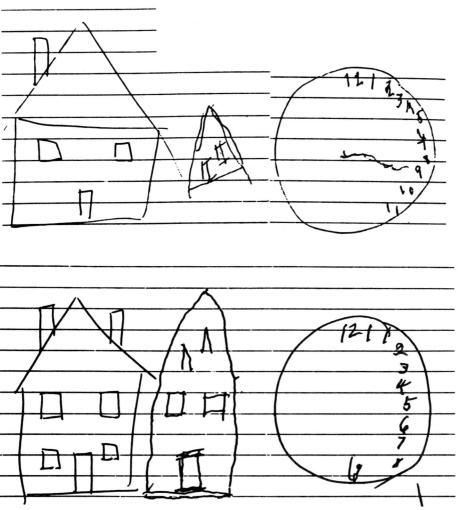

Fig. 18-3. Drawing made by a patient with right parietal lobe damage. The upper drawings were made within 2 days and the lower drawings 9 days after the incident. The watch face drawings on the far right show a neglect of the left half of extrapersonal space contralateral to the cerebral lesion. All the numbers are crowded into the right half of the drawing. The drawing on the far left is the physician's drawing of a house which the patient attempted to replicate. (From Mountcastle, 1976.)

asked to draw a watch face and copy a drawing of a house. He has crowded all the numbers within half the face of the clock showing a total neglect of the contralateral side of extrapersonal space. The name for this bizarre condition is technical, but informative: *amorphosynthesis*, a failure to put the body together. Such names distill the insights of neurologists who, like Hughlings Jackson a century past, can deduce normal function from study of nervous disorder.

Recent experiments by Mountcastle and co-workers (1975) on primates illustrate a key role of the parietal lobe in *selective visual attention*. Monkeys are trained to fixate or to track visually a target, detect a change in a small light carried on the target and upon detection touch the target in order to receive a reward (Fig. 18-4). The activity of single neurons is recorded in parietal cortex during

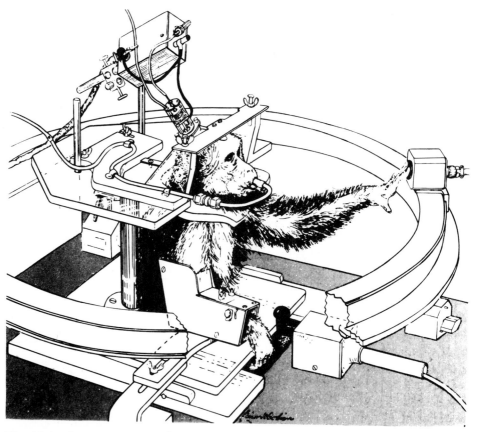

Fig. 18-4. Testing apparatus for studying the activity of parietal cortex neurons during selective visual attention. The animal releases the key with his left hand and then reaches with that arm to touch the lighted switch on the moving carriage. He receives a juice reward when he succeeds in performing the task. Neuronal activity is recorded from parietal cortex by implanted electrodes. (From Mountcastle *et al.*, 1975.)

18. WHY AM I WHAT I AM?

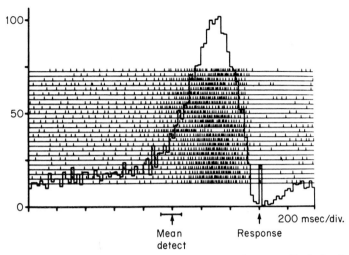

Fig. 18-5. Activity of a projection neuron in the parietal cortex. Each horizontal line is the activity of a single trial of the task. The line illustrates the average change in neural activity over many trials. Neural activity accelerates before release of the detect key (mean detect) reaches a peak as the arm moves toward the target switch and declines before the hand touches the target (response). (From Mountcastle *et al.*, 1975.)

performance of the task. One class of neurons—termed projection neurons—generate commands for initiating and driving a response to completion (Fig. 18-5). This class of cells does not fire to sensory stimuli of any type and the cells are inactive during movements such as aggressive ones. Mountcastle concluded,

> One thing appears certain that there is within area 5 a continually freshened neural image of the position of the limbs and body in space that is particularly sensitive to dynamic changes. Thus, an opportunity is afforded for a running cross-correlation between the commands for certain classes of behavioral acts and the motor components of their execution (Mountcastle, 1976, p. 19).

With further study it was found that fully one-half of the neurons provide commands that direct visual attention. Some of these cells discharge when the animal fixes his gaze upon objects of interest; others fire during smooth pursuit movements as the eyes track an object; still others are involved in saccadic eye movements that bring the object into the visual field. Their activity is conditional and occurs only with fixation of gaze upon objects of strong motivational power that are within or close to the behavioral environment of the animal. These neuronal happenings are in full accord with the ideas derived from parietal lobe lesions which show the neglect is a defect of volition.

We can say then that the parietal lobe generates commands particularly for directed visual attention by calling for selective and conditional fixation of gaze.

This is after all the simplest form of attention. In this way the parietal lobe performs a "matching function" between the neural signals, the nature of objects in the surround and those of our goal or drive states. As Mountcastle summarized:

> Each of us looks outward from the inner universe of his own brain. Each of us is linked outwardly—and thus we each to one another—via a few million sensory nerve channels. These, each single one everlastingly chattering of details, conjointly provide continuous images of the objects and events within perceptive range. Certain of these images are integrated, largely, I believe, in the parietal lobe, into an internal model of the orientation and movement of our own bodies and limbs in surrounding space and in the gravitational field. Loosely linked to that central image is an independent command apparatus, sentient to motivational drives, with governance over manual and visual operations within that intensely personal space scribed by reach of arm and hand and, particularly, for the direction and intensity of visual attention into the world around us (Mountcastle, 1976, p. 41).

The integrated picture from the parietal lobe will be passed forward to the frontal lobe where global strategies of behavior are in the making.

B. The Frontal Lobe—Judgment, Planning and Responsibility

The frontal lobe is the vast territory above the lateral sulcus (or Sylvian fissure) and in front of that of the central sulcus (or Rolando fissure) (see Fig. 18-2). Its great size and tremendous number of direct connections with other parts of the CNS are without doubt the most uniquely human of all aspects of man's nervous system. These structural features are essential for mankind's special attributes. Such features are present, but far less highly developed, in the brains of most other mammals. In certain species, however, such as the chimpanzee, gorilla, whale or elephant, the frontal lobes are extremely large and well fissurated. These animals are now receiving much attention that is long overdue.

The human frontal lobes are extraordinarily well informed on the encyclopedic range of events transpiring in other regions of the nervous system. And they exercise a powerful, highly selective influence over many (fortunately not all) of these occurrences, as we saw in the operation of the motor cortex at the rear of the lobe. The prefrontal lobes make important reciprocal connections to the limbic system. This gives the frontal lobe the unique function of associating cortical sensory information with emotional input from the limbic system.

In front of the motor cortex, a larger region extends to (and includes) the frontal pole. Part of it further elaborates movement patterns. A greater part, however, appears involved in regulating emotional tone, assigning priorities to bodily and environmental demands and stabilizing programs for meeting short-term and long-range goals.

To appreciate the qualities that depend on the frontal lobes, consider the two well-known hallmarks of frontal lobe injury or loss. Over a century ago, a tamping-iron was accidentally blown by dynamite through the cheek and forehead of a railway construction foreman. He miraculously survived this calamity, but underwent a striking deterioration of personality. From an upright, dependable worker he became so profane and irresponsible an individual that he lost his job and spent the rest of his life as a shiftless drifter. His case, beautifully chronicled by the rural doctor who treated his hideous wound and followed his subsequent checkered career, is a classic of nineteenth century American medical literature.

In the past four decades, numerous observations and valuable insights have been added to this first glimpse of frontal lobe function. The new knowledge has come from study of persons who have had frontal lobotomies (lobe removals) or similar neurosurgical procedures for relief of intractable psychosis or unbearable pain (as in terminal stages of cancer). The findings, of course, were obtained in very sick people, under special circumstances and by means of what even then were highly controversial psychosurgical operations. Nevertheless, the results eloquently attest to the importance of these lobes that bulge (and often furrow) our brows and to the critical roles they play in stable, purposeful behavior.

One major deficit noted after injury or surgical isolation of the frontal lobes is diminished anxiety and concern on the part of the affected person. Under certain circumstances, this loss is all too evident in a reduction of that person's ethical standards. Tranquility and indifference, to be sure, were what the surgeons wanted. They were trying to help problem psychotics or to relieve excruciating, unremitting pain. We must remember that such psychosurgery was never taken lightly, but only as a last resort—as an alternative, however crude and empirical, to even greater human suffering in asylums or on the wards. In many patients (unhappily, not all), such operations seemed to bring relief, if only for a while. Today, removal of the frontal lobes or interruption of their connections (all too easily accomplished through tiny holes drilled through the roof of the eye's orbits under local anesthesia) are seldom performed. Better, more predictable and reversible results are possible now with drugs, which can be withdrawn if mistakes are made. In severe cases, where drugs alone are not effective, electrical stimulation (see Chapter 17) (as in the thalamus) may produce a beneficial result.

Another characteristic effect of frontal lobe damage is to lessen an individual's judgment and planning ability. Inappropriate or ill-timed actions occur. Apparently the person can no longer meet changes in the environment, or reconcile life's many conflicting, simultaneous demands and respond to them at the right times and places. Thus one may laugh at something that is not funny, cry at that which is not sad, be unable to plan a meal without forgetting how to cook—even urinate in public while dressed in evening clothes and strolling with a companion to the opera. All these bizarre occurrences have actually happened. Such things do not surprise the neurologists and psychiatrists who care for these patients after their injury or surgery. These are symptoms of the limbic system operating without its highest level of control.

In brief, loss of the frontal poles and their surrounding cortical regions debases a human being. It does not impair intellect, memory or consciousness as much as lesions in certain other parts of the brain do, but it does interfere seriously with ability to respond appropriately in the emotional and social spheres. It reduces morality by lessening worry and care. It impairs the capacity to meet (and reconcile if possible) the pressures of ever-changing internal and external stimuli. A person who has lost the frontal lobes is less likely to persevere at some program of activity in the face of distraction, discomfort or pain. He may also have difficulty in shifting his strategy in the face of changing conditions. The person may do quite well in recognizing the initial strategy, but when it is changed he does poorly. The unfortunate one becomes a "creature of the moment." As a perceptive thinker put it, either the individual has lost the frontal lobes or those lobes have lost hold of the individual. Goals are blurred (though not forgotten), put out of correct order or set aside.

Unlike loss of limbs, sight or speech, injuries which may devastate yet not defeat the human spirit, loss of the frontal lobes is a tragic wound of the stuff that is man. Mercifully, the person is unaware of what is lost.

The temporal lobe has massive intimate connections with the frontal lobe. These two lobes work together on many of the brain's highest functions.

C. The Temporal Lobe—Listening, Dreaming and Remembering

The auditory cortex is a very small region of the temporal lobe that could be covered by a fifty cent piece. It lies on the lower bank of the Sylvian fissure, toward the rear of the lobe (see Fig. 18-2). It adjoins a region where the movements and positions of the head signaled by the inner ear are given further study. The underlying temporal regions elaborate sounds, sights, smells and other experiences in a complex manner. Evidently perception, recording and retrieval of events involve this large, anatomically diversified lobe of the brain. The region is also, as we saw in the limbic system, important in emotional coloration of experience. Striking emotional, hallucinatory and memory disturbances follow destructive or irritative insults (such as those of epilepsy) to this part of the brain. If the damage is near or in the amygdala, there can be overeating, hypersexuality, and excessive placidity or hallucinations of an odor (usually foul), coupled with a fearful feeling of unreality in the environment. If both sides of the brain are involved, there may be loss of recent memory, This severe deficit represents complete inability to commit anything to memory after the time of damage or illness. Long-term memory, however, for events that occurred before the stroke or course of seizures is usually preserved. Intellect also is spared. One man could make witty repartee, play "twenty-one" and manage his business affairs, even though he would forget what he had eaten for breakfast.

Nonverbal visual memory appears particularly affected by loss of the temporal lobes. One test which illustrates this is the so-called recurring nonsense figures (Kimura, 1963). Subjects are tested for their memory of unfamilar designs of geometrical forms. In a pile of cards, these designs appear randomly and the subject is asked to state whether her or she has seen it before. The mean error score in subjects with damage to the right temporal lobe is higher than in normal subjects or those with parietal lobe lesions. Similarly patients with temporal lobe damage have severe difficulties in recognizing portraits they studied 2 minutes earlier. There appears to be interference with visual feature detection and/or recall for higher order inputs. Visual acuity and the topography of visual fields are unaffected.

Stimulation of the temporal lobe during brain surgery calls forth psychical phenomena of a high order. Such responses are not evoked from other parts of the cortex (where only disappointing fragments of functions may be obtained). Hallucinations and illusions unfold in a progressive and dramatic manner, like a motion picture with sound and color. They are based on the person's memories or dreams. Apparently memories of all types—pictures, sounds, melodies, incidents—are accessible to retrieval (not necessarily stored) here in some way. A perceptual illusion is sometimes pronounced: the patient may have a feeling of déjà vu, that something has happened before and is completely familiar, in fact, predictable. There are usually strong emotional colorations to such illusions, which many of us have experienced at some time.

Thus parts of this lobe seem to be involved in the decision to "tape and store" information, as well as in the actual process of recording and storing events, along with their evaluation as agreeable or disagreeable. The "replay" circuits for experiences already "on tape" may survive damage to other components of the recording machinery, but with larger or more generalized types of brain damage long-term memory loss is an inevitable, well-known consequence. Information storage probably does not take place in the temporal lobe alone, even though auditory and olfactory memories appear to draw heavily upon its neurons and connections. As we have stressed, such high functions almost certainly are responsibilities of many brain regions, particularly the thalamus and the many cortical regions it ties together, if not of the whole brain.

In the course of surgical treatment of patients suffering from temporal lobe epilepsy, Wilder Penfield and co-workers at the Montreal Neurological Institute happened upon an astonishing discovery. _Epilepsy_ is a serious self-destructive disease in which the brain goes into uncontrolled electrical discharges. Unless treated, patients become extremely disabled and eventually die. When epilepsy is very severe, one of the treatments is to go into the brain, locate the area generating the seizures and remove it. The brain registers no pain when intruded upon, so the operation can be performed under local anesthesia in awake patients. In order to locate the focus (the location where the seizure originates) a stimulating electrode can be used to apply gentle electric current. This produces the beginning of a potential epileptic discharge and aids the surgeons in locating the focus. It turns out that electrical stimulation also provides remarkable insights into the operational characteristics of the human brain, one of which is called "_flashback_."

As Penfield wrote in his exciting monograph "The Mystery of the Mind,"

> On the first occasion, when one of these "flashbacks" was reported to me by a conscious patient (1933), I was incredulous. On each subsequent occasion, I marvelled. For example, when a mother told me she was suddenly aware, as my electrode touched the cortex, of being in her kitchen listening to the voice of her little boy who was playing outside in the yard. She was aware of the neighborhood noises, such as passing motor cars, that might mean danger to him.
>
> In other cases, different "flashbacks" might be produced from successive stimulations of the same point. Perhaps it may add realism if I describe here one illustrative case briefly.
>
> M.M., a young woman of twenty-six had minor attacks that began with a sense of familiarity followed by a sense of fear and then by "a little dream" of some previous experience. When the right hemisphere was exposed at operation [as shown in Fig. 18-6] I explored the cerebral cortex with an electrode, placing numbered squares of paper on the surface of the brain to show the position each time a positive response was obtained. At point 2 she felt a tingling in the left thumb; at point 3, tingling in the left side of the tongue; at 7 there was movement of the tongue. It was clear then that 3 had been placed on the somatic convolution and 7 on the motor convolution [Fig. 18-6]. It is now obvious that 11 marks the first temporal convolution below the fissure of Sylvius. The stimulating current was increased from two to three volts. The succeeding responses from the temporal lobe were "psychical" instead of sensory or motor. They were activations of the stream of consciousness from the past as follows:
>
> 11—"I heard something, I do not know what it was."
>
> 11—(repeated without warning) "Yes, Sir, I think I heard a mother calling her little boy somewhere. It seemed to be something that happened years ago." When asked to explain, she said, "It was somebody in the neighborhood where I live." Then she added that she herself "was somewhere close enough to hear."
>
> 12—"Yes. I heard voices down along the river somewhere—a man's voice and a woman's calling . . . I think I saw the river."
>
> 15—"Just a tiny flash of a feeling of familiarity and a feeling that I knew everything that was going to happen in the near future."
>
> 17c—(a needle insulated except at the tip was inserted to the superior surface of

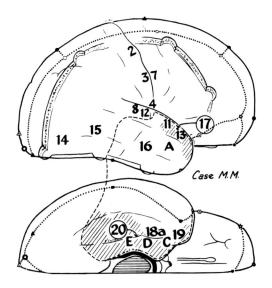

Fig. 18-6. Case M.M. Diagram of the surface of the cerebral cortex and the points where electrical stimulation elicited a particular response (see text). The broken line shows the extent of removal of the temporal lobe in the treatment of focal epilepsy. (From Penfield, 1975.)

the temporal lobe, deep in the fissure of Sylvius, and the current was switched on) "Oh! I had the same very, very familiar memory, in an office somewhere. I could see the desks. I was there and someone was calling to me, a man leaning on a desk with a pencil in his hand."

I warned her I was going to stimulate, but I did not do so. "Nothing."

18a—(stimulation without warning) "I had a little memory—a scene in a play— they were talking and I could see it—I was just seeing it in my memory."

I was more astonished, each time my electrode brought forth such a response. How could it be? This had to do with the mind! (Penfield, 1975, pp. 21–27).

Electrical stimulation of various parts of the human cortex produces a variety of responses (Fig. 18-7).

What about speech, the most characteristic and unique attribute of man-kind? This task is delegated to part of the association cortex.

D. The Association Cortex—Getting It Together in Speech and Language

The *association cortex* consists of extensive territories of gray matter that surround and overshadow the primary and secondary sensory and motor areas. It is concentrated in three major regions: the parietal, occipital and temporal lobes; the territory near the temporal pole (under which the amygdala and hippocampus lie); and the forward part of the frontal lobe (including the frontal pole). We have

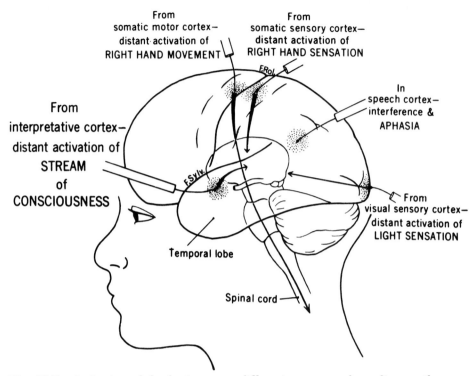

From
somatic motor cortex—
distant activation of
RIGHT HAND MOVEMENT

From
somatic sensory cortex—
distant activation of
RIGHT HAND SENSATION

In
speech cortex—
interference &
APHASIA

From
interpretative cortex—
distant activation of
STREAM
of
CONSCIOUSNESS

From
visual sensory cortex—
distant activation of
LIGHT SENSATION

Temporal lobe

Spinal cord

Fig. 18-7. Activation of the brain causes different responses depending on the area. (From Penfield, 1975.)

already discussed these three regions to some extent: The first in relation to gnostic or knowing functions; the second as it relates to emotion, perceptual matters and memory; and the third as a powerful component of the limbic system. But we have not yet said anything about speech, except that it is not possible until many syntheses of information have taken place. Such syntheses are the major business of the association cortex, and many (if not all) of the above regions are drawn on. Several stand out, as we shall see.

The right and left hemispheres are not alike with respect to certain functions. One of them (more frequently, but not necessarily the left hemisphere) is dominant for speech. In that "talking" hemisphere a focal injury of association cortex can destroy or seriously impair speech and language. Three regions work together on these functions, and any damage that interferes with their team play can diminish linguistic skills. The speech areas are shown in Fig. 18-8. One region, surrounding the auditory cortex in the temporal lobe, is involved in the selection of words from verbal memory. Another, lying in front of the visual area of the occipital lobe, connects with the first and thus allows visual sensations to call up words; it is critically important for reading and writing. A third region lies at some distance from the other two in the frontal lobe. It is necessary for spoken

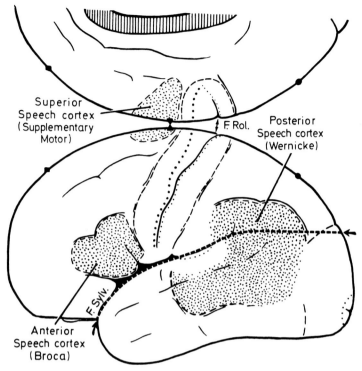

Fig. 18-8. Cortical speech areas of the dominant left hemisphere. (From Penfield and Roberts, *Speech and Brain Mechanisms*, p. 201. Copyright 1959 by Princeton Univ. Press. Reprinted by permission of Princeton Univ. Press.)

language, just as an adjacent region, the hand area of the motor homunculus, is essential for handwriting abilities.

From the above, we can see that speech defects owing to cortical lesions, such as strokes (occlusion of cerebral blood vessels), may involve one's comprehension of spoken or written words, as well as the expression of one's understanding in an easy, meaningful manner, spoken or written. These ongoing and outgoing aspects of communication through language are intimately interwoven in the association cortex. Thus, they are usually both affected by damage to the cortex, in varying degrees relative to one another.

III. Hemispheric Dominance

We already know that each hemisphere is entrusted with the control of one-half of the body, e.g., right motor cortex controls the left side of the body. And, we mentioned above, speech functions are located in one hemisphere. This lateralization is most striking. In fact, the physical or anatomical structure of the brain is asymmetric with respect to speech (Fig. 18-9). In addition, the cerebral hemispheres are specialized in other ways. Each can have its own ideas, thoughts and abilities and seemingly functions separately in many tasks. One is dominant over the other. The dominant one oversees speech, language and certain aspects of math; its subordinate partner, on the other hand, prefers geometry and perhaps reacts a little more spontaneously to situations. One of the exciting frontiers in the behavioral neurosciences is the study of brain function designed to elucidate the rules and relationships between the hemispheres. Next to consciousness itself, hemispheric dominance is the highest level of integration. In man the two cerebral hemispheres are dedicated toward their own purposes but partners in their efforts. Hemispheric dominance seems to be a special attribute of man. Some anatomical asymmetry does exist in chimps. Also, in birds, song is localized primarily in the left hemisphere. In man, however, hemisphere dominance is most developed.

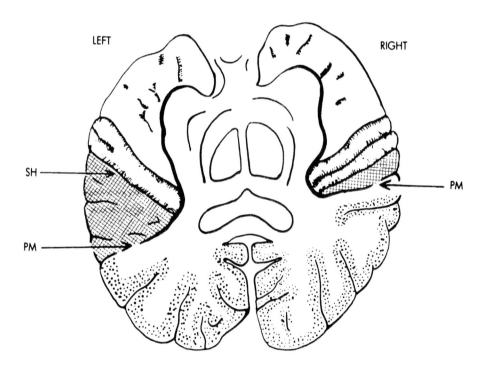

Fig. 18-9. Asymmetry and hypertrophy of human temporal lobes associated with speech. The posterior margin (PM) slopes backward more sharply on the left side and the anterior margin of the sulcus of Heschl (SH) slopes forward more sharply on the left. (From Geschwind and Levitsky, 1968. Copyright by the American Association for the Advancement of Science.)

788   **18. WHY AM I WHAT I AM?**

Moment by moment man's two hemispheres work in close communication and consultation. They are linked by the largest fiber bundle in the brain—the *corpus callosum*—made of about 200 million transverse running fibers interconnecting the two hemispheres. Recent information on the operation of the two cortices comes from a group of patients in which the corpus callosum has been transected as a last resort in the treatment of severe epilepsy after other treatments failed. The corpus callosum is cut but the deep brain stem structures are spared; this operation is called a *commissurotomy* (Fig. 18-10). In commissurotomy patients each hemisphere retains all the cerebral centers which mediate cerebral functions except that each cortex sees only half the world. The visual input, for example, is primarily crossed so the opposite hemisphere receives visual input from only one-half of visual space (see Fig. 18-11). An even simpler situation exists for the input from the hands and legs; the left hand or leg is controlled largely by the right hemisphere, the right by the left hemisphere. Accordingly, the two hemispheres are functionally isolated and can be compared in the same individual in order to discover their functions.

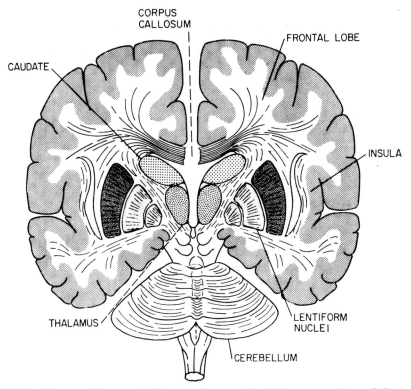

Fig. 18-10. Extent of anatomical separation produced by transection of the corpus callosum. (From Sperry, 1974.)

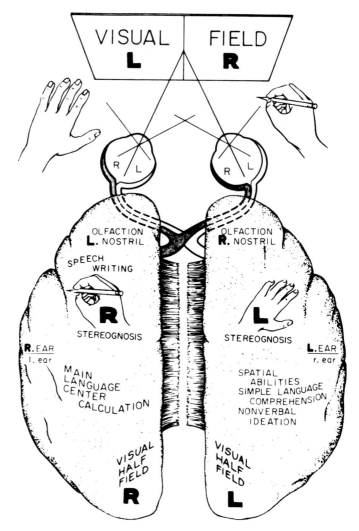

Fig. 18-11. Scheme showing the manner in which the left and right visual fields are projected onto the right and left hemispheres due to partial crossing of the optic nerves. The representation of the sensory inputs is also shown. (From Sperry, 1974.)

On the basis of casual observation, there are no obvious deficits in the behavior of commissurotomy patients. Verbal intelligence, reasoning, perception, motor coordination and personality are similar to the preoperative state. This is, however, only due to the superior computational capacities of the brain, battling and obviously succeeding to an extraordinary degree, to preserve oneness. Detailed testing reveals incredible differences between the two hemispheres (Sperry, 1974; 1977).

A. Verbal Skills

Studies on commissurotomy patients have revealed many new functional relationships in cortical function and confirmed previous data from patients with brain damage on the lateralization of speech. Speech and writing are strongly lateralized and appear in the dominant (left) hemisphere in right-handed subjects. It should be pointed out that in all the subjects studied (approximately 10 patients) the speech centers are located in the left hemisphere. Figure 18-12 shows a sketch of the set-up used for lateralized testing after hemispheric disconnection. The subject fixes his gaze upon a central spot on the screen and on the left or right side a second signal is flashed for a fraction of a second. This flash technique is very important to the success of these experiments: the brief presentation prohibits eye movements and "peeking" by the opposite visual half-field, i.e., hemisphere. The hands are shielded from view. The experimenter can explain various things to the subjects or demonstrate a set of instructions. The word "key" may have just appeared in the right visual field, for example, and the subject has had to use his right hand to retrieve the object just named from among other objects. This he has no trouble doing. The word flashed into the right visual field is passed to the

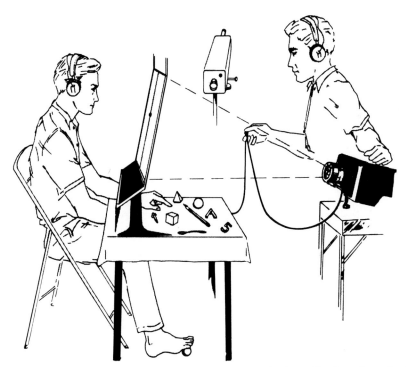

Fig. 18-12. Diagrammatic sketch of the arrangement for lateralized testing after hemispheric disconnection. (From Sperry, 1974.)

left visual cortex and to pathways in the left motor cortex which controls the right hand. If now, however, the experiment is carried out with a flash to the opposite visual field the result is remarkable. The subject can retrieve the key with the left hand. However, he will verbally deny having any knowledge of what is happening! He derives no conscious experience of what is going on from such transactions of the minor hemisphere. In persons where the corpus callosum is intact, interhemispheric transfer compensates and perception is independent of the side of the stimulus.

Is the minor hemisphere really completely mute? Perhaps the subject needs more time to consider the words. Also, can the right hemisphere read sentences? In order to evaluate these possibilities, linguistic abilities have been studied using a stabilized image technique. One eye is covered with a patch while a contact lens is mounted on the other eye with a device that limits the input into one-half of the visual field no matter how the eye is moved. In this way visual instructions can be presented for periods of up to 0.5 hour (Zaidel, 1975). When the minor hemisphere is asked to inspect a picture of a dog, for example, it can correctly select the proper word from a number of choices. Surprisingly the minor hemisphere can show a mental age only 2 years below that of the speaking hemisphere, using a picture vocabulary test. Nouns and verbs are equally recognized (Zaidel, 1976).

The verbal abilities of the minor hemisphere though are limited to simple word recognition. This hemisphere cannot comprehend words in long series. Even after prolonged examination of sentences, the minor hemisphere is unable to fill in a missing word at the end of a sentence or interpret the sentence. For example, when presented with the verbal arrangement: mother loves—nail, baby, brown, stone—the minor hemisphere chooses "baby" only randomly. It is deficient, but not devoid of all linguistic dimensions.

B. Structural Details versus Abstracted Features

Arithmetical operations appear to be predominantly a left (dominant) hemisphere function. The minor hemisphere is unable to perform simple additions except for sums less than 20. In contrast, some geometric operations appear to be processed better in the right hemisphere.

Sperry and co-workers (Franco and Sperry, 1977) tested the split brain patients in a series of cross-modal visual and tactile tests involving different levels and kinds of geometric discriminations. Geometric arrays (see Fig. 18-13) were selected as representative of Euclidian, Affine, projective and topological space. The subjects are presented geometrical forms to inspect. Behind the screen and outside of the patient's view are three geometric forms only one of which conforms with the five item display. After viewing the objects, the subjects are

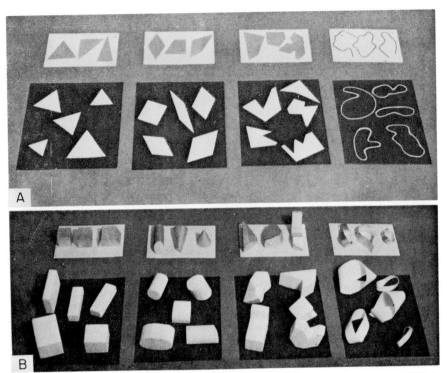

Fig. 18-13. Examples of geometrical arrays. (From Franco and Sperry, 1977.)

instructed to reach behind the screen and select, by hand signal, the one that most resembles the forms viewed. Normal control subjects make only nine mistakes out of some 540 trials. The subjects with commissurotomies, in contrast, show an extreme laterality in their performance. The right hemisphere–left hand system consistently achieves better scores, both in plain and in solid geometry (Fig. 18-14). The right hemisphere is clearly superior in dealing with loosely structured sets of shapes conveying little specific information. It more readily captures the "holistic" or highly abstracted properties of sets independent of structured constraints so that it can deal with equal success with Euclidian and topological tasks. This contrasts to the performance of the left hemisphere which is specialized for highly structured inputs, such as Euclidian figures or linguistic material.

The two hemispheres have mutually complementary functions. A striking revelation of complementary function comes from *chimeric picture studies* (Levy *et al.*, 1972). Chimeric pictures are formed by splitting pictures of a face, for example (Fig. 18-15). The subject fixes on the midpoint of the screen as the combination is flashed around it. When a form from faces 2 and 7 is flashed on the screen, the image in the left visual field (half of 7) is projected to the right

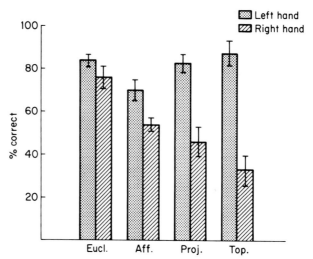

Fig. 18-14. Performance of commissurotomy subjects plotted for different kinds of geometry. Eucl., Euclidean; Aff., Affine; Proj., projective; Top., topological. (From Franco and Sperry, 1977.)

hemisphere and that in the right visual field (half of 2) is projected to the left hemisphere. By the laws of perceptual completion and closure each hemisphere automatically tends to fill in the other half to produce a whole (see Fig. 18-15). The right hemisphere responds to the whole face directly; it can best give information on complex and nondescript patterns such as recognizing the whole face from amongst others. The left hemisphere seems to detect best salient features and details to which verbal labels are easily attached and then used for discrimination and recall. Thus, the dominant left hemisphere responds to faces with verbally identifiable characteristics.

C. Lateralization of Music

Based on lesion studies, musical perception is apparently focused in the right hemisphere, apparently involving the temporal lobe. Patients with lesions of right temporal lobe, for example, perform worse in a tonal memory test. If the subjects are given four or five notes in rapid succession and asked which note is changed in pitch at the second playing, more errors are made after right temporal lobectomy than before. Left temporal lobectomy hardly changes the score (Milner, 1967). Also patients without their temporal lobe are poorer in continuing to hum a traditional tune or in maintaining it (Shankweiler, 1966). This lateralization is in line with the overall notion of the minor hemisphere's abilities in perceptual

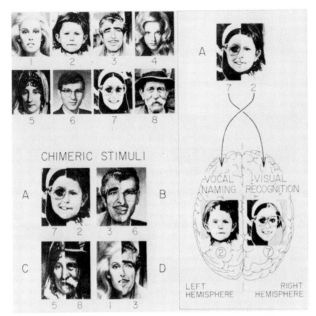

Fig. 18-15. Composite face stimuli for testing hemispheric specialization. (From Levy *et al.*, 1972.)

synthetic insight. Thus the hemispheres work as coordinated specialists each having specialized machinery to deal with tasks.

D. Emotion

Emotional tone is represented in both hemispheres in contrast to feature extraction and other specialized functions. Emotions are promptly transferred from one hemisphere to the other, presumably through intact brain stem mechanisms. Similarly, attentional and alertness properties are projected bilaterally. It appears, though, that the two hemispheres do not respond in an identical manner to emotional stimuli. Responses in the right hemisphere are often more intense and less inhibited than those in the left. For example, the minor hemisphere's reactions include emotional outbursts when a picture of the subject is introduced by surprise in a test series. After an initial six trials with relatively neutral stimuli in which the response had been routine, a middle-aged female patient was presented with a test series of four portraits of herself and asked to choose the one she liked best. The subject exclaimed "Oh no! where did you . . .? What are they?" Cross-leakage apparently was not a factor, since when asked about the contents of the photographs the subject said, "something nice whatever it was" and laughed

(Sperry, 1977). Thus although the emotional content of the response readily crossed to the speaking hemisphere, presumably through the intact brain stem, the major hemisphere clearly remained unaware of the exact nature of the stimuli.

E. Memory and Motor Skills

Long-term memories prior to the commissurotomy are unaffected. However, immediate memory appears impaired (Sperry, 1968, 1974). Especially during the first year and a half after surgery, patients are often unable to remember appointments, telephone messages or where they have put things. Quantitative measures using various tests have amply confirmed that memory deficits exist. The loss persists 4–9 years after surgery, though it may become less severe over time. It is evident that the forebrain commissures play a role in memory consolidation processes in humans (Zaidel and Sperry, 1974).

Similarly, motor performances acquired and highly practiced prior to surgery are well retained, even if they require extreme coordination, e.g., tying of shoe laces, swimming, bicycling, etc. After commissurotomy most new tasks can be acquired and performed as effectively, but the tasks cannot be performed as rapidly. For example, buttoning a shirt is one and a half times slower and operating a machine that requires coordination of both hands is considerably slower (Zaidel and Sperry, 1977). Interhemispheric connections are particularly important for motor output that involves complex intermanual coordination.

F. Development and Plasticity in Hemispheric Dominance

What are the factors which determine hemispheric dominance? Apparently at birth in humans the brain already has an inherent left–right differentiation. According to one recent model, one gene determines which hemisphere will be dominant with the allele for the right hemisphere being recessive. A second gene determines whether hand control or dominance will be contralateral or ipsilateral to the language hemisphere. Ipsilateral is recessive. Thus, there are nine possible genotypes for handedness in man. Presumably the weaker mixed combinations can be more readily reversed by training (Levy and Nagylaki, 1972). In contrast, handedness in rodents—or more appropriately paw preference—does not appear to be genetically determined (Collins, 1969).

Following commissurotomy there appears to be little improvement in most abilities, except in patients where surgery is performed when the patients are young. In one patient, operated upon at age 13, the unifying mechanisms were

796

significantly strengthened some 7 years later. He could, for example, sometimes cross-retrieve with the left hand an item initially identified with the right. He was also able to report verbally the sum, difference or product of two numbers, one flashed to the left and one to the right. One and a half years after surgery, this was impossible. Plasticity mechanisms, such as a reordering of pathways or modification in existing pathways as discussed in Chapter 15, may be involved in this improvement.

When one of the hemispheres is severely damaged at birth, language is always in the intact functioning hemisphere (White, 1961). Effective transfer can occur up to 5 years of age, but the time may extend to as long as 15 years (Obrador, 1964). When transferred, however, speech is defective as are normal functions of the minor hemisphere. The remaining hemisphere apparently has its limits, and it cannot do the jobs normally served by both (McFie, 1961). This certainly indicates in yet another way that hemispheric specialization extends the capabilities of the human brain.

In summary, in split brain man we see that indeed there is a right brain and a left brain. The dominant hemisphere controls speech and writing and calculation. It handles great detail and is the master scholar. It focuses upon detail for which verbal labels are easily attached. Its partner is able to recognize words but cannot decode the meaning of complex sentences. It perceives the whole and is especially talented in dealing with problems which require the visualization of relationships. Its abilities are "holistic" and unitary rather than analytical and fragmentary; they are operational rather than vocal and seem to involve concerted perceptual synthetic insight rather than symbolic or feature by feature sequential reasoning. Thus, the same person will approach a set of problems in different ways like two individuals depending on which hemisphere is in use. The right hemisphere shows more emotion and impulsiveness than its companion, but emotions are not strictly lateralized. Memories and well-practiced motor skills that existed prior to commissurotomy are unchanged by the procedure. Without the corpus callosum, however, memories are difficult to make, and the performance of tasks requiring bilateral skills is slower. We can, thus, see how the corpus callosum is essential in conveying information between the two hemispheres, and how it ties them together and makes a better, more powerful and unified brain.

IV. Toward Unified Behavior

In the previous sections in this chapter, we have seen how various cortical areas are specialized to serve in a vast number of capacities. Even seemingly simple behaviors draw upon many of these capacities. In the course of walking, for example, the brain blends the senses, takes into account the present state of the body—its position and overall state—consults past memories and considers future goals. As we have seen in the course of this text, we understand a great deal about brain mechanism in simple behaviors and about specific aspects of complex behaviors. Certainly we do not as yet, however, understand in detail the interactions between cortical areas in complex behaviors. This is a challenge for the future. We can, though, provide a partial scheme which illustrates the general nature of the transactions as for example in the course of movements.

Figure 18-16 illustrates the general nature of the synthesis in the execution of movement (Allen and Tsukahara, 1974). Association cortex is an important participant in the early phases of evolving movement. In association cortex, the information from various primary sensory cortical areas converges, and it seems that perhaps ideas concentrate there prior to their execution.

Activity from association cortex feeds directly to the motor cortex and as well to the thalamus via the cerebellum and basal ganglia. It appears as if the cerebellum and basal ganglia provide an internal model of actions, a kind of internal substitute for the external world. Motor cortex directs the muscles. Many types of information participate in the programming of movement. Sensory inputs, motivation, behavioral goal, and learned information all play a role. Moreover, many corollary discharges are operating throughout the brain to provide the necessary information in order to provide options and maintain focal action. The cortical areas can converse with each other indirectly or in some cases directly as part of the blend.

The conversation between higher cortical areas is complex indeed. The immense associational pathways (see Chapter 2) and commissural pathways link together cortical areas. Moreover, there are many pathways (often reciprocal) to

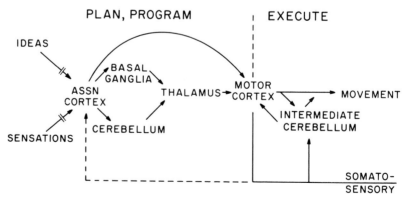

Fig. 18-16. Scheme showing the general pathways in the execution of control of movement. (Modified from Allen and Tsukahara, 1974; Popper and Eccles, 1977.)

thalamic and other areas of the brain. Processing in the cortex is multitiered. It proceeds from primary levels to secondary, tertiary, quarternary and even higher ones. In the visual system, for example, primary visual cortical areas (areas 17, 18, and 19) pass signals directly to parts of the temporal lobe, anterior speech area, prefrontal cortex and limbic system. Thus, at a secondary level of analysis, visual input already has access to speech, memories, emotions and goals, and this is only the beginning. In both the visual and somesthetic system, secondary and tertiary projections are to both frontal and parieto-temporal lobes with cross-linkages. This cascade, the reciprocal connections and higher processing ensure that an appropriate product will result. In its deliberations, the brain uses its resources to act on the present, draw from the past and prepare for the future.

When movement is called for, the motor cortex collects the commands and drives spinal motor neurons which move muscles. The result might be talking, walking or just moving a finger. In turn, the consequences of muscle action are reported back to the brain for approval and revision if necessary. Movements may be exploratory (such as the search for an object in an unknown place) or well-practiced and fairly routine (such as walking). As we have noted in Chapter 11, well-practiced movements appear to draw on central programs which have been built often in the course of a lifetime of experience. These programs appear to be the result of multisynaptic integration. Central programs, though, like all aspects of brain function are subject to revision. Other circuits exist for their control and revision as we mentioned in Chapter 11. The brain takes all into account and produces one unified, coherent product. The product of the nervous system at any instant is indeed focal—we take one action, have one thought, one feeling.

Movement may be stimulus driven or voluntary. Voluntary motion is so common we scarcely think about how remarkable it is. Somehow the brain energizes the neurons appropriate for an action. In man, it has been possible to gain some insight into the processes of voluntary movement by recording potentials from the scalp.

Recall that in Chapter 11 we saw that cortical activity can develop much before an actual movement is expressed. We described an experiment in which monkeys were trained to move a lever in response to visual cues. Neural activity in the motor cortex preceded the actual movement. What happens in the course of voluntary movement? A subject is directed to move his index finger at will; the onset of muscle action is used to trigger a reverse computation of recorded cortical potentials up to 2 seconds preceding the voluntary movement. Cortical potentials are recorded over several trials. About 300 msec prior to the actual movement a potential called the "*readiness potential*" begins to develop in the motor area responsible for movement of the index finger (Kornhuber, 1974). The potential grows until about 50 msec before the muscle response. This is the time required for transmission of impulses from brain to spinal motor neurons to muscle action potentials. The readiness potential reflects the brain's deliberations preceding willed movement. Its slow development appears to be the concentrating of activity. The brain (mind?) gathers activity, draws it to a focus, and when this is large enough it calls forth movement.

Integration proceeds at many levels, and there are phenomena which are well understood, but for which there are no real neural mechanisms. Most research into exploration of the activity of man's brain through the recording of cortical potentials has concentrated on short latency activity which can be related directly to sensory stimuli. Much neural activity, however, follows stimuli at long latency, and many interesting studies have emphasized the types of changes produced by complex events. There are changes as a result of attention, vigilance, habituation, conditioning and even certainty and uncertainty. Those on certainty and uncertainty serve to illustrate some of the remarkable happenings which the brain itself can generate.

In 1963 at a symposium at the convention of the American Psychological Association in Los Angeles, Sutton and co-workers (1965) reported a component of the average evoked potential which appeared, it seemed, only when the sensory stimulus was unanticipated. Tones or lights were delivered as pairs. The first member of the pair served as a cue for the second, which followed after a random interval of 3–5 seconds. In most trials the two stimuli were matched; they were of one modality, tone → tone or light → light. In other trials, the cuing stimulus was followed by an unmatched stimulus—tone → light or light → tone. During the interval between cuing and the test stimulus the subject stated his guess as to the sensory modality of the next stimulus. Evoked potentials were recorded from the scalp.

Figure 18-17 shows the results. The solid tracing is the average evoked response to sound stimuli when the subject was certain it would occur. The dashed tracing is the response to a sound stimulus when the subject was uncertain of its occurrence. There was a dramatic difference in the potentials. The most dramatic difference was in a large positive deflection whose latency came at about 300 msec. This component has come to be called the P-300 wave, and much research has been devoted toward understanding it.

The P-300 wave is a signal generated by the brain itself; it is endogenous activity (Donchin, 1979). Since the sound was the same, the difference in the P-300 potential cannot be due to the sound itself. P-300 is largest in parietal areas and smallest in frontal areas. Subjects must be paying attention to the stimulus in order for it to arise, but the potential is not simply related to attention. P-300 appears to be a function of the subjective probability that individuals assign to events. The more unexpected the stimulus, the more likely it is to elicit P-300. In a sense, P-300 is a surprise potential. The brain is prepared for anything, and it takes special note when its expectations are unfulfilled.

800

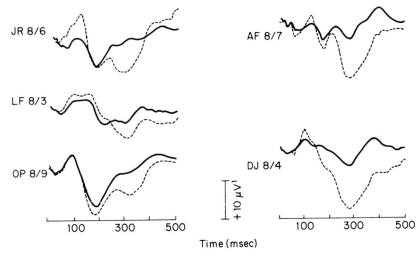

Fig. 18-17. Average wave forms for potentials recorded for certain (solid line) versus uncertain (dashed line) sounds. (From Sutton *et al.*, 1965. Copyright by the American Association for the Advancement of Science.)

Out of the totality of all that the nervous system does emerges total unity, the realization and practice of self. We have a sophisticated consciousness which is perhaps the ultimate mystery of neuroscience.

V. Consciousness

What is meant by consciousness? By consciousness we mean awareness, the kind of experience that is lost when one faints, or is in dreamless sleep, or sinks into a coma. Consciousness will disappear because of a blow on the head, deep anesthesia, or anoxia. Conscious events include all our waking subjective experiences, from a simple pin prick, for example, to an empathy for others' suffering. Consciousness is the inner experience of how things strike us and how we feel about things. Only recently has it been possible to probe into the mysteries of consciousness experimentally.

Let us begin by considering, for the sake of argument, an illustrative example which outlines the nature of the problem in comprehending consciousness and which will allow us to define the two main schools of thought. Consider a young child who is in the process of formulating the beginnings of speech. The child may babble along trying various sounds including "da." This sounds good, he repeats it, and his daddy gets excited. At first the child does not understand but he finds this gets attention and so he repeats the syllable da, da, da. . . . One day when father comes home the child looks up at his father, smiles and says "Dada" (only 2 syllables), consciously realizing the relation between the word and its meaning.

One line of reasoning would postulate that the child learned a complex set of reflexes, and in this way the behavior came about from stimulus induced associations. The child learned in the same way, in principle, as did Pavlov's dogs, by reflexes, (associating events) except the behavior is much more complex. According to this thesis, mind or consciousness is a complex construction emerging as a property of brain mechanisms. Mind is not independent of brain: it is simply a high-order integrative process due to the brain's neural activity. All structural and functional connections integrate to give motor performance. From the component parts and their operation, a complete explanation of behavior including language and consciousness presumably follows. This is the *materialistic position* strongly subscribed to by many. It is the basic assumption of most traditional behaviorist schools of thought and an unwritten law of most neuroscientists. It is highly empirical and has the powerful and certainly uncontested advantage that experiments designed in this framework can be tested with conventional methods. Stimuli are controlled by the experimenter, and the response is measured. Subjective judgment has no place in this approach; it is in fact "blanked out" so far as possible.

On the other hand, the conscious mind can be considered as a causal determinant of higher-level behavior, as a separate entity which is not merely formed by the brain, but which in fact directs the brain. In the example, conscious mind develops a theory and tries it out. Mind activity imposes itself on the process so that it is a causal factor in the behavior. In this view, brain is owned by the self rather than self by the brain. Reflex arcs exist and are probably adequate for automatic and subconscious movements. They will not, however, account for the higher levels of conscious performance of the human brain. Those who subscribe to such a position are considered *dualists*: they believe in a separate, but interacting conscious mind and brain.

At present, there is really no unambiguous way to decide between these two positions or identify a generally accepted intermediate position. On purely scientific grounds, neither position can disprove the other. There are simply not enough facts to allow a decision. The types of neurobiological evidence brought to the firing line, however, are extremely interesting and at the very least shed great light on the complex processing capacities possessed by the human brain and the dilemmas they present. Either brain action explains the mind, or we must deal with two elements, "the self and its brain" (Popper and Eccles, 1977).

A. Brain without Consciousness

Much of the key information currently available about consciousness comes from patients with various disorders. Some disorders result in the dissociation of mental processes and provide revelations into the workings of the mind. A mild form of epilepsy called petit mal is one such example. Epilepsy causes explosive runaway patterns of cell activity called seizures. In *petit mal epilepsy*, the seizure is localized to particular brain areas. In some patients it converts the patient into, as Penfield said "a mindless automaton."

> One patient, whom I shall call A., was a serious student of the piano and subject to automatisms of the type called *petit mal*. He was apt to make a slight interruption in his practicing, which his mother recognized as the beginning of an "absence." Then he would continue to play for a time with considerable dexterity. Patient B. was subject to epileptic automatism that began with discharge in the temporal lobe. Sometimes the attack came on him while walking home from work. He would continue to walk and to thread his way through busy streets on his way home. He might realize later that he had had an attack because there was a blank in his memory for a part of the journey, as from Avenue X to Street Y. If Patient C. was driving a car, he would continue to drive, although he might discover later that he had driven through one or more red lights.
>
> In general, if new decisions are to be made, the automaton cannot make them. In such a circumstance, he may become completely unreasonable and uncontrollable and even dangerous (Penfield, 1975, pp. 39–40).

We have all experienced to some degree the *automaton syndrome*. For example, when we get into a car and take a well-practiced route, the "automaton" delivers us to our destination. However, we can change the destination and deviate our course by an act of intention or mind. We would interpret automaton behavior as an extraordinary display of central programming where particular prerecorded behaviors which are not subject to editing or change are played out. (We have described less elaborate examples of central programming in Chapter 11 on motor systems, as for example in fictive scratching.) Whatever the interpretation, these findings illustrate the immense computerlike qualities of the brain, as it becomes divorced from conscious qualities.

Studies on the localization of such seizures point toward an origin in the brain stem. Thus it appears that seizures in this area will knock out conscious activity but maintain the computerlike qualities of the brain, which in this case runs the central programs. Normally sensory input will have access to motor programs and change them appropriately. In petit mal patients, this action is blocked, and so there is a play out of existing programs without change or awareness.

B. Self or Selves?

Consciousness is generally considered to be a synonym for the self. In the split brain patients, the question has arisen as to whether consciousness has been divided as a result of the operation. This is an important issue because if mind is divided along with brain it follows that it is probably of the substance of brain. As described above (see Section III, D), these patients appear to have some type of "co-consciousness." Both hemispheres have an awareness of the self, although it is more refined in the dominant hemisphere. Initially, this would seem to argue that both hemispheres have their own separate consciousness, but this destroys the doctrine of unity of self. However, as Sperry (1977) has pointed out, it may be that consciousness is normally single and unified, but it is divided when the brain is divided. On the other hand, Popper and Eccles (1977) argue that consciousness resides only in the dominant hemisphere along with language. Their argument is interesting and illustrates the nature of the issue.

> A gedanken experiment reveals the fundamental difference between the responses of the dominant and minor hemispheres. After commissurotomy with left hemisphere dominance the conscious subject has voluntary control of the right forearm and hand, but not of the left, yet the left forearm and hand can carry out skilled and apparently purposive movements. In our gedanken experiment the left hand inadvertently grabs a gun, fires it and kills a man. Is this murder or manslaughter and by whom? If not, why not? But no such questions can be asked if the right hand does the shooting and killing. The fundamental difference between the dominant and minor hemispheres stands revealed on legal grounds. Commissurotomy has split the bihemispheric brain into a dominant hemisphere that is exclusively in liaison with the self-conscious mind and controlled by it and a minor hemisphere that carries out many of the performances previously carried out by the intact brain, but it is not under control by the self-conscious mind. It may be in liaison with a mind, but this is quite different from the self-conscious mind of the dominant hemisphere—so different that a grave risk of confusion results from the common use of the words "mind" and "consciousness" for both entities (Popper and Eccles, 1977, p. 329).

A most startling revelation is that in some cases consciousness actually may shift from one hemisphere to the other. Occasionally, a split brain patient may become so absorbed in a left hemisphere task that the right hemisphere functions become temporarily depressed so that, "one questions whether consciousness may not have shifted entirely to the working hemisphere" (Sperry, 1977). This shift occurs in either direction. However, it is most frequently toward the left or dominant hemisphere.

It is clear that each hemisphere can operate and independently solve problems and maintain to a degree its own conscious awareness. However, cognitive processing is greatly facilitated when the right and left tasks involve a common central background of postural and mental states. Thus the left and right hemispheres are reinforcing in unity. This would tend to argue that there is some commonality or unity even in split brain patients. Conscious awareness tends to be concerned with the focal aspects of cerebral function, and dividing the brain may divide its computerlike capacities. It may be that mind can only partially express itself. That is, when the computer (brain) is uncoupled only part of it can be programmed, so one gets the impression that only half the programmer (conscious mind) exists. However, the programmer shows himself subtly in reinforcing situations.

There is also a form of double awareness in some of the patients in which electrical stimulation to parts of the cortex creates "flashback." The patient is still aware of what is going on in the operating room, yet at the same time he has a "flashback" experience. For example, a young South African patient reported his astonishment to find that "he was laughing with his cousins on a farm in South Africa while he was fully conscious of his presence in the operating room in Montreal" (Penfield, 1975, p. 55).

It is clear that the patient had a conscious experience and yet still knew where he was. This shows that self is not simply composed of a stream of consciousness or experiences (Popper and Eccles, 1977). Moreover if, as is often argued, the brain is about the business of creating the mind by its own action, the result would be mental confusion. The past and the present would be mixed in the ongoing stream of consciousness (Penfield, 1975).

Consciousness in some mysterious way provides direct accurate and personal knowledge of the location of the body. Try holding your arm out and closing your eyes for example. The position of the arm is clearly felt because joint and muscle receptors convey the necessary percepts to mind. Indeed, such conscious information is necessary in order to act rationally. As we have seen, the parietal cortex is in some way necessary for knowing body position, but just how it is involved is unclear. It is particularly curious and significant that in the many attempts and trials to elicit experiences from patients there is no valid evidence that either epileptic discharge or electrical stimulation can activate the mind to alter decisions or bring about an awareness of self for that particular situation (Penfield, 1975). Of course, such negative evidence does not mean that such is not possible. Nonetheless, this argues that these properties are diffuse or perhaps not accessible to electrical activation.

C.   Neural Interactions with Conscious Experience

What are the characteristics of electrical activity that enable it to achieve liaison with conscious experience? Perhaps the simplest form of a conscious experience is simply feeling a skin stimulus, a touch, for example. A conscious sensation in the hand or forearm is also produced by stimulating the appropriate area of the somatosensory cortex. A variety of somatosensory qualities, like touch, pressure, motion, warmth, cold, and of course the tingling qualities of an electric shock (paresthesia), can be experienced. Particular qualities are necessary in order that a cortical stimulus will elicit a conscious experience. Repetitive stimulation (20 to 120 pulses/second) is the most effective stimulus and a minimum period of time (about 500 msec) is required (Fig. 18-18). The time is necessary not simply to elicit neural activity because the neural activity begins quickly, but if the stimulus is cut off prior to the required period the subject does not report feeling anything. Thus, there is a specific temporal requirement in order for a stimulus to enter consciousness. This effect of cortical stimulation contrasts to a skin stimulus, where a single stimulus is quite adequate to elicit feeling. For a skin stimulus as well, however, the long duration of activity is necessary because cortical stimulation will mask the perception of a skin stimulus occurring some 300 msec earlier. The time may be necessary to build up the necessary neural patterns for liaison with consciousness.

A sure sign of uncharted territory is the discovery of the completely unexpected. A cortical stimulus was begun prior to a skin stimulus and with such timing that the end of the cortical stimulus train occurred between the primary evoked response and the late potential of the skin stimulus (Fig. 18-19). One would expect that the conscious experience of the cortical stimulus would precede that of the skin stimulus in the experiment. Not so! The skin stimulus is perceived to have occurred prior to the cortical stimulus. How could this be? Libet (1973, 1978; Libet *et al.*, 1979) suggested that the conscious experience of the skin potential is referred back (*antedated*) to its primary evoked response. The late events after the primary evoked response somehow cause perception to be

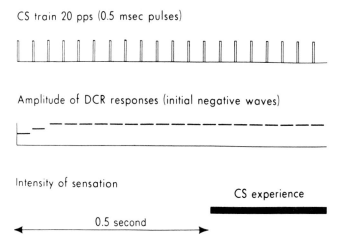

Fig. 18-18. Relationship between a cortical stimulus train (CS) of pulses at liminal (barely perceptible) intensity applied to the cortex and the amplitudes of direct cortical responses (DCR) recorded nearby. The bottom line indicates that no conscious sensory experience is evoked until about 0.5 second has elapsed. (From Libet, 1966.)

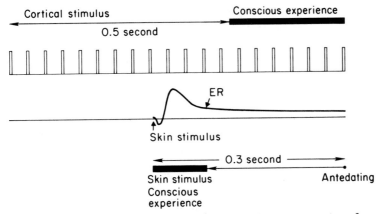

Cortical stimulus

Conscious experience

0.5 second

ER

Skin stimulus

0.3 second

Skin stimulus
Conscious
experience

Antedating

Fig. 18-19. Experimental paradigm used to show antedating properties of a conscious experience. A cortical stimulus requires 0.5 second before it is consciously experienced. A skin stimulus (SS) apparently also requires later evoked responses (ER) in order to be consciously experienced. However, if a skin stimulus is applied just after a cortical stimulus, the skin stimulus is actually felt earlier. The conscious sensation of the skin stimulus is referred back in time.

back-dated. It was suggested that the cortical stimulus is not antedated because it has no primary evoked response.

There are a number of significant conclusions and implications that follow from the experiment described above. It follows that subjective experiences may be temporally dissociated from neural activity. Antedating mechanisms may explain why sometimes you can "act before you know it" in sports, verbal repartee, and other such happenings. The time required for an experience to enter consciousness may serve as a filter to screen out brief inconsequential happenings.

At present there is no real resolution as to the relationship between consciousness and brain. Each position is fraught with uncertainties, and upholding either requires an act of faith. There are no rigorous mechanisms which can stand up against experimental scrutiny. Subjective experiences are difficult to work with by existing scientific methodology. Scientific methodology and approaches where subjective judgments are blanked out will only further support the deterministic position. In other words, an experiment designed to give associative responses may only continue to reveal such relationships. It is necessary to introduce the subjective. How can one obtain such a report from an animal? Nonetheless, there is progress being made, and we can be optimistic more will follow. It is appealing to consider that if the ordering and the integration of neural activity were high enough, consciousness would naturally fall out from existing principles. However, the fact is it has not. Moreover, it is inappropriate to insist that mind and consciousness must derive from existing principles, as it is obvious that all principles are not known. Only a few years ago, for example, we were unprepared to deal with acupuncture. Are there other forms of energy operative in the brain which can act on the assemblies of neural activity? Perhaps there is some type of action whereby decisions are the targets of a force orchestrated by the mind which directs the programming of the various computer-like mechanisms embodied in neural assemblies. It may be as Sherrington concluded: "That our being should consist of two fundamental elements offers, I suppose, no greater inherent improbability than that it should rest on one only" (Sherrington, 1947, p. xx).

Man has always sought to understand himself and no doubt always will. Consciousness, though, is very complex, and like other problems in the neurosciences answers will come at various levels of resolution. The basic issues were posed long ago—brain?, brain, mind? brain, mind, spirit? Answers sometimes do little more than raise other questions. We have as yet only scratched the surface, and unfortunately we have only partial answers. Yet it is now possible to obtain more solid clues than ever before, and this hastens the search.

We could make the mistake of looking too close and never find an entity as pervasive as conscious mind. As one writer said, "the meaning of the message will never be found in the chemistry of the ink" (Stuler, 1977). Science is often equated with reductionism and within this context we may inappropriately erase the pluralistic richness which grows out of subjective experience. To us, our inner feelings are just as real as those directly set by external stimuli which are so easily measured. The challenge of the future is to find an appropriate road into the exploration of the inner world. From where do we derive our sense of dignity, our sense of beauty or morality, our religion, our feelings and compassion for others? We look to the qualities of the conscious mind in order to understand the quality of man. The outcome of this great debate between materialists and dualists is one of great proportions both for individuals seeking to understand themselves more fully and for society in directing the course of the future.

VI. Conclusion

In the cerebral cortex we see the highest level of synthetic analysis. It is there that our view of the world is analyzed, blended with our impressions from within, and the program written for playing out and action. The result of all integration is a knowledge of things (stimuli) in our surroundings which we all identify and describe in similar ways through language, but at the same time ours is an intensely personal view. Mountcastle vividly described the transactions and accomplishments of the brain.

Each of us lives within the universe—the prison—of his own brain. Projecting from it are millions of fragile sensory nerve fibres, in groups uniquely adapted to sample the energetic states of the world about us: heat, light, force, and chemical compositions. That is all we ever know of it directly: all else is logical interference.

Sensory stimuli reaching us are transduced at peripheral nerve endings, and neural replicas of them dispatched brainward, to the great gray mantle of the cerebral cortex. We use them to form dynamic and continually updated neural maps of the external world, and of our place and orientation, and of events, within it. At the level of sensation, your images and my images are virtually the same, and readily identified one to another by verbal description, or common reaction.

Beyond that, each image is conjoined with genetic and stored experiential information that makes each of us uniquely private. From that complex integral each of us constructs at a higher level of perceptual experience his own, very personal, view from within (Mountcastle, 1975. Copyright by Johns Hopkins Univ. Press.).

The visual, auditory and somatosensory cortices process primary sensory stimuli as we have described in earlier chapters. They extract features and make more and more general neural images on the nature of the external world. The motor cortex orchestrates the neuronal patterns which drive spinal motor neurons to move muscles. In the parietal cortex, a bigger and more meaningful self is in the making. The parietal cortex knows about our inner world and matches that with the immediate surround. It oversees our visual attention, for example. The frontal lobe, as we can infer by man's transformation upon its loss, is entrusted with overseeing goals, judgment, planning or we might say seeing to the "stuff" that makes man what he is. Loss of the frontal or parietal lobes does not impair intellectual function or memory. The temporal lobe works in collaboration with other lobes in overseeing higher function. It is important in the emotional coloration of experience. When it is destroyed emotional, hallucinatory and memory disturbances follow. It is involved in "tape and store" as illustrated by the findings that gentle electrical stimulation creates a flashback experience. Association cortex—so-called because many modes and functions converge there—is the center for speech. Loss of the speech cortex or electrical stimulation of it causes aphasia. Speech functions are strongly lateralized and exist in the dominant hemisphere.

In general, the dominant hemisphere is highly verbal and prefers to respond to details to which words are easily attached. It is also very effective in performing mathematics. The minor hemisphere is more concerned with the big picture and has great synthetic insight. It specializes in space and general feature recognition. When interconnected by the corpus callosum the two hemispheres work in harmony: they make a powerful and effective team giving unity to brain and extending its functional capacities.

Recovery from cortical damage is usually most effectively achieved when it is

VI. CONCLUSION   809 time. Once speech centers develop and other areas mature, recovery can occur but not as readily.

Consciousness gives us awareness of self, a greater unity, an identity. Our brain does not tell us the mechanism of its actions. Instead it informs us it is "I" standing, thinking, doing. We feel a subjective and very personal view from within. Consciousness may grow as an emergent property of neuronal activity, or perhaps it is more mysterious arising from where we know not and somehow controlling brain—its computer. The perception of a simple conscious experience, such as a skin sensation, requires a long-duration stimulus as if consciousness builds up. Mind or brain can play with time and perform antedating functions. At present little is known about consciousness, and there is a great deal of lively debate as is so often the case at the frontiers of knowledge. The exploration of the inner world and consciousness is one of the greatest challenges of the future.

In the course of this text, we have gone from neuron to brain to behavior, and with a skip or perhaps a big jump to consciousness. We have explored the action at the neuronal membrane. Channels flicker, opening and closing, permitting ions to generate tiny electrical currents and provide intra- and in some cases interneural communication. At synapses, that "mode of nexus" between neuron and neuron, transmitters carry the message. Synapses are plastic. They record the past and prepare for the future by modifying their transfer functions across well-beaten paths or by growing new pathways for action. Networks and then whole systems are alive with scintillating spatiotemporal patterns of activity, reading and creating neural maps of the external and internal world. Behavior, language and thought flow from the brain's ceaseless activity. The accomplishments are focal, precise and flexible and are designed for each individual. From individual to individual, generation to generation, the nervous system delivers a universe of variation and possibility. The study of behavioral neuroscience holds many mysteries yet untold. It is a young field and an exciting one, which thrives on the many approaches embodied in it. The story is just beginning, and there is great promise and expectation for the future.

Key Terms

Agnosias: A loss of knowledge or awareness of the significance of things.

Amorphosynthesis: A failure to put the body together.

Antedating mechanism: Processes whereby the conscious experience of a stimulus or event precedes its evoked response; the perception is referred back in time.

Association cortex: An area of cortex that surrounds and includes parts of primary and secondary sensory and motor areas; it relates events, perceptual matters, memories, emotions, and it synthesizes aspects of speech.

"Automaton" syndrome: A state in which a person continues to execute a behavior without being aware of it; the syndrome may be triggered by a local seizure.

Commissurotomy: An operation in which the corpus callosum (the fiber tract joining the two cerebral hemispheres) is severed.

Dualistic position: In consciousness, the position that the conscious mind and the brain are separate but interacting entities.

Epilepsy: A brain disorder characterized by convulsive seizures. In *petit mal* epilepsy the seizure is localized to particular brain areas.

Frontal lobe: A lobe of the cerebral cortex located above the lateral sulcus and anterior to the central sulcus; it appears to be critically involved in an individual's judgment and planning ability; stable, purposeful behavior; and other attributes necessary for normal human behavior.

Hemispheric dominance: One cerebral hemisphere is dominant over the other; the dominant one controls speech, writing and calculation.

Hologram: A three-dimensional image produced by interacting light beams.

Materialistic position: In consciousness, the position that the conscious mind is a directly emergent property of the brain as opposed to a separate entity.

Parietal lobe: A lobe of the cerebral cortex located posterior to the central sulcus and anterior to the occipital lobe; it maps the body, blends the senses, and performs a matching function between external objects and goal, or drive, states.

P-300 wave: A potential recorded in humans which occurs about 300 msec after a situation where the stimulus is unexpected.

Readiness potential: A potential which develops in the motor area controlling muscles appropriate to an anticipated, willed movement; the potential is seen about 300 msec prior to the movement.

Temporal lobe: A lobe of the cerebral cortex located ventral to the lateral sulcus; it is thumblike in shape. It contains part of the auditory cortex and is involved in nonverbal, visual memory; stimulation of it produces "flashback," a mental replay of past experiences.

General References

Mountcastle, V. B. (1975). The view from within: Pathways to the study of perception. *Johns Hopkins Med. J.* **136,** 109–131.

Penfield, W. (1975). "The Mystery of the Mind." Princeton Univ. Press, Princeton, New Jersey.

Popper, E. R., and Eccles, J. C. (1977). "The Self and Its Brain." Springer-Verlag, Berlin and New York.

Sperry, R. W. (1974). Lateral specialization in the surgically separated hemisphere. *In* "The Neurosciences: Third Study Program" (F. O. Schmitt and F. G. Worden, eds.), pp. 5–19. MIT Press, Cambridge, Massachusetts.

References

Allen, G. I., and Tsukahara, N. (1974). Cerebrocerebellar communication systems. *Physiol. Rev.* **54**, 987–997.

Collins, R. L. (1969). On the inheritance of handedness. II. Selection for sinistrality in mice. *J. Hered.* **60**, 117–119.

Donchin, E. (1979). Event-related brain potentials: A tool in the study of human information processing. *In* "Evoked Potentials in Behavior" (H. Begleiter, ed.), pp. 13–75. Plenum, New York).

Franco, L., and Sperry, R. W. (1977). Hemispheric lateralization for cognitive processing of geometry. *Neuropsychologia* **15**, 107–114.

Geschwind, N., and Levitsky, W. (1968). Human brain: Left-right asymmetries in temporal speech region. *Science* **161**, 186–187.

Kimura, D. (1963). Right temporal lobe damage. *Arch. Neurol. (Paris)* **8**, 264–271.

Kornhuber, H. H. (1974). Cerebral cortex, cerebellum and basal ganglia: An introduction to their motor functions. *In* "The Neurosciences: Third Study Program" (F. O. Schmitt and F. G. Worden, eds.), pp. 267–280. MIT Press, Cambridge, Massachusetts.

Levy, J., and Nagylaki, T. (1972). A model for the genetics of handedness. *Genetics* **72**, 117–128.

Levy, J., Trevarthen, C., and Sperry, R. W. (1972). Perception of bilateral chimeric figures following hemispheric deconnexion. *Brain* **95**, 61–78.

Libet, B. (1966). Brain stimulation and the threshold of conscious experience. *In* "Brain and Conscious Experience" (J. C. Eccles, ed.), pp. 165–181. Springer-Verlag, Berlin and New York.

Libet, B. (1973). Electrical stimulation of cortex in human subjects, and conscious memory aspects. *In* "Handbook of Sensory Physiology" (A. Iggo, ed.), Vol. 2, pp. 743–790. Springer-Verlag, Berlin and New York.

Libet, B. (1978). Neuronal vs. subjective timing for a conscious sensory experience. *In* "Cerebral Correlates of Conscious Experience" (P. A. Buser and A. Rougeul-Buser, eds.), pp. 69–82. Elsevier, Amsterdam.

Libet, B., Wright, E. W., Feinstein, B., and Pearl, D. K. (1979). Subjective referral of the timing for a conscious sensory experience. *Brain* **102**, 191–222.

McFie, J. (1961). The effects of hemispherectomy on intellectual functioning in cases of infantile hemiplegia. *J. Neurol., Neurosurg. Psychiatry* **214**, 240–249.

Milner, B. (1967). Brain mechanisms suggested by studies of temporal lobes. *In* "Princeton Conference on Brain Mechanisms Underlying Speech and Language" (E. H. Millikan and F. L. Darley, eds.), pp. 122–145. Grune & Stratton, New York.

Mountcastle, V. B. (1975). The view from within: Pathways to the study of perception. *Johns Hopkins Med. J.* **136**, 109–131.

Mountcastle, V. B. (1976). The world around us: Neural command functions for selective attention. *Neurosci. Res. Program, Bull.* **14**, Suppl., 1–47.

Mountcastle, V. B., Lynch, J. C., Georgopolous, A., Sakata, H., and Acuna, C. (1975). Posterior parietal association cortex of the monkey: Command functions for operations within extrapersonal space. *J. Neurophysiol.* **38**, 871–908.

Obrador, S. (1964). Nervous integration after hemispherectomy in man. *In* "Cerebral Localization and Organization" (G. Schattenbrand and C. Woolsey, eds.), pp. 133–154. Univ. of Wisconsin Press, Madison.

Penfield, W. (1975). "The Mystery of the Mind." Princeton Univ. Press, Princeton, New Jersey.

Penfield, W., and Roberts, L., (1959), "Speech and Brain—Mechanisms." Princeton Univ. Press, Princeton, New Jersey.

Popper, K. R., and Eccles, J. C. (1977). "The Self and Its Brain." Springer-Verlag, Berlin and New York.

Shankweiler, D. P. (1966). Effects of temporal-lobe damage on perception of dichotically presented melodies. *J. Comp. Physiol. Psychol.* **62**, 115–119.

Sherrington, C. S. (1947). Foreward to a new edition of "The Integrative Action of the Nervous System" (originally published in 1906). Cambridge Univ. Press, London and New York.

Sperry, R. W. (1968). Mental unity following surgical disconnection of the cerebral hemispheres. *Harvey Lect.* **62**, 293–323.

Sperry, R. W. (1974). Lateral specialization in the surgically separated hemisphere. *In* "The Neurosciences: Third Study Program" (F. O. Schmitt and F. G. Worden, eds.), pp. 5–19. MIT Press, Cambridge, Massachusetts.

Sperry, R. W. (1977). Forebrain commissurotomy and conscious awareness. *J. Med. Philos.* **2**, 101–126.

Stuler, H. (1977). Consciousness from neurons: Where, how, why and so what? *In* "Brain Information Service," Conf. Rep. No. 45, pp. 25–39. BRI Publications Office, University of California, Los Angeles.

Sutton, S., Braren, M., Zubin, J., and John, E. R. (1965). Evoked-potential correlates of stimulus uncertainty. *Science* **150**, 1187–1188.

White, H. H. (1961). Cerebral hemispherectomy in the treatment of infantile hemiphagia. Review of the literature and report of two cases. *Confin. Neurol. Basel* **21**, 1–50.

Zaidel, E. (1975). A technique for presenting lateralized visual input with prolonged exposure. *Vision Res.* **15**, 283–289.

Zaidel, E. (1976). Auditory vocabulary of the right hemisphere following brain bisection or hemidecortication. *Cortex* **12**, 191–211.

Zaidel, E., and Sperry, R. W. (1974). Memory impairment after commissurotomy in man. *Brain* **97**, 263–272.

Zaidel, E., and Sperry, R. W. (1977). Some long-term motor effects of cerebral commissurotomy in man. *Neuropsychologia* **15**, 193–204.

Index

function of, 352
temporal lobe and, 782
Auditory pathway, 58
Auditory space, perception of, 372–377
Auditory system, 27–29, 350–352
alterations of hearing from lesions of, 378–380
brain stem, 384–386
cochlear receptor, 382–384
cortex, 386
VIII nerve fibers, 384
middle ear, 380–381
basic organization of, 352–353
channeling of sound to eardrum and, 355–356
coding for sound frequency and intensity, 362–366
efferent control, 366–367
impedance matching by ossicular system, 356–357
nature of sound and, 354–355
operation of cochlea, 357–360
receptor processes and, 355
transduction from mechanical to electrical signals, 361–362
transmission of sound to cochlea and, 356
dissemination of information in, 29
hearing disorders and, 377–378
modulation in, 30–31
ototoxic drugs, 382, 396
perception of auditory space and, 372–377
perception of sounds and, 367–371
team operations in processing, 29
tonotopic organization of, 29–30
transduction in, 35–36
Automatic behavior syndrome, 632
clinical case, 621–622
Automaton syndrome, consciousness and, 803, 811
Autonomic nervous system (ANS), 53, 58
control functions of, 523–528
functions of, 516–518
neurotransmitters and, 522–523
organization of, 518–522
parasympathetic, 518, 519, 520, 561
sympathetic, 518, 520, 562
Autosomes, 691, 723
Aversion
self-stimulation and, 598–599
taste, 582–583
Avoidance conditioning
brain stimulation and memory and, 317–318
RNA synthesis and, 311
unit studies of, 307

Axon(s), 26, 58, 65, 84–87
of basket cells, 70
boutons en passage (en passant), 68, 671
collaterals of, 65
conduction velocity of, 135–136
electronic conduction in, 122–123
of ganglion cells, 410–411, 420–421
generation of action potential and, 126–134
neurons without, 223
post-ganglionic
parasympathetic, 520–521, 522
sympathetic, 520, 522
propagation of action potential and, 134–137
recovery of ion gradients in, 137, 141
regeneration of, 648, 676–678, 683
of squid, as model system, 256
Axonal outgrowth, of Purkinje cells, 647–648
Axon extension, climbing fibers and, 649–650, 683
Axon hillock, 65, 104, 249
action potentials and, 219–220
Axon sprouting, following damage, 666, 667, 683
Axon trailing, granule cells and, 651, 683
Axoplasm, 85
resistance of, 134
Axoplasmic flow, 98–99, 104
speed of, 99–100

B

Bait shyness, 582, 602
Ballistic movements, 474, 509
Barbiturates, abuse of, 747, 766
Baroreceptors, 525, 560
Basal ganglia, 24, 42, 44, 58
in motor control, 494–496, 798
Basilar membrane, 357, 394
masking and, 371
transduction to electrical signals and, 361–362
Basket cells, 70, 104, 683
of cerebellum, 641, 642–643
differentiation of, 651
synaptogenesis by, 652
Bat, sleeping time of, 614
Bees, hygienic behavior, genetic control of, 690–691, 724
Behavior
consummatory, steering of, 597–598
environmental influences on development of, 711–717
sex-related, genetic and hormonal influences on, 700–708
single gene influences on, 690–692

Homeostasis
    hypothalamus and, 45
    self-stimulation and, 598–599
    stimulation-induced feeding and, 595
Homeostatic behavior, feeding and, 576, 603
Homeostatic hedonism, 600
Horizontal cells, 419, 455
    lateral inhibition and, 420
Hormones, 531–534, 561, *see also* Neuroendo-
        crine system; specific names
    action on brain, 543–547
    adrenal, memory storage and, 327–329
    enzyme induction and, 197
    episodic secretion of, 542–543
    functions of, 529, 535–536, 539
    gonadal, 535–536, 539
    influence on local circuits, 224
    inhibiting, 541
    negative feedback effect of, 540–541
    pituitary, memory storage and, 327–329
    releasing, 539, 541
    sources of, 530, 535
    synthetic, during menopause, 548–549
    types of, 529–530
Horseradish peroxidase (HRP), in axoplasmic
        flow, 100
Hungers, specific, 581–583
Huntington's chorea, GABA-nergic activity in,
        236, 249
γ-Hydroxybutyrate, sleep and, 620
6-Hydroxydopamine, 228, 249, 604
    feeding and, 591, 592, 593
    norepinephrine neurons and, 737
5-Hydroxyindoleacetate, depression and, 742
5-Hydroxytryptophan, sleep and, 619
Hypercolumns, 429, 432, 455
Hypercomplex cells, of visual cortex, 430, 432,
        455
Hyperphagia, 579, 603
    hypothalamic, 589
Hyperpolarization, 122, 147
    inhibition and, 218
    of rods, 415
Hypersomniacs, 620, 632
Hypertonic, 569, 603
Hypoglossal nerve, birdsong and, 720
Hypothalamus, 21, 45, 47
    autonomic functions of, 520
        set point determination, 526–527
        thermoregulatory, 524
    circadian rhythms and, 627
    feeding and, 588, 592–593, 595
    neurochemicals and, 590–592

    satiety, 587, 589–590
        food preferences and, 583
        glucose sensitivity of, 224
        hormonal action on, 543–544, 546
        neurons, accumulation of estrogen by, 708,
            710
Hypotonic, 603
Hypovolemia, 572, 603
Hypoxanthine-guanine phosphoribosyl-
        transferase, deficiency of, 692

I

Illusions, perception of, 439–441
Imipramine, 767
    catecholamine and, 185
    depression and, 739
    serotonin and, 742
Immunohistochemistry, 236, 249
    mapping of cholinergic pathways by, 234
Impedence matching, by ossicular system, 356–
        357, 395
Implants, axonal regeneration and, 676–677
Imprinting, development and, 715, 724
Inactivation mechanism, 167–168
Inbred strains, genetic research and, 693–694, 724
Incus, 356
Induction, nervous system development and,
        640, 659, 684
Inferior colliculus, 27, 29
Information
    needed for movement, 798
    storage, temporal lobe and, 783
Inhibition
    centrally programmed, in locomotion, 485–487
    end product, 188
    lateral, horizontal cells and, 419, 455
    in neuronal integration, 218–221
    permeability and, 165–167
    postsynaptic, habituation and, 271
    presynaptic, habituation and, 271
    reactive, *see* Habituation
Injury, response to, 6
Innervation, degree of, 11
Insects, circadian oscillations in, 624–626
Insomnia, 620, 632
Insulin, 603
    feeding and, 587
    self-stimulation and, 598
Intensity
    of sound, 355
        coding for, 362–365
        presbycusis and, 382

Neuronal signaling, 111–113
Neuroplasm, 97
Neurotransmitters
  in autonomic nervous system, 522–523
  feeding and, 591–592
Neurotransmitter systems, organization in CNS
  distribution of cholinergic neurons, 233–235
  distribution of dopamine pathways, 229–231
  distribution of glycine and GABA neurons, 235–236
  distribution of norepinephrine pathways, 226–228
  distribution of serotonergic pathways, 231–233
  enkephalins and endorphins, 238–243
  glutamate, 236–238
Neurulation, brain development and, 644, 684
Nictitating membrane response, conditioning of, 286–287, 291
Nigrostriatal pathway, 229–231
Nissl substance, 80, 105
Node(s), saltatory conduction and, 136, 148
Node of Ranvier, 86
Norepinephrine, 186, 203
  affective disorders and, 740
  control of releasing hormones by, 541
  distribution of pathways, 226–228
  feeding and, 590–591, 592
  memory storage and, 329–332
  receptor plasticity and, 198
  responses to morphine and, 756–757, 758
  structure of, 736
  synthesis of, 188
  training and, 314
Norepinephrine reward pathways, schizophrenia and, 737, 767
Nucleus(i), 26, 60, 105
  cochlear, 27
  deep auditory, 27, 29
  of hypothalamic cells, estrogen binding by, 710
  of neurons, 78–79
Nutrition, cerebellar development and, 665–666

O

Obesity, 590
  dietary, 583
Occipital lobe, 20
Octopus, life span of, 680
Ocular dominance, depth perception and, 439, 456
Ocular dominance columns, 428–429

early experience and development of, 442–447
Oculomotor system, 472, 474, 510
  saccadic eye movements and, 472
  smooth pursuit tracking and, 473
  vestibulo-ocular reflex and, 473
Odors, 389–390, *see also* Olfactory system
  stereochemical theory of, 390, 394
OFF-center
  of ganglion cells, 419–420, 456
  of lateral geniculate nucleus, 422
Ohm's law, 115, 148
Olfactory bulb, 391–392
Olfactory system, 389–392
Oligodendrocytes, 86
Olivocochlear fibers, 366
  function of, 366–367
ON-center
  of ganglion cells, 418–420, 456
  of lateral geniculate nucleus, 422
Open-loop control, 477, 510
Opiates
  antagonists, 239
  in brain, 238
  memory storage and, 329
Opium, 553
Opium alkaloids, tetrahydropapaveroline and, 762
Opossum, sleep pattern of, 614, 615
Opsin, 416
Optical problems, 407–409
Optic chiasm, 32, 60
Optic nerve, 22, 32, 60, 410–411, 420
Optic radiation, 422
Optic tract, albinism and, 691
Organelles, *see* Mitochondria
Organ of Corti, transduction to electrical signals in, 361–362, 395
Orientation columns, early experience and development of, 447–451
Orientation selectivity
  of complex cells, 430, 456
  of simple cells, 424–427
Osmoreceptors, 570–571, 604
Osmotic pressure, 568, 604
Ossicles, hearing disorders involving, 380, 395
Ossicular system, 355, 356
  impedance matching by, 356–357
Otitis media, 380, 395
Otosclerosis, 380, 395
Oval window, 356, 360, 396
  impedance matching and, 357
Oxytocin, 536–538, 561
  lactation and, 542

Rotational model, 231, 250
Round window, 360, 396

S

Saccadic eye movements, 456, 472, 510
Saltatory conduction, 136, 148
Salty taste, 389
Satiety, 587–589
    brain damage and, 589–592
    self-stimulation and, 598–599
Scala media, 357
    in Meniere's disease, 382
Scala tympani, 357
Scanning, rapid, 433–434, 472, 474
Schizophrenia, 730–731
    clinical description and treatment, 731–733
    dopamine hypothesis, 733–736
    endorphin theory, 737–738
    hypotheses on molecular basis of, 733
    norepinephrine reward pathways and, 737
    transmethylation hypothesis, 736–737
Schwann cells, 86
Scratching, fictive, 481
    ventral spinocerebellar tract and, 481–483
Scratch reflex, organization in spinal animal,
    480–483
Secobarbital, tolerance and, 745
Seconal, 747
Secondary drinking, 568, 604
Seizures, shock-induced, 318
Selective breeding, genetic research and, 694,
    725
Selective visual attention, parietal cortex and,
    778–780
Self-stimulation
    energy balance and, 596
    homeostasis and, 598–599
Sella turcica, 536
Senility, symptoms of, 681
Sensations, magnitude of, 370
Sensitive period
    language development and, 718, 719
    for learning birdsong, 712–715, 725
Sensitivity, of visual receptors, 415
Sensitization, 257, see also Dishabituation
    cellular mechanisms of, 281–282, 291
    dishabituation versus, 272–275
    dual-process theory of habituation and, 278–
    280
Sensory enhancement, 589, 604
Sensory homunculus, 39, 60, 388, 396

Sensory impressions, integration of, 776, 780
Sensory receptors, aging and, 680
Sensory systems, see also specific systems
    spatial fidelity of, 29–30
Septohippocampal pathway, 234, 250
Serotonergic pathways, distribution of, 231–233
Serotonin
    affective disorders and, 742–743
    control of hormones by, 541
    feeding and, 591–592
    morphine dependence and, 757
    quiet sleep and, 619
    structure of, 736
Set point
    cardiovascular, 525–526
    temperature, 524, 562
Sex, genetic determination of, 696–697
Sex chromosomes, 691, 725
Sex-related behavior, development, genetic and
    hormonal influences, 700–708
Sexual desire, marijuana and, 752
Sexual development, mechanism of hormone ac-
    tion in, 708–711
Sexual orientation, of hermaphroditic children,
    sex of rearing and, 702–703
Shock, see Electroconvulsive shock
Sialic acid, in plasma membrane, 78
Silkmoth, circadian rhythm in, 625
Simple cells, of visual cortex, 423–429, 432, 456
Size analysis, visual, 434–438
Size principle, in recruitment order, 466, 510
Skin, see Somesthetic system
Skin stimulus, perception, cortical stimulation
    and, 806–807
Sleep, 6
    active, 333, 613
    chemical substrates of, 617–618
    circadian rhythms and, 622–623
    disorders of, 620–622
    EEG activity during, 299, 613, 633
    episodic hormone secretion during, 542
    hormones and neurotransmitters in, 618–620
    memory modulation and, 333
    neural structures affecting, 616–617
    questions and theories regarding, 610
    quiet, 613, 619
    serotonergic pathways and, 232–233
    species differences in, 613–616
Sleep stages, electrophysiological correlates of,
    611–613
Slow twitch motor units, 465, 510
    recruitment order and, 465–466

          INDEX

drinking and, 568–569
extracellular mechanisms, 572–573, 603
Thought, 5
Threshold
for action potential, 125, 149
in Addison's disease, 548
for amplitude of vibration of basilar membrane, 358
Thyroid gland, 539, 562
Thyroid hormone, cerebellar development and, 651
Thyroid-stimulating hormone (TSH), 536, 539, 562
Thyroid-releasing hormone (TRH), 539, 562
lactation and, 542
Thyroxine, 531, 534, 562
Tinnitus, 382, 396
Tolerance
to alcohol, 761, 768
drugs and, 745
to LSD, 751
to narcotics, mechanisms of, 753–759
Tone decay test, 384
Tonotopic map, 363, 396
Tonotopic organization, 29–30, 61, 396
Traces, see Engrams
Tracking, smooth pursuit, 473, 510
Transduction, 35–36, 61
auditory, 353, 361–362
from mechanical to electrical signal, 361–362
visual, 409–413
cellular feature extractors and, 423–433
lateral geniculate nucleus and, 420–422
primary visual cortex and, 422–423
receptor cells and, 414–417
retinal output characteristics, 417–420
Transfer
binocular, spatial frequency channels and, 437
of memory, 312–313
Transmitters, see also Neurotransmitters; Synaptic transmission
excitation and inhibition and, 166–167
functional role in brain, 243–248
habituation and, 265
inactivation by reuptake, 184–186
release of, 158–161
Traveling wave, 358, 396
Tricyclic antidepressants, 739, 768
affective disorders and, 741
serotonin and, 742
Trigeminal nerve, LH syndrome and, 593
Triple-X syndrome, 699, 725
Trisomy 21, 696

Trophic influences, of nerves, 660–661, 684
tRNA, 79
Troponin, in postsynaptic density, 95, 96
Tryptophan
affective disorders and, 742–743, 767
morphine dependence and, 757
Tuberoinfundibular system, 231
Tuinal, 747
Tumors, of VIII nerve, 384
Tuning curve, of auditory nerve fibers, 363, 396
Turner syndrome, space-form blindness in, 697–699, 725
Tympanic membrane, see Eardrum
Tympanogram, 380, 397
Tyrosine, catecholamine synthesis and, 186
Tyrosine hydroxylase, 186, 187, 203
antidepressant drugs and, 742
catecholamine synthesis and, 188–189
induction of, synaptic plasticity and, 196–198
substantia nigra and, 679, 680

U

Ulnar nerve, 552
Ultradian cycles, 542
sleep and, 614
Unconditional stimulus, see Stimulus, unconditional
Unit studies, of learning, 301–307, 343
Upper airway sleep apnea, dangers of, 621, 633

V

Valium, 747
Vas deferens, opiates and, 239
Vasopressin, 536, 562
memory storage and, 327
Ventral bundle, 228
Ventral lateral nucleus (VL), movement and, 492, 511
Ventral spinocerebellar tract (VSCT), scratch reflex and, 481–483, 511
Ventricles, 21, 61
Verbal skills, hemispheric dominance and, 791–792
Vesicles, synaptic, 88
Vestibulocerebellum, 493, 511
Vestibulo-ocular reflex (VOR), 473, 511
cerebellum in motor control, 493–494
feedback and feedforward control and, 477–479
plasticity of, 496–500

Vestibulospinal reflex, 511
  feedback control and, 477
  vestibulo-ocular reflex compared with, 494
Viscera, 516
  motor control of, 53–54
Vision
  color, 416–417
  foveal, 405
  ganglion cells and, 420
Visual cortex, 21, 22, 32, 402
  cellular feature extractors of, 423–433
  primary, structure of, 422–423
  secondary, depth perception and, 439, 456
Visual pigments, 415–416
Visual radiation, 32, 61
Visual sensations, words and, 786
Visual system, 32, 61, 399–400, *see also*
      Oculomotor system
  crossed connections in, 32, 34
  development and plasticity of, 441–442
    critical period in, 451–452
    ocular dominance columns, 442–447
    orientation columns, 447–451
  eye structure, 404–406
  length and privacy in, 34
  optical problems, 407–409
  perception and, 400–402
    of depth, 438–439
    illusions, 439–441
    rapid scanning, 433–434
    size analysis, 434–438
  precision of, 34–35
  transduction in, 409–413

cellular feature extractors, 423–433
lateral geniculate nucleus, 420–422
primary visual cortex, 422–423
receptor cells, 414–417
retinal output characteristics, 417–420
Vocalization
  in birds and humans, 717–718
  middle ear muscles and, 378
Voltage, 114–116
Voltage clamp technique, 131–132, 149

W

Wakefulness, EEG and, 612
Water, distribution in body, 567–568
Weight regulation, shifts in, 593
White-crowned sparrow, song of, 712
White matter, 21, 61
Wine, soporific effect of, 620
Withdrawal, naloxone-precipitated, brain sites
      of, 758–759
Withdrawal syndrome, heroin and, 746, 768
Wolffian duct system, reproductive system and,
      700, 725
Writing, lateralization of, 791

X

XYY syndrome, occurrence of, 699–700, 725

Z

Zonotrichia leucophrys, song of, 712